T0325386

ANNALS *of* THE NEW YORK ACADEMY OF SCIENCES

DIRECTOR AND EXECUTIVE EDITOR
Douglas Braaten

ASSOCIATE EDITOR
Rebecca E. Cooney

PROJECT MANAGER
Steven E. Bohall

EDITORIAL ADMINISTRATOR
Daniel J. Becker

Artwork and design by Ash Ayman Shairzay

The New York Academy of Sciences
7 World Trade Center
250 Greenwich Street, 40th Floor
New York, NY 10007-2157

annals@nyas.org
www.nyas.org/annals

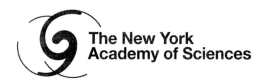

The New York
Academy of Sciences

Published by Blackwell Publishing
On behalf of the New York Academy of Sciences

Boston, Massachusetts
2011

ANNALS *of* THE NEW YORK ACADEMY OF SCIENCES

VOLUME 1232

ISSUE

Barrett's Esophagus

The 10th OESO World Congress Proceedings

ISSUE EDITORS

Robert Giuli,[a] Reza Shaker,[b] and Asad Umar[c]

[a]Deputy Director of OESO, Executive Director of the OESO Foundation, Paris, France. [b]Medical College of Wisconsin, Milwaukee, Wisconsin. [c]National Cancer Institute, Rockville, Maryland.

TABLE OF CONTENTS

Become a Member Today of the New York Academy of Sciences

The New York Academy of Sciences is dedicated to identifying the next frontiers in science and catalyzing key breakthroughs. As has been the case for 200 years, many of the leading scientific minds of our time rely on the Academy for key meetings and publications that serve as the crucial forum for a global community dedicated to scientific innovation.

 Select one FREE Annals volume and up to five volumes for only $40 each.

 Network and exchange ideas with the leaders of academia and industry.

 Broaden your knowledge across many disciplines.

 Gain access to exclusive online content.

Join Online at **www.nyas.org**

Or by phone at **800.344.6902** (516.576.2270 if outside the U.S.).

Focus papers

Ann. N.Y. Acad. Sci. ISSN 0077-8923

ANNALS OF THE NEW YORK ACADEMY OF SCIENCES
Issue: *Barrett's Esophagus: The 10th OESO World Congress Proceedings*

Introduction to *Barrett's Esophagus*

Barrett's Esophagus is the ninth publication on behalf of the World Organization for Specialized Studies on Diseases of the Esophagus (OESO) and the first to benefit from the prestigious cooperation of the New York Academy of Sciences and its scholarly journal of 189 years, *Annals of the New York Academy of Sciences*. This volume is yet another concrete demonstration of the multidisciplinary approach OESO has adopted since its founding.

As with the preceding volumes, the present volume follows The World Conference of the OESO, held in Boston, Massachusetts on August 28–31, 2010. Among the many attractions and benefits of the conference was the unprecedented 36.25 Physician's Recognition Award (PRA) continuing medical education credits granted by the American Medical Association. Similar to previous volumes, the present one is devoted to a single topic of esophagology and was made possible thanks to those who willingly followed the rigid question-and-answer format unique to the OESO conferences. I also send my heartfelt gratitude to those who, in the weeks following the Boston 2010 conference, took time to provide condensed texts corresponding to their replies to questions posed during the plenary sessions. While all the conference participants are not represented in this volume, our appreciation is all the greater to the authors who do appear in its table of contents.

Unlike the preceding conferences, the reader will have three types of access to the enormous wealth of ideas and knowledge that this four-day OESO conference furnished. This volume on Barrett's esophagus is composed of the following:

- Sixteen manuscripts comprising responses given to precise questions by top experts during the plenary sessions. Respecting the original OESO method, these answers were orally delivered in five minutes during the sessions. Now presented in brief syntheses by the authors, these texts are nonetheless complete, with pertinent tables, illustrations, and selected references.
- Fourteen "focus" manuscripts, each composed of responses (fewer than in the plenary sessions) given on a more limited subject during the symposia or topic fora sessions.
- For the first time, thanks to the cooperation between OESO and *Annals of the New York Academy of Sciences*, the contents of all the manuscripts will be accessible on PubMed and ISI, a significant advantage for authors. Because of the unique reach of *Annals* to over 11,000 institutions worldwide, this compilation offers to the scientific community unmatched access to the latest knowledge available on one of the most fascinating subjects in diseases of the upper digestive tract: Barrett's esophagus.

To arouse the reader's interest and easily glide him/her through this mass of information, there is a detailed summary at the beginning of each manuscript that offers a complete glimpse of the responses that follow. To prepare these detailed summaries, I used some of the summaries

doi: 10.1111/j.1749-6632.2011.06072.x
Ann. N.Y. Acad. Sci. 1232 (2011) vii–viii © 2011 New York Academy of Sciences.

written by the "secretaries" assigned to the plenary sessions; I thank them for their contributions. The high-level of expertise shown in this work comes from all who lent their time, seriousness, mastery, and care to their contributions. The thanks of a grateful editor go out to each one of them.

And now, the faithful "troupe" of the current OESO is preparing for the next stage: another world-class scientific event in a dream spot of northern Italy, Lake Como, on "Reflux disease: From the LES to the UES, and beyond."

ROBERT GIULI

Deputy Executive Director of OESO
Executive Director of the OESO Foundation
Paris, France

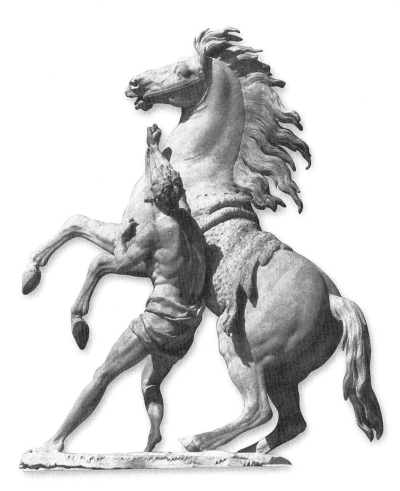

A horse and its rider, sculpted by Coustou, belonging to the group called Horses of Marly on the Champs Elysées in Paris, are the symbol of OESO. They were chosen as a dynamic image of an impetus, that of an entire multidisciplinary organization, and its efforts to master the essential problems still existing in esophageal disease.

Ann. N.Y. Acad. Sci. ISSN 0077-8923

Barrett's esophagus: prevalence–incidence and etiology–origins

Gary W. Falk,[1] Brian C. Jacobson,[2] Robert H. Riddell,[3] Joel H. Rubenstein,[4] Hala El-Zimaity,[5] Asbjørn Mohr Drewes,[6] Katie S. Roark,[7,8] Stephen J. Sontag,[7,8] Thomas G. Schnell,[7,8] Jack Leya,[7,8] Gregorio Chejfec,[7,9] Joel E. Richter,[10] Gareth Jenkins,[11] Aaron Goldman,[12] Katerina Dvorak,[12,13] and Gerardo Nardone[14]

[1]Department of Medicine, Division of Gastroenterology, University of Pennsylvania School of Medicine, Philadelphia, Pennsylvania. [2]Boston University Medical Center, Boston, Massachusetts. [3]Laboratory Medicine and Pathobiology, University of Toronto, Toronto, Ontario, Canada. [4]Veterans Affairs Center for Clinical Management Research, Ann Arbor, MI and Division of Gastroenterology, University of Michigan Medical School, Ann Arbor, Michigan. [5]University Health Network, Toronto General Hospital, Toronto, Ontario, Canada. [6]Department of Gastroenterology, Aalborg Hospital, Aalborg, Denmark. [7]Department of Medicine, Hines Veterans Affairs Hospital, Hines, Illinois. [8]Department of Medicine, Loyola University Medical College, Maywood, Illinois. [9]Department of Pathology, University of Illinois at Chicago, Chicago, Illinois. [10]Temple University, Philadelphia, Pennsylvania. [11]Institute of Life Science, Swansea School of Medicine, Swansea University, Swansea, United Kingdom. [12]Arizona Cancer Center, Tucson, Arizona. [13]Department of Cell Biology and Anatomy, College of Medicine, University of Arizona, Tucson, Arizona. [14]Università degli Studi di Napoli Federico II, Dipartimento di Medicina Clinica e Sperimentale Naples, Napels, Italy

Although the prevalence of Barrett's esophagus (BE) is rising no data exist for racial minorities on prevalence in the general population. Minorities have a lower prevalence than Caucasians, and yet age, smoking, abdominal obesity, and *Helicobacter pylori* are all risk factors. Metabolic changes induced by adipocytokines and the apparently strong association between obesity, central adiposity, and BE may lead to reconsideration of some aspects of the natural history of BE. There is lack of experimental evidence on acid sensitivity and BE, which is hyposensitive compared to esophageal reflux disease. Reactive nitrogen and oxygen species lead to impaired expression of tumor suppressor genes, which can lead to cancer development; thus, antioxidants may be protective. Gastroesophageal reflux disease may be considered an immune-mediated disease starting at the submucosal layer; the cytokine profile of the mucosal immune response may explain the different outcome of gastroesophageal reflux.

Keywords: intestinal metaplasia; BMI; *H. pylori*; palisaded vessels; gastric folds; goblet cells; Barrett's esophagus; duodeno-gastro-esophageal reflux; Bilitec monitoring; bile reflux; oxidative stress; chromosome mutations; interleukins; neoplastic development; esophageal adenocarcinoma; Los Angeles classification

Concise summaries

- Although we do not have data from randomized trials to definitively demonstrate what accounts for the rising incidence of Barrett's esophagus (BE), there are very good epidemiological data to support a role for rising obesity rates and declining *Helicobacter pylori* prevalence. The issue of why BE is less common in Asian countries remains somewhat enigmatic. However, it is not just Asia; BE is rare in the Caribbean, the Middle East, and much of Africa and South America. The ingestion of a high-fat diet with its associated delayed gastric emptying, and possibly oral and salivary carcinogens that are activated in the region of the GE junction, may all play a role.

- BE and esophageal adenocarcinoma are strongly associated with obesity. Obesity likely promotes both symptomatic and asymptomatic gastroesophageal reflux disease (GERD) through mechanical effects, and obese

doi: 10.1111/j.1749-6632.2011.06042.x
1

individuals are likely to behave in ways that also promote GERD. In addition, adipose tissue is metabolically active, and secreted adipokines have been associated with the development of a number of cancers. The rapid rise in incidence in esophageal adenocarcinoma may be due to synergies between these multiple mechanisms of obesity promoting the cancer.

- The natural history of *H. pylori* gastritis is for the inflammation to progress from the antrum into the adjacent corpus. The advancing atrophic front of corpus injury incrementally destroys parietal cells causing further reduction in acid secretion with the eventual development of extensive corpus atrophy. The extent and severity of gastric atrophy, in particular corpus atrophy, determines the patient's risk for GERD following *H. pylori* eradication.

- Indirect and direct evidence exists of acid hyposensitivity in patients with BE compared to other groups of reflux patients. However, in comparison with healthy individuals, the direct evidence is sparse and results conflicting. Not until BE patients have been compared to healthy patients in experimental studies, where the nature of the acid stimulus is controlled, can it be shown if patients with BE are truly acid hyposensitive.

- Patients with BE may have a generalized sensory defect in the esophagus, independent of nervous changes related to the metaplastic mucosa. Hence, the hyposensitivity is a cardinal feature that may bias the clinical evaluation and monitoring of patients with BE, and may be one of several pathogenetic factors in BE to be studied in more detail. Depending on the true prevalence and incidence of BE in children, BE in adults may possibly be congenital—an abnormality of incomplete embryogenesis perhaps related to the cervical inlet patch.

- The role of individual constituents of the gastric reflux in the development of BE and its associated complications still remain uncertain. Gastric acid and pepsin have received the most

attention; however, the development of BE in a few achlorhydric or postgastrectomy patients suggests a possible role for the duodenal contents. The duodenal contents suspected of causing esophageal mucosa injury include bile acids and lysolecithin present in the bile secretions as well as the pancreatic enzymes trypsin. Several studies in humans confirm that a synergy exists between acid and duodeno-gastro-esophageal reflux, which may contribute to the development of esophagitis and possibly BE.

- There is strong evidence that oxidative stress drives neoplastic development in Barrett's tissues. Dietary antioxidant levels appear to prevent neoplastic development and hence support the concept that reactive oxygen species (ROS) are crucial carcinogens in these patients. There is, however, some controversy as to whether dietary antioxidants or antioxidant supplements are the best source of protection. The relative contributions of acid and bile to the generation of these ROS, along with the pathways/enzymes leading to these ROS require further study. DNA damage is one of the most detrimental effects of exposure to toxic, caustic, and harmful agents.

- One of the culprits that elicits a response by the cell to develop defense mechanisms is the DNA damage incurred by bile acid-associated ROS, nitric oxide (NO), and acid-mediated increases in ROS and hydrolysis. These mechanisms of damage become synergistic when bile acids are combined with acid. DNA damage becomes more pronounced and the cells are forced to adapt, incur mutations, and progress through Barrett's to cancer.

- GERD may be considered an immune-mediated disease starting at the submucosal layer. The cytokine profile of the mucosal immune response may explain the different outcome of gastresophageal reflux, the severity of mucosal injury and even the relapse of esophagitis. Finally, this new concept opens the way to the development of new treatment for patients who do not respond to proton pump inhibitors (PPIs), and to the prevention of carcinogenesis.

1. The prevalence of BE in the general population: what do we know?

Gary W. Falk
gary.falk@uphs.upenn.edu

The incidence of BE has increased markedly since the 1970s.[1] This increase was once felt to be due to the increased use of diagnostic upper endoscopy combined with the change in the definition of BE to include shorter segments of columnar-lined epithelium. However, data from the Netherlands[2] suggest that the incidence of BE has increased from 14.3/100,000 person years in 1997 to 23.1/100,000 person years in 2002 in the general population–independent of the number of upper endoscopies.

It is estimated that BE is found in approximately 5–15% of patients undergoing endoscopy for symptoms of GERD. A study of a high-risk patient population (chronic GERD, Caucasian race, age > 50) undergoing endoscopy for symptoms of GERD found BE in 13.2% of the subjects. The prevalence of long segment BE ($\geq$3 cm of intestinal metaplasia) is approximately 5%, whereas that of short segment BE (<3 cm of intestinal metaplasia) is approximately 6–12% in patients undergoing endoscopy in a variety of settings.

BE is predominantly a disease of middle-aged white males. However, it should be kept in mind that approximately 25% of BE patients are women or less than 50 years of age. The prevalence of BE increases until a plateau is reached between the seventh and ninth decades. A variety of risk factors have been identified for the presence of BE, including frequent and long standing reflux episodes, smoking, male gender, older age, and central obesity. Body mass index itself does not appear to be a risk factor for BE, but rather the central obesity characteristic of male pattern obesity.

There have been two population-based studies to address the prevalence of BE in the general population. The first study by Ronkainen *et al.*[3] performed upper endoscopy in a random sample of 1,000 individuals from the adult population in two municipalities from Sweden. BE was found in 1.6% of these individuals: long segment ($\geq$2 cm) in 0.5% and short segment (<2 cm) in 1.1%. Furthermore, only 56% of the individuals had symptoms of GERD. The Loiano-Monghidoro study[4] examined 1,033 adults from two Italian villages that were similar in characteristics to the general Italian populations. BE was

found in 1.3%; 0.2% had long segment BE, whereas 1.1% had short segment BE. Reflux symptoms were reported by 53.8% of the Barrett's patients. Finally, a computer simulation, using the Surveillance Epidemiology and End Results (SEER) database was recently performed[5] in an effort to determine the prevalence of BE in the United States. This study estimated that the prevalence of BE in the general population was 5.6%.

Taken together, the above information suggests that: (1) BE is uncommon in the general population (1.3–1.6%); (2) most of the patients found in the general population have short segments; (3) screening strategies based on reflux symptoms alone will miss almost 50% of Barrett's patients; and (4) current symptom based screening concepts are clearly problematic.

2. Can the reasons for the epidemic rate of rising incidence of Barrett's esophagus be specified?

Brian C. Jacobson
brian.jacobson@bmc.org

To address this question, we must first determine whether the incidence of BE is indeed rising. If there is simply greater use of upper gastrointestinal (GI) endoscopy, there may be a detection bias that explains an increasing number of overall cases of BE (i.e., increased prevalence, but not incidence). However, van Soest *et al.* provide compelling evidence that the incidence is rising by controlling for the use of endoscopy.[1] To explain this rise then, we must consider the various risk factors for BE and determine whether there is more exposure to these risks. The most well-documented risks include increasing age, male gender, Caucasian ethnicity, cigarette use, increased body mass index (BMI), and a lack of *H. pylori* infection. Because the world's male-to-female ratio has not changed recently, and because there have not been significant increases in the relative number of Caucasians, these two risks are unlikely to explain the rising BE incidence. Let us consider the others.

Cigarette use in the United States rose steadily during the early to mid-1900s but has been declining steadily since the 1970s, so on first pass, this seems unlikely to explain the increased incidence of BE. However, if there is a prolonged latency between exposure to cigarettes and development of BE, this could still be an explanation. In this scenario, we would expect a subsequent decline in BE incidence over the next several decades.

Greater age is associated with BE, and the U.S. population is indeed aging, with the so-called "baby boomer" generation now reaching 65 years. Therefore, this growth in the number of relatively older people may be an explanation for the rising incidence. Just as with cigarettes, however, we would expect a decline in BE incidence over the next few decades as the mean population age is expected to fall.

H. pylori infection causes a chronic gastritis that can, after many years, be associated with decreased production of acid. Therefore, it is perhaps not surprising that several studies have documented an inverse association between *H. pylori* infection and BE.[6] It appears that the more virulent strains of *H. pylori* (the CagA-positive strains) may be more relevant here, with one meta-analysis demonstrating an inverse association between CagA-positive *H. pylori* infection and esophageal adenocarcinoma.[7] This relationship was not observed with CagA-negative strains. Epidemiologically, this explanation is attractive, because the rise in BE and esophageal adenocarcinoma in many countries correlates with the decline in *H. pylori* prevalence.

Finally, we must consider the association between greater BMI and BE. This has been well documented among both men and women.[8] There is also a well-documented association between obesity and both symptomatic GERD and esophageal adenocarcinoma.[9] The current "obesity epidemic" that has affected many nations certainly correlates with the observed rise in BE. Whether weight loss can mitigate BE risk has yet to be demonstrated.

In summary, although we do not have data from randomized trials to definitively demonstrate what accounts for the rising incidence of BE, there are very good epidemiological data to support a role for rising obesity rates and declining *H. pylori* prevalence.

3. How do different histologic criteria for Barrett's mucosa affect the prevalence rates of BE in different populations? Why is Barrett's mucosa so uncommon in East Asia?

Robert H. Riddell
rriddell@mtsinai.on.ca

The problem with the definition of BE is that there is no uniformly accepted definition. There are several; however, all insist on one of two endoscopic criteria (region of origin in parentheses):

- Using the lower end of the esophageal palisaded vessels where no biopsy is necessary (Japan), although this has to be modified to >5 mm of palisaded vessels to keep the rate reasonable; or[10]
- 1 cm+ from upper end of the gastric folds—less than this, there is no agreement of where an irregular Z-line stops and short-segment Barrett's begins.[11]

The latter is accompanied by one of three histological criteria:

(1) No histological criteria—the endoscopic appearance is quite sufficient—using either of the two endoscopic criteria stated.
(2) Biopsy of the endoscopically abnormal mucosa confirmed as showing columnar mucosa of any subtype (United Kingdom).[12]
(3) Biopsy with goblet cells (North America and parts of Europe),[13] although this has recently been modified without any sort of general education to include all types of glandular mucosa.[14]

What effect does this have on prevalence? Clearly, the change from "must have goblet cells" to "any columnar lined mucosa" with an appropriate endoscopic picture, must result in an increased prevalence if these criteria are held strictly. However, it is impossible to seriously think that in the whole of North America or much of Europe, one can look at a length of columnar mucosa in the esophagus and not believe that it is BE. Nevertheless, as these patients seem to be at increased risk of getting carcinoma,[15] this seems justified.

The "Japanese" definition of BE is impossible to evaluate until a study is carried out that compares all three potential criteria head to head. Intuitively, where the Japanese criteria are applied in Europe or North America, they seem so sensitive, starting at 5 mm above the gastroesophogeal (GE) junction, that it seems likely that they would result in an even greater prevalence of BE. However, there are no data to suggest that, using these criteria, there is an increased risk of carcinoma, thus the utility of this definition remains unproven.

The issue of why BE is less common in Asian countries remains somewhat enigmatic. However, it is not just Asia; BE is rare in the Caribbean, the Middle East, and much of Africa and South America. If obesity is an issue, then this is not something on which the West has a monopoly, and while the overall BMI may be higher in the West, it is sufficient in other regions for there to be plenty of BE.

The ingestion of a high-fat diet, with its associated delayed gastric emptying, and possibly oral and salivary carcinogens that are activated in the region of the GE junction, may all play a role.[16]

4. In Barrett's patients, does the influence of metabolic changes induced by adipocytokines and the apparently strong association existing between obesity, central adiposity, and BE lead to the need to reconsider some aspects of the natural history of BE or only of GERD?

Joel H. Rubenstein
jhr@umich.edu

Epidemiology of obesity and esophageal adenocarcinoma

It is well documented that the incidence of esophageal adenocarcinoma has been rising dramatically in Westernized countries. Although genetic factors may predispose individuals to esophageal adenocarcinoma, the rapid rate of increase in incidence must be due to nongenetic factors such as behavioral or environmental ones. During the same period of increased incidence of this cancer, there has been a growing epidemic of obesity in Westernized countries. Indeed, obesity has been associated with esophageal adenocarcinoma and BE. Abdominal obesity is a stronger risk factor than total body obesity (as measured by BMI) for both BE and esophageal adenocarcinoma. Furthermore, the risk of neoplastic progression in BE appears to be greater in abdominally obese patients.[17] There are at least three potential explanations for these associations with obesity (Fig. 1): obesity mechanically promotes GERD, the relation of obesity with BE and esophageal adenocarcinoma is confounded by factors promoting GERD, and obesity promotes BE and esophageal adenocarcinoma through circulating adipokines.

Mechanical effect of obesity

A prevalently held hypothesis is that the relation between obesity and esophageal adenocarcinoma is due to a mechanical effect of obesity promoting GERD. Increasing BMI is associated with increased risk of reporting GERD symptoms.[18] Among symptomatic GERD patients, obesity is associated with more severe esophageal acid exposure.[19,20] And weight loss in patients with GERD is associated with improvements in symptoms and healing of erosive esophagitis.[21,22] But these findings could be in part explained by confounding by other factors, such as diet, discussed below. In a cross-sectional study of patients undergoing esophageal manometry for clinical indications, obesity was indeed found to moderately increase intra gastric pressure.[23] However, obesity was also associated with increased intra-esophageal pressure, so the pressure gradient across the EG junction is less strongly associated with obesity. For each 10 cm increase in waist circumference, the pressure gradient across the EG junction increased only 1.5 mmHg. Abdominal obesity was also weakly associated with hiatal hernia formation. In addition to the effect of obesity on the pressure gradient and junctional anatomy, it is also associated with an increased frequency of transient lower esophageal sphincter relaxations.[24] The combinations of these factors might result in substantial reflux.

Is the effect of obesity confounded by factors leading to gastroesophageal reflux?

A number of studies have demonstrated strong associations between obesity and BE or adenocarcinoma

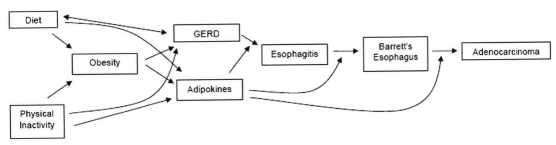

Figure 1. Potential roles of obesity and related factors in Barrett's esophagus.

including after controlling for GERD symptoms,[25–27] but there is potential for residual confounding in these studies, as subjects may have had asymptomatic GERD. Furthermore, the apparent associations could also be confounded by factors that promote both obesity and GERD, such as diet and physical inactivity. The Western style diet (high intake of fat and sweets, low intake of fruits and vegetables) promotes obesity, but features of this type of diet can also directly promote GERD. For instance, obese patients are more likely to eat chocolate, which can promote GERD irrespective of any mechanical effect of their obesity. In fact, in a small study of obese women with GERD, only 6 days of a very low carbohydrate diet improved GERD, suggesting that the baseline diet itself and not obesity, was inducing their symptoms.[28] Although some forms of vigorous physical activity may promote GERD, regular moderate exercise is inversely associated with GERD symptoms, controlling for obesity and dietary intake, but the mechanism for this association is not clear.[29–32]

Potential role of adipokines

Although GERD almost certainly explains at least part of the relation between obesity and BE and esophageal adenocarcinoma, it is unlikely to be the entire explanation. Most patients with GERD symptoms do not have erosive esophagitis, and only a very small minority develop BE. Obesity may play a role in promoting BE and esophageal adenocarcinoma in the setting of GERD. Obesity is associated with a number of other cancers (colon, breast, prostate) for which there is no known mechanical explanation. Adipose tissue is not an inert storage depot, but rather metabolically active, secreting a number of substances termed adipokines (or adipocytokines) that can act from a distance through the circulation, promoting inflammation, insulin resistance, and regulating dietary intake. Visceral adipose tissue appears to be particularly important in these roles. For instance, visceral adipocytes secrete TNF-α, and 50 to 75% of circulating IL-6 in obese subjects may be secreted from omental adipocytes.[33,34] Alterations in circulating levels of a number of adipokines have been associated with the development of other cancers: breast, colon, endometrial, pancreas, and prostate.[35–38] Visceral adipose tissue appears to mediate the effects of obesity on the risk of BE.[39]

Conclusion

BE and esophageal adenocarcinoma are strongly associated with obesity (Fig. 1). Obesity likely promotes both symptomatic and asymptomatic GERD through mechanical effects, and obese individuals are likely to behave in ways that also promote GERD. In addition, adipose tissue is metabolically active, and secreted adipokines have been associated with the development of a number of cancers. The rapid rise in incidence in esophageal adenocarcinoma may be due to synergies between these multiple mechanisms of obesity promoting the cancer. Additional research is needed to elucidate the mechanisms by which adipokines might promote intestinal metaplasia and neoplastic progression.

5. Can it be assessed that the absence of *H. pylori* increases the risk of GERD and, hence, the risk of Barrett's?

Hala El-Zimaity
Hala.el-Zimaity@uhn.on.ca

Chronic GERD is the strongest risk factor associated with Barrett's. Up to 5% of people with longstanding GERD will develop long segment BE, and between 10% and 15% will develop short segment BE. The extent and duration of esophageal acid exposure determines the length of Barrett's mucosa. The question is, "can it be assessed that the absence of *H. pylori* increases the risk of GERD and, therefore, the risk of Barrett's?" The answer to that question seems controversial. Some data suggests *H. pylori* eradication increases the risk of GERD. Other data suggests the opposite. To understand the opposing viewpoints one has to understand the effects of *H. pylori* infection on gastric acid secretion.

The associated injury associated with *H. pylori* gastritis begins at the antrum–corpus junction, specifically at the incisura angularis, with resulting spread of foci up and down the lesser curvature and the anterior and posterior wall. A person's acid secretory status affects both the distribution and severity of *H. pylori* related gastritis (for review, see Ref. 40). In the early stages, *H. pylori*-associated gastritis is antral predominant and oxyntic mucosa acid secretion shows an exaggerated gastrin response to *H. pylori*, an increase enough to cause duodenal ulcer disease in some patients. In this setting, *H. pylori* eradication decreases acid production.[41,42]

With continued inflammation, hypochlorhydria, and achlorhydria develops, which facilitates proximal migration of the bacteria. This allows the development of corpus gastritis, and eventually corpus atrophy. Advanced gastritis (patients with gastric ulcer and the intestinal type gastric cancer) is typically an extensive pan-gastritis (with widespread intestinal metaplasia and hypo or achlorhydria). At this stage, *H. pylori* eradication increases acid secretion.[43] At this stage, *H. pylori* eradication perhaps increases a patient's risk for GERD.

Meta-analysis shows no association between *H. pylori* eradication and the development of new cases of GERD in dyspeptic patients. However, *H. pylori* eradication in cohort studies show a twofold higher risk for developing erosive GERD in patients with peptic ulcer disease, OR 2.04 (95% CI: 1.08–3.85; $P = 0.03$).[44]

The natural history of *H. pylori* gastritis is for the inflammation to progress from the antrum into the adjacent corpus. The advancing atrophic front of corpus injury incrementally destroys parietal cells causing further reduction in acid secretion with the eventual development of extensive corpus atrophy. The extent and severity of gastric atrophy, in particular corpus atrophy, determines the patient's risk for GERD following *H. pylori* eradication.

6. Are patients with BE hyposensitive to acid? And what do sensory abnormalities play in the pathogenesis?

Anne Lund Krarup, Jens Brøndum Frøkjaer, Christian Lottrup, and Asbjørn Mohr Drewes
drewes@smi.auc.dk

To answer if patients with BE are hyposensitive to acid, it is first necessary to decide who to compare with and how the test should be done. To determine if BE patients are hyposensitive, they should be compared to healthy subjects. This is often not done; instead, BE patients are compared to other patients with reflux disease. When testing, acid sensitivity can be addressed directly by examining the response to an experimental acid perfusion, for example, a Bernstein or modified Bernstein test. Indirect evidence can come from pH and impedance studies where the number of refluxes sensed by healthy and patient groups are counted, and the effects of proton pump inhibitor (PPI) treatment to complete symptom control can be assessed. Finally,

the Kalixandra study is a unique source of indirect evidence.

Direct evidence: experimental acid perfusion
In the many studies addressing this issue, patients with BE have mostly been compared to patients with erosive reflux disease (ERD) and not healthy volunteers.

Several studies have demonstrated an acid hyposensitivity in patients with BE when compared to patients with ERD.[45] However, patients with ERD are known to be hypersensitive to acid as well, and comparisons between ERD and BE can therefore not tell us anything of BE versus healthy. The comparison of patients with BE to healthy age and sex matched volunteers has only been examined in studies with fewer than 10 subjects in one of the groups, and the results are conflicting.[46,47] As of now, we do not have sufficient evidence from direct studies of acid sensitivity to conclude if patients with BE are more or less acid sensitive in comparison with healthy controls.

Until experimental acid perfusion studies on a larger patient sample with matching healthy controls are conducted, it is not known if BE patients are truly hyposensitive to acid or only hyposensitive if compared to ERD patients (Fig. 2).

Indirect evidence
Many studies have demonstrated that patients with BE have excessive pathological reflux and that these patients sense fewer reflux events than patients with ERD.[48] Treatment studies in patients with BE have also proven pathological percentage of time with pH below 4 despite complete symptom relief from treatment with PPIs. The third piece of indirect evidence that BE patients are acid hyposensitive came from the Kalixandra study, which found that only 40% of patients with BE reported reflux symptoms at all, but also indicates that only 37% of ERD patients reported symptoms.[3]

All of these pieces of evidence could point in the direction that patients with BE are hyposensitive to acid, but they are still indirect evidence.

Conclusion
Indirect and direct evidence exists of acid hyposensitivity in patients with BE compared to other groups of reflux patients. However, in comparison with healthy individuals the direct evidence is sparse, and results are conflicting. Not until BE patients have

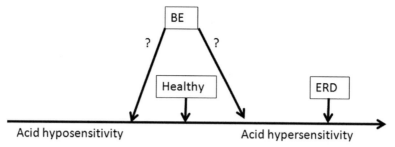

Figure 2. Several studies have demonstrated acid hyposensitivity in patients with BE when compared with ERD. However, in comparisons of BE patients with healthy volunteers, there have only been studies with fewer than 10 subjects in one of the groups, and the results are conflicting. As of now, we do not have sufficient evidence to conclude if patients with BE are more or less acid sensitive in comparison with healthy controls.

been compared to healthy subjects in experimental studies, where the nature of the acid stimulus is controlled (area, volume, and composition of the acid stimulus) can it be shown if patients with BE patients are truly acid hyposensitive.

7. What can we tell about the etiology of BE from experimental testing of the esophagus with multimodal sensory assessment?

Asbjørn Mohr Drewes, Anne Lund Krarup, Christian Lottrup, and Jens Brøndum Frøkjær
amd@mech-sense.com

Assessment of visceral pain

Basic mechanisms in pain processing can be explored by means of human experimental pain models. These models, when applied to healthy volunteers or to patients, provide an important translational link between animal studies and human clinical trials. In clear contrast to clinical pain, experimental pain models allow the possibility of controlling the duration, the intensity and the nature of the pain stimulus. However, as pain is a multidimensional perception it is obvious that the reaction to a single stimulus of a certain modality only represents a limited part of the pain experience and, therefore, a variety of stimulus modalities are required.[49] This was the rational for development of the multimodal pain model for the esophagus.[50]

The main advantage of the model is that it allows a differentiated assessment of the superficial and deep structures of the gut wall, activation of different receptors, nerve fibers and peripheral as well as central pain mechanisms. The model has been

proved to be robust and reliable across experimental sessions. The validity of the model was confirmed in a series of studies where it was used to explore the pathophysiology of esophageal disorders such as erosive and nonerosive reflux disease and noncardiac chest pain. Recently, the model was also used to investigate the sensory system in patients with BE[51] (Fig. 3).

Sensory abnormalities in BE

Several studies have confirmed that patients with BE have pathologic gastroesophageal reflux and slow clearance of acid and other noxious substances from the esophagus. This may be a main factor in the pathogenesis. The reduced clearance could be related to a defect in the afferent (sensory) or efferent (motor) part of the reflex arc leading to fewer secondary contractions. Previous studies have shown

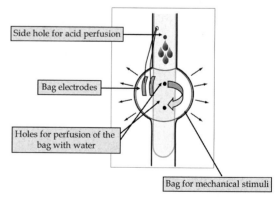

Figure 3. The probe used for multimodal stimulation of the esophagus. The probe allows controlled mechanical, thermal (circulation of heat and cold water with simultaneous measurement of temperature), and electrical stimulation. Furthermore, hyperalgesia of the esophageal mucosa can be evoked with acid (not used in the BE experiment).

that patients with BE have decreased sensation to acid and mechanical stimulation of the esophagus, and, hence, the reduced clearance could be related to a generalized defect in the afferent nerves.[52,53] It is not yet known whether this change in esophageal sensation is a result of the characteristics in the metaplastic mucosa or whether it is present before development of the metaplasia. We hypothesized that patients with BE had primary defects in the afferent signaling (thus leading to reduced acid clearance).

To explore this in detail, we subjected 15 patients and 15 volunteers to mechanical, heat, and electrical stimulation of the metaplastic and normal parts of the esophagus. We found that patients with BE were hyposensitive to heat and partly to mechanical stimulation both in the metaplastic and normal part of esophagus. As the hyposensitivity was present on both segments it was suggested that patients with BE may have a generalized sensory defect in the esophagus independent of nervous changes related to the metaplastic mucosa. Hence, the hyposensitivity is a cardinal feature that may bias the clinical evaluation and monitoring of patients with BE, and may be one of several pathogenetic factors in BE to be studied in more detail.

8. Does BE really develop in adulthood?

Katie S. Roark, Stephen J. Sontag, Thomas G. Schnell, Jack Leya, and Gregorio Chejfec
kroark@lumc.edu

The incidence of BE is increasing. In clinical practice, the true definition of incident Barrett's is the number of patients which actually "develop" Barrett's during a specific time. There have been many speculations as to the reason for the rising incidence. Per review of the current literature, nothing has ever been published regarding when and how long before people go on to actually "develop" BE, which would define the true incidence of this disease.

When BE is diagnosed, did it just recently occur or had it been there for a while but was just recently discovered? Based on an observation that the majority of BE is diagnosed on initial endoscopy and a clinical question of "when does BE actually develop," we set out to determine the true incidencehood of BE.

To find true incidence of this disease, one must observe the replacement of Squam epithelium (Ep-

ith) by intestinal metaplasia (IM). Our data proves that during our 25-year surveillance program for GERD, only 4.6% of patients actually *develop* BE after a negative evaluation for Barrett's. The other 87% are actually *prevalent* Barrett's cases or BE diagnosed on first endoscopy. This makes the true incidence of BE almost negligible after initial normal endoscopy. It raises discussion that Barrett's is most likely present at a much younger age than when initially diagnosed.

The methods we used include our Hines VA GI Database, which contains the data of all procedures performed since January 1979. EGDs were performed by one of three endoscopists (TS, SJS, JL) using the same criteria and definitions. EGD retroflexion was routinely performed to assess the GEJ. Specimens (specs) were taken from all potential BE segments. In general, a minimum of two Bx specs were routinely taken from the SCJ regardless of a "normal" appearance. Histology specs were read by one pathologist (GC). An absolute criterion for BE was intestinal metaplasia (IM) from the tubular esophagus, the Bx had to contain (as one specimen) the squamo-IM junction. To qualify for "Incidence BE," junctional epithelium (J) from the SC junction had to be present on previous Bx at least 12 months before the diagnosis of IM (BE; Fig. 4).

We found that since 1979 1,648 patients (mean age 58 years at first EGD) have been diagnosed to have BE and followed in outpatient surveillance program. Of the 1648 patients, 209 had Barrett's diagnosed 12 months after initial endoscopy. We performed a detailed review of the individual scope report, photos, and diagrams of these patients and found that 53 had squamous (Sq) on initial scope, 79 had no biopsy during their first endoscopy, and 77 (4.6%) had actual junctional epithelium preceding the IM.

We conclude from the data that in our database of 25 years (mean 15.2 years) the documented incidence of BE is at best 0.83% per year, indicating that >99% of BE develops before initial endoscopy.

So, when does BE develop? Depending on the true prevalence and incidence of BE in children, BE in adults may possibly be congenital—an abnormality of incomplete embryogenesis perhaps related to the cervical inlet patch.[54] One thing is for certain, based on our data, Barrett's most likely develops before we look!

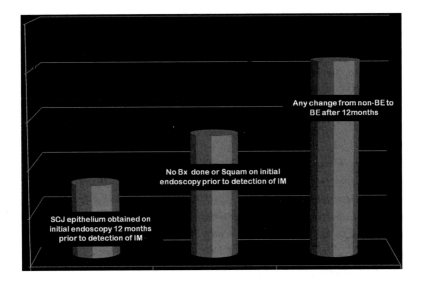

Any change from non-BE to BE after 12 months

No Bx done or Squam on initial endoscopy prior to detection of IM

SCJ epithelium obtained on initial endoscopy 12 months prior to detection of IM

Figure 4.

9. What is the role of duodeno-gastroesophageal reflux in the development of BE?

Joel E. Richter
jrichter@temple.edu

There is now overwhelming evidence supporting the association of GERD and BE. However, the role of individual constituents of the gastric reflux in the development of BE and its associated complications still remain uncertain. Gastric acid and pepsin have received the most attention; however, the development of BE in a few achlorhydric or postgastrectomy patients suggests a possible role for the duodenal contents. The duodenal contents suspected of causing esophageal mucosa injury include bile acids and lysolecithin present in the bile secretions as well as the pancreatic enzymes trypsin.

Although commonly referred to as "bile reflux," it is important to remember that reflux of duodenal contents contain more than just bile. Furthermore, the term "alkaline reflux" is often used interchangeably suggesting that pH 7.0 represents the reflux of duodenal contents into the lower esophagus. However, recent studies have confirmed the inadequacy of pH monitoring under these circumstances.[55] Therefore, duodeno-gastro-esophageal reflux (DGER) is a more appropriate term representing the retrograde reflux of duodenal contents into the stomach with subsequent reflux into the esophagus. The best methodology for measuring DGER has been the Bilitec monitoring system developed in the early 1980s. This is an ambulatory, fiber optic probe that uses the optical property of bilirubin, the most common pigment found in bile, to detect DGER spectrophotometrically, independent of pH.

Using combined 24 pH and Bilitec monitoring, studies of patients with and without complications of BE have found increased reflux of bile and acid into the lower esophagus of both groups as compared to controls.[55,56] Esophageal exposure to both acid and DGER was the most prevalent pattern (Fig. 5) and present in 100% of complicated Barrett's patients, 89% of uncomplicated Barrett's patients, 79% of patients with esophagitis, and 50% of patients with NERD. Furthermore, subsequent studies found that simultaneous esophageal acid exposure to both acid and DGER was the most prevalent reflux pattern, occurring in 95% of patients with BE and 79% of GERD patients.[56] In fact, these authors found a strong correlation ($R = 0.73$) between acid and DGER in controls, reflux patients, and those with BE. Thus, these studies in humans confirm that a synergy exists between acid and DGER, which may contribute to the development of esophagitis and possibly BE.

This was confirmed in a cohort of 392 patients with GERD, where a multivariate analysis found that the presence of a hiatal hernia, increasing body mass index, and GER were important risk factors for the recurrence of esophagitis, but acid exposure was

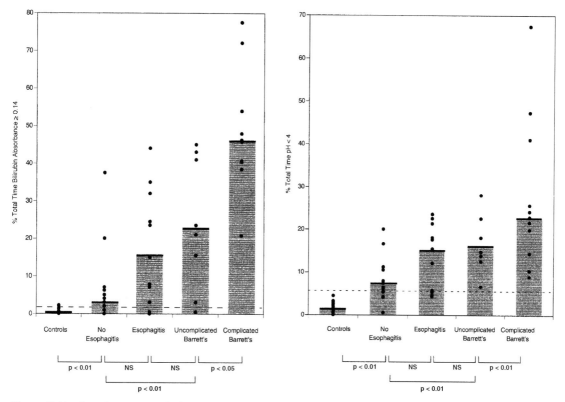

Figure 5. Esophageal exposure to both acid and DGER was the most prevalent pattern and present in 100% of complicated Barrett's patients, 89% of uncomplicated Barrett's patients, 79% of patients with esophagitis, and 50% of patients with NERD.

the principle factor in determining the severity of esophagitis. Similarly, the DGER and acid synergy is important in the development of BE and its complications. Multivariate analysis of two large cohort of patients with DGER identified male gender and exposure to both acid and DGER as important risk factors for BE.[57–59]

10. What is the role of acute and chronic bile acid exposure in reflux induced oxidative stress?

Gareth Jenkins, E. McAdam, N. Rawat, L. Williams, J. Cronin, Z. Eltahir, P. and Griffith, J. Baxter
g.j.jenkins@swansea.ac.uk

Oxidative stress is said to occur when the levels of ROS present in a tissue outweigh the inherent antioxidant defenses, that is dietary antioxidants (vitamin C, etc.) and antioxidant enzymes (glutathione S transferase, superoxide dismutase (SOD), etc.). ROS induced during times of oxidative stress have been implicated in a wide range of diseases such as diabetes, aging, degenerative inflammatory conditions, and of course cancer. In terms of cancer, ROS are known to induce redox sensitive signaling pathways, DNA and chromosome mutations and damage to other macromolecules (proteins, lipids, etc.). These cellular/DNA effects contribute to the neoplastic development of a tissue by increasing cell division rates and introducing genomic instability.

In the premalignant condition BE, oxidative stress has been strongly linked to disease progression (Wetscher *et al.*[60] Dvorak *et al.*[61]). This oxidative stress has been shown to be induced in epithelial cells by exposure of these cells to both bile acid (Jenkins *et al.*[64]) and acid (Zhang *et al.*[74]) components of refluxate. Oxidative stress can also be induced in esophageal tissues by:

1. ROS produced by infiltrating neutrophils during acute inflammatory phases;
2. reductions in antioxidant enzyme levels (GSH, SOD) known to be apparent in Barrett's tissues; and

3. reduced dietary antioxidant levels in the serum of Barrett's patients.

These latter two observations may be due to increased levels of ROS in Barrett's tissues leading to antioxidant depletion. Nonetheless, this state of affairs means that ROS are key players in neoplastic progression in esophageal adenocarcinoma in particular.

Because of the fact that ROS are clearly implicated in BE progression, it would make some sense (and provide some additional evidence) if dietary antioxidant intake protected patients from cancer progression. This is indeed the case, with several patient studies showing an inverse association between dietary intakes of antioxidants and risk of progressing from BE to adenocarcinoma. There is, however, some controversy as to whether dietary antioxidants or antioxidant supplements are the best source of protection. A recent meta-analysis of published studies shows odds ratios of 0.49 for high intakes of dietary vitamin C and 0.46 for high intakes of dietary beta-carotene.[64] Hence, a greater than 50% reduced risk of cancer for those Barrett's patients with high intakes of antioxidants, this clearly supports the hypothesis that oxidative stress drives cancer progression in these patients.

However, there has been limited success in chemoprevention studies in both animal models and Barrett's patients, where surrogate markers of disease progression have been studied (White et al.[65] and Murphy et al.[66]). A recent study highlighted the potential effect of patient heterogeneity on the success of such intervention studies. In a small vitamin C supplement study (1 g/day for 31 days) involving 25 patients, Babar et al.[67] looked at NF-κB activity and cytokine expression levels as surrogate markers in patient tissues, both before and after supplementation. They found that overall there was little effect of supplementation on average levels of NF-κB activity and cytokine expression. However, when looking at individual patients, they noted that within these 25 patients, 8 patients (35%) showed suppression of the markers studied after supplementation, whereas the other patients showed little effects. This perhaps highlights the potential for heterogeneity between these patients to affect the overall results of the study.

For example, for patients who already have high intakes of dietary antioxidants, supplementation with vitamin C will have little effect, whilst for those with low initial intakes, the supplementation may show strong effects. Therefore, in short-term studies, it is always going to be difficult to show a strong effect of supplementation, unless this patient heterogeneity is taken into account. Indeed, patient stratification may be desirable in such studies, as would be longer-term supplementation, where at all possible.

In conclusion, there is strong evidence that oxidative stress drives neoplastic development in Barrett's tissues. Dietary antioxidant levels appear to prevent neoplastic development and hence support the concept that ROS are crucial carcinogens in these patients. However, there are still gaps in our knowledge which need to be filled if we are to better understand the mechanisms involved in neoplastic development, including the source of these ROS in the esophagus, which is still unclear. Indeed the relative contributions of acid and bile to the generation of these ROS, along with the pathways/enzymes leading to these ROS and even the different types of ROS induced, require further study.

11. What is the current understanding of the role of DNA damage induced by bile acids in the development of BE?

Aaron Goldman and Katerina Dvorak
kdvorak@email.arizona.edu

DNA damage is one of the most detrimental effects of exposure to toxic, caustic, and harmful agents. The mechanisms underlying DNA repair are imperfect procedures and the pathological consequences of poor repair processes have been well documented in familial and acquired diseases. Although toxic chemicals from exogenous sources have the ability to produce immense DNA damage within tissue, endogenous chemicals can find their way from the constraints of their normal physiological environment to damage neighboring tissue. The latter case is specifically associated with the development of BE.

BE is a premalignant condition arising in the distal esophagus. It is a condition where metaplastic tissue resembling the columnar epithelium of the intestines, containing goblet cells, replaces normal mucosa. Clinical, animal, and basic studies suggest that BE develops as the consequence of chronic exposure of stomach contents, mainly acid and bile acids, on the squamous epithelium. These endogenous components individually elicit a series of malicious events and together are synergistic within the esophagus, most notably resulting in DNA damage.

Acid alone has the ability to hydrolyze nucleic acid bases causing the liberation of purines and pyrimidines from the sugar backbones on which they reside. This depurination or depyrimidation requires the imperfect process of base excision repair to resolve the missing base within the DNA sequence. As a consequence, incorrectly placed bases can result in the activation of oncogenes, loss of tumor suppressors and onset of pathology.

Bile acids have previously been shown to increase nitric oxide synthase expression and nitric oxide production, generate superoxide radicals via activation of NADPH oxidase (NOX) and perturb the mitochondrial membrane.[68] These responses elicit large amounts of reactive oxygen species (ROS) and reactive nitrogen species (RNS), consequently inducing DNA damage in squamous and BE cells.[69] When bile acids are combined with acid, mimicking the reflux experienced by patients who have BE, the DNA damage elicited by each component of reflux becomes synergistic and results in amplified DNA damage.[70,71] Squamous epithelium is less protected and ill-prepared to manage the onslaught of DNA damage associated with chronic exposure to bile acids and acid.

Squamous cells do not retain sufficient defense mechanisms to ward off ROS, increased extracellular acidity and activation of oncogenic pathways as a result of the synergism elicited by bile acids and acid. Following acute exposures of <10 minutes to bile acids and acid, squamous cells evoke increased DNA damage. As DNA repair takes place, there is likelihood for inefficient repair and mutations can occur. Moreover, in response to DNA damage as a consequence to increased acidity, cells will adapt mechanisms to defend from the insult, developing new cells from progenitor cells that are better adapted to refluxate environment. BE tissue is able to more effectively defend against bile acids and acid exposure.

BE tissue is adapted to an environment containing bile acids and gastric acid. First, mucin secreted by goblet cells provides a protective layer of mucous. Second, BE cells display increased expression of proteins associated with acid removal required for modulation of the extracellular and intracellu-

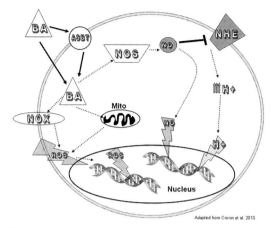

Figure 6. Proposed scheme of bile acid and acid-mediated DNA damage. Bile acids enter the cell or are transported in by ASBT, where they liberate ROS from the mitochondria or through activation of NOX. Activation of NOS leads to inhibition of NHE, increased acidity, and NO-mediated and acid-mediated DNA damage. ASBT, apical sodium-dependent bile acid transporter; BA, bile acid; NOX, NADPH oxidase. Adapted from Ref. 68.

lar acidity, such as Na^+/H^+ exchanger.[70,71] These cells still incur a sufficient amount of DNA damage in response to acid and bile acids, but through their development of acid extrusion pathways such as Na^+/H^+ exchanger, they are able to resist cell death to a greater degree than squamous derived cells under the same conditions.[63,70]

The progression of squamous epithelium in the esophagus to BE metaplasia is a multifaceted process. One of the culprits which elicit a response by the cell to develop defense mechanisms is the DNA damage incurred by bile acid–associated ROS, NO, and acid-mediated increases in ROS (Fig. 6). These mechanisms of damage become synergistic when bile acids are combined with acid. DNA damage becomes more pronounced and the cells are forced to adapt, incur mutations, and progress through Barrett's to cancer.

12. The still unmet needs in esophageal inflammation

Gerardo Nardone

nardone@unina.it

The pathophysiology of GERD is complex, and involves diverse factors, that is, gastric acid secretion, dysfunction of the antireflux barrier, delayed gastric emptying, and abnormalities in esophageal defence mechanisms. How these different factors cause GERD is not well understood, however, they all share one common initiating event: the increased exposure of the esophageal squamous epithelium to gastric contents.

It is generally agreed that gastric content, which consists of acids, pepsin, trypsin, and bile salts, causes caustic and chemical mucosal injury. This process starts at the luminal surface and progresses through the epithelium into the submucosa. Indeed, pepsin breaks junctional proteins and, as a consequence, increases mucosal permeability, thereby making it possible for hydrogen ions and bile to enter the submucosal layer. However, this process results in different outcomes. Indeed, about 60% of patients develop nonerosive esophagitis, 35% erosive esophagitis, and finally about 5% of patients develop complicated esophagitis called "Barrett's esophagus" and adenocarcinoma.

The degree of esophageal mucosa damage does not correlate with the amount of reflux materials and, to date, the exact pathogenetic mechanisms responsible for the diversity of esophageal phenotypes are poorly understood. Although there is a large body of data focusing on damage of the epithelial layer in response to acid, little is known about the molecular events underlying the development of esophageal inflammation.

One of the key steps of the pathogenetic process of GERD is the recruitment and activation of polymorphnuclear cells that, in turn, release ROS and nitric oxide that cause esophageal mucosal damage. Therefore, microbes are among the environmental factors that may contribute to the etiology of GERD. In a recent study of microbiomes from biopsy esophageal samples, Yang *et al.*[72] found that the esophageal microbiome is prevalently constituted by bacteria of the streptococcus genus in normal subjects, and by gram-negative anaerobe/microaerophile bacteria in patients with esophagitis and BE.

Another interesting concept concerns the immune response underlying the esophageal mucosal damage. The esophageal epithelium is embryologically, morphologically, and functionally related to the skin epithelium, which is recognized as a major immunological organ. Therefore, we can consider the esophagus an immunological organ. The reflux of gastric content in the esophagus may activate T cells in the submucosal layer that, in turn, release cytokines and chemokines. Cytokine and chemokine agents, through the recruitment of

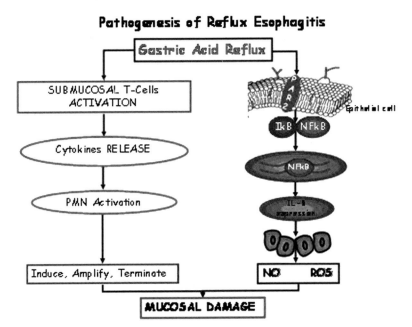

Figure 7. An alternative concept for the development of reflux esophagitis. The reflux of gastric juices does not directly damage the esophagus, but rather stimulates esophageal epithelial cells to secrete chemokines that, in turn, through the recruitment of neutrophils and the release of nitric oxide (NO) and reactive oxygen species (ROS), mediate the damage of esophageal mucosa.

polymorphonuclear cells and the release of inflammatory mediators, may initiate, amplify, and terminate the mucosal damage.[73]

Therefore, esophageal damage starts in the submucosal layer and depends prevalently on cytokine secretion (Fig. 7). Indeed, in a rat model of reflux esophagitis, the inflammatory infiltration occurs early and appears to be prevalently restricted to the submucosal layer; in contrast, mucosal alterations, that is, basal cell proliferation and papillary cell hyperplasia, occur after two weeks.[73]

From a molecular viewpoint, the reflux of gastric contents in the esophagus activates membrane protease activated receptor 2 that in turn induces phosphorylation of IκB and its subsequent degradation. This results in activation of NF-κB and its translocation into the nucleus. At this point, NF-κB, which is involved in various inflammatory conditions through a plethora of genes, upregulates the transcription of IL-8, thereby inducing strong recruitment of neutrophils.[74]

A progressive significant molecular increase of p65 and p50 subunits of NF-κB has been detected in patients with esophagitis and BE. Moreover, IL-8 mRNA expression and mucosal neutrophil infiltration have been reported to be significantly related to the endoscopic severity of reflux esophagitis scored according to the Los Angeles classification.[74] Finally, the mucosal levels of IL-8 were found to be indicative of esophagitis relapse. Taken together these observations suggest that IL-8 is a sensitive marker of esophageal mucosal damage.

A large number of cytokines may be involved in esophageal mucosal injury, for example, IL-1, IL-6, and IL-10, that may affect motility function, fibrosis, cell immune response, and carcinogenesis.[75] In the case of eosinophilic esophagitis, the regulation of the inflammatory-immune response is even more complex and involves IL-5, IL-13, eotaxin, and fibroblast growth factor, which affect muscle cells and fibroblast and may induce motility dysfunction and fibrosis. The cytokine profile may explain the different findings and outcomes of esophageal disease. Fitzgerald *et al.*[76] analyzed bioptic samples of esophageal mucosa, and observed that BE is characterized by a distinct Th2 predominant cytokine profile, that is, IL-4 and IL-10, whereas esophagitis is characterized by a proinflammatory cytokine profile consisting of IL-8, IL-1, IL-6, and IFN-γ.[76]

Therefore, by stimulating submucosal T cells, the reflux of gastric content, as well as environmental agents such as bacteria and food allergens, may induce secretion of cytokines, chemokines, and related inflammatory mediators that can affect fibroblasts, immune cells, muscle cells, and endothelial cells.[78,79] If the inflammatory reaction persists, motility disorders, fibrosis, and even cancer may occur. These recent data are consistent with an alternative concept for the development of reflux esophagitis in which the reflux of gastric juices does not directly damage the esophagus, but rather stimulates esophageal epithelial cells to secrete chemokines that, in turn, mediate the damage of esophageal mucosa.

In conclusion, GERD may be considered an immune-mediated disease starting at the submucosal layer and the cytokine profile of the mucosal immune response may explain the different outcome of gastresophageal reflux, the severity of mucosal injury and even the relapse of esophagitis. Finally, this new concept opens the way to the development of new treatment for patients who do not respond to PPIs, and to the prevention of carcinogenesis.

Conflicts of interest

The authors declare no conflicts of interest.

References

1. Van Soest, E.M., J.P. Dieleman, P.D. Siersema, *et al.* 2005. Increasing incidence of Barrett's esophagus in the general population. *Gut* **54:** 1062–1066.
2. Westhoff, B., S. Brotze, A. Weston, *et al.* 2005. The frequency of Barrett's esophagus in high-risk patients with chronic GERD. *Gastrointest. Endosc.* **61:** 226–231.
3. Ronkainen, J., P. Aro, T. Storskrubb, *et al.* 2005. Prevalence of Barrett's esophagus in the general population: an endoscopic study. *Gastroenterology* **129:** 1825–1831.
4. Zagari, R.M., L. Fuccio, M.A. Wallander, *et al.* 2008. Gastro-esophageal reflux symptoms, esophagitis and Barrett's esophagus in the general population: the Loiano-Monghidoro study. *Gut* **57:** 1354–1359.
5. Hayeck, T.J., C.Y. Kong, S.J. Spechler, *et al.* 2010. The prevalence of Barrett's esophagus in the US: estimates from a simulation model confirmed by SEER data. *Dis. Esophagus.* **23:** 451–457.
6. Wang, C., Y. Yuan & R.H. Hunt. 2009. *Helicobacter pylori* infection and Barrett's esophagus: a systematic review and meta-analysis. *Am. J. Gastroenterol.* **104:** 492–500; quiz 491, 501.
7. Islami, F. & F. Kamangar. 2008. *Helicobacter pylori* and esophageal cancer risk: a meta-analysis. *Cancer Prev. Res.* **1:** 329–338.

8. Jacobson, B.C. *et al.* 2009. Body mass index and Barrett's esophagus in women. *Gut* **58:** 1460–1466.

9. Chow, W.H. *et al.* 1998. Body mass index and risk of adenocarcinomas of the esophagus and gastric cardia. *J. Natl. Can. Inst.* **90:** 150–155.

10. Ogiya, K., T. Kawano, E. Ito, *et al.* 2008. Lower esophageal palisade vessels and the definition of Barrett's esophagus. *Dis. Esophagus.* **21:** 645–649.

11. Sharma, P., J. Dent, D. Armstrong, *et al.* 2006. The development and validation of an endoscopic grading system for Barrett's esophagus: the Prague C&M criteria. *Gastroenterology* **131:** 1392–1399.

12. Playford, R.J. 2006. New British Society of Gastroenterology (BSG) guidelines for the diagnosis and management of Barrett's esophagus. *Gut.* **55:** 442.

13. Wang, K.K. & R.E. Sampliner. 2008. Updated guidelines 2008 for the diagnosis, surveillance and therapy of Barrett's esophagus. *Am. J. Gastroenterol.* **103:** 788–797.

14. Spechler, S.J., R.C. Fitzgerald, G.A. Prasad & K.K. Wang. 2010. History, molecular mechanisms, and endoscopic treatment of Barrett's esophagus. *Gastroenterology* **138:** 854–869.

15. Riddell, R.H. & R.D. Odze. 2009. Definition of Barrett's esophagus: time for a rethink—is intestinal metaplasia dead? *Am. J. Gastroenterol.* **104:** 2588–2594.

16. Winter, J.W., S. Paterson, G. Scobie, *et al.* 2007. N-nitrosamine generation from ingested nitrate via nitric oxide in subjects with and without gastresophageal reflux. *Gastroenterology* **133:** 164–174.

17. Vaughan, T.L., A.R. Kristal, P.L. Blount, *et al.* 2002. Nonsteroidal anti-inflammatory drug use, body mass index, and anthropometry in relation to genetic and flow cytometric abnormalities in Barrett's esophagus. *Cancer Epidemiol. Biomarkers. Prev.* **11:** 745–752.

18. Jacobson, B.C., S.C. Somers, C.S. Fuchs, *et al.* 2006. Body-mass index and symptoms of gastroesophageal reflux in women. *N. Engl. J. Med.* **354:** 2340–2348.

19. El-Serag, H.B., G.A. Ergun, J. Pandolfino, *et al.* 2007. Obesity increases oesophageal acid exposure. *Gut* **56:** 749–755.

20. Crowell, M.D., A. Bradley, S. Hansel, *et al.* 2009. Obesity is associated with increased 48-h esophageal acid exposure in patients with symptomatic gastroesophageal reflux. *Am. J. Gastroenterol.* **104:** 553–559.

21. Kaltenbach, T., S. Crockett & L.B. Gerson. 2006. Are lifestyle measures effective in patients with gastroesophageal reflux disease? An evidence-based approach. *Arch. Internal Med.* **166:** 965–971.

22. Sheu, B.-S., W.-L. Chang, H.-C. Cheng, *et al.* 2008. Body mass index can determine the healing of reflux esophagitis with los angeles grades C and D by esomeprazole. *Am. J. Gastroenterol.* **103:** 2209–2214.

23. Pandolfino, J.E., H.B. El-Serag, Q. Zhang, *et al.* 2006. Obesity: a challenge to esophagogastric junction integrity. *Gastroenterology* **130:** 639–649.

24. Wu, J.C.-Y., L.-M. Mui, C.M.-Y. Cheung, *et al.* 2007. Obesity is associated with increased transient lower esophageal sphincter relaxation. *Gastroenterology* **132:** 883–889.

25. Corley, D.A., A. Kubo, T.R. Levin, *et al.* 2007. Abdominal obesity and body mass index as risk factors for Barrett's esophagus. *Gastroenterology* **133:** 34–41; quiz 311.

26. Edelstein, Z.R., D.C. Farrow, M.P. Bronner, *et al.* 2007. Central adiposity and risk of Barrett's esophagus. *Gastroenterology* **133:** 403–411.

27. Whiteman, D.C., S. Sadeghi, N. Pandeya, *et al.* 2008. Combined effects of obesity, acid reflux and smoking on the risk of adenocarcinomas of the oesophagus. *Gut* **57:** 173–180.

28. Austin, G.L., M.T. Thiny, E.C. Westman, W.S. Yancy, Jr. & N.J. Shaheen. 2006. A very low-carbohydrate diet improves gastroesophageal reflux and its symptoms. *Dig. Dis. Sci.* **51:** 1307–1312.

29. Zheng, Z., H. Nordenstedt, N.L. Pedersen, J. Lagergren, *et al.* 2007. Lifestyle factors and risk for symptomatic gastroesophageal reflux in monozygotic twins. *Gastroenterology* **132:** 87–95.

30. Nocon, M., J. Labenz & S.N. Willich. 2006. Lifestyle factors and symptoms of gastro-oesophageal reflux—a population-based study. *Aliment. Pharmacol. Ther.* **23:** 169–174.

31. Nilsson, M., R. Johnsen, W. Ye, K. Hveem, *et al.* 2004. Lifestyle related risk factors in the aetiology of gastro-oesophageal reflux. *Gut* **53:** 1730–1735.

32. Dore, M.P., E. Maragkoudakis, K. Fraley, *et al.* 2008. Diet, lifestyle and gender in gastro-esophageal reflux disease. *Dig. Dis. Sci.* **53:** 2027–2032.

33. Mohamed-Ali, V., Goodrick S., A. Rawesh, *et al.* 1997. Subcutaneous adipose tissue releases interleukin-6, but not tumor necrosis factor-alpha, in vivo. *J. Clin. Endocrinol. Metab.* **82:** 4196–4200.

34. Fried, S.K., D.A. Bunkin & A.S. Greenberg. 1998. Omental and subcutaneous adipose tissues of obese subjects release interleukin-6: depot difference and regulation by glucocorticoid. *J. Clin. Endocrinol. Metab.* **83:** 847–850.

35. Barb, D., C.J. Williams, A.K. Neuwirth & C.S. Mantzoros. 2007. Adiponectin in relation to malignancies: a review of existing basic research and clinical evidence. *Am. J. Clin. Nutr.* **86:** s858–s866.

36. Erlinger, T.P., E.A. Platz, N. Rifai & K.J. Helzlsouer. 2004. C-reactive protein and the risk of incident colorectal cancer. *JAMA* **291:** 585–590.

37. Kaaks, R. & A. Lukanova. 2001. Energy balance and cancer: the role of insulin and insulin-like growth factor-I. *Proc. Nutr. Soc.* **60:** 91–106.

38. Kumor, A., P. Daniel, M. Pietruczuk, *et al.* 2009. Serum leptin, adiponectin, and resistin concentration in colorectal adenoma and carcinoma (CC) patients. *Int. J. Colorectal Dis.* **24:** 275–281.

39. El-Serag, H.B., P. Kvapil, J. Hacken-Bitar & J.R. Kramer. 2005. Abdominal obesity and the risk of Barrett's esophagus. *Am. J. Gastroenterol.* **100:** 2151–2156.

40. El-Zimaity, H. 2008. Gastritis and gastric atrophy. *Curr. Opin. Gastroenterol.* **24:** 682–686.

41. Derakhshan, M.H., E. El-Omar, K. Oien, *et al.* 2006. Gastric histology, serological markers and age as predictors of gastric acid secretion in patients infected with *Helicobacter pylori*. *J. Clin. Pathol.* **59:** 1293–1299.

42. El-Omar, E., I. Penman, C.A. Dorrian, *et al.* 1993. Eradicating *Helicobacter pylori* infection lowers gastrin mediated acid secretion by two thirds in patients with duodenal ulcer. *Gut* **34:** 1060–1065.

43. El-Omar, E.M., K. Oien, A. El-Nujumi, *et al.* 1997. *Helicobacter pylori* infection and chronic gastric acid hyposecretion. *Gastroenterology* **113:** 15–24.

44. Yaghoobi, M., F. Farrokhyar, Y. Yuan & R.H. Hunt. 2010. Is there an increased risk of GERD after *Helicobacter pylori* eradication?: a meta-analysis. *Am. J. Gastroenterol.* **105:** 1007–1013; quiz 6, 14.

45. Johnson, D.A., C. Winters, T.J. Spurling, *et al.* 1987. Esophageal acid sensitivity in Barrett's esophagus. *J. Clin. Gastroenterol.* **9:** 23–27.

46. Fletcher, J., D. Gillen, A. Wirz & K.E. McColl. 2003. Barrett's esophagus evokes a quantitatively and qualitatively altered response to both acid and hypertonic solutions. *Am. J. Gastroenterol.* **98:** 1480–1486.

47. Miwa, H., T. Minoo, M. Hojo, *et al.* 2004. Esophageal hypersensitivity in Japanese patients with non-erosive gastro-esophageal reflux diseases. *Aliment. Pharmacol. Ther.* **20**(Suppl. 1): 112–7.3.

48. Stein, H.J., S. Hoeft & T.R. DeMeester. 1993. Functional foregut abnormalities in Barrett's esophagus. *J. Thorac. Cardiovasc. Surg.* **105:** 107–114.

49. Drewes, A.M., H. Gregersen & L. Arendt-Nielsen. 2003. Experimental Pain in Gastroenterology. A reappraisal of human studies. *Scand. J. Gastroenterol.* **38:** 1115–1130

50. Drewes, A.M., K.-S. Schipper, G. Dimcevski, *et al.* 2002. Multimodal assessment of pain in the esophagus: a new experimental model. *Am. J. Physiol. Gastrointest. Liver Physiol.* **283:** G95–G103.

51. Krarup, A.L., S.S. Olesen, P. Funch-Jensen, *et al.* 2010. Decreased sensitivity in patients with Barrett's esophagus both in the metaplastic and the normal part of esophagus. *World J. Gastroenterol.* In press.

52. Orr, W.C., C. Lackey, M.G. Robinson, *et al.* 1988. Esophageal acid clearance during sleep in patients with Barrett's esophagus. *Dig. Dis. Sci.* **33:** 654–659.

53. Trimble, K.C., A. Pryde & R.C. Heading. 1995. Lowered esophageal sensory thresholds in patients with symptomatic but not excess gastro-esophageal reflux: evidence for a spectrum of visceral sensitivity in GORD. *Gut* **37:** 712.

54. Avidan, B., A. Sonnenberg, G. Chejfec, *et al.* 2001. Is there a link between cervical inlet patch and Barrett's esophagus? *Gastrointest. Endosc.* **53:** 717–721.

55. Champion, G., J.E. Richter, M.F. Vaezi, *et al.* 1994. Duodenogastresophageal reflux: relationship to pH and importance in Barrett's esophagus. *Gastroenterology* **107:** 747–754.

56. Vaezi, M.F. & J.E. Richter. 1996. Role of acid and duodenogastric reflux in GERD. *Gastroenterology* **111:** 1192–1199.

57. Vaezi, M.F., R.G. La Camera & J.E. Richter. 1994. Bilitec 2000 ambulatory duodenogastric reflux monitoring: studies on its validation and limitations. *Am. J. Physiol.* **30:** 1050–1056.

58. Koek, G.H., D. Sifrim, T. Lerut, *et al.* 2006. Multivariate analysis and association of acid and DGER exposure with the presence of esophagitis, the severity of esophagitis and Barrett's esophagus. **57:** 1056–1064.

59. Campos, G.M., S.R. DeMeester, J.H. Peters, *et al.* 2001. Predictive factors of Barrett's esophagus: multivariate analysis of 502 patients with GERD. *Arch. Surg.* **136:** 1267–1273.

60. Wetscher, *et al.* 1995. *Am. J. Surg.* **170:** 552–557.

61. Dvorak, *et al.* 2006. Bile acids in combination with low pH induce oxidative stress and oxidative DNA damage: relevance to the pathogenesis of Barrett's oesophagus. *Gut* **56:** 763–771.

62. Jenkins, *et al.* 2007. Deoxycholic acid at neutral and acid pH, is genotoxic to oesophageal cells through the induction of ROS: the potential role of anti-oxidants in Barrett's oesophagus. *Carcinogenesis* **28:** 136–142.

63. Zhang, H.Y., K. Hormi-Carver, X. Zhang, *et al.* 2009. In benign Barrett's epithelial cells, acid exposure generates reactive oxygen species that cause DNA double-strand breaks. *Cancer Res.* **69:** 9083–9089.

64. Kubo, *et al.* 2007. Meta-Analysis of Antioxidant Intake and the Risk of Esophageal and Gastric Cardia Adenocarcinoma. *Am. J. Gast.* **102:** 2323–2330.

65. White, *et al.* 2002. *Br. J. Nutr.* **88:** 265–271.

66. Murphy, *et al.* 2008. Neither antioxidants nor COX-2 inhibition protect against esophageal inflammation in an experimental model of severe reflux. *J. Surg. Res.* **145:** 33–40.

67. Babar, *et al.* 2010. Pilot translational study of dietary vitamin C supplementation in Barrett's esophagus. *Dis. Esoph.* **23:** 271–276.

68. Cronin, J., L. Williams, E. McAdam, *et al.* 2010. The role of secondary bile acids in neoplastic development in the esophagus. *Biochem. SoTrans.* **38:** 337–342.

69. Jolly, A.J., C.P. Wild & L.J. Hardie. 2009. Sodium deoxycholate causes nitric oxide mediated DNA damage in esophageal cells. *Free Radic. Res.* **43:** 234–240.

70. Goldman, A.S.M., D. Goldman, G. Watts, *et al.* 2010. A novel mechanism of acid and bile acid-induced DNA damage involving Na+/H+ exchanger: implication for Barrett's esophagus. *Gut* **59:** 1606–1616.

71. Goldman, A., A. Condon, E. Adler, *et al.* 2010. Protective effects of glycoursodeoxycholic acid in Barrett's esophagus cells. *Dis. Esophagus.* **23:** 83–93.

72. Yang, L., X. Lu, C.W. Nossa, *et al.* 2009. Inflammation and intestinal metaplasia of the distal esophagus are associated with alterations in the microbiome. *Gastroenterology* **137:** 588–597.

73. Souza, R.F., X. Huo, V. Mittal, *et al.* 2009. Gastroesophageal reflux might cause esophagitis through a cytokine-mediated mechanism rather than caustic acid injury. *Gastroenterology* **137:** 1776–1784.

74. Yoshida, N., K. Uchiyama, M. Kuroda, *et al.* Interleukin-8 expression in the esophageal mucosa of patients with gastresophageal reflux disease. *Scand. J. Gastroenterol.* **39:** 816–822.

75. Rieder, F., P. Biancani, K. Harnett, *et al.* 2010. Inflammatory mediators in gastresophageal reflux disease: impact on esophageal motility, fibrosis, and carcinogenesis. *Am. J. Physiol. Gastrointest. Liver Physiol.* **298:** G571–G581.

76. Fitzgerald, R.C., B.A. Onwuegbusi, M. Bajaj-Elliott, *et al.* 2002. Diversity in the esophageal phenotypic response to gastro-esophageal reflux: immunological determinants. *Gut* **50:** 451–459.

Ann. N.Y. Acad. Sci. ISSN 0077-8923

ANNALS OF THE NEW YORK ACADEMY OF SCIENCES
Issue: *Barrett's Esophagus: The 10th OESO World Congress Proceedings*

Barrett's esophagus: genetic and cell changes

Rhonda F. Souza,[1] Giancarlo Freschi,[2] Antonio Taddei,[2] Maria Novella Ringressi,[2] Paolo Bechi,[2] Francesca Castiglione,[3] Duccio Rossi Degl'Innocenti,[3] George Triadafilopoulos,[4] Jean S. Wang,[5] Andrew C. Chang,[6] Hugh Barr,[7] Manisha Bajpai,[8] Kiron M. Das,[8] Paul M. Schneider,[9] Kausilia K. Krishnadath,[10] Usha Malhotra,[11] and John P. Lynch[12]

[1]Department of Medicine, University of Texas Southwestern Medical Center and the VA North Texas Health Care System, Dallas, Texas. [2]Department of Medical and Surgical Critical Care–Unit of Surgery and [3]Department of Medical and Surgical Critical Care–Unit of Human Pathology, University of Florence, Florence, Italy. [4]Stanford University School of Medicine, Stanford, California. [5]Division of Gastroenterology, Washington University School of Medicine, Saint Louis, Missouri. [6]Section of General Thoracic Surgery, University of Michigan Health System, Ann Arbor, Michigan. [7]Cranfield University, Gloucestershire Royal Hospital, Gloucester, United Kingdom. [8]Division of Gastroenterology, Department of Medicine, University of Medicine & Dentistry of New Jersey, Robert Wood Johnson Medical School, New Brunswick, New Jersey. [9]Division of Visceral and Transplantation Surgery, Department of Surgery, University Hospital Zurich, Zurich, Switzerland. [10]Department of Gastroenterology and Hepatology, Academic Medical Center, Amsterdam, the Netherlands. [11]Division of Hematology/Oncology, University of Pittsburgh Department of Medicine, Pittsburgh, Pennsylvania. [12]Department of Medicine, Gastroenterology, University of Pennsylvania, Philadelphia, Pennsylvania

The following includes commentaries on how genetic code of Barrett's esophagus (BE) patients, the mechanisms for GERD-induced esophageal expression of caudal homeobox, and the development of Barrett's metaplasia are increasingly better known, including the role of stromal genes in oncogenesis. Additional lessons have been learned from *in vitro* models in nonneoplastic cell lines, yet there are limitations to what can be expected from BE-derived cell lines. Other topics discussed include clonal diversity in Barrett's esophagus; the application of peptide arrays to clinical samples of metaplastic mucosa; proliferation and apoptosis of Barrett's cell lines; tissue biomarkers for neoplasia; and transcription factors associated with BE.

Keywords: Barrett's esophagus; IGF-1R genotype; intestinal metaplasia; Hox genes; bile; mitogen-activated protein kinase; adenocarcinoma; p16; p53; CDKN2A; TP53; villin; mAb Das-1; BAR-T cells; CDX-1gene; CDX-2 gene; NF-κB; Hedgehog pathway; BMP-4

Concise summaries

- The mechanisms for GERD-induced esophageal expression of caudal homeobox and development of Barrett's metaplasia are better known, as is the genetic code of Barrett's patients, but there is not a specific genetic code predictive of Barrett's esophagus (BE). There is an upregulation of embryological pathways that are silenced in the late and postembryonic phase; the role of stromal genes in oncogenesis, as shown in rat models, as well as the lessons learned from *in vitro* models in nonneoplastic cell lines are helpful to understand the natural history of the disease. The clonal diversity in BE must be emphasized, but there are limitations to what can be expected from BE-derived cell lines. *In vitro* experiments with cells in culture should be viewed as preliminary, and will need to be confirmed by *ex vivo* studies with whole Barrett's tissues that include elements of the stroma. Ultimately, *in vivo* longitudinal studies will need to confirm the pathways to neoplasia. Novel *in vitro* models demonstrate that benign Barrett's epithelial cells can change phenotype expression following exposure to acid and bile. The study of proteomics will probably result in an unparalleled understanding of BA carcinogenesis and will not only be helpful in identifying BE patients at risk for progression, but they will also be critical in better defining tumor stage. The complete transformation of normal esophageal squamous cells into intestinal type cells might be through a cooperative interaction of BMP-4 and CDX-2.

doi: 10.1111/j.1749-6632.2011.06043.x

- In nondysplastic Barrett's cells, acid exposure decreases proliferation and causes a slight increase in apoptosis. In contrast, bile salt exposure does not induce apoptosis in *ex vivo* cultures of nondysplastic Barrett's cells. Levels of the tumor suppressor and transcription factor are frequently increased with progression to HGD and may be useful markers for adenocarcinoma, but this is a mutated form that is transcriptionally inactive.

---

1. Is there a specific genetic code predictive of BE to be considered as a useful tool in epidemiologic studies?

Rhonda F. Souza

rhonda.souza@utsouthwestern.edu

BE develops through metaplasia, which is the process whereby one adult cell type replaces another. In the esophagus, the normal esophageal squamous epithelium becomes replaced by specialized intestinal epithelium that is characteristic of BE. In a general Swedish population, the prevalence rate of BE was found to be 1.6%.[1] Data from the United States suggest that familial Barrett's accounts for 7.3% of cases, whereas the vast majority of cases are considered sporadic.[2]

Familial Barrett's esophagus

Familial BE is defined as having a first- or second-degree relative with BE, esophageal adenocarcinoma (EAC), or adenocarcinoma of the gastresophageal junction.[2] Recent data generated from 881 "familial Barrett's" families suggest that there is inheritance of one or more rare autosomal dominant susceptibility alleles in these families.[2] However, no specific genetic code indicative of familial BE has been identified yet.

Sporadic Barrett's esophagus

The main risk factors for BE are advanced age, male gender, white ethnicity, obesity, and gastresophageal reflux disease (GERD). Of these risk factors, the ones that have been investigated for genetic variation as a predictor of BE include GERD and obesity. GERD is a major risk factor for BE.

So maybe rather than BE being an inherited condition, perhaps GERD is the inherited condition in these patients. In support of such a hypothesis, a number of studies have found a clustering of symptomatic GERD among relatives of patients with BE, suggesting that in Barrett's families there may be a genetic component for GERD. However, one study has also reported a clustering of symptomatic GERD among relatives of GERD patients without BE, which refutes this hypothesis.[3]

Regardless, no specific genetic code indicative of familial GERD has been identified yet. Even if there was an inherited predisposition to GERD, this would still not explain why only a minority of GERD patients develop BE. So perhaps there is another mechanism whereby GERD causes a minority of patients to develop BE. Gastresophageal reflux clearly leads to reflux esophagitis. In a minority of GERD patients, this inflammation can heal with the development of Barrett's metaplasia (BM). So it is conceivable that genetic alterations in the reflux-mediated inflammatory response may predict which GERD patients develop BE. In fact, there are a number of studies suggesting that patients with BE maybe genetically predisposed to more severe inflammation in response to reflux.[4]

Obesity is the other risk factor, which has been investigated for genetic variation as a predictor of BE. Although it is not entirely clear exactly how obesity contributes to the development of BE, one way might be to increase GERD. Another way may be to mediate signaling through the pro-proliferative insulin and insulin-like growth factor pathways. In fact, obese patients with BE may be genetically predisposed to enhanced signaling via these pathways by alterations in the IGF-1R. In one study, blood from obese patients with and without BE was analyzed for the presence of a pro-proliferative IGF-1R genotype.[5] The investigators found that there was no difference between obese patients with BE and those without GERD or BE in the frequency of the wild-type genotype for IGF-1R.[5] In contrast, they found that obese patients with BE were more likely to have a pro-proliferative IGF-1R genotype than obese patients without GERD or BE.[5]

Conclusion

Is there a specific genetic code predictive of BE to be considered a useful tool in epidemiological studies? The answer is NO.

2. What is the role of developmental signaling pathways in the mechanisms by which GERD may induce the esophageal expression of Caudal homeobox (Cdx) genes that mediate the development of BM?

Giancarlo Freschi, A. Taddei, M.N. Ringressi, V. Ceccherini, F. Castiglione, D.R. Degl'Innocenti, and P. Bechi
giancarlo.freschi@unifi.it

To determine the molecular mechanisms responsible for BM, it is important to understand how tissue types are specified during normal development. A specific set of transcription factors, like Hox genes or Cdx genes specifying intestine and signaling molecules, are important regulators of tissue type during embryogenesis.

Particularly CDX2, a homeobox gene, has a role in the development of the gastrointestinal tract. In fact, CDX2 has been shown to be an important transcriptional regulator in maintenance of normal adult small intestine and colonic epithelium and has been shown to activate other intestinal differentiation genes, including MUC2.

Cdx genes in BE
CDX2 is not expressed in normal esophageal mucosa but is abundantly re-expressed in intestinal metaplastic mucosa in the esophagus, and immunohistochemical staining studies have confirmed that the CDX2 protein is overexpressed in human BM.[6] Animal studies have suggested that gastresophageal reflux may enhance CDX2 expression in rat esophageal keratinocytes and studies of CDX2 gene expression in human esophageal biopsy specimens reveal an increase at each step in the development of BE.[7]

Although *in vitro* studies have demonstrated increased CDX2 promoter activity, RNA and protein expression, and upregulation of downstream target genes, Cdx regulation is an incompletely understood process, but it probably involves complex interactions among key signaling pathways, morphogenetic factors, and transcription factors involved in regulating embryonic development and in maintaining the homeostasis of adult tissues. Literature suggests that many developmental signaling pathways, like Wnt, BMP, transforming growth factor-β, hedgehog, notch, NF-κB, and

other growth factor pathways play an important role in this process.[8]

Bone morphogenetic proteins (BMPs) are a group of growth factors now considered to constitute a group of pivotal morphogenetic signals, orchestrating tissue architecture throughout the body http://en.wikipedia.org/wiki/Bone_morphogenetic_protein-cite_note-1. They are an important factor in the progression of colon cancer and, conversely, overactivation of BMP signaling following reflux-induced esophagitis provokes BE and is thus instrumental in the development of adenocarcinoma in the proximal portion of the gastrointestinal tract. Supporting this contention, recent studies suggest that GERD may cause esophageal stromal cells to express BMP-4, one of the key players in early morphogenesis of the esophagus, which promotes the change from squamous to columnar epithelium.

Notch
Notch is translocated to the nucleus where it interacts with transcription factors to become a transcriptional activator and then can modulate the expression of Notch target genes that regulate cell fate decisions. The hypothesis is that exposure of esophageal cells to the bile acid, deoxycholic acid (DCA), results in inhibition of the Notch pathway, with alterations in its downstream effectors and induction of CDX2 expression.

NF-κB
Recent evidence suggests that the transcription factor nuclear factor κB may be a candidate factor linking inflammation to cancer because it plays a central role in the inflammatory cascade and has been linked to cancer development. NF-κB is found at increasing levels from normal esophagus to esophagitis and from BM to EAC. NF-κB has been shown to be integral to the regulation of two homeobox genes, caudal type homeobox transcription factors (CDX) 1 and 2. There is now increasing evidence of a link between NF-κB and the CDX genes, suggesting a mechanism by which inflammation could induce metaplasia.[9]

Wnt
The Wnt-signaling pathway is essential in many biological processes and numerous studies of this pathway over the past years have led to the identification of several novel components. CDX2 has been shown to be a downstream target of WNT, and the

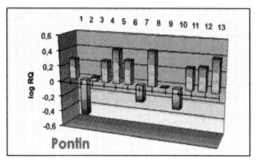 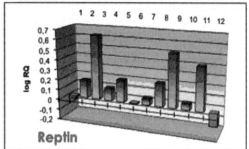

Figure 1. Relative expression of pontin and reptin genes in BM with respect to normal esophageal mucosa.

cytoplasmic accumulation and nuclear translocation of β-catenin, a transcription factor, represents a key step in the activation of the pro-oncogenic canonical WNT pathway.

Here, in comparison to normal, GERD, or BM tissues, β-catenin was found to be overexpressed in about one-third of EA tissues. Of particular interest were several significant associations between the expression of β-catenin and CDX2 in esophageal tissues, suggesting a central role for the WNT/CDX2 pathway in the molecular pathogenesis of EA. In the absence of the signal, action of the destruction complex (CKIα, GSK3β, APC, and Axin) creates a hyperphosphorylated β-catenin, which is a target for ubiquitination and degradation by the proteosome. Binding of Wnt leads to stabilization of hypophosphorylated β-catenin, which interacts with TCF/LEF proteins in the nucleus to activate transcription.[10] β-catenin activity is further modulated by other factors. Among these there is pontin and reptin.

Pontin and reptin

Pontin (Ruvb1) and reptin (Ruvb2) are highly conserved components of multimeric protein complexes important for chromatin remodeling and transcription. They interact with many different proteins, including c-myc and β-catenin, and thus potentially modulate different pathways. In other words, pontin and reptin are Wnt-signaling interaction partners that antagonistically modulate β-catenin transcriptional activity.

Personal data

From our previous analyses using real-time PCR on rectal carcinoma samples, we observed that the expression of pontin is clearly more prevalent than that of reptin. We performed the same study on BE samples, and the results were inconsistent for pontin, whereas reptin expression appeared to be more prevalent in the various BM samples (Fig. 1).

We have begun to check BM biopsies for the expression of other key transcription factors known to effect intestinal differentiation, especially HOX genes (HoxD locus in particular). Significant differences exist for some of the genes, both in BM compared to a normal esophagus and compared to simple esophagitis (Fig. 2). This confirms our opinion, as well as that of many other researchers, that a single transcription factor like CDX2 is probably

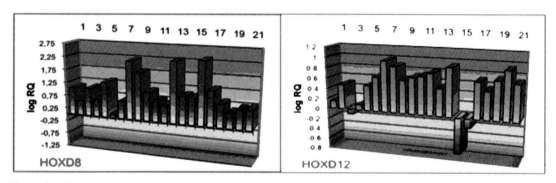

Figure 2. Relative expression of HOXD8 and HOXD12 genes in BM with respect to normal esophageal mucosa.

not solely responsible for a change as dramatic as that of BE, and that the homeobox gene network (HOX and CDX) acts just like an integrated circuit, with yet unexplored potential.

Although these data are very interesting, they are merely speculative and observational and obviously needs to be backed up with functional correlations with other types of experiments.

Conclusions

From recent findings, it has become apparent that in BM there is upregulation of embryological pathways that are silenced in the late and postembryonic phase. Identification of CDX2 as a key transcriptional regulator, and studies dissecting its activation are rapidly evolving, as is our understanding of its potential pathogenesis. The interaction of different components (Wnts, BMPs, Shh) is required for proper morphogenesis of the intestine but also for cdx gene expression and thus for BM. Future investigation of these factors is fundamental to further delineate the enigma of BM and to develop novel molecular therapeutic strategies aimed at preventing or reversing this premalignant condition. These additional studies may be warranted in several areas, especially how signaling pathways and transcription factors (such as CDX1, CDX2, and HOX genes) may interact with each other to mediate the development of BM (Fig. 1).

3. What model systems are likely to show the impact of acid and bile on gene expression of the esophagus *in vivo*?

George Triadafilopoulos
vagt@stanford.edu

Thus far there have been two settings in which research has been done to address the question of acid and bile on gene expression. The first setting has been various cell culture systems, the latter, an *ex vivo* tissue culture Barrett's tissues, and both have been extensively used.

In one of many examples using cell lines, and to explore mechanisms whereby acid reflux might contribute to carcinogenesis in BE, Souza *et al.*, studied the effects of acid on the mitogen-activated protein kinase (MAPK) pathways, cell proliferation, and apoptosis in a Barrett's adenocarcinoma cell line (SEG-1).[11] SEG-1 cells were exposed to acidic media for three minutes, and the activities of three MAPKs

(ERK, p38, and JNK) were determined. Proliferation was assessed using flow cytometry; cell growth and apoptosis were assessed using cell counts and an apoptosis ELISA assay. They found that acid-exposed SEG-1 cells exhibited a significant increase in proliferation and total cell numbers, and a significant decrease in apoptosis. These effects were preceded by a rapid increase in the activities of ERK and p38, and a delayed increase in JNK activity.

In a classic example of *ex vivo* experiments, and because acid is a major component of refluxate, Fitzgerald *et al.*[12] investigated its effects *ex vivo* on cell differentiation as determined by villin expression, and on cell proliferation, as determined by tritiated thymidine incorporation and proliferating cell nuclear antigen expression. To mimic known physiological conditions, endoscopic biopsies of normal esophagus, BE, and duodenum were exposed, in organ culture, to acidified media (pH 3–5) either continuously, or as a one hour pulse and compared with exposure to pH 7.4 for up to 24 hours. Before culture, villin expression was noted in 25% of metaplasia samples, and increased after 6 or 24 hours of continuous acid to 50% or 83% of metaplasia, respectively. Increased villin expression correlated with ultrastructural maturation of the brush border. In contrast, an acid-pulse followed by culture at pH 7.4, did not alter villin expression in BE. Moreover, continuous acid exposure blocked cell proliferation in BE, whereas, an acid-pulse enhanced cell proliferation, as compared to pH 7.4. Based on their *ex vivo* findings, the authors proposed a model in which the diverse patterns of acid exposure *in vivo* might contribute to the observed heterogeneity and unpredictable progression to neoplasia of BE. However, both these types of models carry inherent limitations, and they do not address acid and bile reflux on metaplasia *in vivo*. One of their key limitations is the noninvolvement of the stroma in such experiments, because it plays an increasingly important role in Barrett's carcinogenesis.[13]

A small animal endoscopy in a rat model of BE has been recently described and it appears promising in the *in vivo* study of gene expression in this disease.[14] The model allows the performance of surveillance, classification of mucosal patterns, for observation of the onset of intestinal metaplasia, and monitoring the progression of neoplastic transformation. Advantages of the model include (1) the

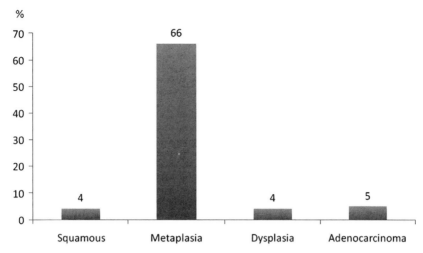

Figure 3. Esophageal histology at 36 weeks in an animal model of Barrett's carcinogenesis that allows for dynamic assessment of acid and bile exposure on gene expression *in vivo*.

esophago-gastro-jejunal anastomotic procedure is easy to perform; (2) it allows reflux of both acid and bile to occur and alter the biological behavior of BE; (3) gastric function, weight, and nutritional status are preserved; and (4) there is a high rate of animal survival and ability to achieve rapid gain in body weight. Figure 3 reveals esophageal histology at 36 weeks in the model.

Souza *et al.* also examined the ability of acid to activate the MAPK pathways *in vivo* in patients with BE.[11] MAPK activation was studied in biopsy specimens taken from patients with BE before and after esophageal perfusion for three minutes with 0.1N HCl. In these patient experiments, acid exposure significantly activated the MAPK pathways in the metaplastic epithelium.

The clonal evolution model in BE has recently evolved.[15] The concept of an initial single clone that evolves and accumulates genetic defects, has now been replaced by another model, in which multiple defective clones progress independently or together into malignant transformation. This latter model has been substantiated by recent *ex vivo* studies by Leedham *et al.*,[16] who aimed to assess clonality at a much higher resolution by microdissecting and genetically analyzing individual crypts. Determination of tumor suppressor gene loss of heterozygosity patterns, p16 and p53 point mutations, were carried out on a crypt-by-crypt basis. Cases of contiguous neosquamous islands and columnar metaplasia with esophageal squamous ducts were identified. Tissues were isolated by laser cap-

ture microdissection and genetically analyzed. Individual crypt dissection revealed mutation patterns that were masked in whole biopsy analysis. Dissection across esophagectomy specimens demonstrated marked clonal heterogeneity, with multiple independent clones present. The authors identified a p16 point mutation arising in the squamous epithelium of the esophageal gland duct, which was also present in a contiguous metaplastic crypt, whereas neo squamous islands arising from squamous ducts were wild-type with respect to surrounding Barrett's dysplasia. They concluded that by studying clonality at the crypt level they demonstrated that Barrett's heterogeneity arises from multiple independent clones, in contrast to the selective sweep to fixation model of clonal expansion previously described. They also suggested that the squamous gland ducts situated throughout the esophagus are the source of a progenitor cell that may be susceptible to gene mutation resulting in conversion to Barrett's metaplastic epithelium. Additionally, these data suggested that wild-type ducts might be the source of neo squamous islands.

In conclusion, *in vitro* experiments with cells in culture should be viewed as preliminary and will need to be confirmed by *ex vivo* studies with whole Barrett's tissues that include elements of the stroma. Ultimately, *in vivo* longitudinal studies will need to confirm the pathways to neoplasia. Further, tissue heterogeneity is common in Barrett's epithelia and reflects evolution of multiple mutated clones.

4. What are the limitations of currently available Barrett's cell lines?

Jean S. Wang
jeanwang@wustl.edu

Cell lines serve as useful preclinical models of human disease and play an important role in research on BE and EAC because of the limited availability of patient samples and animal models. There are currently ten authenticated EAC cell lines (FLO-1, KYAE-1, SK-GT-4, OE19, OE33, JH-EsoAd1, OACP4C, OACM5.1, ESO26, and ESO51) that have been verified to be derived from human EACs.[17] Recent technology using telomerase has now allowed for the immortalization of Barrett's cells. There are currently three cell lines derived from patients with BE and high-grade dysplasia and two cell lines derived from patients with nondysplastic BE.[18,19]

One of the major limitations of cell lines has been contamination. It is estimated that up to one-third of all cell lines have an origin other than what was expected due to cross-contamination and mislabeling of cultures. Recently, four commonly used EAC cell lines were identified as being contaminated and confirmed to be other tumor types.[17] In fact, these cell lines actually represented lung cancer, colorectal cancer, gastric cancer, and esophageal squamous cell carcinoma cell lines. Therefore, it is very important to always authenticate cell lines by using DNA fingerprinting techniques such as short tandem repeat profiling or mutation analysis.

Another limitation is that we do not know how similar or representative the cultured cells are compared to the original cells. Barrett's mucosa *in vivo* is likely composed of a mosaic of different clonal populations. Over time, clonal evolution and the dynamics between these multiple clones may be important in the neoplastic progression to adenocarcinoma.[20] However, with a cell line, it is not possible to evaluate the interaction between multiple clones.

Furthermore, artificial selection pressure during the creation of the cell line may result in the propagation of rare clones that have adapted successfully to the cell culture conditions, and it is possible that these clones may not be representative of the biology of the original esophageal tissue. The immortalization procedures alone may affect the growth behavior of cells. In addition, during the creation and propagation of the cell line, there may be *ex vivo* acquisition of genetic or epigenetic alterations.

Finally, another limitation with cell lines is that it is difficult to replicate the natural *in vivo* environment. BE is thought to develop through a multifactorial process that involves not only genetic and epigenetic factors, but also interactions between other important contributors in the microenvironment such as chronic inflammation and the complex physiology behind acid and bile reflux in conjunction with esophageal dysmotility. It is also difficult to simulate the impact of various lifestyle factors such as obesity, diet, and smoking, which may interact and contribute to the development of BE or EAC. Other unknown factors not yet discovered within the microenvironment may also interact with the Barrett's cells and evaluating cell lines alone would not allow for the study of these interactions.

To overcome some of the disadvantages of standard monolayer cell cultures, recently there has been the development of innovative 3D culture systems. These systems are multilayered structures which mimic the tissue microenvironment by using a monolayer of epithelial cells overlaid on a special ECM gel enriched with collagen and fibroblasts.[21] These models allow for the assessment of tumor cell interaction with stromal components and are a promising new technology that may help to overcome some of the limitations seen with standard cell lines.

5. How is clonal diversity in BE recognized?

Andrew C. Chang
andrwchg@umich.edu

While a number of molecular events have been identified in the neoplastic progression from BM to dysplasia and thence adenocarcinoma, the cellular origin of BM, as well as the mechanisms that drive the development of tumor heterogeneity, remain a matter of considerable debate. Clarification of the extent of clonal diversity that exists within dysplastic or malignant Barrett's epithelium might provide further insight into these questions.

Tumor genetic heterogeneity may arise from the development of genetic instability, which can lead to alterations that confer an advantage in terms of survival or proliferation. While clonal diversity appears to correlate with genetic instability, such diversity is not equivalent to genetic instability but, instead, is "a function of both the generation and selection of mutations."[22] Assessment of clonal diversity at different stages of tumorigenesis can provide an indication of the origins of tumor heterogeneity.[23]

Premises for the development of tumor heterogeneity include the cancer stem cell hypothesis and clonal evolution.[23] In the cancer stem cell hypothesis pluripotent epithelial stem cells differentiate into either squamous or intestinal-type columnar epithelium, depending on the exposure to local stresses such as gastresophageal refluxate.[24] If there is more than one progenitor cell population, tumor heterogeneity may develop as a result of ongoing and diverging cellular proliferation and differentiation. In the process of clonal evolution,[25] malignancy arises in a population of cells as a result of progressive accumulated genetic changes. Such changes can confer either an advantage or disadvantage in terms of survival or proliferation during natural selection.[23]

Although tumor heterogeneity has been evaluated widely in terms of specific genetic events or histologic descriptors, in 2006, Maley *et al.* quantified the clonal diversity of esophageal biopsies obtained from patients with BE using methods of molecular evolutionary biology.[26] Using systematic sampling across segments of BE, tissue biopsies from 268 subjects were analyzed for DNA content, changes in microsatellite length (shifts), and/or loss of heterozygosity (LOH) at 9p and *CDKN2A* or *TP53* sequence mutations. In addition to segment length and number of clones, diversity was measured by mean pairwise divergence, defined as the number of loci showing molecular differences (e.g., LOH) divided by the number of informative (normal heterozygote) loci, or by the Shannon diversity index to integrate the number and abundance of clones.[26] During mean follow-up of 4.4 years, EAC developed in 37 subjects.

A number of diversity measures were predictive for the development of EAC, particularly the number of clones (RR 1.40, 95% CI 1.13–1.73), mean pairwise divergence (RR 1.45, 95% CI 1.08–1.95), and Shannon index (RR 3.10, 95% CI 1.37–7.01), as determined by 9p LOH, correcting for *TP53* LOH and abnormal DNA content. In multivariate analysis, the best predictive model for the development of adenocarcinoma included mean pairwise divergence and the number of clones.

To explore this further, this research group demonstrated that increasing clonal diversity, as determined by several other diversity measures, was associated with increased risk for developing EAC. In particular, they found that diversity found even at evolutionarily neutral loci, specifically 9q and 17q, was as strongly associated with progression to adenocarcinoma as at loci where genetic alterations might confer a selective advantage, suggesting that clonal diversity alone can be predictive for the progression to adenocarcinoma regardless of the underlying molecular defect.[22]

Merlo *et al.* caution that novel but low abundance "minority clones" might not be readily detectable when utilizing tissue biopsies to determine clonal diversity.[22] Leedham *et al.* suggest that precise compartmental localization (i.e., laser-capture microdissection) can be used to evaluate more precisely the clonal nature of individual crypts.[27] This group observed considerable crypt-to-crypt clonal heterogeneity that otherwise might be obscured by analysis of whole biopsy samples. Their findings lend further credence to the concept that BE may develop as a result of a number of molecular events occurring in parallel, rather than being due to progressive stepwise accumulation of genetic heterogeneity.

While the steps that lead to the development of tumor heterogeneity and clonal diversity remain obscure, further elucidation of these mechanisms for the pathogenesis of Barrett's-associated adenocarcinoma could direct more specific antineoplastic therapy and improved clinical management.

6. How can the clonality study by individual crypt dissection demonstrate that Barrett's epithelium heterogeneity results from multiple individual clones?

Hugh Barr
hugh.barr@glos.nhs.uk

Despite years of active research, the histiogenesis of BE, a metaplastic condition of the lower esophagus, remains essentially unknown. Over many years, hypotheses have been generated and explored. One area of direct interest are the esophageal gland ducts. These are lined in the proximal two-thirds by a cuboidal epithelium, and undergo a transition to a stratified squamous epithelium as they approach the lumen. It has been suggested that pluripotential stem cells may be located distally in the duct. These become exposed, inflamed with ulceration, and then heal with selective differentiation into an

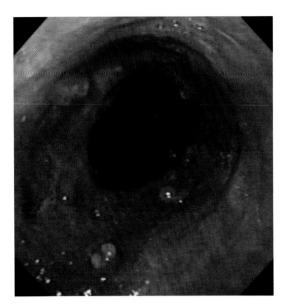

Figure 4. An endoscopic picture of multifocal high-grade dysplasia in Barrett's esophagus.

acid-resistant columnar phenotype. They then migrate to the surface replacing the squamous lining. This is similar to Wright's "ulcer-associated cell lineage" (UACL), a glandular differentiation occurring at sites of intestinal ulceration.[28]

In addition, there is yet to be a consensus on the the clonal evolution, clonal interaction, and neoplastic degeneration, and these subjects remain very controversial issues. It may be that neoplasia develops through clonal selection which sweeps through the Barrett's segment.[29,30] Nevertheless, BE is an excellent area to examine and develop models and systems to examine the progression to cancer. However, much of the work has been based on large biopsy samples—heterogeneous samples taken at multiple segments (Fig. 4).

Recently, Leedham *et al.*[31] have contributed to the histogenesis debate by examining in detail individual crypts for genetic changes. The specimens were obtained from endoscopic resection specimens and whole esophageal resection specimens from endoscopic resection and esophagectomy specimens. The Figure shows an endoscopic picture of multifocal high-grade dysplasia. Individual laser capture micro-dissection was performed and tumor suppressor genes, loss of heterozygosity, p16 and p53 point mutations were examined on individual crypts within these resected specimen. In addition they examined neosquamous islands and metapla-

sia within the esophageal gland ducts. They clearly identified mutation patterns that had been hidden in whole biopsy analysis.

Clonal heterogeneity was identified, and p16 mutations were seen in the esophageal gland duct and its associated metaplastic crypt. It appears that BE may arise from multiple independent clones and is very heterogeneous.

They also suggested that squamous gland ducts could be the source of the metaplastic cells. This confirms earlier morphological three dimensional histological studies that have found continuity between human esophageal gland ducts and Barrett's mucosa. There was a gradual transition of the morphological features of the cells lining the duct: normal cuboidal cells, lining the basal aspect of the duct, into metaplastic cells as the duct opens onto the mucosal surface. This previously demonstrated a definite interrelationship between the two structures. However, identifying the direction of migration is difficult.[32]

7. What lessons can be learned from the influence of environmental factors on various *in vitro* models and the cellular phenotype(s) of the nonneoplastic Barrett's cell line about pathogenesis of Barrett's epithelium and its progression to neoplasia?

Manisha Bajpai and K.M. Das
bajpaima@umdnj.edu

Epidemiology indicates a strong relationship between gastroesophageal reflux disease (GERD) and EAC. Barrett's epithelium is an intestinal type of columnar metaplasia that replaces normal squamous epithelium of the distal esophagus secondary to chronic GERD.

Barrett's epithelium is a major risk factor for development of EAC, causing a 30–125-fold increased risk in GERD patients complicated with BE. In BE, such morphologic changes can be recognized with a spectrum by pathologists as metaplasia–dysplasia–adenocarcinoma (MDA). The esophageal squamous epithelium is exposed to a dynamic environment where the differentiation process is modulated by the gastro-duodenal refluxate and GERD.

Various *in vitro* (nonneoplastic Barrett's cell lines, Barrett's adenocarcinoma cell lines, normal human esophageal epithelial cells, and *in vivo*

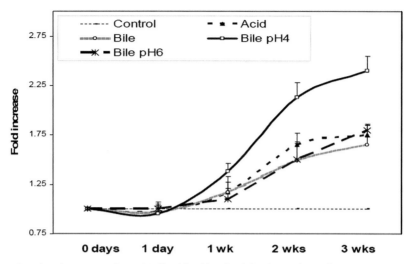

Figure 5. Effect of continued treatment of BAR-T cells with acid and/or bile salt on colonic phenotype expression.

[rodent]) models have been used for the study of pathogenesis of Barrett's epithelium to columnar metaplasia. Acid and assorted components of bile have been implicated in the process of metaplasia of native esophageal squamous epithelium. Presence of pluripotent stem cells, induction of NF-κB, CDX-2 (caudal homeo-box gene) expression, villin expression, and mucin-secreting cells, all favor the resemblance of metaplastic Barrett's epithelium to intestinal epithelium. However, there is limited knowledge regarding the cellular phenotype(s) of this metaplastic process.

We utilized a nonneoplastic, telomerase-immortalized Barrett's cell line (BAR-T) that has key histochemical features of benign Barrett's epithelium.[33] With intact p53 and p21 cell cycle checkpoints, this cell line is ideal for studies on morphologic, phenotypic, and molecular changes under the influence of environmental factors such as acid and bile.

It is a heterogeneous cell line positive for CK4 a marker for squamous, CK 8/18, mAb Das-1, villin, and mucin, all markers indicative of intestinal type of epithelium. Monoclonal antibody Das-1 is a specific marker for colonic epithelium and incomplete type of gastricintestinal metaplasia, type II and III[34], and it does not react with small intestinal enterocytes and complete type or type I (intestinal metaplaisa). However mAb Das-1 reacts with Barrett's epithelium with almost 100% sensitivity and speci-ficity suggesting that Barrett's epithelium is colonic phenotype of metaplasia.[35]

We observed an increase in the columnar, and particularly colonic phenotype (mAbDas-1 positive) cells (Fig. 5),[36] when BAR-T cells were exposed to acid and/or bile (glycocheno-deoxycholic acid, GCDA 200μM) individually or in combination at different pH, particularly at pH4, for five minutes each day for up to three weeks. The CK4 phenotype did not change.[36]

We hypothesized that prolonged, repeated exposure of BAR-T cells to A + B may further induce intestinal phenotype and lead to tumorigenicity. In a systematic, prospective analysis over the course of 65 weeks, we demonstrated that following daily exposure to A + B for a brief period of five minutes per day, BAR-T cells showed progressive morphological, molecular, and biological changes.

Morphological changes between untreated and A + B treated cells were evident from 34 weeks. The treated cells grew as round or oval cells in clumps and displayed acini-like formation (Fig. 6B). Untreated cells remained spindle shaped and evenly dispersed on the culture plate (Fig. 6A). Changes in p53 expression as well as p53 target genes, MDM2, PERP, and p21, were consistent with a transformed phenotype. Loss of anchorage dependence was observed around 54 weeks of A + B treatment. The A + B treated cells could form foci after overconfluent on culture dishes (Figs. 6C and D), grow on

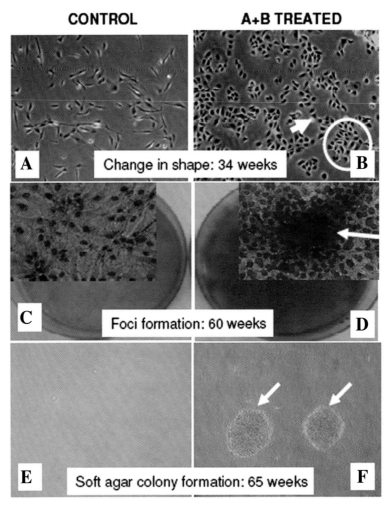

Figure 6. Progressive tumorigenic changes in BAR-T cells upon chronic exposure to A + B.

soft agar (Figs. 6E and F), and form tumors in nude mice.[37]

Conclusion

The novel *in vitro* model demonstrates that benign Barrett's epithelial cells can change phenotype expression following exposure to acid and bile. This phenotype change occurs in favor of columnar phenotype and particularly colonic (incomplete-type) of metaplasia in BAR-T cells similar to *in vivo* situation3. This *in vitro* model further demonstrates that continued exposure to acid and bile for longer duration may cause transformation of benign Barrett's epithelium to neoplasia.[37] BAR-T cells seem to closely reproduce the pathophysiologic progression of Barrett's epithelium and thus can be utilized as an "*in vitro*" model to study the phenotypic

and molecular changes in the pathogenesis of Barrett's epithelium /EAC, to evaluate gene targets and chemo-therapeutic candidates for treatment of Barrett's epithelium and to impede its progression to EAC.

8. What insight into the molecular process of Barrett's esophagus can be expected by applying peptide arrays to clinical samples of metaplastic mucosa?

Georg Lurje, P. Kambakamba, C. Soll, M. Bueter, and P.M. Schneider
paul.schneider@usz.ch

BE development is a multistep process that starts with the mucosal injury of the squamous epithelium of the distal esophagus by gastroesophageal reflux disease (GERD) and progresses through intestinal metaplasia and dysplasia to invasive Barrett's adenocarcinoma (BA). Approximately 10% of patients diagnosed with BE ultimately progress from metaplasia to dysplasia and subsequently to BA. Routine endoscopic surveillance of patients with BE is an expensive practice due to the low rate of progression to EAC in patients without dysplasia. Identification of factors predicting progression to EAC would substantially help to improve screening and surveillance programs especially for patients with BE without dysplasia. While most efforts have been directed at genetic and epigenetic changes within the MDA sequence, little is known about the protein changes that occur in the progression of the disease.

Genomic-based approaches to biomarker development include the measurements of expression of full sets of mRNA and genomic DNA, such as serial analysis of gene expression (SAGE) levels,[38] large-scale gene expression arrays,[39] and genomic polymorphisms.[40] As proteins are often subject to proteolytic cleavage or posttranslational modifications, such as phosphorylation or glycosylation, studies of differential mRNA expression are informative, but do not necessarily correlate with associated protein expression or activity within a given cell. Even though several potential biomarkers have been described over the last decades, none of them have been validated in a population based-study.

It is becoming increasingly apparent that disease progression is largely driven by complex pathways, and analysis of one single genetic or protein marker is unlikely to precisely predict progression of disease with sufficient resolution and reproducibility. The human proteome—like the proteomes of all organisms—is dynamic, changing constantly in response to the needs of the body and differs widely between people depending on factors such as age, gender, diet, level of exercise, and sleep cycle. The proteome also changes in response to cancer and other nonmalignant diseases, making the proteome of great interest to cancer researchers. The science of proteomics—the study of the totality of proteins within a given cell, tissue, or oganism—may therefore provide novel insights for the next level of molecular inquiry that is represented by functional genomics and proteomics.

Two-dimensional gel electrophoresis has been the mainstay of electrophoretic technology for a decade and is a commonly used tool for separating proteins. In many cases, two-dimensional gel electrophoresis evaluates whole-cell or tissue protein extracts. The use of narrow, immobilized pH gradients for the first dimension has increased resolving power for the detection of low-abundance proteins. Radioactive or fluorescent labeling and silver staining allows visualization of hundreds of proteins in a single gel.

Over the past decade, advances in mass spectrometry (MS) and bioinformatics have improved our ability to discriminate cancer-specific peptides. As such, an MS-enhanced, high-resolution, two-dimensional (2D), polyacrylamide gel electrophoresis approach has been applied to further improve detection and separation of proteins at a wide range of pH gradients maximizing the number of separated proteins to up to 2000 proteins using a matrix-assisted laser desorption/ionization, time-of-flight and tandem mass spectrometry (MALDI TOF MS) technology.

Utilizing this technology, a recent study by Peng *et al.* identified protein upregulation of ErbB3, Dr5, cyclin D1, as well as several members of the zinc finger protein family, in eight BAs and four normal mucosal control samples.[41] Interestingly, these proteins were validated in an independent set of 39 BA tissue samples by reverse-transcriptase PCR (RT-PCR) and immunohistochemistry (IHC), suggesting a critical role of these proteins in BA carcinogenesis.[41] Another recent study by De Godoy and coworkers, used advanced computational proteomics to compare essentially all endogeneous proteins in haploid yeast cells to their diploid counterparts, suggesting that system-wide, precise quantification directly at the protein level will help to open new perspectives in postgenomics and system biology.[42] Although standards need to be agreed upon for what determines the validity of a biomarker, now that the draft of the human genome has been completed, the field of proteomics is emerging to tackle vast protein networks that both control, and are controlled by, the information encoded by the genome.

The study of proteomics will probably result in an unparalleled understanding of BA carcinogenesis and will not only be helpful in identifying BE patients at risk for progression, but will also be critical in better defining tumor stage, identifying novel therapeutic targets, and measuring response to therapy, thus tailoring a targeted and effective therapy to the molecular profile of both the patient and the tumor while minimizing and avoiding life-threatening toxicity.

9. Can active cell-signaling pathways in BE be delineated?

Kausilia K. Krishnadath and F. Milano
k.k.krishnadath@amc.uva.nl

Several research groups have been performing studies to elucidate the role of CDX-2, a key intestinal transcription factor involved in both physiological and aberrant processes, such as intestinal metaplasia, in BE. One relevant study was recently performed by H. Kazumori and others, where it was demonstrated that administration of bile and acids to esophageal squamous cell lines increases the CDX-2 gene transcriptional activity. In this study they found, as well as in a rat surgical model, that expression of CDX-2 and mucin-2, a direct target of CDX-2, is increased upon bile and acid injury. They hypothesized that this increased transcriptional activity is mediated by NF-κB.[43] In a study last year, the group of R. Souza *et al.* confirmed these finding esophageal primary cultures of BE patients.[44]

A few years after the 2006 study, the group of Kazumori *et al.* performed another study where they observed that CDX-1, belonging to the same family of CDX-2 transcription factors, is expressed in a surgical rat model. Bile and acid exposure of esophageal cell lines and rat esophageal primary keratinocytes increased the promoter activity of CDX-1 transcription factor, and overexpression of CDX-1 in HET1A esophageal squamous cell line induced expression of mucin-2, an intestinal specific marker. The conclusion from this study was that CDX-1 and CDX-2, in the case of bile and acid injury in the esophageal wall, autoregulate themselves and interregulate each other.[45]

In 2008, Stairs and colleagues published interesting data in the journal *PloS One*, where they showed that EPC2-hTERT normal esophageal keratinocytes, after transfection with c-myc and CDX-1, show upregulation of mucin 5A, another pivotal BE marker, and of intestinal metaplasias, in a subset of cells. Moreover, clonal gene expression of several markers of BE, such as CDX-1, CDX-2, mucin2, mucin 5a, and CK20, is observed after microarray performed on patient material.[46] In none of these studies, however, was it demonstrated which mech-

anism determines exactly the development of an intestinal phenotype.

Interestingly, D. Wang and others published important data about the involvement of the hedgehog pathway in the development of BM. Namely, they looked at the expression of this pathway by microarray in BE and found expression of sonic hedgehog (SHH), namely. In functional studies, they observed that treatment of HET1A cells with BMP-4 induces expression of SOX-9, a transcription factor found in paneth cells and stem cells of the intestinal crypt. SOX-9, in turn, can upregulate expression of deleted in malignant brain tumors 1 (DMBT1), an extracellular matrix protein sufficient to induce a columnar-like phenotype in mice. They concluded the study with the hypothesis that bile and acid injury in the esophageal wall determines the upregulation of aberrant SHH expression, which, in turn, upregulate BMP-4, and subsequently SOX-9.[47] However, once more, it was not possible to observe the development of a specialized type of intestinal epithelium, as seen in BE.

In 2005, in a study performed by our group, we used SAGE and found that BMP-4 is uniquely expressed in BE as compared to squamous epithelium.[48] Here, we performed another study, whose results were published in 2007. We found that exposure of primary esophageal keratinocytes to BMP-4 induces upregulation of pSMAD 1, 5, 8, a downstream target of BMP-4, and by carrying out microarray on these cells, we could observe a shift of the gene expression pattern of the normal esophageal cells toward that of BE cells. At the protein level, we observed that a switch of cytokeratins expression pattern, toward those specifically expressed in BE columnar cells, could be achieved. However, we could not observe upregulation of intestinal specific genes, such as mucin 2 and villin 1.[49]

The concluding hypothesis of this study was that BMP-4 is needed to initiate the transformation of the normal esophageal cells into columnar cells, but it is not sufficient to determine an entire shift of the cells into an intestinal phenotype. Presently, we are working on further defining these mechanisms, and we hypothesize that the complete transformation of normal esophageal squamous cells into intestinal type of cells might be through a cooperative interaction of BMP-4 and CDX-2.

10. What characteristics of Barrett's cell lines are related to proliferation and apoptosis?

Rhonda F. Souza

rhonda.souza@utsouthwestern.edu

Traditional models that have been used to study proliferation and apoptosis in BE include human adenocarcinoma cell lines grown in culture, and human esophageal biopsy specimens grown in *ex vivo* organ culture. However, neither of these models is ideal for studying proliferation and apoptosis in benign Barrett's epithelial cells. Human adenocarcinoma cells have sustained numerous poorly characterized genetic abnormalities, and they are cancer cells, which have altered rates of proliferation and apoptosis. Human esophageal biopsies grown *ex vivo* contain diverse and uncharacterized cell types, so they are not useful for studies to address proliferation or apoptosis specifically in Barrett's epithelial cells. To improve upon the traditional models of BE, we and others have established telomerase-immortalized nondysplastic Barrett's epithelial cell lines from endoscopic biopsy specimens from patients with BE.[50] These cells are immortalized by telomerase expression but are not transformed.[50]

Characteristics of proliferation in Barrett's cells
Proliferation of Barrett's epithelial cells has been studied in response to acid exposure using cultures of Barrett's-associated adenocarcinoma cells and Barrett's esophageal biopsies. In these *in vitro* models, acid exposure has been shown to increase proliferation.[51,52] However, using nondysplastic Barrett's epithelial cells (BAR-T), we have reported very different effects of acid on proliferation. Cell number was significantly decreased by a 10-min exposure to acid in three Barrett's epithelial cell lines.[53] Using flow cytometry, we determined the effects of acid specifically on cell proliferation. At two hours following a 10-min exposure to acid, we found that there were slightly more cells in G1 and significantly less cells in S phase in the acid treated group compared to controls.[4] By four hours, we found significantly more cells in G1 and significantly less cells in S phase in the acid treated group compared to control suggesting that acid decreases proliferation by causing a delay in cell cycle progression at the G1-S cell cycle checkpoint.[53] Subsequent data from our laboratory have demonstrated that acid caused DNA double strand breaks due to generation of intracellular reactive oxygen species suggesting that the antiproliferative effects of acid are in response to genetic damage.

Characteristics of apoptosis in Barrett's cells
We have also reported that a 10-minute exposure to acid induces a small (1%), but statistically significant increase in apoptosis in Barrett's epithelial cells.[53] Apoptosis of Barrett's epithelial cells has also been studied in response to bile acid exposure using *ex vivo* cultures of esophageal squamous and Barrett's esophageal biopsies.[54] In these models, exposure to the unconjugated bile acid DCA increased apoptosis in the esophageal squamous biopsies, but not in the BE biopsies, suggests that the Barrett's epithelial cells resist apoptosis in response to bile acid exposure.[54]

Conclusions
In nondysplastic Barrett's cells, acid exposure decreases proliferation and causes a slight increase in apoptosis. In contrast, bile salt exposure does not induce apoptosis in *ex vivo* cultures of nondysplastic Barrett's cells.

11. Are there tissue biomarkers that can stratify risk for future neoplasia in BE?

Usha Malhotra, A. Atasoy, A. Zaidi, K. Nason, B.A. Jobe, and M. Gibson

malhotrau@upmc.edu

BE is one of the most significant known risk factors for development of EAC. The proportion of patients with BE progressing to EAC is small, thus there are continuous efforts to stratify these patients accurately to focus rigorous surveillance on a high risk group in a cost effective manner. Clearly, the available clinical and endoscopic criteria are not highly predictive and this has led to increasing interest in biomarkers. Early Detection Research Network (EDRN) has proposed five phases of biomarker evaluation[55] as illustrated in Table 1. Various biomarkers have been studied in context of Barrett's progression and are in different phases of development.

DNA content abnormalities (aneuploidy/tetraploidy)
Multiple studies have evaluated DNA content abnormalities due to structural and or numerical changes in chromosome numbers. They have shown

Table 1. Phases of biomarker development

1	Identification
2	Cross-sectional studies for validation and standardization of assay
3	Case-control studies to confirm expression
4	Prospective longitudinal studies
5	Population-based studies

variable relative risk of progression with one phase 4 study showing a five year cumulative cancer rate of 28%.[56] DNA content abnormalities are one of the most widely studied markers of progression in subjects with BE, but technical challenges with flow cytometry, in addition to need for special media, has limited widespread application.

Tumor suppressor loci abnormalities
p53, a well-known tumor suppressor, has been shown to be frequently inactivated in Barrett's carcinoma progression. There is convincing evidence that supports p53 LOH as a fairly accurate predictive marker.[57] Evaluation of p53 LOH requires genotyping that is currently limited to the research setting. Immunohistochemistry has been proposed to be an alternative means of evaluation but is not as accurate. Thus, despite high predictive power, clinical use has been a challenge.

p16 hypermethylation
Epigenetic silencing of p16 is one of the most common abnormalities reported in BE. Its high prevalence has led to its evaluation in multiple studies, but predictive power has been found to be low.[58] It has been proposed that this may be the initial event creating an environment conducive for further accumulation of genetic changes and eventually leading to the progression to carcinoma.

Other biomarkers of interest
Cyclin D1, aberrant methylation of tumor suppressor genes: RUNX3 and HPP1, HEr2/Neu, c-myc, COX2, EGFR, survivin, caspase 3, and E-cadherin. To address the initial question, there are tissue biomarkers that may help in risk stratification, but none of them are equipped for widespread clinical use.

Future directions
With increasing availability of compelling information on various biomarkers, there has been an interest in evaluation of panels combining clinical features, endoscopic criteria, and molecular biomarkers as tools of risk stratification.

12. Is there one transcription factor that shows a significant increase in the progression from BM to adenocarcinoma?

John P. Lynch
lynchj@mail.med.upenn.edu

The basis for this question likely emerges from what is currently understood or suspected regarding the pathogenesis of BE.[59] Presently, one model for BE holds that ectopic expression of transcription factors and growth factors normally associated with the intestine and colon contributes to the emergence of the intestinal metaplasia. A number of transcription factors have been identified with prominent roles in BE pathogenesis including C, Gli (SHH), Smad (BMP4), Sox9, and NF-κB. The criteria by which these factors were identified include (1) they are not normally expressed in the esophagus; (2) they are nearly universally detected in BE tissues; (3) they have prominent roles in intestinal development or cellular responses to inflammation; and (4) for many of these factors there is experimental data from cell culture and animal models demonstrating their contribution to promoting intestinal metaplasia.[59]

The question is, then, can we identify a transcription factor or factors that meet similar criteria and that are equally important for transforming BE cells into neoplastic adenocarcinoma cells? A review of the literature finds a number of microarray and other genetic studies of EACs that have identified candidate factors. Most of these studies compared gene expression patterns in BE tissues and EACs, and suggested *increased* expression of Sox9, ERG3, ERG4, c-Myc, COX2, DNMT3b, RARa, SPARC, and Wnt/β-catenin are all associated with progression from BE to EAC.[60] One problem with these candidates is that all are expressed in BE without dysplasia, only their levels are increased with progression to cancer. This seems unsatisfactory, since none would appear to have the same dramatic transforming effect as those factors associated with BE pathogenesis; none are presently being utilized as a marker predicting disease progression.

However, one transcription factor does meet these stringent criteria in an unexpected way, and

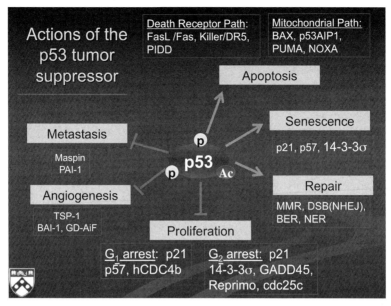

Figure 7. Functions of the tumor suppressor and transcription factor p53. The p53 gene targets are indicated with their associated tumor-suppressor functions.

that factor is p53. p53 is a transcription factor and a well-known tumor suppressor. The genes targeted by p53 perform many tumor–suppressor functions, including growth arrest, induction of DNA repair, induction of apoptosis, induction of cell senescence, and the prohibition of cell metastasis and angiogenesis (Fig. 7).[61] The actions of these many gene targets serve to inhibit five of the six hallmark features of cancer cells identified by Hanahan and Weinberg in their seminal review of the subject.[62] Thus, mutation and inactivation of p53 disrupts these many tumor–suppressor qualities and advances the neoplastic transformation of a cell. Consistent with this, p53 is typically normal in BE cells but frequently mutated in BE with high-grade dysplasia and in EAC.[63]

One other feature of p53 should be noted here. MDM2 is a ubiquitin ligase and an important p53 target gene. MDM2 normally ubiquinates p53, shunting it to the proteosome for degradation. In cells with normal p53, induction of MDM2 acts to feedback and limit p53 levels. However, when p53 is mutated, it cannot induce MDM2, and therefore levels of mutant p53 remain elevated. This is why immunohistochemistry for p53 in BE tissues is being studied as a marker for predicting disease progression.[63] Those tissues that have acquired a mutant p53 will often have elevated p53 levels eas-

ily detected by immunohostochemistry. And those cells with p53 mutations are at an advanced stage in their transformation to cancer.

In summary, with regard to the question: is there one transcription factor that shows a significant increase in the progression from BM to adenocarcinoma? The answer to this is: it is a trick question. Levels of the tumor suppressor (and transcription factor) p53 are frequently increased with progression to HGD and EAC, and may be a useful marker predicting likely progression to adenocarcinoma. However, this is a mutated form that is transcriptionally inactive. Loss of p53 function confers many hallmark features for neoplasia, and undoubtedly contributes to progression of BE cells to EAC.

Conflicts of interest

The authors declare no conflicts of interest.

References

1. Ronkainen, J., P. Aro, T. Storskrubb, *et al.* 2005. Prevalence of Barrett's esophagus in the general population: an endoscopic study. *Gastroenterology* **129:** 1825–1831.
2. Chak, A., H. Ochs-Balcom, G. Falk, *et al.* 2006. Familiality in Barrett's esophagus, adenocarcinoma of the esophagus, and adenocarcinoma of the gastresophageal junction Cancer Epidemiol. *Biomarkers Prev.* **15:** 1668–1673.

3. Trudgill, N.J., K.C. Kapur & S.A. Riley. 1999. Familial clustering of reflux symptoms. *Am. J. Gastroenterol.* **94:** 1172–1178.

4. Moons, L.M., J.G. Kusters, J.H. Van Delft, *et al.* 2008. A proinflammatory genotype predisposes to Barrett's esophagus. *Carcinogenesis* **29:** 926–931.

5. Macdonald, K., G.A. Porter, D.L. Guernsey, *et al.* 2009. A polymorphic variant of the insulin-like growth factor type I receptor gene modifies risk of obesity for esophageal adenocarcinoma. *Cancer Epidemiol.* **33:** 37–40.

6. Souza, R.F., K.Krishnan & S.J. Spechler. 2008. Acid, Bile and CDX: the ABCs of making Barrett's metaplasia. *Am. J. Physiol. Gastrointest. Liver Physiol.* **295:** 211–218.

7. Fitzgerald, R.C. 2006. Molecular basis of Barrett's esophagus and esophageal adenocarcinoma. *Gut.* **55:** 1810–1820.

8. Kazumori, H., S. Ishihara & Y. Kinoshita. 2009. Roles of caudal-related homeobox gene Cdx1 in esophageal epithelial cells in Barrett's epithelium development. *Gut.* **58:** 620–628.

9. Peters, J.H. & N. Avisar 2010. The molecular pathogenesis of Barrett's esophagus: common signaling pathways in embryogenesis metaplasia and neoplasia. *J. Gastroint. Surg.* **14**(Suppl 1): S81–S87.

10. Vaninetti, N., L. Williams, L. Geldenhuys, *et al.* 2009. Regulation of CDX2 expression in esophageal adenocarcinoma. *Mol. Carcinog.* **48:** 965–974.

11. Souza, R.F., K. Shewmake, L.S. Terada & S.J. Spechler. 2002. Acid exposure activates the mitogen-activated protein kinase pathways in Barrett's esophagus. *Gastroenterology* **122:** 299–307.

12. Fitzgerald, R.C., M.B. Omary, G. Triadafilopoulos. 1996. Dynamic effects of acid on Barrett's esophagus. An *ex vivo* proliferation and differentiation model. *J. Clin. Invest.* **98:** 2120–2128.

13. Saadi, A., N.B. Shannon, P. Lao-Sirieix, *et al.* 2010. Stromal genes discriminate preinvasive from invasive disease, predict outcome, and highlight inflammatory pathways in digestive cancers. *Proc. Natl. Acad. Sci. U. S. A.* **107:** 2177–2182.

14. Lu, S., A.W. Lowe, G. Triadafilopoulos, *et al.* 2009. Endoscopic evaluation of esophago-gastro-jejunostomy in rat model of Barrett's esophagus. *Dis. Esophagus.* **22:** 323–330.

15. Merlo, L.M., L.S. Wang, J.W. Pepper, *et al.* 2010. Polyploidy, aneuploidy and the evolution of cancer. *Adv. Exp. Med. Biol.* **676:** 1–13.

16. Leedham, S.J., S.L. Preston, S.A. Mcdonald, *et al.* 2008. Individual crypt genetic heterogeneity and the origin of metaplastic glandular epithelium in human Barrett's esophagus. *Gut.* **57:** 1041–1048.

17. Boonstra, J.J., R. Van Marion, D.G. Beer, *et al.* 2010. Verification and unmasking of widely used human esophageal adenocarcinoma cell lines. *J. Natl. Cancer Inst.* **102:** 271–274.

18. Jaiswal, K.R., C.P. Morales, L.A. Feagins, *et al.* 2007. Characterization of telomerase- immortalized, non-neoplastic, human Barrett's cell line (BAR-T). *Dis. Esophagus* **20:** 256–264.

19. Palanca-Wessels, M.C., A. Klingelhutz, B.J. Reid, *et al.* 2003. Extended lifespan of Barrett's esophagus epithelium transduced with the human telomerase catalytic subunit: a useful in vitro model. *Carcinogenesis* **24:** 1183–1190.

20. Maley, C.C., P.C. Galipeau, J.C. Finley, *et al.* 2006. Genetic clonal diversity predicts progression to esophageal adenocarcinoma. *Nat. Genet.* **38:** 468–473.

21. Okawa, T, C.Z. Michaylira, J. Kalabis, *et al.* 2007. The functional interplay between EGFR overexpression, hTERT activation, and p53 mutation in esophageal epithelial cells with activation of stromal fibroblasts induces tumor development, invasion, and differentiation. *Genes. Dev.* **21:** 2788–2803.

22. Merlo, L.M., N.A. Shah, X. Li, *et al.* 2010. A comprehensive survey of clonal diversity measures in Barrett's esophagus as biomarkers of progression to esophageal adenocarcinoma. *Cancer Prev. Res.* **3:** 1388–1397.

23. Michor, F. & K. Polyak. 2010. The origins and implications of intratumor heterogeneity. *Cancer Prev. Res.* **3:** 1361–1364.

24. Barbera, M. & R.C. Fitzgerald. 2010. Cellular origin of Barrett's metaplasia and esophageal stem cells. *Biochem. Soc. Trans.* **38:** 370–373.

25. Nowell, P.C. 1976. The clonal evolution of tumor cell populations. *Science* **194:** 238.

26. Maley, C.C., P.C. Galipeau, J.C. Finley, *et al.* 2006. Genetic clonal diversity predicts progression to esophageal adenocarcinoma. *Nat. Genet.* **38:** 468–473.

27. Leedham, S.J., S.L. Preston, S.A.C. Mcdonald, *et al.* 2008. Individual crypt genetic heterogeneity and the origin of metaplastic glandular epithelium in human Barrett's esophagus. *Gut* **57:** 1041–1048.

28. Wright, N.A. Migration of the ductular elements of Gut-associated glands gives clues to the histogenesis of structures associated with responses to acid hypersecretory state: The origins of "gastric metaplasia in the duodenum of specialised mucosa of Barrett's esophagus and pseudopyloric metaplasia. *Yale J. Biol. Med.* **69:** 147–153.

29. Fitzgerald, R.C. 2008. Dissecting out the genetic origins of Barrett's esophagus. *Gut* **57:** 1033–1034.

30. Maley, C.C., P.C. Galipeau, X. Li, *et al.* 2004. The combination of genetic instability and clonal expansion predicts progression to esophageal adenocarcinoma. *Cancer Res.* **64:** 7629–7633.

31. Leedham, S.J., S.L. Preston, S.A.C. Mcdonald, *et al.* 2008. Individual crypt genetic heterogeneity and origin of metaplastic glandular epithelium in human Barrett' esophagus. *Gut* **57:** 1041–1048.

32. Coad, R.A., A.C. Woodman, P.J. Warner, *et al.* 2005. On the histogenesis of Barrett's esophagus and its associated squamous islands: a three-dimensional study of their morphological relationship with native esophageal gland ducts. *J. Pathol.* **25:** 388–394.

33. Jaiswal, K.R., C.P. Morales, L.A. Feagins, *et al.* 2007. Characterization of telomerase- immortalized, non-neoplastic, human Barrett's cell line (BAR-T). *Dis. Esophagus.* **20:** 256–264.

34. Mirza, Z.K., K.K. Das, J. Slate, *et al.* 2003. Gastric intestinal metaplasia as detected by a monoclonal antibody is highly associated with gastric adenocarcinoma.*Gut.* **52:** 807–812.

35. Das, K.M., I. Prasad, S. Garla & P.S. Amenta. Detection of a shared colon epithelial epitope on Barrett epithelium by

a novel monoclonal antibody. *Ann. Intern. Med.* **120:** 753–756.

36. Bajpai, M., J. Liu, X. Geng, *et al.* 2008. Repeated exposure to acid and bile selectively induces colonic phenotype expression in a heterogeneous Barrett's epithelial cell line. *Lab Invest* **88:** 643–651.

37. Das, K.M., Y. Kong, M. Bajpai, *et al.* 2010. Transformation of benign barrett's epithelium by repeated acid and bile exposure over 65 weeks: a novel in-vitro model. *Int. J. Cancer.* **22.**

38. Xi, H., S.E. Baldus, U. Warnecke-Eberz, *et al.* 2005. High cyclooxygenase-2 expression following neoadjuvant radiochemotherapy is associated with minor histopathologic response and poor prognosis in esophageal cancer. *Clin. Cancer Res.* **11:** 8341–8347.

39. Luthra, R, T.T. Wu, M.G. Luthra, *et al.* 2006. Gene expression profiling of localized esophageal carcinomas: association with pathologic response to preoperative chemoradiation. *J. Clin. Oncol.* **24:** 259–267.

40. Lurje, G., J.M. Leers, A. Pohl, *et al.* 2010. Genetic variations in angiogenesis pathway genes predict tumor recurrence in localized adenocarcinoma of the esophagus. *Ann. Surg.* **251:** 857–864.

41. Peng, D., E.A. Sheta, S.M. Powell, *et al.* 2008. Alterations in Barrett's-related adenocarcinomas: a proteomic approach. *Int. J. Cancer* **122:** 1303–1310.

42. de Godoy, L.M., J.V. Olsen, J. Cox, *et al.* 2008. Comprehensive mass- spectrometry-based proteome quantification of haploid versus diploid yeast. *Nature* **455:** 1251–1254.

43. Kazumori, H., S. Ishihara, M.A. Rumi, *et al.* 2006. Bile acids directly augment caudal related homeobox gene Cdx2 expression in oesophageal keratinocytes in Barrett's epithelium. *Gut.* **55:** 16–25.

44. Huo, X., H.Y. Zhang, X.I. Zhang, *et al.* Acid and bile salt-induced CDX2 expression differs in esophageal squamous cells from patients with and without Barrett's esophagus. *Gastroenterology* **139:** 194–203 e191.

45. Kazumori, H., S. Ishihara & Y. Kinoshita. 2009. Roles of caudal-related homeobox gene Cdx1 in oesophageal epithelial cells in Barrett's epithelium development. *Gut.* **58:** 620–628.

46. Stairs, D.B., H. Nakagawa, A. Klein-Szanto, *et al.* 2008. Cdx1 and c- Myc foster the initiation of transdifferentiation of the normal esophageal squamous epithelium toward Barrett's esophagus. *PLoS One* **3:** e3534.

47. Wang, D.H., N.J. Clemons, T. Miyashita, *et al.* Aberrant epithelial- mesenchymal Hedgehog signaling characterizes Barrett's metaplasia. *Gastroenterology* **138:** 1810–1822.

48. van Baal, J.W., F. Milano,A. Rygiel, *et al.* 2005. A comparative analysis by SAGE of gene expression profiles of Barrett's esophagus, normal squamous esophagus, and gastric cardia. *Gastroenterology* **129:** 1274–1281.

49. Milano, F., J.W. Van Baal, N.S. Buttar, *et al.* 2007. Bone morphogenetic protein 4 expressed in esophagitis induces a columnar phenotype in esophageal squamous cells. *Gastroenterology* **132:** 2412–2421.

50. Jaiswal, K.R., C.P. Morales, L.A. Feagins, *et al.* 2007. Characterization of telomerase-immortalized, non-neoplastic, human Barrett's cell line (BAR-T) Dis. *Esophagus.* **20:** 256–264.

51. Hong, J., M. Resnick, J. Behar, *et al.* 2010. Acid-induced p16 hypermethylation contributes to development of esophageal adenocarcinoma via activation of NADPH oxidase NOX5-S. *Am. J. Physiol. Gastrointest. Liver Physiol.* **299:** G697-G706.

52. Fitzgerald, R.C., M.B. Omary & G. Triadafilopoulos. 1996. Dynamic effects of acid on Barrett's esophagus. An ex vivo proliferation and differentiation model. *J. Clin. Invest.* **98:** 2120–2128.

53. Zhang, H.Y., X. Zhang, K. Hormi-Carver, *et al.* 2007. In Non-neoplastic Barrett's epithelial cells, acid exerts early antiproliferative effects through activation of the Chk2 pathway. *Cancer Res.* **67:** 8580–8587.

54. Dvorakova, K., C.M. Payne, L. Ramsey, *et al.* 2005. Apoptosis resistance in Barrett's esophagus: ex vivo bioassay of live stressed tissues. *Am. J. Gastroenterol.* **100:** 424–431.

55. Pepe, M.S., R. Etzioni, Z. Feng, *et al.* 2001. Phases of biomarker development for early detection of cancer. *J. Natl. Cancer Inst.* **93:** 1054–1061.

56. Rabinovitch, P.S., G. Longton, P.L. Blount, *et al.* 2001. Predictors of progression in Barrett's esophagus: baseline flow cytometric variables. *Am. J. Gastroenterol.* **96:** 3071–3083.

57. Reid, B.J., L.J. Prevo, P.C. Agalipeau, *et al.* 2001. Predictors of progression in Barrett's esophagus II: baseline 17p (p53) loss of heterozygosity identifies a patient subset at increased risk for neoplastic progression. *Am. J. Gastroenterol.* **96:** 2839–2848.

58. Maley, C.C., P.C. Galipeau, X. Li, *et al.* 2004. The combination of genetic instability and clonal expansion predicts progression to esophageal adenocarcinoma. *Cancer Res.* **64:** 7629–7633.

59. Stairs, D.B., J. Kong, & J.P. Lynch, Cdx genes, inflammation, and the pathogenesis of intestinal metaplasias, In *Molecular Biology of Digestive Organs.* K. Kaestner, Ed. In Press, Elsevier.

60. Hormi-Carver, K. & R.F. Souza. 2009. Molecular markers and genetics in cancer development. *Surg. Oncol. Clin. N. Am.* **18:** 453–467.

61. Farnebo, M., V.J. Bykov, & K.G. Wiman. 2010. The p53 tumor suppressor: a master regulator of diverse cellular processes and therapeutic target in cancer. *Biochem. Biophys. Res. Commun.* **396:** 85–89.

62. Hanahan, D. & R.A. Weinberg. 2000. The hallmarks of cancer. *Cell* **100:** 57–70.

63. Prasad, G.A., *et al.* Predictors of progression in Barrett's esophagus: current knowledge and future directions. *Am. J. Gastroenterol.* **105:** 1490–1502.

Ann. N.Y. Acad. Sci. ISSN 0077-8923

Barrett's esophagus: clinical features, obesity, and imaging

Eamonn M. M. Quigley,[1] Brian C. Jacobson,[2] Johannes Lenglinger,[3] Joel H. Rubenstein,[4] Hashem El-Serag,[5] Michele Cicala,[6] Richard W. McCallum,[7] Marc S. Levine,[8] and Richard M. Gore[9]

[1]Alimentary Pharmabiotic Centre, Department of Medicine, Clinical Sciences Building, Cork University Hospital, Cork, Ireland. [2]Section of Gastroenterology, Boston University Medical Center, Boston, Massachusetts. [3]Department of Surgery, Medical University of Vienna, Vienna, Austria. [4]Veterans Affairs Center for Clinical Management Research, Ann Arbor, Michigan and Division of Gastroenterology, University of Michigan Medical School, Ann Arbor, Michigan. [5]Sections of Gastroenterology and Health Services Research, The Houston Veterans Affairs Medical Center and Baylor College of Medicine, Houston, Texas. [6]Dipartimento di Malattie dell'Apparato Digerente, Campus Bio-Medico University, Rome, Italy. [7]Department of Internal Medicine, Paul L. Foster School of Medicine, Texas Tech University Health Sciences Center, El Paso, Texas. [8]Department of Radiology, Hospital of the University of Pennsylvania, Philadelphia, Pennsylvania. [9]Department of Radiology, North Shore University Health System, Evanston Hospital, University of Chicago, Evanston, Illinois

The following includes commentaries on clinical features and imaging of Barrett's esophagus (BE); the clinical factors that influence the development of BE; the influence of body fat distribution and central obesity; the role of adipocytokines and proinflammatory markers in carcinogenesis; the role of body mass index (BMI) in healing of Barrett's epithelium; the role of surgery in prevention of carcinogenesis in BE; the importance of double-contrast esophagography and cross-sectional images of the esophagus; and the value of positron emission tomography/computed tomography.

Keywords: Gastroesophageal reflux disease; Barrett's esophagus; adiponectin; lectin; esophageal adenocarcinoma; BMI; serum leptin; inflammation; diabetes; ghrelin; IGF-1; IGF binding protein; esophagography; esophagitis; central obesity; esophageal reflux; gastric banding; PET/CT; fluoro deoxyglucose

Concise summaries

- The major value of the barium study in patients with reflux symptoms is its ability to stratify them into various risk groups for Barrett's esophagus (BE) to determine the relative need for endoscopy and biopsy.

- Recent advances in multidetector computed tomography (MDCT), now allow routine visualization of the entire esophagus in a single breath-hold. Positron emission tomography/computed tomography (PET/CT) is not sufficiently sensitive and specific enough to differentiate BE from other benign disorders, but with technical improvements, may help detect malignant transformation and even dysplasia in patients with this disorder.

- It is striking that although retrospective studies tend to confirm an association with increasing length of the BE segment, this has not, in general, been borne out in prospective studies.

Excess body fat does raise one's risk of complicated gastroesophageal reflux disease (GERD), including BE, and centralized fat is the predominant risk factor. However, whether this is true for both men and women equally remains unclear. Specific effects of central obesity, independent of body mass index (BMI), on reflux mechanisms potentially include elevated intragastric pressure and a disruption of the esophago-gastric junction (EGJ) integrity, but data are still scarce. There is substantial reason to suspect that circulating adipokines may promote BE.

- Alterations in levels of circulating factors related to obesity, including adipokines directly secreted from adipose tissue, are likely involved in the development of BE and neoplastic progression. Visceral fat is metabolically active, and has been strongly associated with low serum levels of potentially protective (e.g., adiponectin), or proinflammatory cytokines (e.g., interleukin-1 β,

doi: 10.1111/j.1749-6632.2011.06044.x

interleukin-6, and tumor necrosis factor-α), which may play a role in the development of BE.

- However, although the prevalences of erosive esophagitis and BE are both associated with

- BMI, there are no compelling data to suggest that healing rates are affected by BMI.
- Surgical treatment of obesity has positive effect on GERD and its complications, e.g., BE.

---

1. Do particular clinical factors influence the development and extent of BE?

Eamonn M. M. Quigley
e.quigley@ucc.ie

BE presents a formidable challenge to the clinician and endoscopist: on the one hand, its predilection to progress to adenocarcinoma of the esophagus has been widely publicized, whereas on the other, there is no doubt that, amidst a worldwide epidemic of GERD, BE has become very frequent. If, as indicated by a recent community survey from Sweden, for example, BE may be found among 2% of the general population, many of whom are asymptomatic, we have a very considerable challenge indeed, as only a very tiny minority of such individuals will ever progress to adenocarcinoma. It is self-evident that population screening for BE is not going to be a cost effective approach;[1] what we need is a strategy that will permit the identification, at an appropriately early stage, of that subgroup who are at risk for progression. Can clinical features assist in either predicting the presence of BE or, more importantly, its risk for progression to cancer?

At endoscopy, BE is almost always identified in the context of chronic reflux disease and a hiatal hernia; it must be remembered that these individuals have been selected on the basis of chronic and often troublesome symptoms, a factor that has tended to bias the outcome of many studies in this area. The findings of the study by Chak and colleagues tend to confirm these clinical impressions: in comparison to GERD patients without BE, patients with BE (or adenocarcinoma of the esophagus or EGJ), were more likely to be male, older, obese, smokers, and drinkers of alcohol. It must be conceded that many of these associations were modest. BE subjects also tended to have more frequent and severe heartburn but no significant relationship between BE and duration of symptoms was evident. The strongest predictor of BE or related cancers (odds ratio 6.4) was, however, a family history of BE, or adenocarcinoma of the esophagus or EGJ.[2] Relationships between symptomatic GERD and BE have been the subject of a recent meta-analysis,[3] which dissects the interaction between GERD and BE further. Although confirming a relationship between GERD symptoms and long-segment BE, they found no association with short-segment BE. This is more bad news; if short-segment BE is an important entity with a predilection to progression, looking for GERD symptoms will not be helpful in identifying it.

The lack of sufficient numbers did not permit Chak and colleagues to differentiate between those with BE alone and those who had progressed to cancer.[2] To address this all important issue, Prasad and colleagues have recently performed a comprehensive systematic review of predictors for progression in BE and their results are not very encouraging.[4] Yes—age, male gender, and length of BE segment were linked to progression to adenocarcinoma but the association was weak. Although obesity was identified as an independent risk factor for the development of adenocarcinoma of the esophagus, in Lagergren and his colleagues' study based on the Swedish national data base,[5] there was not, as yet, in the judgment of Prasad and colleagues, compelling evidence to link obesity with BE progression. As in their examination of many other clinical and demographic factors (age, tobacco and alcohol use, acid suppression), Prasad and colleagues found the data limited, fraught with methodological issues (small sample sizes, study design, method, and extent of follow-up) and often conflicting with regard to both the direction and magnitude of the effect. Among endoscopic features, BE segment length does confer some, albeit inconsistent, relationship with progression. It is striking that although retrospective studies tend to confirm an association with increasing length of the BE segment, this has not, in general, been borne out in prospective studies.

Although we may think that we can identify clinical features that indicate whether a given individual may harbor BE, these very same features do not appear to be very helpful in helping us to make the much more important prediction: who is at risk for progression through dysplasia to adenocarcinoma. Recent meta-analyses, while revealing hints of what may be relevant, have also identified the important short-comings of existing data and should encourage all involved in this area to collaborate in large prospective studies of the natural history of this common condition; only then will be able to truly identify those clinical features that can help us to select patients for endoscopic surveillance with the expectation that we will truly impact on mortality from adenocarcinoma of the esophagus.

2. What is the respective influence of BMI and body fat distribution on the development of BE?

Brian C. Jacobson
brian.jacobson@bmc.org

It has been well established that an elevated BMI is associated with symptomatic GERD, erosive esophagitis, BE, and esophageal adenocarcinoma. Recently, investigators have begun to ask whether the actual distribution of body fat is more important than just having an excess amount. For example, it appears that central adiposity (also called "visceral adiposity") is important for the development of BE.[6] Such central body fat could be causing more severe GERD simply through mechanical factors, such as a greater gastroesophageal pressure gradient.[7] It also appears that central obesity may elicit more frequent transient lower esophageal sphincter relaxations.[8] Finally, excess centralized fat is associated with a greater likelihood of a hiatal hernia. All of these factors play a role in the pathogenesis of GERD.

However, investigators have also begun to wonder about the role of adipocytokines, peptides produced by adipose tissue that have several effects on cell growth, apoptosis, and other potentially neoplastic factors. It is interesting to note that adipocytokines, such as adiponectin and leptin, are produced predominantly by visceral fat, the very fat that seems associated with BE. Men tend to have greater amounts of visceral fat than women, a fact that correlates nicely with the observation that men are twice as likely as women to develop BE and six or seven times as likely to progress to esophageal adenocarcinoma compared to women.

Investigators have noted an association between serum leptin and BE in men, with greater levels cor-

relating with higher risk for BE.[9] Interestingly, an inverse association was noted between serum leptin and BE in women, arguing that there may be gender differences in how body fat imparts risk for BE. It is possible that central fat plays a dominant role in the genesis of BE in men, but that other BMI-associated factors predominate in women. For example, peripheral fat (nonvisceral fat) is the predominant source of estrogens in postmenopausal women, and estrogens are associated with a greater risk of symptomatic GERD.[10]

In summary, it appears that excess body fat does raise one's risk of complicated GERD, including BE, and that centralized fat is the predominant risk factor. However, whether this is true for both men and women equally remains unclear.

3. Can it be said that central obesity may worsen acid reflux leading to BE? If so, by what mechanisms?

Johannes Lenglinger
johannes.lenglinger@meduniwien.ac.at

The continuous rise of the prevalence of both obesity and GERD in Western societies over the last three decades suggests a link between these conditions. The aim of this article is to provide a short overview of literature investigating the effects of central obesity on esophageal acid exposure and mechanisms potentially increasing reflux and thus leading to BE.

A significantly higher prevalence of reflux related symptoms in overweight and obese subjects was found in 7 of 9 cross-sectional surveys included in a meta-analysis of papers based on validated or structured questionnaires.[11] Pooled data from these studies showed an adjusted odds ratio (OR) for reflux symptoms of 1.43 (95% CI 1.16–1.77) in subjects with a BMI of 25–29.9 and 1.94 (95% CI 1.47–2.57) in individuals with a BMI $\geq$ 30. Jacobson *et al.* found an almost linear increase in the OR for frequent reflux symptoms with body mass BMI in women participating in the Nurses' Health Study.[12] (Table 1).

An increase of esophageal acid exposure in overweight and obese patients has been described for subjects with and without symptoms suggestive of GERD. In most comparative studies, patients were stratified by BMI. Data on a specific role of central obesity are scarce. In a study of 206 patients undergoing 24-hour esophageal pH-monitoring by

Table 1. Adjusted ORs (95% confidence interval) based on data of 2,306 women reporting heartburn and/or acid regurgitation at least once a week and 3,904 asymptomatic women, adjusted for age, smoking status, total activity, daily caloric intake, intake of alcohol, coffee, tea, and chocolate, use of postmenopausal hormone therapy, use of antihypertensive or asthma medication, and presence or absence of diabetes mellitus[11]

OR	0.67	1.0	1.38	2.2	2.43	2.92	2.93
(95% CI)	(0.48–0.93)		(1.13–1.67)	(1.81–2.66)	(1.96–3.01)	(2.35–3.62)	(2.24–3.85)
BMI	<20.0	20.0–22.4	22.5–24.9	25.0–27.4	27.5–29.9	30.0–34.9	≥35.0

El-Serag *et al.*, waist circumference (WC) and BMI were positively correlated with parameters of acid reflux.[13] As an example, for each unit increase of BMI, 2.76 more reflux episodes in the postprandial period were encountered ($P < 0.001$).

A 1 cm increase of WC was associated with 0.85 more reflux episodes ($P = 0.002$). In a multivariable linear regression model including both BMI (as categorical variable) and WC (as continous variable) a BMI ≥ 30 was no longer associated with any parameter of acid exposure.

Potential mechanisms of how central obesity worsens acid reflux include a temporary or permanent disruption of the EGJ integrity and elevated intragastric pressure, resulting in an elevated gastroesophageal pressure gradient. In a high-resolution manometry study of 285 patients Pandolfino *et al.* found a significant correlation of BMI and WC with intragastric pressure (inspiration, BMI ($r = 0.57$), WC ($r = 0.62$) $P < 0.0001$; expiration, BMI ($r = 0.58$), WC ($r = 0.64$), $P < 0.0001$).[7] Furthermore a weaker, but still significant correlation of the separation of lower esophageal sphincter and crural diaphragm with BMI ($r = 0.17$, $P < 0.005$) and WC ($r = 0.21$, $P < 0.001$) could be demonstrated.

In a case control study of 197 patients newly diagnosed with specialized intestinal metaplasia and 418 GERD controls, a high waist to hip ratio (male ≥ 0.9, female ≥ 0.8) increased the risk for visible BE (adjusted OR 1.9, 95% CI 1.0–3.5) and long segment BE (adjusted OR 4.1, 95% CI 1.5–11.4) independent of BMI.[14]

In summary, it can be said that obesity is associated with a higher prevalence of reflux symptoms, increased esophageal acid exposure, and prevalence of BE. Specific effects of central obesity, independent of BMI, on reflux mechanisms potentially include elevated intragastric pressure and a disruption of the EGJ junction integrity, but data are still scarce. The association of anthropometric data with BE requires further study as well, as this has important implications for screening.

4. What is the impact of proinflammatory adipocytokines and metabolic syndrome on the development of Barrett's mucosa?

Joel H. Rubenstein
jhr@umich.edu

There is substantial reason to suspect that circulating adipokines may promote BE. In brief, obesity is associated with both BE and esophageal adenocarcinoma. Although this is likely partly explained by a mechanical effect promoting GERD, and by dietary habits that promote GERD, obesity is also associated with a number of other cancers for which no known mechanical mechanism exists. It is increasingly recognized that adipose tissue is not an inert storage compartment, but rather metabolically active, secreting a number of substances. It is believed that those other cancers are promoted by adipokines secreted from adipose tissue, or other circulating factors. Adipokines secreted from visceral adipose appear to be particularly involved in inflammation. For instance, visceral adipocytes secrete TNF-α, and 50–75% of circulating IL-6 in obese subjects may be secreted from omental adipocytes.[15,16] Inflammation is believed to be intrinsic to the development of BE.

The rapid rise in incidence of esophageal adenocarcinoma might be explained by synergies in the multiple mechanisms by which obesity might promote this cancer (mechanical plus humoral). The potential roles for adipokines and other circulating factors in the development of BE and esophageal adenocarcinoma are just beginning to be explored. Here, I summarize the currently available data for some of the leading factors under consideration.

Diabetes and insulin resistance

Increased visceral fat is associated with insulin resistance. Insulin resistance is associated with a chronic inflammatory state,[17] and elevated insulin levels stimulate cell growth and inhibit apoptosis.[4] Hyperinsulinemia has been associated with the development of cancers of the colon, pancreas, and endometrium.[18] In a case-control study utilizing national Veterans Health Administration data, we found no evidence for an association between diabetes mellitus with a combined outcome of adenocarcinoma of the lower esophagus or gastric cardia.[19] However, we were not able to examine the effects on the risk of adenocarcinoma of the esophagus separately from the risk of gastric cardia in that study. Since then, diabetes was associated specifically with EAC in a population-based study.[20] However, the effect of diabetes appeared to be partially attenuated by GERD symptoms, tobacco use, and BMI. Given the body of evidence supporting a role of insulin resistance in other epithelial cancers, further research on its role in BE is warranted.

Adiponectin

Adiponectin is a peptide secreted primarily by visceral adipocytes. Circulating levels are paradoxically inversely related to obesity, and are lower in men than women. Low levels have been associated with increased risk of cancers of the stomach, colon, prostate, breast, and uterus.[21] Receptors specific for adiponectin are found in the esophageal mucosa, and adiponectin can induce apoptosis and inhibit proliferation in cell lines of esophageal adenocarcinoma.[22,23] In a pilot study, we found a trend toward lower blood levels of adiponectin in patients with BE compared to patients undergoing upper endoscopy for other indications.[24]

However, in a separate, larger study, we found no such association with total adiponectin levels.[25] Adiponectin circulates in various multimers, each with specific actions. The low molecular weight (LMW) form appears to be antiinflammatory, and the high molecular weight form is proinflammatory. We found that a high ratio of LMW to total adiponectin was strongly inversely associated with the presence of BE, compared to GERD controls, including after adjustment for abdominal obesity.[25] The specific roles of the molecular weight isoforms of adiponectin in the development of BE deserve further study.

Leptin

Leptin is a peptide secreted by primarily by adipocytes; it acts to signal satiety to the brain. Most obese humans are resistant to this signal, and have elevated circulating leptin levels. In addition to its effects on satiety, leptin stimulates proliferation and inhibits apoptosis in cell lines of esophageal adenocarcinoma.[26] Blood levels have been correlated with an increased risk of colorectal cancer.[27] Elevated leptin has also been directly associated with the presence of BE among men, including after adjustment for GERD and obesity.[9] However, an inverse association with BE was found in women. The reason for these discordant findings is unclear. In a smaller study composed mostly of men, no association was found between plasma leptin and BE.[28] BE was associated with elevated gastric fundus levels of leptin, controlling for BMI, compared to patients with esophagitis or to patients undergoing upper endoscopy for other indications. Therefore, intralumenal leptin, rather than circulating leptin, may be more important for its effect on esophageal mucosa.

Ghrelin

Ghrelin is a peptide secreted by the gastric fundus. It signals to the brain to stimulate appetite. Most obese humans have suppressed circulating levels of ghrelin—that is, they continue to eat despite low levels. In a cell line of esophageal adenocarcinoma, ghrelin inhibited COX-2 and IL-1β expression induced by TNF-α.[22] A small study found that very elevated levels of circulating ghrelin (>3.2 ng/mL) were protective against the development of esophageal adenocarcinoma, but only among overweight subjects.[29] The investigators noted a threshold effect, with no effect at lower concentrations.

Insulin-like growth factor axis

In addition to its insulin-like effects via the insulin receptor, insulin-like growth factor one (IGF-1) stimulates proliferation and inhibits apoptosis in many tissues via the IGF-1 receptor, including in esophageal epithelium and intestinal crypts.[30–33] Insulin enhances the synthesis of IGF-1, and hyperinsulinemia and obesity are associated with increased levels of free IGF-1[18,34] Most circulating IGF-1 is bound to IGF binding protein-3 (IGFBP-3), and bound IGF-1 is inactive.[35] IGFBP-3 inhibits cell growth and is proapoptotic.[36] IGF functions primarily in paracrine and autocrine manners, making it difficult to study epidemiologically. However, polymorphisms of the genes encoding IGFs and the IGF receptors have been associated the risk of BE and esophageal adenocarcinoma.[37–39] Elevated circulating IGF-1 levels have been associated with esophageal adenocarcinoma.[40]

Conclusions

Alterations in levels of circulating factors related to obesity, including adipokines directly secreted from adipose tissue, are likely involved in the development of BE and neoplastic progression. Research in this field is relatively new, and many questions remain unanswered.

5. May body fat distribution in men, where visceral obesity is more common, be an explanation for the high incidence of BE in this population?

Hashem El-Serag
hasheme@bcm.tmc.edu

There are gender-related differences in the distribution of GERD and its potential complications including BE. GERD symptoms seem to be equally prevalent between men and women; erosive esophagitis is more common among men,[41] BE is much more common in men (70–80%),[42] whereas esophageal adenocarcinoma is dominated by men[43] (Fig. 1).

Differences in obesity do not explain gender differences. Abdominal obesity explains some of the epidemiological features of BE and esophageal adenocarcinoma. The distribution of body fat tends to be more visceral than truncal in high-risk groups for BO including Caucasians (compared with African Americans), and men (compared with women).[44] Two recent case-control studies have shown abdominal diameter measured as WC to be a risk factor of BE independent of BMI, whereas the association between BMI and BE disappeared after adjustment of abdominal diameter.[6,45] These studies indicate that abdominal fat is possibly the key factor linking obesity and BE.

Only one study reported the association between WC and the risk of BE in men and women separately. Edelstein *et al.* in a case-control study (193 BE cases and 211 non-BE controls) conducted in the United States reported higher risk estimates for large WC and BE in men with an odds ratio of 5.9 (95% confidence intervals 1.8–19.4) than in women with an odds ratio of 2.9 (95% confidence intervals 8–11.0).[6] The other three studies that examined the association between obesity and BE risk did not convey useful information on the differences between men and women. One study was conducted exclusively in men,[46] the second had no abdominal obesity measurements,[47] and third matched case and controls on gender.[45]

The leading hypothesis is that abdominal obesity promotes gastroesophageal reflux through increased pressure stress and anatomical disruption of the gastroesophageal junction.

Obese individuals may experience extrinsic gastric compression by surrounding adipose tissue leading to increase intragastric pressures and subsequent relaxation of the lower esophageal sphincter, thus facilitating abnormal reflux (Fig. 2). A study of 285 patients[7] analyzed the relationship between obesity, pressure stresses on the OGJ, and the morphology of the OGJ pressure segment itself using a solid-state manometric assembly with 36 circumferential sensors spaced at 1 cm intervals. Intragastric pressure, as well as gastroesophageal pressure gradient, during both expiration and inspiration was significantly higher in obese and overweight patients compared with those with a normal BMI. WC was an independent risk factor for increased intragastric pressure, whereas BMI was no longer significantly associated with pressure independent of waist. The associations were stronger in men than women. These changes lead to increased reflux across

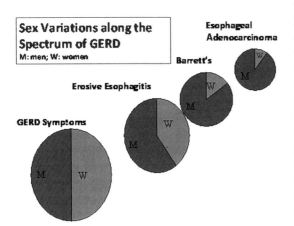

Figure 1. GERD symptoms seem to be equally prevalent between men and women, whereas erosive esophagitis is more common in men,[41] BE is much more common in men (70–80%),[42] and esophageal adenocarcinoma is dominated by men.

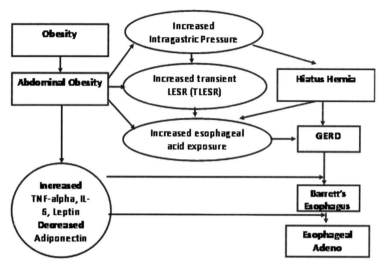

Figure 2. The relationship between obesity, pressure stresses on the OGJ, and reflux disease.

the lower esophageal sphincter with subsequent increased esophageal exposure to gastroduodenal contents. We conducted a cross-sectional study of 206 consecutive patients undergoing 24-hour pH-metry who were not on acid-suppressing medications.[13] Both BMI > 30 and high WC were associated with a significant increase in acid reflux episodes, long reflux episodes (>5 min), time with pH < 4, as well as a calculated summary score. The association between obesity and esophageal acid exposure also became attenuated when adjusted for WC suggesting that the latter may mediate a large part of the effect of obesity. Finally, visceral fat is metabolically active, and has been strongly associated with low serum levels of potentially protective (e.g., adiponectin), or proinflammatory cytokines (e.g., interleukin-1β, interleukin-6, and tumor necrosis factor-α), which may play a role in the development of BE.

6. Does BMI induce a difference in healing erosive esophagitis or Barrett's epithelium?

Brian C. Jacobson
brian.jacobson@bmc.org

The short answer is "no." We generally do not monitor the natural healing rate of erosive esophagitis, and this has certainly not been correlated with BMI. Healing rates have been monitored in the setting of clinical trials evaluating the efficacy of acid-mediating agents. However, these studies were never primarily designed to specifically look for an association between BMI and healing rates. Another, perhaps more fruitful, way to think about this question is to ask whether BMI is associated with the efficacy of acid-mediating agents. For example, one can think about whether excess body fat can affect the pharmacokinetics of these drugs. However, despite theoretical reasons why BMI might have some association with the distribution or metabolism of acid-mediating agents, there is no published evidence suggesting any important differences in the pharmacokinetics of acid-mediating agents and BMI?[48]

Despite this, have there been well-established clinical differences observed in patient response rates to proton pump inhibitors (PPIs) or histamine type 2 receptor antagonists (H2RAs) based upon BMI? Again, the answer is no. For example, in one pooled analysis with a total of 2,458 subjects from three randomized controlled trials of PPIs in nonerosive reflux disease, BMI was not predictive for patient response.[49] Further, no clear association was seen in *post hoc* analyses of PPI studies in both erosive and nonerosive reflux disease specifically asking if response rates differed by BMI.[50–51]

Therefore, although the prevalences of erosive esophagitis and BE are both associated with BMI,[52] there are no compelling data to suggest that healing rates are affected by BMI.

Ann. N.Y. Acad. Sci. 1232 (2011) 36–52 © 2011 New York Academy of Sciences.

7. Is it likely that intraabdominal fat is a risk marker of GERD, BE, and adenocarcinoma? What are the means by which obesity may (also) promote carcinogenesis in BE patients?

Michele Cicala, Silvia Cocca, and
Michele Pier Luca Guarino
m.cicala@unicampus.it

Obesity has increased considerably in the last few decades, with a prevalence from 15% in 1976–1980 to 32% in 2003–2004 in the United States and in several parts of Europe and Asia. The health implications of obesity are relevant, affecting almost every apparatus. Obesity and GERD, as well as GERD complications, such as BE and adenocarcinoma, are clearly related.[45,53]

The finding that increased abdominal fat, rather than a high BMI value, is strongly associated with GERD and BE has been well established. In a hospital-based study, the increase in visceral, rather than subcutaneous, fat, assessed at computerized tomography (CT) scan, has been shown to be an independent and strong risk factor for BE.[53] Furthermore, data from a case control study in which patients with an incidental diagnosis of BE were compared both with controls and patients with GERD, have provided further support to the hypothesis that abdominal obesity, in terms of abdominal circumference, is a risk factor of BE and is associated with severe GERD symptoms.[2] Another measure of abdominal girth, the waist to hip ratio, more than the BMI, seems to be strongly associated, irrespective of symptom severity, with the presence of BE and, in particular, with long-segment Barrett's metaplasia.[6]

A positive association between increased abdominal diameter and the risk of esophageal adenocarcinoma, but not *cardia* or squamous cell carcinoma, has recently been demonstrated by Kubo *et al.*[54] These findings might explain the higher risk of BE and adenocarcinoma in white men, who are more commonly affected by abdominal obesity.

A potential limitation of all case-control studies is the difficulty in establishing a temporal association between exposure and outcome, for instance between the onset and duration of obesity and the endpoint, the disease. Moreover, observational studies are subject to several other confounding factors, and the effect of weight loss on the development of the disease has not yet been established.

In summary, given all these limitations, intraabdominal fat could likely be considered a risk marker of GERD, BE and adenocarcinoma; however, further research is mandatory to obtain direct evidence of this pathway.

Another important question concerns the means by which obesity may also promote carcinogenesis in BE patients. It is known that metabolic effects of obesity, particularly abdominal obesity, may also contribute to carcinogenesis. Fat, located in the visceral compartment, induces changes in hormone production such as adiponectin and leptin, insulin and IGFs, and in cytokine production, all of which are able to affect cellular proliferation and apoptosis.[55] Several studies, have demonstrated that increased serum levels of leptin, a cytokine discovered in 1994 as a regulator of body weight and energy balance, are directly correlated with onset of various tumors and with an increased risk of BE.[55] On the other hand, levels of adiponectin, that are usually inversely associated with the risk of malignancies related to obesity, are found to be lower in obese patients than in normal weight patients.[55] As a result of this impaired metabolic activity the increased production of fatty acids, leading to insulin resistance and result in hyperinsulinemia, may have a direct effect upon insulin receptors as well as an effect mediated by decreasing IGF binding proteins, thus increasing IGF bioavailability, both of which result in reduced apoptosis and increased cell proliferation. Finally, abdominal obesity could also play a role in the development of BE by increasing intragastric pressure and, therefore, promoting reflux. Surprisingly, evidence confirming this pathway is still weak.[53]

Further investigations on the endocrine effects of adipose tissue and its potential role in carcinogenesis are now mandatory.

8. Does surgery for obesity result in better control of GERD and risk of malignancy in BE?

Reza A. Hejazi and Richard W. McCallum
richard.mccallum@ttuhsc.edu

The prevalence of GERD is markedly higher in overweight and obese individuals as compared to those with normal BMI,[56] since GERD itself is now recognized as an obesity-related comorbidity.

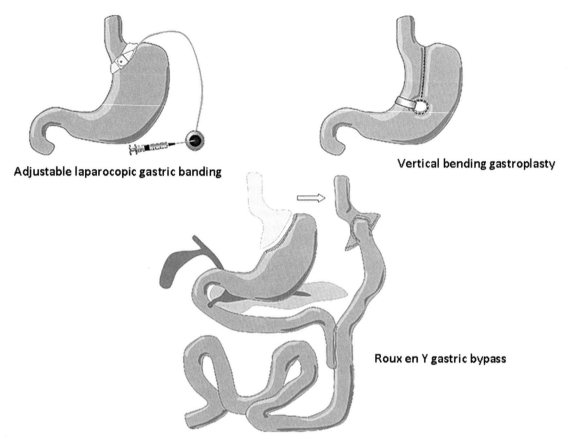

Adjustable laparocopic gastric banding

Vertical bending gastroplasty

Roux en Y gastric bypass

Figure 3. Adjustable laparoscopic gastric banding; Vertical banding gastroplasty; Roux en Y gastric bypass. Adapted from De Groot *et al.*[58] and with permission from John Wiley and Sons.

Bariatric surgery actually has become a widely accepted form of treatment for severe obesity, and several studies have demonstrated a significant reduction in GERD symptoms and medication utilization, as well as weight and metabolic comorbidity, including diabetes, hypertension and dyslipidemia.[57] The different techniques for performing bariatric surgery have variable effects on GERD and subsequently on the risk of BE. Roux en Y gastric bypass (Fig. 3), as the most performed bariatric operation in the United States, was found in majority of studies to have a positive effect on GERD symptoms.[3] Vertical banding gastroplasty as a restrictive procedure, on the other hand, has no change or even, based on some reports, may cause an increase of GERD.[58] Although laparoscopic adjustable gastric banding might have a beneficial effect, the results of this procedure are still conflicting.[3] Preoperative selection of GERD patients, as well as em-

ploying the most beneficial procedure, are the goals. The good news here is that the resolution of Barrett's disease and atypia of the esophageal epithelial after gastric bypass and laparoscopic gastric bypass/LAP-BAND were reported in just two cases.[59] After laparoscopic placement of adjustable gastric banding, Barrett's esophagus could be a rare (one case) but not unexpected complication, and the incidence of it is still unknown.[60]

Conclusions

GERD is common problem in obese and overweight populations. Surgical treatment of obesity has positive effect on GERD and its complications, such as BE.

Roux en Y gastric bypass has the most favorable impact on GERD symptoms, although certain restrictive procedures such as laparoscopic gastric bypass/LAP-BAND have also been reported to have some postive effects on Barrett's disease and esophageal dysplasia.

9. What is the role of double-contrast esophagography in the diagnosis and screening for BE in patients with reflux symptoms?

Marc S. Levine
marc.levine@uphs.upenn.edu

The classic radiologic features of BE consist of a mid-esophageal stricture or ulcer, often associated with a sliding hiatal hernia and GER.[61] These strictures typically appear as ring-like constrictions or as tapered areas of narrowing below the level of the aortic arch. However, strictures are actually more common in the distal esophagus in patients with BE, so most cases do not fit the classic description of a high stricture or ulcer.[62] A reticular mucosal pattern has also been described as a relatively specific sign of BE on double-contrast esophagograms, particularly if located just distal to a midesophageal stricture.[62] However, a reticular mucosal pattern is present on barium studies in only 5–30% of all patients with BE.

Other morphologic findings of reflux disease, such as hiatal hernias, GER, reflux esophagitis, and peptic strictures, can be detected on double-contrast studies in the vast majority of patients with BE, but these findings frequently occur in patients with uncomplicated reflux disease.[63] Thus, those radiographic findings that are relatively specific for BE are not sensitive, and those findings that are more sensitive are not specific. As a result, double-contrast esophagography has traditionally been thought to have limited value for diagnosing BE.

Gilchrist *et al.* introduced a novel approach for the diagnosis of BE on double-contrast esophagography by stratifying patients based on specific radiologic criteria.[64] Patients who were classified at high risk for BE because of a high stricture or ulcer or a reticular mucosal pattern were almost always found to have this condition, so endoscopy and biopsy should be performed in this group for a definitive diagnosis. A larger group of patients were classified at moderate risk for BE because of esophagitis or strictures in the distal esophagus; 16% of these patients were found to have BE, so the decision for endoscopy in this group should be based on the severity of symptoms, age, and overall health of the patients (i.e., whether they are reasonable candidates for surveillance). However, the majority of patients were classified as low risk for BE because of the absence of esophagitis or strictures in the esophagus; many of these patients were found to have mild reflux esophagitis, but less than 1% had BE, so these patients can be treated empirically for their reflux symptoms without need for endoscopy. Thus, the major value of the barium study in patients with reflux symptoms is its ability to stratify them into these various risk groups for BE to determine the relative need for endoscopy and biopsy.[64,65]

10. Cross-sectional imaging in the detection of BE

Richard M. Gore, Kiran H. Thakrar, Geraldine M. Newmark, Uday K. Mehta, and Jonathan W. Berlin
rgore@uchicago.edu

Upper gastrointestinal endoscopy and barium esophagography are the primary means of evaluating patients with known or suspected esophageal pathology.[65,66] Although these examinations superbly depict the esophageal mucosa, they are limited by their inability to directly image the esophageal wall and surrounding adventitia, fat, and lymph nodes. Recent advances in MDCT now allow routine visualization of the entire esophagus in a single breath-hold with thin collimation and isotropic voxels. This allows the production of high-quality multiplanar reformations and 3D reconstruction images. The sensitivity of MDCT in the evaluation of esophageal disease is further enhanced by proper distention of the esophagus by the oral administration of effervescent granules and water and optimally timed administration of intravenous contrast material.

Although detection of the actual metaplastic columnar epithelium of BE is beneath the spatial resolution of MDCT, there are a number of secondary features that help suggest diagnosis, especially of long segment, circumferential disease.

MDCT is superb in the identification of hiatal hernias (Fig. 4). There is extension of a portion of the proximal stomach or other abdominal contents into the lower mediastinum. An abnormally wide

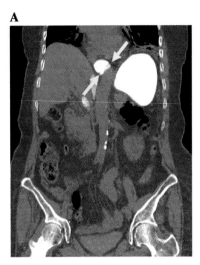
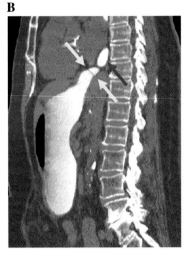

Figure 4. MDCT scan in a patient subsequently proven to have Barrett's esophagus. (A) Coronal and (B) sagittal reformatted images demonstrate a hiatal hernia and Schatzki's ring (yellow arrows). Note the gastroesophageal reflux (red arrow).

esophageal hiatus with increased separation of the esophagus and diaphragmatic crura is often present.

MDCT can also document the presence of gastroesophageal reflux (see Fig. 4) however this is less reliably detected than by conventional barium esophagrams and nuclear medicine reflux studies. Oral contrast material is routinely given for abdominal and pelvic CT scans and this contrast material may be visualized in the distal esophagus and can show the presence of a stricture or Schatzki's ring.

MDCT is superb in depicting mural thickening (Fig. 5) of the esophagus and the diagnosis can be confidently made in patients with a well-distended esophagus. Mural thickening of the esophagus as shown on MDCT is nonspecific and can be seen in a variety of benign and malignant disorders including: reflux esophagitis, infectious esophagitis, tuberculosis, radiation esophagitis, eosinophilic esophagitis, BE, Crohn's disease of the esophagus, achalasia, scleroderma, diffuse esophageal spasm, esophageal pseudodiverticulosis, adenocarcinoma of the esophagus, squamous cell carcinoma of the esophagus, lymphoma of the esophagus, and esophageal metastases.[67]

Five mm is a useful threshold for esophageal wall thickening in patients with esophagitis. Indeed, some 55% of all patients with esophagitis have an esophageal wall thickness of 5 mm or greater on MDCT. Benign or malignant tumors of the esophagus are usually manifested on CT by focal, asymmetric thickening of the esophageal wall, whereas mural thickening in esophagitis is concentric and circumferential, and usually involves a relatively long segment of the esophagus.[67]

Some 20% of patients with esophagitis may also demonstrate mural stratification, in which the axially imaged esophagus has a target appearance. This is caused by the combination of mucosal enhancement and a hypodense submucosa. In the small bowel and colon, the target sign almost always indicates benign disease associated with submucosal edema resulting from inflammation, infection, or ischemia.

Other clues to esophageal pathology include the distribution of intraluminal air on MDCT. Intraluminal air is normal in the esophagus, but distention of more than 10 mm at a fixed point, such as the carina, is uncommon. Any segment over 20 mm should be considered abnormal. The normal lower esophageal sphincter should be closed. In the upper 30% of the esophagus (to about the top of the aortic arch) and from 61% to 75% of the length of the esophagus (behind the base of the heart) less than 5% of the lumina are larger than 10 mm in diameter.[68]

The greatest luminal dimensions and variation occur in the area between where the diaphragm first appears and where the esophagus enters the abdomen. Here, 15 mm should the upper limits

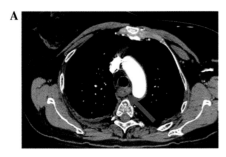

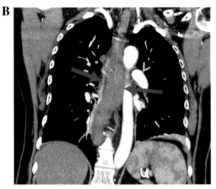

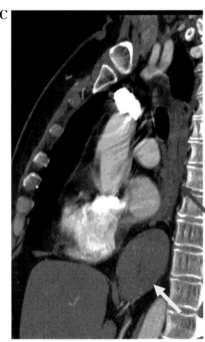

Figure 5. MDCT scan in a patient with reflux esophagitis and a long segment of Barrett's esophagus proven by endoscopic biopsy. (A) Axial, (B) coronal reformatted, and (C) sagittal reformatted images show a large hiatal hernia (yellow arrows) associated with a long segment of mural thickening of the esophagus (red arrow). (A) Submucosal edema produces the target appearance of the axially imaged esophagus.

of normal. An air–fluid level on any section of the esophagus is abnormal.[68]

In summary, the following constellation of findings should raise the possibility of BE or at least esophagitis on MDCT: hiatal hernia, mural thickening of the esophagus in a symmetric, circumferential manner, the target sign, too much intraluminal air, air-fluid levels, foodstuffs or tablets in the esophagus. These CT findings should be carefully searched for on pulmonary embolism and thoracic aortic dissection MDCT scans performed on patients with chest discomfort. A minority number of these patients will ultimately be shown to have significant esophageal pathology.

11. Can PET/CT differentiate BE from other benign esophageal disorders?

Richard M. Gore, Kiran H. Thakrar, Geraldine M. Newmark, Uday K. Mehta, and Jonathan W. Berlin
rgore@uchicago.edu

Combined PET/CT with fluorine[18] fluorodeoxyglucose (FDG) is a hybrid device that fuses structural information provided by multidetector CT with the functional imaging provided by PET (Fig. 6). This technique improves the radiologic assessment of normal anatomic structures and pathological lesions. Cellular FDG uptake is predominantly related to expression of the protein glucose transport 1. This protein is ubiquitously expressed in almost all cell types, but its over expression in dysplastic and malignant tissue is quite frequent and leads to intracellular accumulation of FDG, which is visualized on PET. The high lesion to background contrast and whole body data acquisition on FDG PET represent critical advantages over CT and MRI, where contrast between pathologic and normal structures may be limited. FDG PET has been developed to quantitatively assess local glucose metabolism. PET can help differentiate benign and malignant tumors, determine the degree of malignancy, evaluate the effectiveness of chemotherapy and/or radiotherapy, and help predict prognosis. Indeed FDG PET has been used to screen for malignancies.[69]

FDG PET is a well-accepted method for the detection and staging of a number of malignancies including lung, breast, colorectal, and esophageal

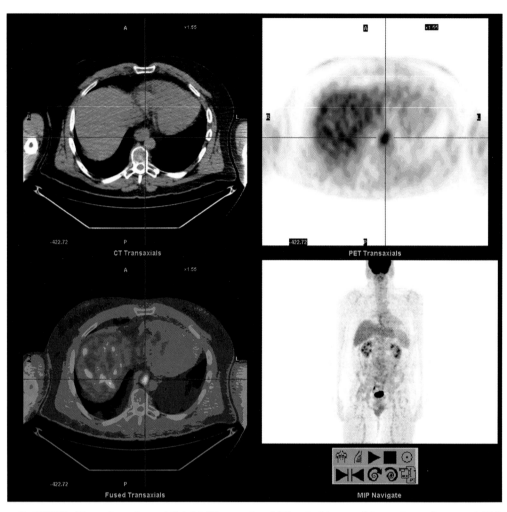

Figure 6. PET/CT of Barrett's esophagus. (A) Axial, (B) coronal, and (C) sagittal images of the esophagus show mural thickening of the esophagus on the CT (white arrow), increased metabolic activity on PET (red arrow), mural thickening of the esophagus and increased metabolic activity on the PET/CT (yellow arrow), and increased metabolic activity on coronal scanogram (black arrow) components of the examination.

cancer. The applications of FDG PET in the clinical diagnosis of BE have not been established.

Preliminary experimental work has demonstrated the efficacy of high-resolution PET scanning to examine the degree and time dependency of changes in FDG uptake in rat esophageal tissues during the esophageal reflux injury carcinogenic progression pathway. FDG accumulation is significantly elevated in esophageal tissues three and six month (correlating to BE with high grade dysplasia and early adenocarcinoma) than that at one week and one month (reflux esophagitis), and this accumulation corresponds

to the histopathologically observed progression of squamous epithelium to hyperplasia to metaplasia and onto adenocarcinoma. This early work suggests that FDG PET scanning may play an important role in the assessment of a subset of patients that are at risk for the esophagitis to metaplasia to dysplasia to esophagitis-adenocarcinoma sequence.[70]

Nonspecific esophageal uptake is a common finding when interpreting PET/CT studies and is usually due to reflux esophagitis. This is not surprising considering that about 15% of the population suffers from reflux disease. These benign lesions,

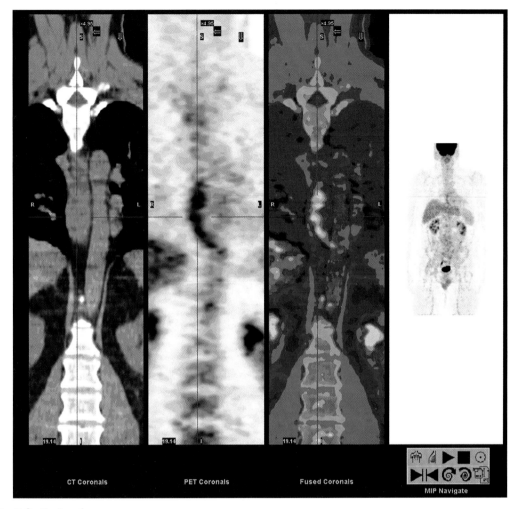

CT Coronals   PET Coronals   Fused Coronals

MIP Navigate

Figure 6. *Continued*

however, can resemble early esophageal malignancies. The clinical challenge is that, on the one hand, the only chance for cure of esophageal carcinoma is its early detection, and, on the other hand, the rate of false positives among nonspecific esophageal uptake is too high to recommend further evaluation with endoscopy in all of those cases. Therefore, the differentiation between early malignant and benign lesions has important clinical implications.[71,72]

The differential diagnosis of increased FDG uptake on PET CT includes: reflux esophagitis, infectious esophagitis, radiation esophagitis, BE, primary and secondary achalasia, scleroderma, diffuse esophageal spasm, intramural pseudodiverticulosis, tuberculosis, Crohn's disease, adenocarcinoma, squamous cell carcinoma, lymphoma, and metastases.

When evaluating abnormal PET CT findings of the esophagus, Roedl *et al.*[73] have suggested closely interrogating the scans for the following features: esophageal thickness, focality and location of the lesion, eccentricity of the esophageal thickening, and degree of metabolic activity-standard uptake value. Roedl *et al.* found no significant differences in esophageal thickness on CT and location of the lesion between the 36 early malignant and the 66 benign lesions. However, higher SUV, greater lesion focality, and greater eccentricity of the mural thickening are significantly increased in the early malignant group when compared with benign lesions.[73]

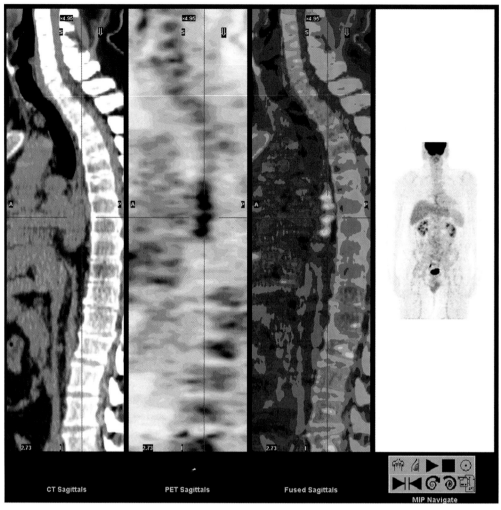

Figure 6. *Continued*

At the present time, PET CT is not sufficiently sensitive and specific enough to differentiate BE from other benign disorders but, with technical improvements, may help detect malignant transformation and even dysplasia in patients with this disorder.

Conflicts of interest

The authors declare no conflicts of interest.

References

1. Quera, R., K. O'Sullivan & E.M. Quigley. 2006. Surveillance in Barrett's oesophagus: will a strategy focused on a high-risk group reduce mortality from oesophageal adenocarcinoma? *Endoscopy* **38:** 162–169.
2. Chak, A., T. Lee, M.F. Kinnard, *et al.* 2002. Familial aggregation of Barrett's oesophagus, oesophageal adenocarcinoma, and oesophagogastric junctional adenocarcinoma in Caucasian adults. *Gut.* **51:** 323–328.
3. Taylor, J.B. & J.H. Rubenstein. 2010. Meta-analyses of the effect of symptoms of gastroesophageal reflux on the risk of Barrett's esophagus. *Am. J. Gastroenterol.* **105:** 1730–1737.
4. Prasad, G.A., A. Bansal, P. Sharma & K.K. Wang. 2010. Predictors of progression in Barrett's esophagus: current knowledge and future directions. *Am. J. Gastroenterol.* **105:** 1490–1502.
5. Lagergren, J., R. Bergström & O. Nyrén. 1999. Association between body mass and adenocarcinoma of the esophagus and gastric cardia. *Ann. Intern. Med.* **130:** 883–890.
6. Edelstein, Z. *et al.* 2007. Central adiposity and risk of Barrett's esophagus. *Gastroenterology* **133:** 403–411.
7. Pandolfino, J. *et al.* 2006. Obesity: a challenge to esophagogastric junction integrity. *Gastroenterology* **130:** 639–649.

8. Wu, J. *et al.* 2007. Obesity in associated with increased transient lower esophageal sphincter relaxation. *Gastroenterology* **132:** 883–889.

9. Kendall, B.J. *et al.* 2008. Leptin and the risk of Barrett's oesophagus. *Gut.* **57:** 448–454.

10. Jacobson, B. *et al.* 2008. Postmenopausal hormone use and symptoms of gastroesophageal reflux. *Arch. Intern. Med.* **168:** 1–7.

11. Hampel, H., N.S. Abraham & H.B. El-Serag. 2005. Meta-analysis: obesity and the risk for gastroesophageal reflux disease and its complications. *Ann. Intern. Med.* **143:** 199–211.

12. Jacobson, B.C., S.C. Somers, C.S. Fuchs, *et al.* 2006. Body-mass index and symptoms of gastroesophageal reflux in women. *N. Engl. J. Med.* **354:** 2340–2348.

13. El-Serag, H.B., G.A. Ergun, J. Pandolfino, *et al.* 2007. Obesity increases oesophageal acid exposure *Gut.* **56:** 749–755.

14. Edelstein, Z.R., M.P. Bronner, S.N. Rosen & T.L. Vaughan. 2009. Risk factors for Barrett's esophagus among patients with gastroesophageal reflux disease: a community clinic-based case-control study. *Am. J. Gastroenterol.* **104:** 834–842.

15. Mohamed-Ali, V., S. Goodrick, A. Rawesh, *et al.* 1997. Subcutaneous adipose tissue releases interleukin-6, but not tumor necrosis factor-alpha, in vivo. *J. Clin. Endocrinol. Metab.* **82:** 4196–4200.

16. Fried S.K., D.A. Bunkin & A.S. Greenberg. 1998. Omental and subcutaneous adipose tissues of obese subjects release interleukin-6: depot difference and regulation by glucocorticoid. *J. Clin. Endocrinol. Metab.* **83:** 847–850.

17. Festa, A., R. D'Agostino Jr, G. Howard, *et al.* 2000. Chronic subclinical inflammation as part of the insulin resistance syndrome: the Insulin Resistance Atherosclerosis Study (IRAS). *Circulation* **102:** 42–47.

18. Kaaks, R. & A. Lukanova. 2001. Energy balance and cancer: the role of insulin and insulin-like growth factor-I. *Proc. Nutr. Soc.* **60:** 91–106.

19. Rubenstein, J.H., J. Davis, J.A. Marrero & J.M. Inadomi. 2005. Relationship between diabetes mellitus and adenocarcinoma of the oesophagus and gastric cardia. *Aliment. Pharmacol. Ther.* **22:** 267–271.

20. Neale, R.E., J.D. Doecke, N. Pandeya, *et al.* 2009. Does type 2 diabetes influence the risk of oesophageal adenocarcinoma? *Br. J. Cancer* **100:** 795–798.

21. Kelesidis, I., T. Kelesidis & C.S. Mantzoros. 2006. Adiponectin and cancer: a systematic review. *Br. J. Cancer* **94:** 1221–1225.

22. Konturek, P.C., G. Burnat, T. Rau, *et al.* 2008. Effect of adiponectin and ghrelin on apoptosis of barrett adenocarcinoma cell line. *Dig. Dis. Sci.* **53:** 597–605.

23. Ogunwobi, O.O. & I.L. Beales. 2008. Globular adiponectin, acting via adiponectin receptor-1, inhibits leptin-stimulated oesophageal adenocarcinoma cell proliferation. *Mol. Cell. Endocrinol.* **285:** 43–50.

24. Rubenstein, J.H., A. Dahlkemper, J.Y. Kao, *et al.* 2008. A pilot study of the association of low plasma adiponectin and Barrett's esophagus. *Am. J. Gastroenterol.* **103:** 1358–1364.

25. Rubenstein J.H., J.Y. Kao, R.D. Madanick, *et al.* 2009. Association of adiponectin multimers with Barrett's esophagus. *Gut* **58:** 1583–1539.

26. Ogunwobi, O., G. Mutungi & I.L. Beales. 2006. Leptin stimulates proliferation and inhibits apoptosis in Barrett's esophageal adenocarcinoma cells by cyclooxygenase-2-dependent, prostaglandin-E2-mediated transactivation of the epidermal growth factor receptor and c-Jun NH2-terminal kinase activation. *Endocrinology* **147:** 4505–4516.

27. Stattin, P., A. Lukanova, C. Biessy, *et al.* 2004. Obesity and colon cancer: does leptin provide a link? *Int. J. Cancer* **109:** 149–152.

28. Francois, F., J. Roper, A.J. Goodman, *et al.* 2008. The association of gastric leptin with oesophageal inflammation and metaplasia. *Gut* **57:** 16–24.

29. de Martel, C., T.D. Haggerty, D.A. Corley, *et al.* 2007. Serum ghrelin levels and risk of subsequent adenocarcinoma of the esophagus. *Am. J. Gastroenterol.* **102:** 1166–1172.

30. Vinayek, R., L.S. Pichney, U. Tantry, *et al.* 1994. Characterization of insulin-like growth factor I receptors in human esophageal epithelial cells. *Am. J. Physiol.* **267:** G105–G114.

31. Jimenez, P., A. Lanas, E. Piazuelo & F. Esteva. 1998. Effect of growth factors and prostaglandin E2 on restitution and proliferation of rabbit esophageal epithelial cells. *Dig. Dis. Sci.* **43:** 2309–2316.

32. Tchorzewski, M.T., F.G. Qureshi, M.D. Duncan, *et al.* 1998. Role of insulin-like growth factor-I in esophageal mucosal healing processes. *J. Lab. Clin. Med.* **132:** 134–141.

33. Lund, P.K. 1999. IGFs and the digestive tract. In Roberts C.T., Rosenfeld R.G., Eds.: 517–544. *The IGF System: Molecular Biology, Physiology, and Clinical Applications.* Totowa, NJ: Humana Press.

34. Renehan, A.G., J. Frystyk & A. Flyvbjerg. 2006. Obesity and cancer risk: the role of the insulin-IGF axis. *Trends Endocrinol. Metab.* **17:** 328–336.

35. Yu, H. & T. Rohan. 2000. Role of the insulin-like growth factor family in cancer development and progression. *J. Natl. Cancer Inst.* **92:** 1472–1489.

36. Leroith, D., W. Zumkeller & R.C. Baxter, Eds. 2003. *Insulin-like Growth Factors.* Landes Bioscience/Eurekah.com; New York. Georgetown, TX.

37. Macdonald K, G.A. Porter, D.L. Guernsey, *et al.* 2009. A polymorphic variant of the insulin-like growth factor type I receptor gene modifies risk of obesity for esophageal adenocarcinoma. *Cancer Epidemiol.* **33:** 37–40.

38. Hoyo, C., J.M. Schildkraut, S.K. Murphy, *et al.* 2009. IGF2R polymorphisms and risk of esophageal and gastric adenocarcinomas. *Int. J. Cancer* **125:** 2673–2678.

39. McElholm, A.R., A-J McKnight, C.C. Patterson, *et al.* 2010. A population-based study of IGF axis polymorphisms and the esophageal inflammation, metaplasia, adenocarcinoma sequence. *Gastroenterology* **139:** 204–12.e3.

40. Sohda, M., H. Kato, T. Miyazaki, *et al.* 2004. The role of insulin-like growth factor 1 and insulin- like growth factor binding protein 3 in human esophageal cancer. *Anticancer Res.* **24:** 3029–3034.

41. El-Serag, H.B., N.J. Petersen, J. Carter, *et al.* 2004. Gastroesophageal reflux among different racial groups in the United States. *Gastroenterology* **126:** 1692–1699.

42. Falk, G.W., P.N. Thota, J.E. Richter *et al.* 2005. Barrett's esophagus in women: demographic features and

progression to high-grade dysplasia and cancer. *Clin Gastroenterol. Hepatol.* **3:** 1089–1094.

43. Pohl, H. & H.G. Welch. 2005. The role of overdiagnosis and reclassification in the marked increase of esophageal adenocarcinoma incidence. *J. Natl. Cancer Inst.* **97:** 142–146.

44. Weinsier, R.L., G.R. Hunter, B.A. Gower, *et al.* 2001. Body fat distribution in white and black women: different patterns of intraabdominal and subcutaneous abdominal adipose tissue utilization with weight loss. *Am. J. Clin. Nutr.* **74:** 631–636.

45. Corley, D.A., A. Kubo, T.R. Levin, *et al.* 2007. Abdominal obesity and body mass index as risk factors for Barrett's esophagus. *Gastroenterology* **133:** 34–41.

46. El-Serag, H.B., P. Kvapil, J. Hacken-Bitar, *et al.* 2005. Abdominal obesity and the risk of Barrett's esophagus. *Am. J. Gastroenterol.* **100:** 2151–2156.

47. Smith, K.J., S.M. O'brien, B.M. Smithers, *et al.* 2005. Interactions among smoking, obesity, and symptoms of acid reflux in Barrett's esophagus. *Cancer Epidemiol. Biomarkers Prev.* **14**(11 Pt 1): 2481–2486.

48. Jacobson, B.C. 2008. Body mass index and the efficacy of acid-mediating agents for GERD. *Dig. Dis. Sci.* **53:** 2313–2317.

49. Talley, N.J. *et al.* 2006. Predictors of treatment response in patients with non-erosive reflux disease. *Aliment Pharmacol. Ther.* **24:** 371–376.

50. Sharma, P. *et al.* 2007. Effect of Obesity on Symptom Resolution in Patients with Gastroesophageal Reflux Disease (GERD). *Am. J. Gastroenterol.* **102:** S139–140 [abstract].

51. Vakil, N. *et al.* 2007. Is Obesity the Cause of Reduced Healing Rates in Advanced Grades of Erosive Esophagitis (EE)? *Am. J. Gastroenterol.* **102:** S445.

52. Hampel, H., N. Abraham & H. El-Serag. 2005. Meta-analysis: Obesity and the risk for astroesophageal reflux disease and its complications. *Ann. Intern. Med.* **143:** 199–211.

53. El Serag H.E. 2008. The association between obesity and GERD: a review of the epidemiological evidence. *Dig. Dis. Sci.* **53:** 07–12.

54. Kubo, A., D.A. Corley, *et al.* 2006. Body mass index and adenocarcinomas of the esophagus or gastric cardia: a systematic review and meta-analysis. *Cancer Epidemiol. Biomarkers Prev.* **15:** 872–878.

55. Thompson, O.M., S.A.A. Beresford, Kirket E.A., *et al.* 2010. Serum Leptin and Adiponectin Levels and Risk of Barrett's Esophagus and Intestinal Metaplasia of the Gastroesophageal Junction. *Obesity* **18:** 2204–2211.

56. Hampel, H., N.S. Abraham & H.B. El-Serag. 2005. Meta-analysis: obesity and the risk for gastroesophageal reflux disease and its complications. *Ann. Intern. Med.* **143:** 199–211.

57. Buchwald, H., Y. Avidor, E. Braunwald, M.D. Jensen, *et al.* 2004. Bariatric surgery: a systematic review and meta-analysis. *JAMA* **292:** 1724–1737.

58. De Groot, N.L., J.S. Burgerhart, P.C. Van De Meeberg, de D.R. Vries, *et al.* 2009. Systematic review: the effects of conservative and surgical treatment for obesity on gastro-oesophageal reflux disease. *Aliment. Pharmacol. Ther.* **30:** 1091–1102.

59. Chang, C.G. & E. Perez. 2009. Case reports—resolution of Barrett's disease and esophageal epithelial atypia after gastric bypass and LAP-BAND. *Obes. Surg.* **19:** 1597–1598.

60. Varela, J.E. 2010. Barrett's esophagus: a late complication of laparoscopic adjustable gastric banding. *Obes. Surg.* **20:** 244–246.

61. Robbins, A.H., J.A. Hermos, E.M. Schimmel, *et al.* 1977. The columnar-lined esophagus: analysis of 26 cases. *Radiology* **123:** 1–7.

62. Levine M.S., H.Y. Kressel, D.F. Caroline, *et al.* 1983. Barrett esophagus: reticular pattern of the mucosa. *Radiology* **147:** 663–667.

63. Chen, Y.M., D.W. Gelfand, D.J. Ott, *et al.* 1985. Barrett esophagus as an extension of severe esophagitis: analysis of radiologic signs in 29 cases. *Am. J. Roentgenol.* **145:** 275–281.

64. Gilchrist, A.M., M.S. Levine, R.F. Carr, *et al.* 1988. Barrett's esophagus: diagnosis by double-contrast esophagography. *Am. J. Roentgenol.* **150:** 97–102.

65. Levine, M.S. 2008. Gastroesophageal reflux disease. In *Textbook of Gastrointestinal Radiology*, 3rd ed. R.M. Gore & M.S. Levine, Eds.: 337–357. WB Saunders. Philadelphia.

66. Gore, R.M., J.W. Berlin, F.H. Miller, *et al.* 2010. Esophageal cancer. In *Imaging in Oncology*. J.E. Husband & R.H. Reznek, Eds.: 127–158. Informa Healthcare. London.

67. Berkovich, G.Y., M.S. Levine & W.T. Miller. 2000. CT findings in patients with esophagitis. *Am. J. Roentgenol* **175:** 1431–1434.

68. Schraufnagel, D.E., J.C. Michel, T.J. Sheppard, *et al.* 2008. CT of the normal esophagus to define the normal air column and its extent and distribution. *Am. J. Roentgenol* **191:** 748–752.

69. Kajander, S., A. Saraste, H. Ukkonen & J. Knuuti. 2010 Anatomy and function: PET-CT. *EuroIntervention* **6**(Suppl G): G87–G93.

70. Li, Y., C. Woodall, Wo J.M., *et al.* 2008. The use of dynamic positron emission tomography imaging for evaluating the carcinogenic progression of intestinal metaplasia to esophageal adenocarcinoma. *Cancer Invest.* **26:** 278–285.

71. Israel, O., N. Yefremov, R. Bar-Shalom, *et al.* 2005. PET/CT detection of unexpected gastrointestinal foci of 18F-FDG uptake: incidence, localization patterns, and clinical significance. *J. Nucl. Med.* **46:** 758–762.

72. Kamel, E.M., M. Thumshirn, K. Truninger, *et al.* Significance of incidental 18F-FDG accumulations in the gastrointestinal tract in PET/CT: correlation with endoscopic and histopathologic results. *J. Nucl. Med.* **45:** 1804–1810.

73. Roedl, J.B., R.R. Rolen, K. King, *et al.* 2008 Visual PET/CT scoring for nonspecific 18F-FDG uptake in the differentiation of early malignant and benign esophageal lesions. *Am. J. Roentgenol.* **191:** 515–521.

Ann. N.Y. Acad. Sci. ISSN 0077-8923

ANNALS OF THE NEW YORK ACADEMY OF SCIENCES

Issue: *Barrett's Esophagus: The 10th OESO World Congress Proceedings*

Barrett's esophagus: endoscopic diagnosis

Norihisa Ishimura,[1] Yuji Amano,[2] Henry D. Appelman,[3] Roberto Penagini,[4] Andrea Tenca,[4] Gary W. Falk,[5] Roy K.H. Wong,[6] Lauren B. Gerson,[7] Francisco C. Ramirez,[8] J. David Horwhat,[9] Charles J. Lightdale,[10] Kenneth R. DeVault,[11] Giancarlo Freschi,[12] Antonio Taddei,[12] Paolo Bechi,[12] Maria Novella Ringressi,[12] Francesca Castiglione,[12] Duccio Rossi Degl'Innocenti,[12] Helen H. Wang,[13] Qin Huang,[14] Andrew M. Bellizzi,[15] Mikhail Lisovsky,[16] Amitabh Srivastava,[16] Robert H. Riddell,[17] Lawrence F. Johnson,[18] Michael D. Saunders,[19] and Ram Chuttani[20]

[1]Department of Gastroenterology, Shimane University Hospital, Shimane, Japan. [2]Division of Gastrointestinal Endoscopy, Shimane University Hospital, Shimane, Japan. [3]Department of Pathology, University of Michigan, Ann Arbor, Michigan. [4]Università degli Studi and Fondazione IRCCS "Ca Granda," Milan, Italy. [5]Division of Gastroenterology, University of Pennsylvania School of Medicine, Philadelphia, Pennsylvania. [6]Walter Reed Army Medical Center/National Naval Medical Center, Uniformed Services University of Health Sciences, Bethesda, Maryland. [7]Stanford University School of Medicine, Stanford, California. [8]Mayo Clinic, Scottsdale, Arizona. [9]Gastroenterology Service, Walter Reed Army Medical Center, Washington, District of Columbia. [10]Columbia University Medical Center, New York, New York. [11]Department of Medicine, Mayo Clinic College of Medicine, Jacksonville, Florida. [12]Department of Medical and Surgical Critical Care, Unit of Surgery, University of Florence, Florence, Italy. [13]Department of Pathology, Beth Israel Deaconess Medical Center and Harvard Medical School, Boston, Massachusetts. [14]Department of Pathology, VA Boston Healthcare System and Harvard Medical School, West Roxbury, Massachusetts. [15]Department of Pathology, Brigham and Women's Hospital, Harvard Medical School, Boston, Massachusetts. [16]Pathology Department, Dartmouth Hitchcock Medical Center, Lebanon, New Hampshire. [17]University of Toronto, Mount Sinai Hospital, Toronto, Ontario, Canada. [18]Division of Gastroenterology & Hepatology, University of Alabama, Birmingham, Alabama. [19]University of Washington Medical Center, Seattle, Washington. [20]Beth Israel Deaconess Medical Center, Harvard Medical School, Boston, Massachusetts

This collection of summaries on endoscopic diagnosis of Barrett's esophagus (BE) includes the best endoscopic markers of the extent of BE; the interpretation of the diagnosis of ultra-short BE; the criteria for endoscopic grading; the sensitivity and specificity of endoscopic diagnosis; capsule and magnifying endoscopy; narrow band imaging; balloon cytology; the distinction between focal and diffuse dysplasia; the techniques for endoscopic detection of dysplasia and the grading systems; and the difficulty of interpretation of inflammatory or regenerative changes.

Keywords: gastroesophageal junction; C&M criteria; palisade vessels; ultrashort segment; Prague criteria; focal islands; narrow band imaging; Barrett's esophagus; endoscopic diagnosis; PPV; ACG guidelines; capsule endoscopy; PillCam; string capsule; trimodal imaging; high resolution endoscopy; chromoendoscopy; specialized intestinal metaplasia; magnification endoscopy; chromoendoscopy; NBI; specialized columnar epithelium; neoplastic progression; Vienna Classification System; 5-ALA sensitization; protoporphyrin; PpIX; confocal laser endomicroscopy

Concise summaries

- A new modification may be necessary for the Prague C&M criteria, taking into account the technical difficulty for the definition of gastroesophageal junction (GEJ) by endoscopic landmarks. However, the reliability of the Prague criteria, evaluated by a measure of interobserver agreement for recognizing different lengths of Barrett's esophagus (BE) and the position of the GEJ indicated by the proximal margin of the gastric folds was very satisfactory.

- Ultra-short segment Barrett's mucosa (USSBE) or intestinal metaplasia (IM) at the junction is common. To put it under surveillance comes with excessive demands, and it should be ignored.

- Contrast endoscopy appears to be the most practical way to detect islands of IM after

doi: 10.1111/j.1749-6632.2011.06045.x

ablation. Endomicroscopy has potential but is less practical for this goal. Acetic acid chromoendoscopy has good potential but is not widely used. Utilizing the ACG guidelines, the positive predictive value (PPV) of endoscopically identifying BE would vary considerably depending on the number of biopsies obtained and the length of the Barrett's epithelium. Further advances in video capsule endoscopy technology, allowing for even better visualization of the Z-line and possible tissue acquisition, could render the performance parameters of this technique favorable compared to standard upper endoscopy.

- String capsule endoscopy (SCE), allowing controlled movement within the esophagus, seems to have better accuracy in the diagnosis of BE. Narrow band imaging (NBI) has changed the approach to Barrett's in specialized centers in that it allows a more detailed view and mapping of the affected segment. It is used as an adjunct to conventional white-light endoscopy for targeted investigation of suspicious areas.
- However, trimodal imaging is still unable to be considered superior to random four-quadrant biopsies (4QB) taken with standard endoscopy with regard to detection of lesions.
- Current evidence shows that autofluorescence-based strategies are still expensive, not widely available, nonstandardized, and even in expert hands suffer from an unacceptably high false positive rate to make it viable at this time. Balloon cytology has low sensitivity but high specificity to detect low-grade dysplasia in BE. A new type of mechanical balloon and ancillary molecular study may improve the sensitivity of this technique.
- DNA ploidy determination appears to be a powerful method for determination of cancer risk and progression in BE-related disease and can be carried out by improved image cytometry that is easier to use and more reliable than flow cytometry (FC). With histology as the gold standard, balloon cytology has been found to have low sensitivity, but reasonable to high specificity. There is a need to minimize the discrepancies in interpretation of morphologic dysplasia between Western and Japanese pathologists and to reach a uniform consensus on the nomenclature of neoplastic precursor lesions.
- Endoscopic FED gives a comparable result to that obtained with four quadrants biopsies taken every 1 cm. High-resolution (HR) endoscopy has likely become the default standard imaging technique for best selection of biopsies and endoscopic diagnosis of dysplasia.

---

1. What is the most consistent landmark for the endoscopic diagnosis of BE? What are the best markers of the distal extent of endoscopic BE by use of standard equipment?

Norihisa Ishimura and Yuji Amano
amano@med.shimane-u.ac.jp

A reliable diagnosis of BE depends on the accurate endoscopic recognition of the anatomic landmarks at the GEJ and squamocolumnar junction (SCJ). To standardize the objective diagnosis of endoscopic BE, the Prague C&M criteria was proposed by a subgroup of the International Working Group for the Classification of Oesophagitis (IWGCO).[1] In this system, the landmark for the GEJ is the proximal end of the gastric folds, not the distal end of palisade vessels, which are used to endoscopically identify the GEJ in Japan. Although the Prague C&M criteria are clinically relevant, an important shortcoming of this system may be failure to identify short segment BE (SSBE),[2] a lesion that is found frequently in most Asian countries, including Japan.

Our aim was to compare the diagnostic yield for BE when using the gastric folds versus palisade vessels as a landmark for the GEJ, and we evaluated interobserver diagnostic concordance.[3]

Eighty-four endoscopists classified 30 patients with BE by viewing projected endoscopic photographs. The endoscopists were asked to identify the GEJ, first by using palisade vessels as a landmark and then by using the gastric folds. Endoscopists were divided into groups according to years in practice as an endoscopist, presence, or absence of board certification from the Japan Gastroenterological Endoscopy Society, and whether they had taken any special endoscopic training courses on GERD. The κ coefficient of reliability was calculated for each group.

Results

Of the 30 cases, 17 had clearly visible palisade vessels, whereas the vessels could not be found in 13 cases. In 17 cases with clearly visible palisade vessels, the κ value was 0.16, an unacceptably low value of concordance over chance agreement. The value of trained endoscopists was significantly higher than that of nontrained endoscopists. In 13 cases where gastric folds were used as a landmark of GEJ, the κ values were lower than those in palisade vessels criteria. Trained endoscopists also showed a higher κ value than nontrained endoscopists. To assess the effectiveness of the systematic education and training about the Prague C&M criteria, the same trained endoscopists were thoroughly explained this criteria, and the same test was repeated two months later. As a result, the diagnostic concordance significantly increased from 0.17 to 0.35 after the education and training about the criteria and the use of the proximal end of gastric folds as a landmark. In the evaluation by the still photographs, gastric folds showed a higher κ value than palisade vessels as a landmark of the GEJ.

The most important weakness of proximal ends of gastric folds is that the diagnostic concordance is low in SSBE, which is difficult to identify the proximal end of gastric folds. Moreover, the position of the proximal margin of the gastric fold can easily change by altering the degree of air deflation with endoscopy (Table 1).

Palisade vessels can be found easily when the lower esophagus is adequately distended. However, the visual identification of palisade vessels may be disturbed by several factors including mucosal inflammation, dysplastic changes, and the presence of a thick double muscularis mucosa. Insufficient extension and inadequate stretch of the esophagus under conscious sedation may also disturb the identification of palisade vessels. Thus, neither of the landmarks of GEJ—gastric folds and palisade vessels—are the ideal, for different reasons, and are difficult to identify accurately and consistently in all patients with BE.[4]

Table 1. Technical difficulty for definition of GEJ by endoscopic landmarks

Endoscopic landmark of GEJ	Technical difficulty
Proximal ends of gastric folds (C&M criteria)	The position can easily change by air deflation Unable to recognize the fold in cases with severe atrophic gastritis
Distal ends of palisade vessels (Japanese criteria)	Difficult to identify when inflammation and dysplastic change are present Insufficient distention of the lower esophagus under conscious sedation may disturb the identification of the vessels

Conclusion

A new modification may be necessary for the C&M criteria, as more accurate and suitable criteria for both patients with long segment BE (LSBE) and SSBE. Also, systematic education and training are important to improve the diagnostic consistency in patients with SSBE, especially for less experienced endoscopists.

2. Is the diagnosis of USSBE beneficial for patient care?

Henry D. Appelman
appelman@umich.edu

To answer this question, we need to know the definition of USSBE. This seems to be the same as IM, identified by the presence of goblet cells, at the GEJ, on the columnar side of the SCJ.[5] To satisfy this definition, does the SCJ have to be normal or can it be exaggerated? This is not clear. Because this junction region is so small, a tiny patch of IM in a biopsy from the junction may be either on the esophageal or on the gastric cardiac side, and there is no way to tell from the microscopic exam.

According to the 2008 American College of Gastroenterology (ACG) Practice Parameters Committee definition, BE is "a change in the distal esophageal epithelium of any length that can be recognized as columnar type mucosa at endoscopy and is confirmed to have IM by biopsy of the tubular esophagus."[6] This is somewhat different from the 2006 definition from the British Society of Gastroenterology in which BE is defined as "an endoscopically apparent area above the esophagogastric junction that is suggestive of Barrett's, which is supported by the finding of columnar-lined esophagus on histology."[7] In this definition, the presence of goblet cells are not a requirement for diagnosis, presumably because limited sampling may miss them. However, USSBE does not satisfy either the American or British endoscopic requirements for the diagnosis of Barrett's mucosa, so it does not deserve to be given the Barrett name.

How common is USSBE? About 15% of people with normal-appearing SCJs have IM, so this clearly is not seen endoscopically.[8] About a third or more of people with jagged, irregular, or especially prominent SCJs have IM. This irregularity or especial prominence can be seen endoscopically, so, perhaps, this may be considered to be a modification of the endoscopic requirements for Barrett's mucosa. However, if these data are correct, then it is likely that millions of people have USSBE.

Barrett's mucosa is only important because it has a cancer risk, so does USSBE have a cancer risk comparable to that of typical Barrett's mucosa? Some studies suggest that the length of columnar-lined esophagus of Barrett's mucosa is a significant risk factor in the development of dysplasia and carcinoma. One study indicates that the risk for adenocarcinoma in patients with short segment Barrett's is not substantially lower than that in long segment disease, although the results of that study did suggest a small increase in risk for neoplastic progression with increasing segment length. In this study, seven patients had IM at the junction—that is, USSBE—without endoscopic Barrett's mucosa, and no cancers were detected during over 23 person years of follow-up.[9] Therefore, there seems to be no data proving that IMGEJ has a cancer risk comparable to long segment Barrett's mucosa or even short segment Barrett's mucosa. In fact, there is no data proving that USSBE has any increased cancer risk.

What is the downside for labeling a patient as having Barrett's mucosa based simply on IM at the junction? First, there is the patient's anxiety because of perceived cancer risk, which then leads to the need for repeat surveillance endoscopy and biopsy.

Insurability problems are superimposed, and, in addition, it is commonly difficult to find that IM at subsequent endoscopy and biopsy.

In summary, USSBE or IM at the junction is common. To put it under surveillance comes with excessive demands on our medical resources including endoscopists, biopsies, and pathologists to interpret the biopsies. It does not satisfy any of the definitions of Barrett's mucosa because it does not have the endoscopic findings. It does not have an established cancer risk, and it is difficult to find at subsequent endoscopies. These facts lead to this obvious conclusion: USSBE, also known as IM at the GEJ, should be ignored.

3. What is the value of the Prague C&M criteria for standardization of the endoscopic grading of BE and its progression over time?

Roberto Penagini and Andrea Tenca
roberto.penagini@unimi.it

Validated endoscopic descriptions of BE are lacking. The International Working Group for the Classification of Oesophagitis (IWGCO) has recently validated criteria for the endoscopic description of BE.[2] These criteria are called the Prague C&M because they were developed during the United European Gastroenterology Week in Prague and are based on measurement of both circumferential (C) and maximal (M) extent of metaplasia (Fig. 1). In the original paper, criteria were externally validated by 29 expert endoscopists. The reliability coefficient (RC), a measure of interobserver agreement, for recognizing different lengths of BE (C&M values), and the position of the GEJ indicated by the proximal margin of the

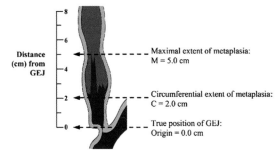

Figure 1. The Prague C&M criteria by the International Working Group for the Classification of Oesophagitis (IWGCO).[2] With permission from Elsevier.

gastric folds were very good, ranging from 0.88 to 0.94. Recognition of $\leq$1 cm of BE was, however, only slightly reliable (RC of 0.21). Recently, criteria have also been validated by 16 gastroenterology trainees and RCs were similarly high, ranging from 0.93 to 0.97.[10] These data show that the Prague C&M criteria can reliably be used in clinical practice both by experts and trainees after adequate teaching. A recent study in Japan has highlighted the importance of training on Prague criteria and has shown that the RC of 25 experienced endoscopists for identification of the GEJ was poor when assessed without training and it improved markedly after training.[3]

Considering that validation of the Prague criteria has been done using video clips or still photographs, another study from Japan involving experienced endoscopists has suggested that RC for recognizing the position of the GEJ is less during live endoscopy than with still photographs.[4] A study by Kinjo *et al.* has questioned the use of the proximal margin of gastric fold for identification of the GEJ in the Japanese population where gastric folds are less visible because of a high prevalence of atrophic gastritis.[11] In this population, the lower limit of the palisade vessels (using HR endoscopy [HRE]) has been suggested to be a more reliable indicator. Finally, ongoing studies will assess whether the Prague C&M criteria have an impact on overall patients' outcome.

4. What are the means of detecting focal islands of SIM not visible at conventional endoscopy?

Gary W. Falk
gary.falk@uphs.upenn.edu

There are two scenarios where one is trying to address focal islands of IM. The first is an attempt to detect IM within the mosaic of columnar epithelium that is characteristic of a typical BE segment. The second is to detect islands of IM after endoscopic ablation by any of a variety of different methods. The current tools available to accomplish this task are chromoendoscopy, contrast endoscopy, and confocal endomicroscopy.

Methylene blue[12] is a vital stain that selectively diffuses into the cytoplasm of absorptive epithelium of the small intestine and colon. The presence of staining in the esophagus indicates the presence of IM. However, there is no agreement on application technique in terms of the concentration, volume, and "dwell time" for methylene blue chromoendoscopy and interpretation of staining is subjective. Methylene blue chromoendoscopy[12] also adds additional procedure time. A recent meta-analysis found that methylene blue chromoendoscopy resulted in no incremental yield when compared to random biopsies for the detection of IM, high-grade dysplasia, or early cancer.

On the other hand, application of acetic acid[13] in conjunction with magnification endoscopy[14] can enhance the detection of IM both before and after ablation therapy. However, this requires pit pattern interpretation and magnification endoscopic techniques, thereby making this method of uncertain clinical utility.

A variety of optical imaging enhancements have been developed to allow for detailed inspection of the mucosal and vascular surface patterns. NBI[15] involves the placement of optical filters that narrow the band width of white light to blue light. This allows for detailed imaging of the mucosal and vascular surface patterns in BE without the need for chromoendoscopy. There are also two postprocessing software-driven systems to accomplish similar visualization (I-scan and FICE). A recent systematic review found that NBI has a sensitivity of 77–100% and a specificity of 79–94% for the detection of IM. The overall accuracy is estimated to be approximately 88–96%. There are a number of unresolved issues regarding NBI, including the use of multiple classification schemes for mucosal and vascular patterns, image interpretation based on still images instead of real time endoscopy, the use of optical versus electronic zoom, and the use of study populations enriched with early neoplasia in tertiary care centers.

Confocal laser endomicroscopy (CLE)[16] is a new endoscopic imaging technique that allows for subsurface imaging and *in vivo* histologic assessment of the mucosal layer during standard white light endoscopy. It is a potential ideal small field imaging technique that optimally should be used with a "red flag" method to target image acquisition. The main goal of endomicroscopy is to distinguish neoplastic from nonneoplastic tissue in "real time" and thus provide the potential for decreased number of biopsies. However, there are also clear criteria that may distinguish IM from gastric type metaplasia at the time of endoscopy that may be helpful in the future. Two different platforms are available: a scope-based device that is integrated into the distal tip of the endoscope and a probe-based device that can be inserted through a standard endoscope. Both devices require administration of an intravenous fluorescence agent, fluorescein.

In summary, contrast endoscopy appears to be most practical way to detect islands of IM after ablation. Endomicroscopy has potential but is less practical and too time consuming for this goal. Acetic acid chromoendoscopy has good potential but is not widely used.

5. What is the sensitivity–specificity of the endoscopic diagnosis of BE?

Roy K.H. Wong
Roy.Wong@us.army.mil

This question will be rephrased to ask: "what is the positive predictive value of diagnosing Barrett's esophagus at endoscopy?" This definition would relate to endoscopies which reveal tongues or long columns of columnar appearing epithelium within the esophagus that when biopsied reveal either columnar epithelium or intestinal dysplasia.

The PPV would be calculated by the formula: true histologically proven BE positives/endoscopically suspected BE. The PPV would depend on the definition of BE. According to the British Society of Gastroenterology,[7] any histologically proven columnar epithelium within the esophagus would be considered BE, whereas the ACG Guidelines[6] define BE as requiring IM within the columnar appearing epithelium.

Utilizing these criteria, there would be a much higher PPV for BE with the British definition. For LSBE, it would be 100%; whereas for SSBE, it would probably be greater than 95% with difficulty differentiating a very short segment of BE also known as cardia IM (CIM), esophagogastric junction specialized IM (EGJ-SIM), and ultra-short segment BE from a normal SCJ.

Utilizing the ACG guidelines, the PPV of endoscopically identifying BE would vary considerably depending on the following factors: (1) the number of biopsies obtained and (2) length of the Barrett's epithelium[17]; whether the biopsies were obtained from areas of esophagitis or visually uninflamed columnar epithelium.

Studies by Harrison *et al.*[17] indicate that the more biopsies obtained, the greater the likelihood of identifying BE. For practical purposes, the optimal number of biopsies that should be taken is eight per procedure with a likelihood of identifying IM in 67.9%. If only four biopsies are obtained, 34.7% would be positive for IM. Another factor that is associated with a higher yield is the length of the columnar epithelium.[18] As the length of the tongue or column of columnar epithelium increases, the likelihood of identifying IM will also increase. In histological studies, the IM was proximal, located mainly next to the SCJ with fundic and cardia cells noted

Table 2. Positive predictive value of identifying BE with SIM

Author	n	EGJ-SIM (prevalence)	SSBE (PPV)	LSBE (PPV)
Winters *et al.*[76] (Gastro)	97			50%
Cameron *et al.*[77] (Gastro)	27		37%	
Johnston *et al.*[78] (AJG)	172	7%	9.4%	100%
Weston *et al.*[79] (AJG)	237		48%	
Trudguill *et al.*[80] (Gut)	120	18%		
Pereira *et al.*[81] (Gut)	75	25%	61.3%	
Hackelsberger *et al.*[82] (Gut)	423	13.4%	44%	88%
Eloubeidi *et al.*[18] (AJG)	146		25%	55%
Hirota *et al.*[83] (Gastro)	889		54%	73%
Harrison *et al.*[17] (AJG)	296		Mixed group (1–11 cm, mean = 4 cm) 16 Bx = 100%, 8 Bx = 67.9%, 4 Bx = 34.7%	

in the mid- and proximal portion of the columnar lined esophagus. Finally, biopsies obtained from esophagitis had a lower likelihood of identifying BE by 12%.[19]

The calculated PPV for SSBE ranged from 9.4% to 61.3% and for LSBE 50% to 100% for LSBE (Table 2).

6. Is capsule endoscopy an accurate enough tool for BE screening in clinical practice?

Lauren B. Gerson
lgerson@stanford.edu

Wireless video capsule endoscopy (VCE) was approved by the Food and Drug Administration in 2001 as an adjunctive aid for the detection of small bowel disorders. Because patients ingest the capsule in the standing position and the small bowel VCE captures two frames per second, the traditional VCE often does not capture images of the esophagogastric junction. Developed in 2004, the esophageal capsule, or PillCam ESO (Given Imaging, Ltd., Duluth, GA, USA), captures 14 frames per second whereas the patient ingests the capsule in a supine position and then gradually resumes the sitting position during a 5-minute period.[20] Usage of the first generation PillCam ESO demonstrated excellent sensitivity and specificity for the detection of erosive esophagitis and BE in a preliminary study of 106 patients (93 with GERD, 13 with BE).[21] However, the results may have been biased by the usage of a *post hoc* adjudication committee and BE was not confirmed by biopsy. A second blind prospective trial demonstrated a sensitivity of 67% for BE detection comparing PillCam ESO to standard esophagogastroduodenoscopy (EGD).[22] Using these performance parameters, two cost-effectiveness models were unable to conclude that the usage of esophageal capsule endoscopy (ECE) was cost-effective in the screening of BE.[23,24] The main reason for these findings were that the detection rates of BE were modeled to be 70% for ECE compared to 85% with EGD, in addition to a 50% poor visualization rate of the EGJ, which would lead to an upper endoscopic examination and increase the cost of the EGD arm.

A second generation esophageal capsule, ESO-2, was released by Given Imaging in 2007 with a 30% increase in the frame capture rate from 14 to 18 frames per second, advanced optics with three lenses instead of one lens, and expansion of field of view from 140° to 169°.[25] To maximize visualization of the EGJ and reduce the presence of bubbles, the standardized ingestion protocol (SIP) was published by Gralnek *et al.* and included having the patient lie on his/her right side during capsule ingestion while sipping 5–10 ml of water every 30 seconds.[25] A subsequent clinical trial in 28 subjects using the SIP protocol and ESO-2 demonstrated visualization of the Z-line in 75% of subjects, and sensitivity of 100% with specificity of 74% for BE detection.[26] The agreement between ESO-2 and EGD for description of the Z-line was 86% ($\kappa = 0.68$).

A 2009 meta-analysis[27] including nine studies with 618 patients undergoing primarily the first generation ECE demonstrated a pooled sensitivity and specificity of ECE for BE detection of 77% and 86% compared to 78% sensitivity and 90% specificity for EGD. Usage of SCE in one study demonstrated sensitivity of 78% with specificity of 83%.[28] The authors concluded that upper endoscopy should remain the preferred modality in the evaluation of patients with suspected BE.

Therefore, although the usage of ECE has been demonstrated to be an acceptable screening modality for the presence of esophageal varices,[29] it is not possible in most regions of the United States to obtain insurance authorization in order to perform an ECE study in a patient for evaluation of GERD and/or screening for BE. Given the superior performance parameters with usage of the ESO-2 and SIP protocol, however, further clinical studies may be able to add to the encouraging results from the initial study using ESO-2. In addition, further advances in VCE technology allowing for even better visualization of the Z-line and possible tissue acquisition, could render the performance parameters of VCE favorable compared to standard upper endoscopy.

7. Should SCE, allowing controlled movement within the esophagus, have better accuracy in the diagnosis of BE?

Francisco C. Ramirez
FRami36715@aol.com

The major drawbacks of the ECE device in its current form that may affect the accuracy of the images and thus the diagnosis of an esophageal

Table 3. Performance characteristics of string capsule endoscopy (SCE) for the diagnosis of Barrett's esophagus when using esophagogastroduodenoscopy (EGD; visual) and intestinal metaplasia (IM) as the gold standard

	Sensitivity	Specificity	PPV	NPV	Accuracy
SCE (visual)	78%	89%	86%	83%	84%
EGD (IM)	87%	69%	59%	91%	75%
SCE (IM)	94%	79%	79%	96%	84%

PPV, positive predictive value; NPV, negative predictive value.

condition, BE in this case, include (1) esophageal transit time, which often is too short and in about 5% may be too prolonged, but, more importantly, is unpredictable with reported ranges from 1 to 1,678 sec; (2) the challenge of the Z-line visualization and its relationship to the gastro-esophageal junction; (3) the potential and frequent interference of the images with bubbles and secretions and the inability to clean the lens(es); and (4) the "snapshot" phenomenon that refers to the inherent inability to reexamine any area of interest multiple times and when in doubt. The data regarding the performance characteristics of wireless capsule endoscopy in the diagnosis of BE have been reported recently in the form of a meta-analysis.[32] The pool sensitivity and specificity were found to be 77% and 86%, respectively for all studies analyzed. The pooled sensitivity and specificity of capsule endoscopy when EGD was used as the gold standard were 78% and 90%, and when IM was used as the gold standard, were 78% and 73%, respectively (the low specificity was thought to be the result of a study published in abstract form only). SCE was designed by attaching a tethering device (composed of

strings, or strings with a sleeve) to the small bowel or the esophageal capsule devices for circumventing the drawbacks outlined above and its feasibility initially tested for BE[30] and esophageal varices.[31] The control of the capsule device through strings converts a physiological-dependent into an operator-dependent procedure. The addition of the real time viewer makes the procedure easier and more efficient. An additional feature allows its retrieval and, after discarding the tethering device and sterilization or high-grade disinfection, to reuse the capsule and thus render the procedure cost-effective.

The data of SCE of 100 consecutive patients[28] referred for screening of BE and when using IM as the gold standard are summarized in Table 3.

So, going back to the question: should SCE, allowing controlled movement within the esophagus, have better accuracy in the diagnosis of BE? The answer is not only that it should, but, it does. However, the data need to be validated.

8. What attitude should be adopted when there are no visible abnormalities in a patient?

John David Horwhat
John.david.horwhat@us.army.mil

One can appreciate that the ability to diagnose Barrett's when encountering a columnar-lined esophagus at endoscopy is not a straightforward task, so what is meant by "no visible abnormalities?" First, we must acknowledge that what we see when we perform endoscopy is greatly influenced by a host of factors, including our training and the prejudices, biases, and experiences that we have had in our practices (Table 4). Too often, what we see is

Table 4. Comparison of imaging techniques

Modality	Availability	Cost	Ease of use	Utility
Indigo carmine	+++	+	+++	++/+++
Methylene blue	+++	+	++	+/++
Acetic acid	+++	+	+++	+++
High definition endoscopy	++	++	+++	+++
Narrow band imaging (zoom)	+/++	++	++	+++
Autoflourescence imaging	+	+++	+	++
Trimodal endoscopy	+	+++	+	++/+++

what we expect to see, and we can certainly miss subtle abnormalities if our eyes are not calibrated or trained to detect them. In fact, what is not visible or conspicuous to one endoscopist may be a glaring abnormality to another. One needs only to compare adenoma detection rates between colonoscopists to gain an understanding of how similar physicians can achieve different outcomes.

Further, we should acknowledge that looking is not the same as seeing, and you need to know what you are looking at. This includes an understanding of the appearance and proper interpretation of findings at simple white light endoscopy. Very subtle changes in the surface texture or color may be overlooked if one fails to clean surface mucus with proper irrigation, take the time to insufflate or let the lumen quiet after peristalsis. Just as one might overlook a flat adenoma in the colon, we need to be aware for subtleties when examining patients with a columnar-lined esophagus. Clearly, if one has the ability to perform surface enhancement with acetic acid and/or magnify the image, the endoscopist must have a complete understanding of, and ability to, interpret both the normal and abnormal vascular and pit patterns of the mucosa before stating there are no visible abnormalities.

Next, one must know how best to employ existing technologies to see the mucosa. We realize that not all of us currently have or will be able to justify the purchase of equipment to perform advanced imaging techniques. And even if we do have these scopes in our centers, not all of us will have been properly trained in the interpretation of images taken with narrow band or multiband endoscopy or the application of red flag technology such as autofluorescence to avoid high false positive rates. Certainly, we cannot expect all the world's Barrett's patients to only be treated at centers of excellence that do have this capability. So what can the rest of us do?

Indigo carmine, as shown by a multicenter study of 56 patients, had a sensitivity and specificity in the 83–88% range and negative predicitive value (NPV) of 98% for HGD.[32] A recent meta-analysis reviewing work done with methylene blue concluded that there is really no significant incremental yield over random biopsies for the detection of SIM or dysplasia with this agent.[15] Acetic acid scores favorably in being cheap, readily available and easy to use. A recent study from Longcroft-Wheaton *et al.* demonstrated

a 95.5% sensitivity and a near perfect correlation with final histology ($r = 0.98$) when using acetic acid for guiding targeted biopsies using HR white light endoscopy.[33] HRE is hard to describe by itself because the bulk of the literature speaks to HR NBI or HR acetic acid and not merely the incremental gain of HR compared to standard endoscopy.

To consider narrow band and multiband imaging, we need to acknowledge that the published work with this technology is almost entirely with magnification using 240 series Olympus endoscopes not available in the United States. With autofluorescence and trimodal endoscopy, we shift toward modalities that are still very much confined to a few centers of excellence—namely Amsterdam; Nottingham, UK; Jacksonville, Florida; and Rochester, Minnesota. Even within these centers, there remains difficulty in finding the best application and interpretation of this technology. Experts from these centers convened to determine how to reduce false positives seen with autoflourescence by trying to determine what endoscopic features were most predictive of early neoplasia in AF-positive areas. The best they could accomplish was moderate agreement with a κ ranging from 0.49 to 0.56.[34] This statement is not meant to impugn their efforts or the technology, but merely to show that we are still quite far away from realizing the best way to employ this technology.

So, what current guidance can we take from the experts? A recent multicenter study has demonstrated that trimodal imaging is still unable to be considered superior to random 4QB taken with standard endoscopy with regard to detection of lesions.[35] This study, from the group of four centers of excellence previously mentioned, used an HR trimodal Olympus system versus standard endoscopy with an Olympus 140 or 160 series instrument. Although the targeted yield of endoscopy was improved with autofluorescence, the problem of false positives remained, and even using NBI to try and reduce the false positives was problematic in that 17% of HGD and cancer lesions were erroneously classified as nonsuspicious by NBI. In addition, a study from the Weisbaden, Germany group studied high- and low-risk Barrett's groups with HR acetic acid targeted biopsies versus standard 4QB.[36] Interestingly, although the targeted exams were superior, their final statement was that they do not advocate abandoning 4QB outside of a setting such as exists within their highly specialized center with rigorous quality control measures in place.

In summary, the attitude that should be taken for the patient with no visible abnormalities is one of high-quality white light endoscopy. Ideally, we would all like to have HR as our standard instruments, but while we wait for this, we should at least aim to enhance our knowledge of the interpretation of normal—at a minimum, teaching ourselves and our trainees what the normal and abnormal pit and vascular patterns look like. One should learn how to optimally use the technology you currently have, but if not fortunate enough to have enhanced imaging capability, surface enhancement with cheap, readily available materials like acetic acid can be used. The current evidence shows that autofluorescence-based strategies are still too expensive, not widely available, nonstandardized, and even in expert hands suffer from an unacceptably high false positive rate to make it viable at this time. That leaves the majority of us in the United States with learning how to interpret unmagnified NBI images, learning how to better appreciate subtleties for targeted biopsies and remembering to always, always, always, take four-quadrant random biopsies to make sure we do not miss the forest for the trees.

9. What can be expected from magnifying endoscopy associated with NBI for the detection of SIM in BE?

Charles J. Lightdale
cjl18@columbia.edu

High-resolution white light endoscopy

Modern endoscopes use HR digital systems using charge-coupled devices (CCD) in the endoscope tip with greater than 1,000,000 pixels compared to the 300,000 of prior standard endoscopes. Combined with high-definition television monitors with 1,080 scanning lines compared with the standard analog 576 lines, HRE provides an extraordinary clear and detailed moving image.[37]

Magnification endoscopy

HREs also are generally equipped with an electronic zoom system that provides some magnification, routinely to 1.5×. However, magnification endoscopes are available using optical zoom system with mechanically adjusted lens systems for much greater magnification without loss of resolution. The difficulty is that focal length decreases with increasing magnification, which can make it difficult to keep images in focus even with the use of transparent endoscope caps to stabilize the target tissue. The maximal efficiency of these systems is in combination with chromoendoscopy.[38]

Optical chromoendoscopy

Optical chromoendoscopy sometimes called virtual image enhanced endoscopy provides an instant "virtual" contrast applied with the push of a button. Thus, optical chromoendoscopy offers a fast clean alternative to dye-spraying or physical chromoendoscopy. The Olympus system called NBI uses filtered light for this effect, whereas other systems use digital postprocessing.[37,38]

Narrow band imaging

In this system, filters alter the illuminating light, decreasing the red component, and allowing only narrow bands of blue (390–445 nm) and green light (530–550 nm) to illuminate the mucosal surface. These short wavelengths penetrate the mucosa only superficially, improving the view of mucosal surface patterns and highlighting vasculature.[15]

NBI and magnification in BE

Nondysplastic specialized IM (SIM) under NBI and magnification shows a regular tubular, ridged, or villous pattern with branching elongated vessels. Norimura *et al.* recently described an appearance of characteristic "light blue crests" in a beautifully illustrated article.[39] Mannath *et al.* recently published a meta-analysis using NBI for detection of SIM, finding a high sensitivity of 0.95 in six pooled studies, whereas specificity was low at 0.65.[40] Magnification with NBI has improved visualization of the squamo-columnar junction (Z-line) and small tongues of SIM in very short BE, and has helped detect small islands of SIM for biopsy or ablation.

10. Can association of NBI with HRE lead to a change in the current practice of random biopsies in Barrett's patients?

Kenneth R. DeVault
devault.kenneth@mayo.edu

In the United States, the diagnosis of BE requires the endoscopic appearance of columnar mucosa extending into the tubular esophagus along with histological confirmation of specialized columnar epithelium (SCE) in biopsies from that mucosa. On the other hand, many patients with the appearance of short segment BE, and even some with what appears to be long segment BE, will not have SCE on random biopsies.[41] Whether this is due to the patient not having BE or whether it represents sampling error has not been clear. In addition, in regards to finding dysplasia, some patients will have dysplasia on one endoscopy and not on subsequent exams,[6] which also could be due to sampling error.

Among the several methods of enhancing the mucosal view, NBI is simple, widely available, and may improve the yield of esophageal biopsies for both SCE and dysplasia.[42] Based on these and other data, we would suggest that NBI does increase the yield of SCE over random biopsies, but would still do a similar number of biopsies as have been suggested for nontargeted exams (at least four biopsies for each 2 cm of Barrett's appearance).

Difficulties in finding dysplasia in a patient with BE remains a challenging proposition. A study where patients underwent both standard resolution endoscopy and HR/NBI was recently reported by Wolfsen *et al.*[43] In that study, NBI and standard endoscopy found the same grade of dysplasia in 82% of patients, but a higher grade of dysplasia was noted 18% of patients with combined HR/NBI. In no cases did standard endoscopy find a higher grade of dysplasia than HR/NBI and there were less biopsies required in the HR/NBI study. This study has resulted in our center suggesting a careful HR/NBI evaluation of all BE patients with targeted biopsies. We still add additional random biopsies in most cases to equal at least the total minimal number suggested in the so-called Seattle protocol (four-quadrants for every 1 cm).

In summary, NBI has changed the approach to Barrett's in specialized centers in that it allows a more detailed view and mapping of the affected segment. Whether this change in practice will be widely adopted remains to be seen.

11. Can NBI be considered a tool for routine clinical practice?

Giancarlo Freschi, Antonio Taddei, Maria Novella Ringressi, Vega Ceccherini, Francesca Castiglione, Duccio Rossi Degl'Innocenti, and Paolo Bechi
giancarlo.freschi@unifi.it

When NBI was introduced, endoscopists were fascinated by the possibility of detecting the pathology in real time by simply pressing a switch, such as taking a picture. In 2006, Sharma *et al.*[44] published an editorial with a compelling title, "*Barrett's esophagus—see more, biopsy less!*" The question in the title obviously concerns the diagnosis of GERD, and its pathological consequences, in normal endoscopy units rather than in highly specialized BE centers.

To compare our performances to the data presented in literature and to answer the question, we analyzed 200 consecutive EGDS performed in GERD patients and evaluated the effectiveness of NBI with respect to:

- recognition of esophagitis cases (distinguishing NERD from true esophagitis);
- detection of Barrett's metaplasia; and
- detection of esophageal dysplasia (low or high grade) or adenocarcinoma. All the images were correlated with histology results.

Concerning recognition of esophagitis, previous studies have found that fewer than 40% of GERD patients have positive upper endoscopy findings. The utility of the NBI magnification system as a diagnostic tool for GERD has been explored increasingly focusing whether the changes on observed mucosal and vascular patterns correlate with histology. Sharma and Fock found that a significantly higher proportion of GERD patients had changes easy to observe using NBI, such as:

- the number, dilation, and tortuosity of intrapapillary capillary loops (IPCL);
- the presence of microerosions;
- an increase in vascularity at the SCJ; and
- columnar islands in distal esophagus.

Our experience of using NBI to diagnose erosive esophagitis, observing the parameters previously described, in 162 consecutive EGDS performed on patients with clinical symptoms indicating GERD, reveals that the improvement in diagnosis of esophagitis after NBI observation compared with simply white light observation was of nearly 25% ($P < 0.01$). However, to date, there is still a need for prospective randomized controlled trials to validate the mucosal and vascular patterns seen in the above studies.

Detection of Barrett's metaplasia

Theoretically, NBI has the advantage of allowing the endoscopist to make an *in vivo* diagnosis, without the need for random biopsies. In recent years, several studies[44–46] have led to different classifications of patterns suggesting IM. These studies have described and classified patterns of mucosal and vascular morphology in BE based on magnification endoscopy associated with NBI, focusing on the recognition of IM in columnar-lined esophagus. Unfortunately, the classifications proposed in these studies consist in many different categories hampering implementation of NBI in daily practice. Some classifications use up to six categories for mucosal patterns, and others also require the description of the vascular pattern in multiple categories. In other words, although the available results from the studies describing the changes seen under NBI endoscopy for BE appear promising, the lack of a sufficiently validated and standardized classification scheme is one of the main limitations to the diffusion of the use of NBI for detecting BE and dysplasia. To improve the practicality of NBI in BE, some authors have proposed a more simplified classification in which only the (ir)regularity of the mucosal and vascular patterns are described. Our group used this simple classification for detection of BM in clinical practice. We had 89 NBI images for 38 patients in areas indicating columnar metaplasia from white light observation. The results were a good sensitivity (90%), but only 78% for specificity with 83% for PPV (Fig. 2, left).

Diagnosis of dysplasia or neoplasia

The current practice of endoscopic surveillance in patients with BE has limitations. Biopsies are performed randomly and sample only 4% to 6% of the surface area of the metaplastic epithelium. Preliminary results from a randomized, controlled crossover showed that, as compared with a strategy of performing 4QB every 2 cm, the use of targeted biopsies with narrow-band imaging identified similar proportions of patients with metaplastic lesions (85% with each procedure) and neoplastic lesions (71% with targeted biopsies and 55% with 4QB, but involved fewer biopsy specimens per procedure [3.6 versus 7.6, $P < 0.001$]).[44,51] But this is not the case when identifying dysplasia or carcinoma in BE patients through a simple endoscopy procedure, so that many experts conclude that it is questionable whether magnification endoscopy in combination with NBI at this time is ready to replace histological sampling for differentiating dysplastic from non-dysplastic Barrett's tissues. Also, for the detection of early Barrett's neoplasia, only two studies with conflicting results have investigated NBI for this indication. Both studies, however, have considerable drawbacks that may impede their validity. Our limited experience confirms the uncertainty concerning NBI's potential in diagnosis of dysplasia (sensibility: 80%; specificity: 78%; PPV: 60%; Fig. 2, right).

Conclusion

The available studies regarding the use of NBI in detecting GERD, SIM, and dysplasia or neoplasia appears promising and, presently, NBI is used as an adjunct to conventional white light endoscopy for targeted investigation of suspicious areas.

The main limitations of the NBI system include:

- the learning curve associated with the new technology (the reported studies have been performed in very high-risk BE patients by endoscopists very experienced in the care of such patients, but the widespread applicability of this technique is unknown);
- the lack of sufficiently validated and standardized classification schemes for the NBI patterns observed in various conditions; and

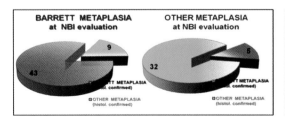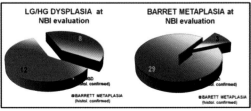

Figure 2. Personal data: results in NBI endoscopic detection of Barrett's metaplasia.

- the limited number of randomized controlled trials investigating NBI compared with conventional white light endoscopy.

Further large-scale studies are also required to address these limitations before NBI can be recommended as a primary method of screening or follow-up for Barrett's esophagus in routine practice.

12. What is the sensitivity–specificity of balloon cytology in detecting low-grade dysplasia?

Helen H. Wang
hwang@bidmc.harvard.edu

Although it is a wonderful idea to screen with nonendoscopic balloon cytology for dysplasia in patients with BE, data on this subject are limited by the fact that most studies of balloon cytology were conducted in high-risk regions of China for esophageal squamous cell carcinoma. In addition, the diagnosis of low-grade dysplasia in BE is controversial even on histology as cases are often overdiagnosed and its prevalence is underestimated.[47]

With histology as the gold standard, balloon cytology has been found to have low sensitivity (20–55%), but reasonable to high specificity (66–100%).[48–50] The higher sensitivity results were based on studies that involved using a new mechanical balloon for 50% of the study subjects, which apparently increased cellular yield and thus sensitivity.[49]

Despite its low sensitivity when compared to histology, based on an outcome/follow-up study,[51] balloon cytology was useful for risk stratification of esophageal cancer, including glandular lesions. Ancillary molecular studies on cytologic specimens have been investigated to determine its value. When appropriate probes, such as for 8q24 (*C-MYC*), 9p21 (*P16*), 17q12 (*HER2*), and 20q13, were used, fluorescence *in situ* hybridization (FISH) indeed significantly improved the sensitivity in the detection of dysplasia in patients with BE.[52]

In summary, balloon cytology has low sensitivity but high specificity to detect low-grade dysplasia in BE. New types of mechanical balloons and ancillary molecular study may improve the sensitivity of balloon cytology.

13. Despite the promising value of FC in detecting aneuploidy of G2/tetraploidy on cytological specimens, cost, and restricted availability of this technique represent limitation of its wide clinical use

Qin Huang
Qin.huang@va.gov

FC uses laser technology to measure the DNA content of cells in suspension that pass through a laser beam. The reliability of this method for detection of DNA aneuploidy associated with Barrett's esophagus and Barrett's esophageal adenocarcinoma (BEA) has been questioned for its low sensitivity and poor reproducibility. In biopsies of Barrett's esophagus, DNA aneuploidy detected by FC was considered to be a better marker than histology for assessing prognosis by some investigators,[53] a conclusion that could not be confirmed by others.[54]

In BEA, conventional karyotyping and comparative genomic hybridization studies have showed that aneuploidy with widespread chromosomal and DNA abnormalities are present in almost all BEA tumors. However, previous reports using FC have shown that up to 31% of BEA cases were diploid and negative for DNA aneuploidy.[53–56] For example, in one recent study by standard FC in archival formalin-fixed, paraffin-embedded resection tissues with histopathology-confirmed 42 BEA tumors,[55] FC detected DNA aneuploidy in only 71% of cases; the remaining 29% were diploid and negative for aneuploidy. In the cases with DNA aneuploidy, FC showed the qualitative evidence of DNA aneuploidy and failed to identify severe aneuploidy and high DNA heterogeneity fractions in 32% of cases and 9N exceeding rates in 51%. These parameters are the markers for high risk of cancer progression and were missed by FC. In addition to the low sensitivity of DNA aneuploidy detection and failure of identification of high-risk cases with DNA ploidy abnormalities, the reproducible rate of DNA ploidy by FC in different parts of the same tumor was only 50%.[55] This apparent sampling error is not acceptable clinically.

This poor reliability of FC in detection of DNA aneuploidy in BEA results from intrinsic technical errors due to inclusion of all cells in suspension into calculation of DNA content. Another source of errors is biopsy sampling, a problem associated with all biopsies. By FC, the cell suspension sample should have at least 20% of neoplastic cells with a total number of over 10,000 cells for an effective analysis.[56] This requirement may not be practical for FC to meet in a small biopsy tissue sample.

In conclusion, recent data indicate that DNA ploidy analysis by FC in a biopsy or resection tissue specimen is qualitative, insensitive, poorly reproducible, and lacks quantitative information such as heterogeneity index and 9N exceeding fractions for disease progression. These shortcomings along with technical flaws and high cost prevent its wide clinical applications. However, DNA ploidy determination appears to be a powerful method for determination of cancer risk and progression in Barrett esophagus-related disease and can be carried out by improved image cytometry that is easier to use and more reliable than FC.[57]

14. What is unstable aneuploidy? Is it a marker for neoplastic progression?

Andrew M. Bellizzi
abellizzi@partners.org

What is aneuploidy?

Aneuploidy, most simply put, refers to an abnormal number of chromosomes. The aneuploid phenotype reflects genomic, and more specifically chromosomal, instability and is commonly observed across the broad range of human tumors. Although the proximate cause of aneuploidy is abnormal mitotic segregation, the ultimate causes are poorly understood. In addition to being a biomarker for neoplastic progression, aneuploidy may be mechanistically involved, by increasing the dosage of oncogenes, decreasing the dosage of tumor suppressor genes, and by serving as a source of genetic diversity on which natural selection acts.[58] Aneuploidy is assessed by DNA FC and image cytometry on tissue sections.

Aneuploidy and neoplastic progression in BE

Aneuploidy represents one of the best-studied and most powerful predictors of neoplastic progression in BE. Reid *et al.* (Seattle Barrett's Esophagus Research Program) found that 9/13 (69%) patients with aneuploid or increased G2/tetraploid populations on initial FC developed high-grade dyspla-

sia (HGD) or adenocarcinoma (AdCa) on follow up (mean 34 months). This included two patients with biopsies initially negative for dysplasia and five patients in the indefinite/low-grade dysplasia category. In contrast, 0/49 (0%) patients without a flow abnormality progressed to HGD or AdCa.[53] In a larger study from the same group, constituting their experience with a prospective surveillance cohort of 307 patients, 42 of whom developed cancer, Rabinovitch *et al.* reported the relative risk (RR) of aneuploidy for the development of AdCa at 5.9. They also showed that the distribution of aneuploidies is bimodal, with "triploid," and "near-diploid" aneuploidies. "Triploid" aneuploidy, which they defined as a DNA content >2.7N, is an especially high-risk lesion with an RR of 9.5.[59]

What is unstable aneuploidy?

The term "unstable aneuploidy" is ill-defined, and in fact, a *PubMed* search for the terms "unstable aneuploidy" and either "esophagus" or "Barrett's" returns three results, only one of which actually uses the term "unstable aneuploidy" in the manuscript text. Although Yu *et al.* do not formally define "unstable aneuploidy," they refer to the "appearance of newer clones of severer aneuploidy" and state that "increased scatter of cells, including elevation of the 5N exceeding fraction may represent *unstable aneuploidy*." They report the results of high-fidelity DNA histograms (image cytometry on formalin-fixed, paraffin-embedded tissue sections) in normal controls (nl), BE, negative for dysplasia (neg), low-grade dysplasia (LGD), HGD, and AdCa. Data for each case include ploidy, heterogeneity index (a measure of the "scatter of cells"), and 5N exceeding fraction. They found "markedly elevated" heterogeneity index values and 5N exceeding fractions >5% in 0% of nl, 5% of neg, 32% of LGD, 50% of HGD, and 88% of AdCa. Interestingly, 69% of neg cases demonstrated at least mild aneuploidy.[60]

Is unstable aneuploidy a marker of neoplastic progression?

Aneuploidy is common in BE and can be seen in cases even without dysplasia. It would be of interest to learn the follow up on the cases in the Yu *et al.* study negative for dysplasia but with "severe" DNA content abnormalities. From the Seattle Barrett's Cohort, it is clear that aneuploidy is a marker for neoplastic progression and that not all aneuploidies confer the same risk. Although the concept of "unstable aneuploidy" is ill-defined, it can be conceived of as "progressive aneuploidy" or "aneuploidy conferring increased risk." Yu *et al.*'s cross-sectional study was not positioned to answer the earlier question, which remains a testable hypothesis.

15. How should extent of dysplasia be histologically defined? How should precise distinction between "focal" and "diffuse" dysplasia be made?

Mikhail Lisovsky and Amitabh Srivastava
Mikhail.Lisovsky@Hitchcock.org

Detection of dysplasia in BE is the current gold standard for identification of patients at high-risk for progression to esophageal adenocarcinoma (EA). However, the natural history of BE patients with low-grade dysplasia (LGD) and high-grade dysplasia (HGD) remains uncertain and the individual risk of progression to EA is difficult to quantify. Extent of dysplasia may correlate with the risk of progression to EA, but testing of this hypothesis is compounded by the absence of a uniformly accepted method for evaluation of the extent of dysplasia. Any proposed method for measuring extent of dysplasia in BE must be objective and reproducible, in order for it to be validated across different studies, and be easily applicable in routine clinical practice.

Extent of dysplasia in BE as a risk factor for EA has been evaluated in only a few studies, thus far, using variable definitions.[61–63] The study by Buttar *et al.*[61] defined focal HGD as one focus of ≤ 5 dysplastic crypts in one fragment and diffuse HGD as ≥ 5 dysplastic crypts in one fragment or more than one fragment with HGD.[61] The primary endpoint was a histologic diagnosis of EA on follow-up. Diffuse HGD had a 3.5-fold increase in the risk of progression to EA compared to focal HGD, when adjusted for endoscopic nodularity. Endoscopic nodularity was present in 34% of diffuse HGD, only 6% of focal HGD and was associated with a 2.5 times higher risk of EA when adjusted for extent of dysplasia. Thus, extent of HGD and endoscopic nodularity were both independent predictors of progression to EA. Not all HGD patients were treated with esophagectomy in this study and, therefore, the possibility of undiagnosed EA could not be completely ruled out.[61]

In 2003, Dar *et al.* studied 42 patients treated with esophagectomy for a diagnosis of HGD.[62] They defined focal HGD as dysplasia present at one level and diffuse HGD as dysplasia present at more than one level of the BE segment.[62] The extent of HGD, as defined by their own criteria, and by those of Buttar *et al.*, did not predict presence of EA in the esophagectomy specimen.[61,62]

Extent of both LGD and HGD as a predictor of progression to EA was analyzed in a more recent study by Srivastava *et al.*[63] All biopsies were scored for the total number of crypts and the total number of crypts with LGD or HGD which provided a measure of percentage of dysplastic crypts with LGD or HGD in each biopsy. The primary endpoint of this retrospective longitudinal study was a histologic diagnosis of EA. The patients who progressed to cancer had a significantly higher mean percentage of total dysplastic crypts and crypts with LGD but not HGD. The authors also defined focal dysplasia as dysplasia present in one fragment, and diffuse dysplasia as dysplasia present in more than one fragment, regardless of the level of the BE segment. Using this definition, diffuse LGD or combined LGD and HGD was significantly associated with progression to EA. The focal and diffuse definitions of Buttar *et al.* and Dar *et al.*, when applied to this data set, did not predict progression to EA.

In view of the conflicting data discussed earlier, an objective and standardized approach to evaluate the extent of dysplasia is needed. We favor abandoning the use of "focal" and "diffuse" dysplasia to assess extent of dysplasia because any proposed definition will be arbitrary. We propose that the extent of dysplasia be evaluated using a four part approach that will allow a more objective assessment of extent of dysplasia in patients with BE: (1) studies evaluating extent of dysplasia as a predictor of progression to EA should report the number of biopsies obtained from flat mucosa and those taken from areas of endoscopic abnormality to avoid a sampling bias. Estimation of dysplasia extent should be performed and reported separately for flat mucosa and endoscopic abnormality. (2) When only a single biopsy fragment is involved with dysplasia, the number and percentage of crypts with LGD, HGD, or combined LGD and HGD should be provided. (3) If more than one fragment from the same level is positive for dysplasia, then the total number of fragments, the number of fragments with dysplasia, and the grade(s) of dysplasia should be recorded. (4) Finally, the number of levels in a BE segment positive for dysplasia and the grade(s) of dysplasia should be recorded.

Using this approach, the data across relevant studies on this subject can be easily compared and allow correlation of accurately defined groups of extent of dysplasia with risk of progression to EA. This may eventually lead to detection of a threshold that enables meaningful stratification of BE patients with dysplasia into those at low and high risk of progression to EA.

16. What are the differences between the main categorization systems used for grading dysplasia in BE?

Robert H. Ridddell
rriddell@mtsinai.on.ca

It needs to be appreciated that these two systems were "invented" for completely different reasons. The IBD-C was created in the early 1980s to try to resolve numerous issues causing problems at that time.[64] These included (1) no definition or criteria for dysplasia; (2) three grades of dysplasia in general use—mild, moderate, and severe, which may or may not include carcinoma *in situ* (CIS); (3) ambiguity of terminology in use because terms such as "dysplasia," "mild dysplasia," and "atypia" were all used for both reactive and neoplastic changes; (4) the clinical implications of these diagnoses were unclear; and (5) for all of these reasons there could be no attempt to determine reproducibility.

The resulting classification did the following: dysplasia was defined as an unequivocally neoplastic proliferation and any grade could give rise directly to an invasive carcinoma. The classification system included four categories, each of which also had clinical implications that, until recently, also applied to BE, as follows:

- Negative: continue surveillance;
- Indefinite: early rebiopsy following Rx if possible;

- LGD: early rebiopsy or consider colectomy; and
- HGD: consider colectomy.

Note: There were only two grades of dysplasia, so that "mild," "moderate," and "severe" dysplasia ceased to exist, and were (and still are) now obsolete terms. It was also found to be fairly reproducible, especially when no or HGD were present.

The aim of the VCS was to develop a common worldwide terminology for gastrointestinal epithelial neoplasia. In practice, this expanded to become a classification and grading system for both dysplasia (noninvasive) and invasive neoplasia, whereas the concepts, principles, and definition of dysplasia system were accepted from the 1983 publication. Its objectives were to minimize the widely recognized discrepancies in interpretation of morphologic dysplasia between Western and Japanese pathologists; and to reach a uniform consensus on the nomenclature of neoplastic precursor lesions.

The resulting classification system was as follows[65] with the IBD-C shown on the right.

Category 1: Negative for neoplasia/dysplasia	Negative
Category 2: Indefinite for neoplasia/dysplasia	Indefinite
Category 3: Noninvasive low-grade neoplasia (low-grade adenoma/dysplasia)	Low grade
Category 4: Noninvasive high-grade neoplasia	High grade
4.1: High-grade adenoma/dysplasia	
4.2: Noninvasive carcinoma (carcinoma *in situ*)∗	
4.3: Suspicion of invasive carcinoma	
Category 5: Invasive neoplasia	
5.1: Intramucosal carcinoma (lamina propria)	
5.2: Submucosal carcinoma or beyond	

In practice, there was a minor change in terminology, and the addition of several categories after high-grade dysplasia.

17. What can be expected from the endoscopic detection of dysplasia using 5-ALA sensitization and illumination with blue light?

Lawrence F. Johnson
lfjmd@bellsouth.net

The compound 5-amino levulinic acid (5-ALA) is a prodrug that may be given orally or topically and is absorbed by the mucosa and metabolized to protoporphyrin IX (PpIX), a photo sensitizer. Because the degradation enzyme of PpIX, ferrochelatase, is deficient in dysplastic tissue, PpIX accumulates, and in blue light fluoresces. In turn, this fluorescence provides the endoscopist an opportunity to visually distinguish dysplastic tissue/adenocarcinoma with its intense fluorescence from that of normal tissue, and thereby, to perform target biopsies as opposed to random 4QB taken every one or two centimeters.[66–68]

This special fluorescent illumination was accomplished through a standard endoscope. To excite the PpIX, a filtered xenon lamp using blue light at a wave length of (380–460 nm) was connected to the scope, and in turn the ocular part of the scope was connected to a camera controller that sent either an image with white or the blue excitation light to the video monitor.[68]

The proof of the above concept was established by Endligher *et al.*,[66] who looked at sensitivity, specificity, and positive and negative predictive values determined from the presence or absence of dysplasia in fluorescent or nonfluorescent tissue using different doses of 5-ALA (Fig. 3). As shown, sensitivity occurred in the 80–100% range with the 10 and 20 mg/kg, dose respectively, and specificity much less (56% and 51%, respectively). However, the negative predictive value was high in both groups (90–100%, respectively). That is, if the mucosa was fluorescence-negative, no dysplasia was found—an endoscopically helpful and clinically relevant finding in the surveillance of patients with BE. Based on these results, the authors recommended a randomized prospective clinical trial to demonstrate the benefit of endoscopic FED compared to the standard technique of white light endoscopy with

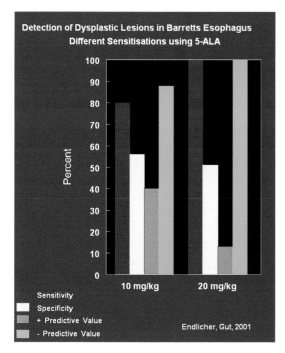

Figure 3. Sensitivity, specificity, and positive and negative predictive values determined from the presence or absence of dysplasia in fluorescent or nonfluorescent tissue using different doses of 5-ALA (from Endlicher *et al.*[66]).

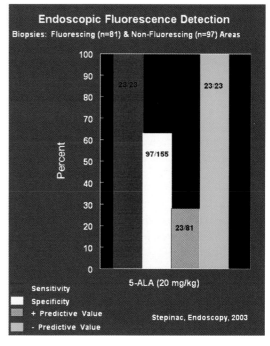

Figure 4. Comparable sensitivity, specificity, and positive and negative values were obtained for dysplasia found in fluorescing and nonfluorescing mucosal areas as reported by Endlicher *et al.*[66]

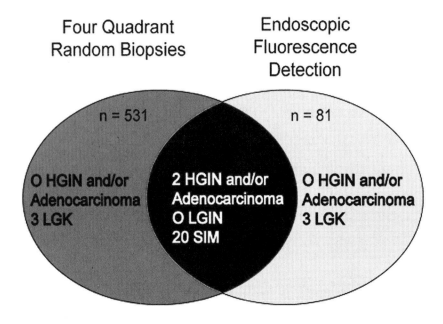

Comparison (28 patients)

Four Quadrant Random Biopsies

Endoscopic Fluorescence Detection

n = 531

n = 81

O HGIN and/or Adenocarcinoma 3 LGK

2 HGIN and/or Adenocarcinoma O LGIN 20 SIM

O HGIN and/or Adenocarcinoma 3 LGK

Stepinac, Endoscopy, 2003

Figure 5.

random biopsies taken every 1–2 cm in four quadrants in patients with BE.

The above proposed randomized clinical trial was completed and published by Stepinac *et al.*[68] In their study involving 28 patients, the authors used endoscopic fluorescence with 5-ALA to target biopsies for dysplasia and compare them to those obtained randomly using white light (four quadrants every 1 cm). Again, comparable sensitivity, specificity, and positive and negative values were obtained for dysplasia found in fluorescing and nonfluorescing mucosal areas as reported by Endlicher *et al.*[66] (Fig. 4). Most importantly, in the comparison between 4QB obtained every 1 cm and those that used endoscopic FED, both techniques gave comparable diagnostic accuracy (Fig. 5). However, endoscopic FED achieved that result with only 81 biopsies as opposed to 531 for the conventional white light technique that took random biopsies from four-quadrants every 1 cm.[68]

Wanting to eliminate the human eye from qualitatively determining fluorescence versus nonfluo-

rescence, Bland *et al.*[2] used a laser spectrograph system that measured fluorescence intensity at 635 nm and compared both the presence or absence of dysplasia and fluorescence intensity from the mucosa immediately before the biopsies were obtained. As expected, high-grade dysplasia had protoporphyrin fluorescence intensity significantly greater than that found in non-dysplastic Barrett's epithelium. Interestingly, sometimes nodular dysplastic mucosa sometimes had less PpIX fluorescence intensity than the surrounding mucosa with high-grade dysplasia. This inconsistency in detection was overcome by establishing a fluorescence intensity ratio of 635 nm/480 nm, which permitted nodular high-grade dysplasia to be differentiated from non-dysplastic tissue with 100% sensitivity and specificity.

In summary, PpIX fluorescence appears useful for identifying areas of high-grade dysplasia so that target biopsies might be obtained in patients with BE. In support of this assertion, endoscopic FED gives a comparable result compared to that obtained with four-quadrants biopsies taken every 1 cm;

however, with fewer biopsies, and, by implication, less time.

18. What is the technique that allows for best selection of biopsies and *endoscopic* diagnosis of dysplasia?

Michael D. Saunders
mds@u.washington.edu

Current recommended endoscopic surveillance of BE using the Seattle protocol, 4QB taken every 1–2 cm of the Barrett's segment has limitations. These include difficulty in visualizing early neoplastic lesions with standard white light endoscopy, that random biopsies may sample on approximately 5% of the Barrett's mucosa, and that the dysplasia can have a patchy and focal distribution.[69] These limitations have ignited a search for an adjunctive imaging tool to detect and target areas of dysplasia. Ideally, this tool or technique would reliably detect early neoplasia, decrease the already low pretest probability of dysplasia, and, in the absence of neoplasia, enable risk stratification comparable to current histology (i.e., no dysplasia versus low grade).[69] To date, no technique has fulfilled these ideal criteria and, therefore, cannot yet replace the need for random 4QB. Advanced imaging techniques that have been evaluated for the detection of Barrett's dysplasia are summarized below with their respective advantages and current limitations (Table 5).

NBI and CLE have been shown to be more accurate than random biopsies, requiring fewer total biopsies, in detecting and targeting dysplasia in high-risk patients (those with known or suspected dysplasia).[70,71] However, the overall yield of dysplasia per patient is not changed. Furthermore, the sensitivity of these techniques is decreased in patients at lower risk for dysplasia, who are the majority of Barrett's patients.[70]

Endoscopic trimodal imaging (ETMI),[56,71,75] which includes HRE, autofluorescence (AF), and NBI has been recently compared to standard white light endoscopy with random 4QB in high-risk patients with suspected early Barrett's cancer and no endoscopically visible abnormality.[72] No significant difference was observed in overall yield per patient of dysplasia. AF imaging improved targeted detection of early Barrett's cancer compared to standard endoscopy. NBI decreased false positives but was associated with a false negative rate of 17%. Similar results were seen in a separate community-based study involving intermediate risk patients.[73]

Summary

HRE has likely become the default standard imaging technique for best selection of biopsies and *endoscopic* diagnosis of dysplasia. ETMI (AFI) and CLE improve the targeted detection of dysplasia in high-risk patients. However, no current technique can

Table 5. Advanced imaging techniques for detection of dysplasia in Barrett's esophagus

Imaging technique	Comment
High-resolution, white-light endoscopy (HRE)	• Becoming the standard
Narrow band imaging (NBI)	• Yield similar to routine biopsies but with fewer biopsies
	• Difficulty with pattern recognition
Autofluorescence imaging (AFI)	• Improves detection of dysplasia
	• High false positive rates
Endoscopic trimodal imaging (high resolution endoscopy, autofluorescence, NBI)	• Improves targeted detection of dysplasia in high-risk patients
Confocal laser endomicroscopy (CLE)	• *In vivo* imaging with subcellular resolution of focal areas
	• Image interpretation
Magnification endoscopy	• No comparisons with standard endoscopy
	• Tedious to use
Chomoendoscopy	• Varying results in RCTs
	• Lack of standardization of technique

Adapted from Sharma *et al.*[2]

at this time replace random 4QB, particularly in low-to-intermediate risk patients, for detection of dysplasia.

19. What are the criteria to differentiate inflammatory or regenerative changes from dysplasia?

Ram Chuttani
rchuttan@bidmc.harvard.edu

Key issues
- A wide spectrum of atypia exists in patients with Barrett's and persistent reflux.
- Regenerative changes may be extreme, especially in mucosa adjacent to the neo-SCJ or in areas of active inflammation and ulceration.
- These changes may lead to overdiagnosis of dysplasia.[74,75]

What is seen pathologically in inflammation?
- Cytologic features of inflammation and preservation of crypt architecture. In severe inflammation—crypt budding, branching, atrophy, crowding, distortion, or even cystic changes may be seen.
- There may be nuclear stratification particularly at the bases of crypts, but occasionally also at the surface.

Inflammation versus dysplasia
- Regenerating cells contain nuclei with smooth membranes, normal nuclear/cytoplasmic ratio, and variable number of normal mitosis.
- Dysplastic cells show nuclear pleomorphism, loss of cell polarity, and markedly increased nuclear/cytoplasmic ratio.
- Regenerating cells contain nuclei with smooth membranes, normal nuclear/cytoplasmic ratio, and variable number of normal mitosis.
- Dysplastic cells show nuclear pleomorphism, loss of cell polarity, and markedly increased nuclear/cytoplasmic ratio.

How to differentiate inflammation from dysplasia?
- Although in inflammation, some changes of increased nuclear/cytoplasmic ratio, hyperchromacity, and slight loss of polarity and pleomorphism may be present, tufting of surface cells helps distinguish from dysplasia.

- In inflammation, goblet cells, both normal and dystrophic, are common.
- In inflammation, cytoplasmic mucin may be depleted but the crypt cells show a progressive increase in mucin close to or at the luminal surface.
- The surface maturation is exhibited by preservation of nuclear/cytoplasmic ratio and decrease in nuclear stratification in the upper level of the crypts.
- The degree of atypia related to regenerative changes decreases in mucosa more distant from the inflammation.

Acknowledgments

The authors thanks Professor Raj K. Goyal and Professor John Hayes for assistance of the manuscript preparation.

Conflicts of interest

The authors declare no conflicts of interest.

References

1. Armstrong, D. 2004. Review article: towards consistency in the endoscopic diagnosis of Barrett's oesophagus and columnar metaplasia. *Aliment Pharmacol. Ther.* **20**(Suppl. 5): 40–47.
2. Sharma, P., J. Dent, D. Armstrong, *et al.* 2006. The development and validation of an endoscopic grading system for Barrett's esophagus: the Prague C&M criteria. *Gastroenterology* **131**: 1392–1399.
3. Amano, Y., N. Ishimura, K. Furuta, *et al.* 2006. Which landmark results in a more consistent diagnosis of Barrett's esophagus, the gastric folds or the palisade vessels? *Gastrointest. Endosc.* **64**: 206–211.
4. Ishimura, N., Y. Amano & Y. Kinoshita. 2009. Endoscopic definition of esophagogastric junction for diagnosis of Barrett's esophagus: importance of systematic education and training. *Digest Endsc.* **21**: 213–218.
5. Fléjou, J.F. & M. Svrcek. 2007. Barrett's oesophagus—a pathologist's view. *Histopathology.* **50**: 3–14.
6. Wang, K.K. & R.E. Sampliner. 2008. Updated guidelines 2008 for the diagnosis, surveillance and therapy of Barrett's esophagus. *Am. J. Gastroenterol.* **103**: 788–797.
7. Playford, R.J. 2006. New British Society of Gastroenterology (BSG) guidelines for the diagnosis and management of Barrett's oesophagus. *Gut* **55**: 442–443.
8. Spechler, S.J. 1997. Short and ultrashort Barrett's esophagus—what does it mean? *Semin. Gastrointest. Dis.* **8**: 59–67.
9. Rudolph, R.E., T.L. Vaughan, M.E Storer, *et al.* 2000. Effect of segment length on risk for neoplastic progression in patients with Barrett esophagus. *Ann. Intern. Med.* **132**: 612–620.

10. Vahabzadeh, B., A.B. Seetharam, M.B. Cook, *et al.* 2010. Validation of the Prague C&M criteria for the endoscopic grading of Barrett's esophagus among gastroenterology trainees: a multicenter study. *Gastrointest. Endosc.* **71:** AB156.

11. Kinjo, T., C. Kusano, I. Oda, *et al.* 2010. Prague C&M and Japanese criteria: shades of Barrett's esophagus endoscopic diagnosis. *J. Gastroenterol.* In press.

12. Ngamruengphong, S., V.K. Sharma & A. Das. 2009. Diagnostic yield of methylene blue chromoendoscopy for detecting specialized intestinal metaplasia and dysplasia in Barrett's esophagus: a meta-analysis. *Gastrointest. Endosc.* **69:** 1021–1028.

13. Guelrud, M. & I. Herrera. 1998. Acetic acid improves identification of remnant islands of Barrett's epithelium after endoscopic therapy. *Gastrointest. Endosc.* **47:** 512–515.

14. Guelrud, M., I. Herrera, H. Essenfeld & J. Castro. 2001. Enhanced magnification endoscopy: a new technique to identify specialized intestinal metaplasia in Barrett's esophagus. *Gastrointest. Endosc.* **53:** 559–565.

15. Curvers, W.L., F.J. Van Den Broek, J.B. Reitsma, *et al.* 2009. Systematic review of narrow-band imaging for the detection and differentiation of abnormalities in the esophagus and stomach. *Gastrointest. Endosc.* **69:** 307–317.

16. Kiesslich, R., L. Gossner, M. Goetz, *et al.* 2006. In vivo histology of Barrett's esophagus and associated neoplasia by confocal laser endomicroscopy. *Clin. Gastroenterol. Hepatol.* **4:** 979–987.

17. Harrison, R., I. Perry, W. Haddadin, *et al.* 2007. Detection of intestinal metaplasia in Barrett's esophagus: an observational comparator study suggests the need for a minimum of eight biopsies. *Am. J. Gastroenterol.* **102:** 1154–1161.

18. Eloubeidi, M.A. & D. Provencal. 1999. Does this patient have Barrett's esophagus? The utility of predicting Barrett's esophagus at the index endoscopy. *Am. J. Gastro.* **94:** 937.

19. Hanna, S., A. Rastogi, A.P. Weston, *et al.* 2006. Detection of Barrett's esophagus after endoscopic healing of erosive esophagitis. *Am. J. Gastro.* **101:** 1416–1420.

20. Koslowsky, B., H. Jacob, R. Eliakim, *et al.* 2006. PillCam ESO in esophageal studies: improved diagnostic yield of 14 frames per second (fps) compared with 4 fps. *Endoscopy* **38:** 27–30.

21. Eliakim, R., V.K. Sharma, K. Yassin, *et al.* 2005. A prospective study of the diagnostic accuracy of PillCam ESO esophageal capsule endoscopy versus conventional upper endoscopy in patients with chronic gastroesophageal reflux diseases. *J. Clin. Gastroenterol.* **39:** 572–578.

22. Lin, O.S., D.B. Schembre, K. Mergener, *et al.* Blinded comparison of esophageal capsule endoscopy versus conventional endoscopy for diagnosis of Barrett's esophagus in patients with chronic gastroesophageal reflux. *Gastrointest. Endosc.* In press.

23. Gerson, L. & O.S. Lin. 2007. Cost-benefit analysis of capsule endoscopy compared with standard upper endoscopy for the detection of Barrett's esophagus. *Clin. Gastroenterol. Hepatol.* **5:** 319–325.

24. Rubenstein, J.H., J.M. Inadomi, J.V. Brill & G.M. Eisen. 2007. Cost utility of screening for Barrett's esophagus with esophageal capsule endoscopy versus conventional upper endoscopy. *Clin. Gastroenterol. Hepatol.* **5:** 312–318.

25. Gralnek, I.M., R. Rabinovitz, D. Afik & R. Eliakim. 2006. A simplified ingestion procedure for esophageal capsule endoscopy: initial evaluation in healthy volunteers. *Endoscopy* **38:** 913–918.

26. Gralnek, I.M., S.N. Adler, K. Yassin, *et al.* 2008. Detecting esophageal disease with second-generation capsule endoscopy: initial evaluation of the PillCam ESO 2. *Endoscopy* **40:** 275–279.

27. Bhardwaj, A., C.S. Hollenbeak, N. Pooran & A. Mathew. 2009. A meta-analysis of the diagnostic accuracy of esophageal capsule endoscopy for Barrett's esophagus in patients with gastroesophageal reflux disease. *Am. J. Gastroenterol.* **104:** 1533–1539.

28. Ramirez, F.C., R. Akins & M.R. Shaukat. 2008. Screening of Barrett's esophagus with string-capsule endoscopy: a prospective blinded study of 100 consecutive patients using histology as the criterion standard. *Gastrointest. Endosc.* **68:** 25–30.

29. Gerson, L.B. 2009. Screening for esophageal varices: is esophageal capsule endoscopy ready for prime time? *J. Clin. Gastroenterol.* **43:** 899–901.

30. Ramirez, F.C., M.S. Shaukat, M.A. Young, *et al.* 2005. Feasibility of string wireless capsule endoscopy in diagnosisn Barrett's esophagus. *Gastrointest. Endosc.* **61:** 641–646.

31. Ramirez, F.C., Hakim S, E. Tharalson, *et al.* 2005. Feasibility and safety of string wireless capsule endoscopy in the diagnosis of esophageal varices. *Am. J. Gastroenterol.* **100:** 1065–1071.

32. Sharma, P., N. Marcon, S. Wani, *et al.* 2006. Non-biopsy detection of intestinal metaplasia and dysplasia in Barrett's esophagus: a prospective multicenter study. *Endoscopy* **38:** 120–1212.

33. Longcroft-Wheaton, G.A., M. Duku, R. Mead, *et al.* 2010. Acetic acid spray is an effective tool for the endoscopic detection of neoplasia in patients with Barrett's esophagus. *Clin. Gastroenterol. Hepatol.* **8:** 843–847 [Epub 2010 Jun 30].

34. Curvers, W.L., R. Singh, M.B. Wallace, *et al.* 2009. Identification of predictive factors for early neoplasia in Barrett's esophagus after autofluorescence imaging: a stepwise multicenter structured assessment. *Gastrointest. Endosc.* **70:** 9–17 [Epub 2009 Apr 25].

35. Curvers, W.L, L.A. Herrero, M.B. Wallace, *et al.* Endoscopic tri-modal imaging is more effective than standard endoscopy in identifying early-stage neoplasia in Barrett's esophagus. *Gastroenterology* **139:** 1106–1114.

36. Pohl, J., O. Pech, A. May, *et al.* 2010. Incidence of macroscopically occult neoplasias in Barrett's esophagus: are random biopsies dispensable in the era of advanced endoscopic imaging? *Am. J. Gastroenterol.*

37. Kiesslich, R. & H. Tajiri. 2010. Advanced Imaging in Endoscopy. In *Gastroenterological Endoscopy*. 2nd ed. M. Classen, G.N.J. Tytgat & C.J. Lightdale, Eds.: 21–35. Thieme. Stuttgart/New York.

38. Elta, G. & K.K, Wang, Eds. 2009. Enhanced endoscopic imaging. *Gastrointest. Endosc. Clin. N. Am.* **19:** 193–314.

39. Norimura, D., H. Isomoto, T. Nakayama, *et al.* 2010. Magnifying endoscopic observation with narrow band imaging for specialized intestinal metaplasia in Barrett's esophagus

with special reference to light blue crests. *Dig. Endosc.* **22**: 101–106.

40. Mannath, J., V. Subramanian, C.J. Hawkey & K. Ragunath. 2010. Narrow band imaging for characterization of high grade dysplasia and specialized intestinal metaplasia in Barrett's esophagus: a meta-analysis. *Endoscopy* **42**: 351–359.

41. Kim, S.L., J.P. Waring, S.J. Spechler, *et al.* 1994. Diagnostic inconsistencies in Barrett's esophagus. Department of Veterans Affairs Gastroesophageal Reflux Study Group. *Gastroenterology* **107**: 945–949.

42. Goda, K., H. Tajiri, M. Ikegami, *et al.* 2007. Usefulness of magnifying endoscopy with narrow band imaging for the detection of specialized intestinal metaplasia in columnar-lined esophagus and Barrett's adenocarcinoma. *Gastrointest. Endosc.* **65**: 36–46.

43. Wolfsen, H.C., J.E. Crook, M. Krishna, *et al.* 2008. Prospective, controlled tandem endoscopy study of narrow band imaging for dysplasia detection in Barrett's Esophagus. *Gastroenterology* **135**: 24–31.

44. Sharma, P., A. Bansal, S. Mathur, *et al.* 2006. The utility of a novel narrow band imaging endoscopy system in patients with Barrett's esophagus. *Gastrointest. Endosc.* **64**: 167–175.

45. Kara, M.A., M. Ennahachi, P. Fockens, *et al.* 2006. Detection and classification of the mucosal and vascular patterns (mucosal morphology) in Barrett's esophagus by using narrow band imaging. *Gastrointest. Endosc.* **64**: 155–166.

46. Singh, R., G.K. Anagnostopoulos, K. Yao, *et al.* 2008. Narrow-band imaging with magnification in Barrett's esophagus: validation of a simplified grading system of mucosal morphology patterns against histology. *Endoscopy* **40**: 457–463.

47. Curvers, W.L., F.J. ten Kate, K.K. Krishnadath, *et al.* 2010. Low-grade dysplasia in Barrett's esophagus: overdiagnosed and underestimated. *Am. J. Gastroenterol.* **105**: 1523–1530.

48. Falk, G.W., R. Chittajallu, J.R. Goldblum, *et al.* 1997. Surveillance of patients with Barrett's esophagus for dysplasia and cancer with balloon cytology [see comments]. *Gastroenterology* **112**: 1787–1797.

49. Pan, Q.J., M.J. Roth, H.Q. Guo, *et al.* 2008. Cytologic detection of esophageal squamous cell carcinoma and its precursor lesions using balloon samplers and liquid-based cytology in asymptomatic adults in Linxian, China. *Acta. Cytol.* **52**: 14–23.

50. Saad, R.S., L.K. Mahood, K.M. Clary, *et al.* 2003. Role of cytology in the diagnosis of Barrett's esophagus and associated neoplasia. *Diagn. Cytopathol.* **29**: 130–135.

51. Liu, S.F., Q. Shen, S.M. Dawsey, *et al.* 1994. Esophageal balloon cytology and subsequent risk of esophageal and gastric-cardia cancer in a high-risk Chinese population. *Int. J Cancer* **57**: 775–780.

52. Fritcher, E.G., S.M. Brankley, B.R. Kipp, *et al.* 2008. A comparison of conventional cytology, DNA ploidy analysis, and fluorescence in situ hybridization for the detection of dysplasia and adenocarcinoma in patients with Barrett's esophagus. *Hum. Pathol.* **39**: 1128–1135.

53. Reid, B.J., P.L. Blount, C.E. Rubin, *et al.* 1992. Flow-cytometric and histological progression to malignancy in Barrett's esophagus: prospective endoscopic surveillance of a cohort. *Gastroenterology* **102**(4 Pt 1): 1212–1219.

54. Sikkema, M., M. Kerkhof, E.W. Steyerberg, *et al.* 2009. Aneuploidy and overexpression of Ki67 and p53 as markers for neoplastic progression in Barrett's esophagus: a case-control study. *Am. J. Gastroenterol.* **104**: 2673–2680.

55. Huang, Q., C. Yu, X. Zhang & R.K. Goyal. 2008. Comparison of DNA histograms by standard flow cytometry and image cytometry on sections in Barrett's adenocarcinoma. *BMC Clin. Pathol.* **8**: 5.

56. Shankey, TV., P.S. Rabinovitch, B. Bagwell, *et al.* 1993. Guidelines for implementation of clinical DNA cytometry. International Society for Analytical Cytology. *Cytometry* **14**: 472–477.

57. Yu, C.G., Q. Huang, M. Klein & R.K. Goyal. 2007. Quantitative targeted DNA index analysis in Barrett's mucosa, dysplasia and carcinoma. *Lab. Invest.* **87**: 466–472.

58. Merlo, L.M., L.S. Wang, J.W. Pepper, *et al.* 2010. Polyploidy, aneuploidy and the evolution of cancer. *Adv. Exp. Med. Biol.* **676**: 1–13.

59. Rabinovitch, P.S., G. Longton, P.L. Blount, *et al.* 2001. Predictors of progression in Barrett's esophagus III: baseline flow cytometric variables. *Am. J. Gastroenterol.* **96**: 3071–3083.

60. Yu, C., X. Zhang, Q. Huang, *et al.* 2007. High-fidelity DNA histograms in neoplastic progression in Barrett's esophagus. *Lab. Invest.* **87**: 466–472.

61. Buttar, N.S., K.K. Wang, T.J. Sebo, *et al.* 2001. Extent of high-grade dysplasia in Barrett's esophagus correlates with risk of adenocarcinoma. *Gastroenterology* **120**: 1630–1639.

62. Dar, M.S., J.R. Goldblum, T.W. Rice & G.W. Falk. Can extent of high grade dysplasia in Barrett's oesophagus predict the presence of adenocarcinoma at oesophagectomy? *Gut* **52**: 486–489.

63. Srivastava, A., J.L. Hornick, X. Li, *et al.* 2007. Extent of low-grade dysplasia is a risk factor for the development of esophageal adenocarcinoma in Barrett's esophagus. *Am. J. Gastroenterol.* **102**: 483–493.

64. Riddell, R.H., H. Goldman, D.F. Ransohoff, *et al.* 1983. Dysplasia in inflammatory bowel disease: standardized classification with provisional clinical applications. *Hum. Pathol.* **14**: 931–968.

65. Schlemper, R.J., R.H. Riddell, Y. Kato, *et al.* 2000. The Vienna classification of gastrointestinal epithelial neoplasia. *Gut* **47**: 251–255.

66. Endlicher, E., R. Knuechel, T. Hauser, *et al.* 2001. Endoscopic fluorescence detection of low and high grade dysplasia in Barretts oesophagus using systemic or local 5-aminolevulinic acid sensitization. *Gut* **48**: 314–319.

67. Bland, S., T.D. Wang & K.T. Schomacker. 2002. Detection of high-grade dysplasia in Barretts esophagus by spectroscopy measurement of 5-aminolevulinic acid-induced protoporphyrin IX fluorescence. *Gastrointestinal. Endoscopy* **56**: 478–487.

68. Stepinac, T., C. Felley & P. Jornod. 2003. Endoscopic fluorescence detection of intraepithelial neoplasia in Barrett's esophagus after oral administration of aminolevulinic acid. *Endoscopy* **35**: 663–668.

69. Bisschops, R. & J. Bergman. 2010. Probe-based confocal laser endomicroscopy. Scientific toy or clinical tool? *Endoscopy* **42**: 487–489.

70. Sharma, P. 2009. Barrett's esophagus. *N. Engl. J. Med.* **361:** 2548–2556.

71. Wallace, *et al.* 2010. Preliminary accuracy and interobserver agreement for the detection of intraepithelial neoplasia in Barrett's esophagus with probe-based confocal laser endomicroscopy. *Gastrointest. Endosc.* **72:** 19–24.

72. Curvers, *et al.* 2010. Endoscopic tri-modal imaging is more effective than standard endoscopy in targeting early-stage neoplasia in Barrett's esophagus. *Gastroenterology* **139:** 1106–1114.

73. Curvers, *et al.* 2011. Endoscopic trimodal imaging versus standard video endoscopy for detection of early Barrett's neoplasia: a multicenter, randomized, crossover study in general practice. *Gastrointest. Endosc.* **73:** 195–203.

74. Odze, R.D. 2006. Diagnosis and grading of dysplasia in Barrett's esophagus. *J. Clin. Pathol.* **59:** 1029–1038.

75. Goldblum, J.R. 2003. Barrett's esophagus and Barret's related dysplasia. *Mod. Pathol.* **16:** 316–324.

76. Winters, C., T.C. Spurling, S.J. Chobanian, *et al.* 1987. Barrett's esophagus: A prevalent occult complication of gastroesophageal reflux disease. *Gastroenterology* **92:** 118–124.

77. Cameron, A.J., C.T. Lomboy, M. Pera, *et al.* 1995. Adenocarcinoma of the esophagogastric junction and Barrett's esophagus. *Gastroenterology* **109:** 1541–1546.

78. Johnston, M., A. Hammond, W. Laskin, *et al.* 1996. The prevalence and clinical characteristics of short segments of specialized intestinal metaplasia in the distal esophagus on routine endoscopy. *Am. J. Gastroenterol.* **1:** 1507–1511.

79. Weston, A., P. Krmpotich, W. Makdisi, *et al.* 1996. Short segment Barrett's esophagus: Clinical and histological features, associated endoscopic findings, and association with gastric intestinal metaplasia. *Am. J. Gastroenterol.* **91:** 981–986.

80. Trudgill, N.J., S.K. Suvarna, K.C. Kapur, *et al.* 1997. Intestinal metaplasia at the squamocolumnar junction in patients attending for diagnostic gastroscopy. *Gut* **41:** 585–589.

81. Pereira, A.D., A. Suspiro, P. Chaves, A. Saraiva, L. Glória, J.C. de Almeida, C.N. Leitão, J. Soares, F.C. Mira. 1998. Short segments of Barrett's epithelium and intestinal metaplasia in normal appearing oesophagogastric junctions: the same or two different entities? *Gut* **42:** 659–662.

82. Hackelsberger, T.G., G. Manes, J.E. Dominguez-Munoz, A. Roessner & P. Malfertheiner. 1998. Intestinal metaplasia at the gastroesophageal junction: Helicobacter pylori gastritis or gastrooesophageal reflux disease? *Gut* **43:** 17–21.

83. Hirota, W.K., T.M. Loughney, D.J. Lazas, C.L. Maydonovitch, V. Rholl & R.K.H. Wong. 1999. Specialized intestinal metaplasia, dysplasia and cancer of the esophagus and esophagogastric junction: prevalence and clinical data. *Gastroenterology* **116:** 277–285.

Ann. N.Y. Acad. Sci. ISSN 0077-8923

ANNALS OF THE NEW YORK ACADEMY OF SCIENCES
Issue: *Barrett's Esophagus: The 10th OESO World Congress Proceedings*

Barrett's esophagus: histology and immunohistology

Hugh Barr,[1] Melissa P. Upton,[2] Roy C. Orlando,[3] David Armstrong,[4] Michael Vieth,[5] Helmut Neumann,[6] Cord Langner,[7] Elizabeth L. Wiley,[8] Kiron M. Das,[9] Octavia E. Pickett-Blakely,[10] Manisha Bajpai,[9] Peter S. Amenta,[9] Ana Bennett,[11] James J. Going,[12] Mamoun Younes,[13] Helen H. Wang,[14] Antonio Taddei,[15] Giancarlo Freschi,[15] Maria Novella Ringressi,[15] Duccio Rossi Degli'Innocenti,[16] Francesca Castiglione,[16] and Paolo Bechi[15]

[1]Cranfield University, Gloucestershire Royal Hospital, Gloucester, United Kingdom. [2]University of Washington Medical Center, Seattle, Washington. [3]University of North Carolina School of Medicine at Chapel Hill, Chapel Hill, North Carolina. [4]Division of Gastroenterology and Farncombe Family Digestive Health Research Institute, McMaster University Medical Centre, Hamilton, Ontario, Canada. [5]Institute of Pathology, Klinikum Bayreuth, Bayreuth, Germany. [6]Medical Clinic, University of Erlangen, Erlangen, Germany. [7]Institute of Pathology, Medical University Graz, Graz, Austria. [8]Division of Surgical Pathology, Department of Pathology, University of Illinois Medical Center, Chicago, Illinois. [9]UMDNJ-Robert Wood Johnson Medical School, New Brunswick, New Jersey. [10]Hospital University of Pennsylvania, Philadelphia, Pennsylvania. [11]Department of Anatomic Pathology, Cleveland Clinic Main Campus, Cleveland, Ohio. [12]Institute of Cancer Sciences, University of Glasgow and Department of Pathology, Glasgow Royal Infirmary, Glasgow, Scotland, United Kingdom. [13]Department of Pathology and Immunology, Baylor College of Medicine, Houston, Texas. [14]Department of Pathology, Beth Israel Deaconess Medical Center, Harvard Medical School, Boston, Massachusetts. [15]Unit of Surgery, Department of Medical and Surgical Critical Care, University of Florence, Italy. [16]Unit of Human Pathology, Department of Medical and Surgical Critical Care, University of Florence, Italy

The following on histology and immunohistology of Barrett's esophagus (BE) includes commentaries on the various difficulties remaining in reaching a consensus on the definition of BE; the difficulties in the characterization of intestinal and cardiac mucosa, and in the role of submucosal glands in the development of BE; the importance of a new monoclonal antibody to recognize esophageal intestinal mucosa; the importance of pseudo goblet cells; the best techniques for the endoscopic detection of Barrett's epithelium; and the biomarkers for identification of patients predisposed to the development of BE.

Keywords: ACG guidelines; BSG guidelines; epithelium; intestinal metaplasia; esophageal microanatomy; cytokeratin 7; cytokeratin 20; CDX2; reflux esophagitis; submucosal glands; Montreal Working Group; Prague criteria; cardiac mucosa; oxyntic cells; goblet cells; gastroesophageal junction; adenocarcinoma; pseudogoblet cells; esophageal glands; four-quadrant biopsies; MUC2; villin; Das-1; immunohistochemistry

Concise summaries

- There are still several challenges to achieving consensus on the definition of Barrett's esophagus (BE). The element of proximal extension must be based on an accurate, reproducible endoscopic identification of the gastroesophageal junction (GEJ). All metaplasia in the columnar lined esophagus may already be partway on the path to cancer. In addition, the progression to cancer of patients with no goblet cells and goblet cells appears to be similar. Intestinal metaplasia (IM) of both the

- esophagus and the cardia share many features, with respect to expression of certain antigens.

- There is currently no immunohistochemical marker that is specific to assist in defining the anatomic site of the biopsy or resection sample.

- Despite experimental observations on animals suggesting that BE can develop from an alternative source in an esophageal environment made noxious by reflux, they does not preclude the cell of origin for BE in humans being derived from the ducts of the submucosal glands (SMGs).

doi: 10.1111/j.1749-6632.2011.06046.x

- There is not yet consensus on the definition of BE. The element of proximal extension must be based on an accurate and reproducible endoscopic identification of the GEJ. Cardiac mucosa can be abnormal and metaplastic and can progress to dysplasia and adenocarcinoma, but the frequency is unknown.
- The type of GEJ adenocarcinomas and the male:female ratio are different from those with a profile of Barrett's mucosa, thus suggesting differences in the mechanism of cancer development and the role IM as a marker of cancer risk.
- Metaplasia of colonic phenotype may occur at the distal esophagus in the absence of histological BE and may progress to BE. Therefore, Das-1 monoclonal antibody reactivity may be a useful marker in the identification of BE at an early stage when chemopreventive strategies may be effective.
- It is essential for the pathologist to be aware of the presence of "pseudogoblet" cells or goblet mimickers that, in the absence of true intestinal-type goblet cells, do not seem to have a predictive value in neoplastic progression. Systematic biopsy appears to be a sound method for identifying IM defined by the presence of goblet cells. However, if the definition of BE is revised to include glandular mucosae without goblet cells, then less comprehensive biopsy strategies may be as effective in establishing the diagnosis, and detection of dysplasia will be even more important.
- The use of biomarkers may help confirm the diagnosis. Problems arise, however, if these markers are applied indiscriminately to all esophageal or esophagogastric junction biopsies endoscopically suspected of being BE.
- Although CDX2 and MUC-2 are both definite markers of IM, they cannot be used to identify patients at risk of BE because they do not seem to be expressed in any of the earlier steps of reflux disease.

---

1. Is the histological presence of IM to defiantly included in the definition of BE?

Hugh Barr
hugh.barr@glos.nhs.uk

The diagnosis of BE is dependent on endoscopic and histopathological criteria. The identification of patients at risk of neoplastic progression with "bad Barrett's" is vital. Currently, the guidelines produced by the American College of Gastroenterology[1] and the British Society of Gastroenterology differ.[2]

The American College of Gastroenterology definition states that the change in the distal esophageal epithelium of any length that can be recognized as columnar type mucosa at endoscopy and is confirmed to have IM by biopsy of the tubular esophagus. These guidelines recognize that the yield of IM decreases as the segment of columnar lining shortens and fewer biopsies are taken. Repeat endoscopy and biopsy are often necessary to establish the presence of IM. Very few patients with long segment Barrett's have no goblet cells on biopsy. It is also common not to see these cells in patients with segments less than 1 cm in length. It is also clear that intestinalization is heterogeneous and focal.[1]

The British Society of Gastroenterology definition states that any portion of the normal squamous lining replaced by a metaplastic columnar epithelium that is visible macroscopically. To make a positive diagnosis of a segment of columnar metaplasia of any length, it must be visible endoscopically above the esophago-gastric junction and confirmed, corroborated, or in keeping with histology:

(i) *Confirmed:* native esophageal structures are present with juxtaposition to metaplastic glandular mucosa, whether intestinalized or not;
(ii) *Corroborative:* this could potentially still represent incomplete IM in the stomach;
(iii) *In keeping:* gastric type mucosa of either fundic or cardiac type; and
(iv) *No evidence:* esophageal type squamous mucosa with no evidence of glandular epithelium.[2]

Liu *et al.*[3] have shown that of 68 patients with columnar metaplasia, 22 patients had no goblet cells identified, and 46 contained goblet cells in their biopsies. In both groups, there were chromosomal and genetic instability, and DNA content abnormalities. There were no significant differences between these cellular DNA abnormalities between the

Table 1. Progression to cancer of patients with intestinal metaplasia or not on biopsy

	Number of patients	Cancer progression
Kelty *et al.*[4]		
12 year follow-up		
Intestinal metaplasia	379	4.5%
No intestinal metaplasia	309	3.6%
Gatenby *et al.*[5]		
Registry data		
Intestinal metaplasia	612	3.1%
No intestinal metaplasia	322	3.2%

two groups. Both were significantly different from gastric controls. Thus, all metaplasia in the columnar-lined esophagus may already be part way on the path to cancer. In addition, the progression to cancer of patients with no goblet cells and goblet cells appears to be similar (Table 1).[4,5]

It appears that all columnar metaplasia in the distal esophagus has neoplastic potential. Guidelines will need to be formulated in the context with this new knowledge and guidelines should be harmonized internationally.

2. Can IM in the esophagus be reliably distinguished from IM in cardiac mucosa?

Melissa P. Upton

mupton@u.washington.edu

Can IM in the esophagus be reliably distinguished from IM in cardiac mucosa? The answer is sometimes, but not always, for the following reasons.

The precise site where the esophagus ends and stomach begins cannot always be determined endoscopically or histologically. There is controversy regarding how best to identify the GEJ at endoscopy. In Japan, the preference is to use the palisade vessels as the landmark, but this is not reliable in Western series, which may reflect differences in body habitus of the patients or in endoscopic technique. The Prague criteria use the reference point of the proximal extent of the rugal folds, but there are challenges in interpretation, especially in ultra-short segment BE, due to irregularity of the squamocolumnar junction and the motion of the junction in real time in a living patient. Thus, endoscopic biopsy specimens are provided to pathologists with, at best,

"estimates" of location when taken from the GEJ or distal esophagus.

What microanatomic features can define the location of IM detected in biopsy and endoscopic mucosal resection samples?

Specific microanatomic features are seen in the esophagus but not in the stomach. These include SMGs and their ducts, squamous epithelium, and duplication of the muscularis mucosae.[6] Depending on sampling, identification of these structures on histology permits the pathologist to locate the specimen as esophageal. Other histologic features more often seen in biopsies from esophagus include multilayered epithelium, the presence of hybrid glands with IM at the mucosal surface and other morphology below, crypt disarray, incomplete IM, and extensive IM. When a biopsy sample has more than one of these features, there is increased sensitivity and sensitivity to predict that the biopsy is from the esophagus; when four to five of these features are seen, the sensitivity and specificity of assigning location as esophageal are 85% and 95%, respectively.[7]

Is there a background of helicobacter pylori (HP) gastritis?

Biopsies from gastric antrum and body are essential to evaluate the context of background gastric histology. "Short-segment" IM at the GEJ in a setting of intestinalized pan-gastritis and HP infection is likely HP-related cardiac IM rather than related to chronic reflux, but some patients with HP gastritis may also have reflux esophagitis. Helicobacter organisms may be seen on hematoxylin and eosin (H&E) or special stains but might not be detected in chronic and extensively intestinalized cases.

Is there a difference in expression of cytokines, comparing esophageal IM with cardia IM?

Ormsby and associates at the Cleveland Clinic Foundation studied 31 surgical resection or biopsy specimens from long segment BE and 13 gastric cardia biopsies with IM, obtained by retroflexing the endoscope within 5 mm of a normal appearing squamocolumnar junction.[8] They identified a "BE specific staining pattern" of strong expression of Cytokeratin 7 by surface and glandular epithelium, along with weak superficial CK20 staining. This BE pattern was not seen in any of the gastric IM specimens.[8] However, this staining pattern has not been consistently reproduced in other hands. Glickman and associates reported in 2001 a study of cases of short segment BE, long segment BE, IM at GEJ, IM in gastric antrum in HP gastritis, normal non-metaplastic GEJ, and normal antrum. The Barrett's-type CK pattern defined by the Ormsby group was seen in LSBE, SSBE, and IMGEJ, and in 14% of IM in gastric antrum in HP cases in their hands. El-Zimaity *et al.* reported (also in 2001) that eight of 23 patients with cardia IM had the Ormsby "BE pattern." In a review summarizing results of 16 studies with 46 comparisons using cytokeratin staining, approximately half of the studies reported results that supported the Ormsby finding, but the other half rejected the specificity of CK7/20 staining to separate IM of BE from IM of cardia.[9] Consequently, given the variability of reported results, pathologists in most institutions are not applying these stains in clinical practice to differentiate esophageal IM from cardiac IM.

Are there other markers that can assist in differentiating esophageal IM from cardia IM?

Das-1 antibody recognizes goblet cells in colonic mucosa, and it can be seen in mucosa of BE even without goblet cells. It is an interesting marker that may be an early sign of IM, but it is also seen in cardiac glands with IM. CDX2 (caudal-type homeobox 2) is a master switch for intestinalization that is expressed in BE with and without goblet cells. It appears to be an early marker of intestinalization that can be detected before intestinal features, such as goblet cells or production of acidic mucin, can be seen on routine histology; however, it is also expressed in gastric IM. Antibodies against mucins (MUCs), Hepar-1, CD-10 may be useful for identification of IM, but they do not improve detection over histology, and they do not appear to assist in discerning if a biopsy is from the esophagus or the cardia. There are many individual studies of various immunohistochemical markers, summarized in several recent reviews, and none appears specific for differentiating esophageal IM from cardia IM.[10]

In summary, in 2010, IM of both the esophagus and the cardia share many features, with respect to expression of certain antigens. There is currently no immunohistochemical marker that is specific to assist in defining the anatomic site of the biopsy or resection sample. Careful histologic examination, with attention to certain microanatomic features, appears to be the most sensitive and specific method to determine the location of biopsies, and clear endoscopic-pathologic correlation remains the gold standard of clinical practice.

3. Is there evidence for a role of the esophageal SMGs in the origin of BE?

Roy C. Orlando
rorlando@med.unc.edu

BE is an esophageal lesion that develops in the distal esophagus of patients with reflux esophagitis. In this respect, it is likely a form of adaptive protection because its biology appears to provide greater protection against acid injury than does native esophageal stratified squamous epithelium.[11] Among the data that support this scenario are the greater frequency of the lesion in subjects with gastroesophageal reflux disease (GERD) than in the general population without GERD, its emergence in distal esophagus in those with reflux esophagitis and in the proximal esophageal segment following esophagectomy in those with esophagogastrostomy, and documentation in animal models of reflux esophagitis showing replacement of eroded squamous epithelium with Barrett's specialized columnar epithelium.[12]

The origin of the cell(s) that give rise to BE is unknown. However, since the characteristic morphology of BE requires the presence of goblet cells, and goblet cells are not normally present in any tissue adjacent to esophageal epithelium, the cell of origin must be pluripotential and capable of adapting to the noxious environment. The candidate tissues from which the pluripotential cell is derived include (a) gastric cardiac epithelium; (b) esophageal stratified squamous epithelium; and (c) the epithelium lining the ducts of the esophageal SMGs.

The case for the cell of origin in BE being from the ducts of the esophageal SMGs include the following:

1. Location: the ducts of the SMGs are widely distributed along the length of the human esophagus, as is evident by their visualization when dilated in patients with intramural pseudodiverticulosis;
2. Morphology: the morphology of the ducts of the SMGs varies from simple columnar in the lower two-third nearest the acini to stratified squamous in the upper one-third nearest the

lumen which indicates that it has the intrinsic capacity for generation of both squamous and columnar phenotypes; and[13]

3. Observation: experimental models of reflux esophagitis in the canine, an animal whose esophagus contain SMGs, have shown continuity between the ducts of the SMGs and the surface generation of Barrett's specialized columnar epithelium.[14] Moreover the generation of BE in this model occurs in the lower esophagus even when the damaged/resected areas are not in continuity with gastric mucosa.[15]

The most challenging observation that argues against the cell of origin in BE being derived from the ducts of the esophageal SMGs is that experimental models of reflux esophagitis in the rat, an animal whose esophagus is devoid of SMGs, have also been shown to develop Barrett's specialized columnar epithelium. While this observations suggests that BE can develop from an alternative source in an esophageal environment made noxious by reflux, it does not preclude the cell of origin for BE in humans being derived from the ducts of the SMGs.

4. Is there a consensus on the definition of BE?

David Armstrong
armstro@mcmaster.ca

A diagnosis of BE is predicated on the presence of metaplastic columnar epithelium, extending proximally from the GEJ, leading to replacement of the original esophageal squamous epithelium.[1]

The criterion that the columnar epithelium should extend proximally from the GEJ, necessarily excludes columnar islands found in the proximal esophagus but it should not exclude islands of columnar epithelium located in the distal esophagus. However, although there is good general agreement on the principle that BE represents columnar metaplasia, a precise definition remains tantalizing elusive.[1] The diagnosis of BE requires the endoscopic identification of an abnormal area of epithelium in the distal esophagus, but it is generally agreed that the diagnosis should then be confirmed histologically.

On this basis, the Montreal working group proposed the term "endoscopically suspected esophageal metaplasia" (ESEM) to describe endoscopic findings consistent with BE that await histological evaluation.[16] The American College of Gastroenterology guidelines state that "BE is a change in the distal esophageal epithelium of any length that can be recognized as columnar type mucosa at endoscopy and is confirmed to have IM by biopsy of the tubular esophagus."[1]

However, there is, by no means, universal agreement that IM is a prerequisite for the diagnosis of BE,[1] and, for this reason, the Montreal working group proposed that BE be diagnosed when biopsies from ESEM show columnar epithelium with the rider that the presence or absence of intestinal-type metaplasia should also be specified.[16]

There are several challenges to achieving consensus on the definition of BE. One major challenge is that it can be difficult to locate the GEJ precisely; if this cannot be achieved, it will be difficult to know whether any columnar epithelium has, indeed, been replaced by squamous epithelium. Another major challenge arises from uncertainty as to the malignant potential of different types of columnar epithelium; specifically, there is no consensus as to whether the absence of intestinal-type metaplasia is sufficient to conclude that there is negligible risk of developing esophageal adenocarcinoma.[1] The final major challenge arises because it is clear that there can be marked disparity between endoscopic findings and histological findings.[16]

The endoscopic detection of ESEM and a precise description that includes a standardized measure of its endoscopic extent[16] requires recognition of the squamocolumnar junction (SCJ) and the GEJ as well as their location, for example, in relation to the distance from the incisors or the dental arcade. The importance of accurate and reproducible endoscopic identification of the GEJ was acknowledged in the development of the Prague C&M Criteria.[17] The proximal limit of the gastric folds, the distal esophageal pinch (attributable to the lower esophageal sphincter), and the distal limit of the esophageal palisade vessels[18] were all considered as potential landmarks of the GEJ. In the validation of the Prague Criteria, the reliability coefficients of 0.88 and 0.78, respectively were reported for identification of the proximal limit of the gastric folds and the pinch in the distal esophagus.[17] This excellent inter observer agreement on identification of the GEJ was not, however, matched in a similar study that reported markedly lower kappa values for identification of the palisade vessels (0.16) and the tops of the gastric folds (0.12: pre-education; 0.35: post-education).[18]

For patients with columnar metaplasia, the risk of esophageal adenocarcinoma is greater for those who have intestinal-type metaplasia.[1] However, the detection of intestinal-type metaplasia is dependent upon the extent of the ESEM and on the number of biopsies taken; it has been proposed that eight biopsies may be needed to assess adequately for intestinal-type metaplasia.[1] Thus, the absence of documented intestinal-type metaplasia may not be sufficient to exclude a diagnosis of BE. Obtaining adequate numbers of biopsies and ensuring that the biopsies are acquired from the area of interest can also be a challenge, particularly if the area of interest is small, as in short segment BE. For example, less than one third of biopsies obtained in a study of patients with reflux disease showed histological features consistent with the area that had been targeted.[19] This, along with regional heterogeneity in the columnar epithelium, may explain the discrepancies, noted previously, between endoscopic and histological findings in patients with ESEM.[16]

In conclusion, there is not yet consensus on the definition of BE although there is, perhaps, agreement that the term, BE, describes columnar metaplasia, extending proximally from the GEJ to replace esophageal squamous epithelium.[16] Histological confirmation that the abnormal endoscopic appearances are, indeed, indicative of columnar metaplasia is consistent with this definition with the caveat that the element of proximal extension must be based on an accurate, reproducible endoscopic identification of the GEJ.

The Prague C&M criteria, currently, provide the best-validated GEJ landmarks, although they are not infallible;[17] however, inter-observer agreement studies have not, to date, provided adequate support for the use of other landmarks.[18] The biggest barrier to achieving consensus on the definition of BE relates to the risk of esophageal adenocarcinoma. If BE is defined as the replacement of esophageal squamous epithelium by metaplastic columnar epithelium, it should not be difficult to achieve consensus on the definition although the diagnosis may still be difficult in individuals with very small areas of columnar metaplasia. If, however, the definition of BE encompasses the malignant potential attributable to the metaplasia, it will be very difficult to achieve consensus. The number and location of biopsies required for an accurate assessment of the cancer risk is unknown; similarly, the risks attributable to different types of metaplasia are unknown as are the effects of treatment, age, environmental, and genetic factors. Furthermore, in practice, the diagnosis is influenced by social factors such as the patient's financial or health insurance status.[1] Clearly, BE is important because of the risk of malignancy; however, if it is defined by this risk, it will remain very difficult, if not impossible, to achieve consensus on the definition of BE.

5. Is cardia mucosa always abnormal and of metaplastic origin? Can it progress to dysplasia and adenocarcinoma?

Michael Vieth, Helmut Neumann, and Cord Langner
Vieth.LKPathol@uni-bayreuth.de

Cardia mucosa is rather ill-defined. It consists of foveolar epithelium and mucous glands but can contain oxyntic cells as well and differs from pure oxyntic mucosa by the notion that cardia epithelium appears rather atrophic. Since no strict and widely accepted histopathological definition of cardia mucosa exists, one has to accept cardia mucosa as being kind of a transitional epithelium between the squamous epithelium of the distal esophagus and the columnar epithelium of the proximal stomach, which is present in virtually every individual. Data available are weak also due to the fact that there is no precise definition in terms of gross anatomy. The mean length reported in the literature varies between 0.314 mm and 1.8 mm,[20,21] probably depending on the selected population. Of note, cardia mucosa may not be detected in some individuals, but in general it is believed to lengthen with age and can be found in fetuses, kids, toddlers, and adults with and without reflux disease. According to experimental data, development of a cardia-like mucosa can be induced by reflux promoting operation in baboons. Moreover, cardia mucosa was documented to occur proximal to the anastomosis after cardia resection in the majority of individuals within a follow-up period of 3–88 months.[22] In this study the length varied between 0.3 and 7 cm.

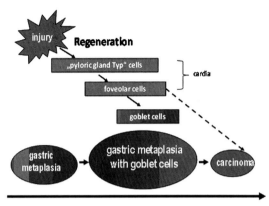

Figure 1. Gut regenerative cell lineage on morphogenesis of columnar metaplasia within the distal esophagus, modified after Hattori *et al.*[23]

The concept of gut regenerative cell lineage includes stem cell driven regeneration induced by epithelial injury and followed by the appearance of deep gastric mucous glands (pyloric type cells) and foveolar type of cells (gastric surface epithelium). Together, these two components are nothing else than cardia-like mucosa. Later on, goblet cells may appear[23] (Fig. 1).

Recently, a thorough literature review demonstrated that not all Barrett adenocarcinomas showed goblet cell-containing epithelium right next to the tumor, but cardia-like epithelium was observed in a considerable amount of cases.[24] There was no significant association with the size of the tumor but with the length of the Barrett's segment. In addition, these columnar segments without goblet cells and without neoplasia show molecular abnormalities similar to goblet cell-containing epithelium,[25] indicating that individuals without goblet cells in a columnar segment may have a risk of malignant transformation.

Thus, available data are confusing:

- On the one hand, it is possible that cardia epithelium within the proximal stomach (however that is defined) represents a physiological condition; it may even become longer with age, indicating adaptive rather than metaplastic change.
- On the other, cardia-like epithelium proximal to the gastro-esophageal junction (however that is defined) has to be regarded a meta-

plastic condition with risk of malignant transformation (that is much lower than in cases with goblet cells as it looks at the moment.) Adopting data on the carcinogenic role of IM in the stomach to the esophagus, the risk of malignant transformation of columnar metaplasia (in the distal esophagus) with goblet cells may be at least five to six times higher compared to cases with columnar metaplasia lacking goblet cells, but in fact, we do not know.

Clinical implications are not clear at the moment. In particular, we do not know what to do with individuals that show endoscopic columnar-lined esophagus but no goblet cells. An inflationary increase of the diagnosis "BE" is possible.

In conclusion, the questions addressed above can be answered as follows:

- Yes, cardia mucosa can be abnormal and metaplastic, but not in all cases (depending also on the definition of the gastro-esophageal junction); and
- Yes, cardia mucosa can progress to dysplasia and adenocarcinoma, but the frequency is unknown.

6. What is the significance of microscopic foci of specialized IM at the GEJ?

Elizabeth L. Wiley
ewiley@uic.edu.

IM is a known risk factor for development of adenocarcinoma (AdCa) of distal esophagus, distal stomach, and gallbladder. The degree of risk of AdCa developing in the setting of IM of the esophagus varies with the length of esophagus that has undergone columnar metaplasia.[26] Long segment BE has greater risk of AdCa than short segment. Stein[26] suggests that ultra-short segment Barrett's or small foci of IM at the GEJ, may carry an elevated but lesser risk of carcinoma than either short segment and long segment Barrett's mucosa.

Case reports, such as Gangarsosa's report of two patients with foci of IM at the GEJ in which one developed invasive carcinoma in follow-up, indicate that increased risk of development of AdCa may exist for patients with small foci of IM at the GEJ.[27] Siewert,[28] in his review of 1002 patients with AdCa of the GEJ found differences in the patient population and tumor type by precise tumor location. AdCa of the distal esophagus (DE) had co-existing IM in 75%, and nearly 80% of tumors had intestinal growth pattern. Only 10% of tumors arising at the GEJ had coexisting IM and more than half had diffuse type AdCa; but since only 14% of GEJ tumors were pT1 tumors, any preexisting foci of IM may have been overrun by the carcinomas. There was also a difference in the patient population. There was a 9:1 male to female ratio for DE AdCa, whereas GEJ tumors had a 5.4:1 male to female ratio.

Tytgat,[29] in his review of several studies, found a 6 to 24% incidence of IM at the GEJ in symptomatic patients undergoing upper gastrointestinal endoscopy. In the same group of studies, short segment BE had a slightly lower incidence (2–12%). Although Tytgat[29] suggests that the incidence of IM at the GEJ may be higher in the general population, the exact difference has not been established. At the author's university medical center, a large group of patients undergo upper endoscopy for complaints other than GERD. Review of pathology for Quality Assurance showed that in a one-year period, 2% of patients without complaints of gastritis, GERD, or history of Barrett's had a new diagnosis of IM on biopsy of the DE, and IM was found in 9% of those who were biopsied at the GEJ. For comparison, 5% of DE, and 7% of GEJ biopsies of patients with symptoms of GERD had newly diagnosed IM, and 4% of DE and 12% of GEJ biopsies of patients with symptoms of gastritis were diagnosed with IM. Eleven AdCas were diagnosed during the same one-year period, only two of which were associated with a history of Barrett's, and none of the remaining nine had presenting complaints of GERD or gastritis.

In summary, there is a low incidence of IM in the distal esophagus and at the GEJ junction. This incidence varies with symptoms; patients with GERD have a higher incidence of IM in the DE, whereas patients without symptoms of GERD have a higher incidence of IM at the GEJ. Indirect evidence shows an elevated risk of AdCa for patients with IM at the GEJ, but the degree of elevation of risk is unknown. The type of GEJ AdCa and the male to female ratio are different than those with a profile of Barrett's mucosa;[2] this suggests differences in the mechanism of cancer development and the role IM as a marker of cancer risk.

7. Is the monoclonal antibody, mAb Das-1 likely to help in early recognition of IM of the esophagus?

Kiron M. Das, Octavia E. Pickett-Blakely, Manisha Bajpai, and Peter S. Amenta
daskm@umdnj.edu

Adenocarcinoma of the esophagus (EAC) has the highest rate of increase among all cancers in the U.S. and in the Western World. The incidence has increased approximately 400% over the last 25 years. Barrett's epithelium, a specialized columnar metaplasia of the distal esophagus/gastro-esophageal junction (GEJ) from chronic GERD, is a precursor to EAC.

Chronic gastritis from H. Pylori leads to gastric intestinal metaplasia (GIM), which predisposes to gastric cancer, which is a leading cause of cancer-related deaths in Asian countries. There appears to be a special phenotype known as incomplete or colonic phenotype (also known as Type II or Type III) that is strongly associated with Barrett's epithelium/EAC and GIM/gastric carcinoma.[30,31] Early detection of Barrett's epithelium and GIM is essential to identify high risk patients with chronic GERD and chronic gastritis to institute appropriate surveillance and treatment.

We developed a monoclonal antibody named mAb Das-1 (also called 7E12H12, IgM isotype) that reacts with the colonic epithelium but not with any other gastrointestinal tract epithelium; including columnar epithelium of small intestine and stomach and squamous epithelium of the esophagus (Fig. 2).[32] However, mAb Das-1 reacts with Barrett's epithelium and adenocarcinoma arising from Barrett's epithelium with 95% sensitivity and 100% specificity (Fig. 2).[30] It does not react with normal esophageal or gastro-esophageal junction mucosa. This has been confirmed by three independent groups of investigators[4] who reported a 90–100% sensitivity and specificity of mAb Das-1 in the detection of Barrett's epithelium. Subsequently, we demonstrated that mAb Das-1 can detect metaplasia before the appearance of histological Barrett's epithelium suggesting the existence of a "Pre-Barrett's" stage.

IM of the stomach can be divided into complete or small intestinal and incomplete or colonic type (Type II or III) based on the staining pattern with alcian blue/high iron diamine (AB/HID) and

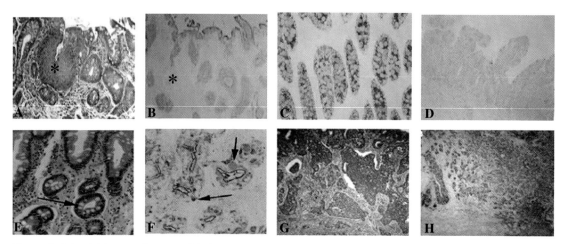

Figure 2. (A) and (B) are serial sections of the biopsy specimen from a patient with BE. (A) H&E stain showing squamo-columnar junctional mucosa from the EGJ with columnar metaplasia with presence of goblet cells. (B) mAb Das-1 reactivity is present in all the glands, including both goblet and nongoblet cells. Squamous epithelium is identified by (*) that did not stain with mAb Das-1. (C) and (D) show immunoperoxidase staining of colon (C) and small intestine (D), respectively, as positive and negative control for mAb Das-1. mAb Das-1 reactivity is restricted to colon epithelium, both goblet and absorptive cells. Small-intestinal epithelium did not react with mAb Das-1. Serial sections of formalin fixed paraffin embedded biopsy tissue from a patient with gastric intestinal metaplasia (GIM) without carcinoma (E & F) and another patient with gastric carcinoma (G and H). Hematoxylin-eosin staining (E) and (G) and immunoperoxidase assay with mAb Das-1 (F and H). mAb Das-1 stained both goblet cells (shorter arrow) and metaplastic nongoblet cells (longer arrow) in the glands (F). Intense cytoplasmic staining of the cancer cells with mAb Das-1 is clearly evident in the gastric carcinoma (H) (original magnification 160×).

differences in goblet cell glycoprotein composition. The complete or colonic phenotype appears to carry the highest preneoplastic potential. The colonic phenotype of metaplasia as detected by mAb Das-1 has been reported in stomach, particularly associated with gastric carcinoma.[31] Ninety-three percent of gastric intestinal metaplasia that stained positive for mAb Das-1 was associated with gastric cancer. Although normal small intestinal epithelium does not react with mAb Das-1, small intestinal cancer reacts with the antibody.[33] These findings demonstrate the potential of mAb Das-1 antibody to detect preneoplastic changes in the esophagus, stomach, and small intestine.

We rather serendipitously discovered the reactivity of mAb Das-1 against Barrett's epithelium and demonstrated that this antibody reacts with Barrett's epithelium with high sensitivity and specificity.[30] The reactivity in Barrett's epithelium is present in the goblet cells (GC), as well as in nongoblet cells[30] in the same glands (Fig. 2B). The reactivity to mAb Das-1 indicates that the metaplastic change in Barrett's epithelium is of colonic phenotype, includes the entire gland, and is independent of the presence of morphologically evident typical goblet cells. mAb Das-1 also reacts with 100% of adenocarcinoma of

the esophagus, but does not react with squamous cell carcinoma.[30]

Early detection of columnar metaplasia at the distal esophagus/GEJ in GERD in the absence of histological Barrett's epithelium

In several studies, we and others demonstrated the presence of mAb Das-1 reactive cells at the distal esophagus in patients with GERD symptoms in the absence of histological Barrett's epithelium. The mAb Das-1 reacted with "cardia-type" columnar epithelium located at the distal esophagus, and not with gastric cardia-epithelium. In one study, mAb Das-1 reactivity in the IM of the gastroesophageal junction (IM-GEJ) was reported to be 100%.[34] Following complete histological ablation of Barrett's epithelium by laser therapy, persistence of mAb Das-1 reactivity was found to be a better predictor of recurrence.[35] One hundred percent of cardia-type mucosa reactive to mAb Das-1 after complete "endoscopic and histologic ablation" of Barrett's epithelium had recurrence of Barrett's epithelium.

We recently completed a prospective study of 262 patients with chronic GERD symptoms who had endoscopy and 4-quadrant biopsies from the distal esophagus/GEJ. Sixteen percent of these patients

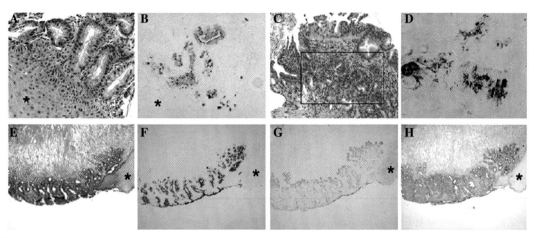

Figure 3. Serial sections of a biopsy specimen from squamo–columnar junction of a patient with initial biopsy that shows mAb Das-1 positive (panel B), but histology with mild esophagitis only (panel A). Panels (C) and (D) show repeat endoscopic biopsy specimen from three-and-a-half years later, showing BE with severe dysplasia (identified by the rectangle). The patient subsequently had endomucosal resection. (E)–(H) show H&E, mAb Das-1, Cdx-2, and AB/HID stains, respectively. *Indicates squamous epithelium.

with GERD had mAb Das-1 reactivity without histological evidence of Barrett's epithelium/IM. A subset of 11 of these mAb Das -1 positive patients had histological diagnosis of esophagitis ($n = 8$) and three had reportedly normal mucosa. These patients were prospectively followed for up to four years with serial upper endoscopies at one to three year intervals. Of the 11 patients with mAb Das-1 reactivity in the absence of IM, two developed Barrett's epithelium. One of the two patients that developed Barrett's epithelium subsequently developed Barrett's epithelium with high grade dysplasia after three and a half years (Fig. 3). These data together suggest that metaplasia of colonic phenotype may occur at the distal esophagus in the absence of histological Barrett's epithelium and may progress to Barrett's epithelium. Therefore, mAb Das-1 reactivity may be a useful marker in the identification of BE at an early stage when chemopreventive strategies may be effective. Immunoperoxidase staining with mAb Das-1 can be performed easily with a serial histologic sections parallel to H&E.

These *in vivo* observations are also supported by the novel *in vitro* model we recently reported.[35] Exposure of the hTERT transfected, immortalized, benign Barrett's cell line (BAR-T) to HCL (pH4) (A) and bile salt (200 μm glycochenodroxycholic acid) (B) for 5 min/day for two weeks, BAR-T cells show a two- to threefold increase in colonic phenotype cells that react to mAb Das-1.[36] Furthermore, long-term

daily exposure (65 weeks) to A + B causes transformation of benign BAR-T cells to neoplastic cells as evident by foci formation, distinct colonies in soft agar and formation of tumor in nude (nu/nu) mice.[37]

8. What is the frequency of cells showing a similarity with intestinal goblet cells on biopsies and their influence on false diagnosis of Barrett's metaplasia?

Ana Bennett
benneta@ccf.org

Not uncommonly, cardiac-type gastric mucosa may contain foveolar cells with barrel-shaped or distended cytoplasmic vacuoles resembling goblet cells. These distended gastric foveolar cells are also called "pseudogoblet" cells and represent a potential source of error in the diagnosis of BE. Fortunately, these mimics usually stain less intensely than true goblet cells with Alcian blue at pH 2.5, and pseudogoblet cells are generally arranged in linear contiguous stretches without intervening columnar cells.[38–40] Pseudogoblet cells contain a hazy, ground glass appearance to their cytoplasmic mucin (Fig. 4). Esophageal glands and gland ducts are another source of confusion about Alcian blue-positive cells. If they are sampled at all, these glands and ducts are usually located within the deeper

Pseudogoblet cells ➡

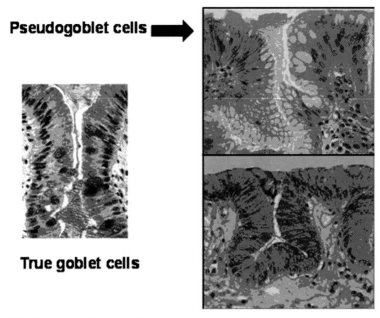

True goblet cells

Figure 4. Pseudogoblet cells contain a hazy, ground glass appearance to their cytoplasmic mucin.

portions of endoscopic biopsies in either the lamina propria or submucosa. They are characteristically intensely and diffusely Alcian blue positive at pH 2.5, but differentiation from true columnar metaplasia is not difficult because esophageal glands have a rounded or lobular configuration similar to minor salivary glands, and are located deep in the mucosa and submucosa. The ducts draining these glands may have a mucinous or transitional-type epithelium and may also contain Alcian blue-positive cells. The contiguous Alcian blue-positive cells within a duct-like structure and/or coexistent transitional-type epithelium and/or identification of the actual esophageal glands being drained by the duct, usually permit distinction from Barrett's metaplastic epithelium.

A correct diagnosis is essential to spare patients life-long surveillance anxiety and avoid possible inability to obtain medical insurance. Few data are available on the frequency of pseudogoblet cells in esophageal biopsies. In a recent study,[41] initial biopsies of 78 patients with diagnosis of BE, negative for dysplasia and a mean follow-up of 72 months were reviewed, intestinal-type goblets cells were identified in 56 (72%) of the cases. In the remaining twenty-two cases, only pseudogoblet cells were identified in 12 cases and 10 cases, although originally diagnose as BE did not show either pseudogob-

let cells or true goblet cells. Furthermore, only the presence of intestinal-type goblet cells was associated with significant risk of dysplasia ($P = 0.008$). One patient with pseudogoblet cells was diagnosed with dysplasia after 146 months of follow-up compared with 21 (35%) patients with intestinal-type goblet cells that developed dysplasia on follow-up.[41]

It is essential for the pathologist to be aware of the presence of "pseudogoblet" cells or goblet mimickers, which in the absence of true intestinal-type goblet cells do not seem to have a predictive value in neoplastic progression.

9. Are systematic four-quadrant biopsies the safest way to detect Barrett's epithelium?

James J. Going
gqxa02@udcf.gla.ac.uk

Paull *et al.*[43] described three types of columnar mucosa in Barrett's esophagus (BE), proximal to the lower esophageal sphincter: one resembling gastric fundic mucosa with parietal and chief cells; one resembling gastric cardia mucosa, with mucous glands; and a distinctive type with mucous glands and goblet cells.

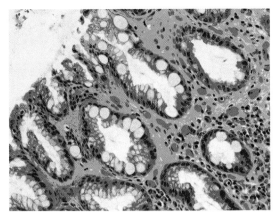

Figure 5. Intestinal metaplasia with goblet cells: until recently, this has been taken as defining feature in Barrett's esophagus. If future work sustains the proposal that cancer risk may be significantly elevated without goblet cells, their importance as a risk marker will diminish.

The answer to the title question depends on whether mucosa with IM defined by goblet cells (IM with GC) is regarded as essential for the diagnosis of BE (Fig. 5). That IM with goblet cells *is* essential for a diagnosis of BE has been generally held in the United States and widely, but not universally, in the UK and elsewhere, including Japan. This definition is motivated by the belief in a strong association between IM with goblet cells and dysplasia and increased risk of progression to invasive adenocarcinoma; and that glandular metaplasia alone, in the absence of goblet cells, is not associated with the same elevated cancer risk. After a number of years during which this view has generally been accepted, the evidence for it has begun to be questioned.

Notably, Takubo *et al.*[44] describe a weaker than expected association between IM with goblet cells and early Barrett's adenocarcinoma, which appeared in their cases to arise on a background of cardia-like glandular mucosa. In addition, Odze *et al.*[45] have pointed out that even in the absence of goblet cells, there may be evidence of intestinal differentiation, including expression of intestinal markers MUC2, DAS1, CDX2, and Villin. Also, recent studies suggest that chromosomal and DNA content abnormalities are not different between metaplastic esophageal glandular mucosa with and without goblet cells, in keeping with a risk of neoplastic progression similar in both.

In the West of Scotland, it is rare for a long segment Barrett's esophagus (LSBE) patient to have

no histological IM with goblet cells.[46] Of thirty-two randomly selected and systematically biopsied LSBE patients, the cumulative probability of IM being present at any level was about 90%, and 100% overall. On the other hand, other studies have found a lower prevalence of IM, which may be a function of age.

If the endoscopist thinks there is a long segment Barrett's mucosa, and the histopathologist can demonstrate glandular mucosa in a locus considered to be esophageal by the endoscopist but no IM, often, but not always, the reason will be too few biopsies. For as long as IM with GC is taken to define BE, a minimum of 4-quadrant biopsies will be required before BE could be excluded. Things are less clear cut in SSBE, but, here too, a 4-quadrant biopsy would be a reasonable diagnostic minimum, except perhaps in the case of an isolated mucosal tongue.

This question is related to whether or not systematic 4-quadrant biopsy is the most effective way to diagnose *dysplastic* Barrett's mucosa, not Barrett's *per se*. A (nonrandomized) comparison[47] of two biopsy approaches at Glasgow Royal Infirmary over nine years began in 1995 when a group of surgeons adopted a systematic biopsy approach, while medical gastroenterologists adhered to nonsystematic protocols. Two demographically similar cohorts each of 180 patients were compared. Prevalance of dysplasia was 18.9% with systematic biopsy but only 1.6% with random biopsy. Only 2.2% of systematically biopsied patients developed incident LGD after a median of 62 months compared with 6.6% of nonsystematically biopsied patients after a median of 36 months. These data are in keeping with a relatively low incidence of genuinely new dysplasia: most BE patients have had BE for a long time by the time of their index endoscopy. The relatively high prevalence of dysplasia is not unexpected given the high incidence of esophegeal adenocarcinoma in Scotland.

In summary, systematic biopsy appears to be a sound method for identifying IM defined by the presence of goblet cells in columnar-lined esophagus (BE). However, if the definition of BE is revised to include glandular mucosae without goblet cells, then less comprehensive biopsy strategies may be as effective in establishing the diagnosis; if so, detection of dysplasia (or a validated surrogate risk marker) will be even more important.

10. Can the exact role of biomarkers for the diagnosis of BE be defined?

Mamoun Younes and Helen H. Wang
myounes@bcm.edu

BE, or Barrett's metaplasia, is a condition in which the normal squamous lining of the esophagus is replaced by columnar epithelium. Paul and his colleagues classified BE on the basis of histologic appearance into three types: cardiac, fundic, and specialized columnar with intestinal type goblet cells. However, only the intestinal type with goblet cells has so far been definitively associated with increased risk of progression to esophageal adenocarcinoma. Currently, in the United States, histologic documentation of intestinal type columnar epithelium with goblet cells is required for the diagnosis of BE.

The diagnosis of BE is made by identifying intestinal-type goblet cells on routine hematoxylin and eosin (H&E) stained sections of esophageal biopsies. Several molecular markers have been shown to be expressed in BE by immunohistochemistry (IHC); these include MUC2,[48] which stains the goblet cells; hepatocyte antigen,[49] which stains the absorptive cells; villin,[50] which stains the brush border that incidentally may be lacking in some cases of BE; Das-1,[51] which stains goblet cells; and CDX2,[52] which stains cells with intestinal differentiation including goblet and absorptive cells. As expression of these markers was found to correlate very well with "IM" in BE, their clinical utility is limited.

In a few cases, pathologists who may not feel confident making a diagnosis of BE because of a suboptimal H&E stain, orientation of the biopsy tissue, quality of the section preparation, or presence of rare cells that are equivocal for being intestinal-type goblet cells, the use of biomarkers may help confirm the diagnosis. Problems arise, however, if these markers are applied indiscriminately to all esophageal or esophagogastric junction biopsies endoscopically suspected of being BE. Figure 1 illustrates two such examples. In Figure 6A, IHC for CDX2 shows scattered cells that slightly resemble, but are not typical of full-blown intestinal-type goblet cells (arrows). Here, positive nuclear staining for CDX2 confirms an "intestinal" phenotype. In Figure 6B, none of the columnar epithelial cells at the squamo–columnar junction even slightly resem-

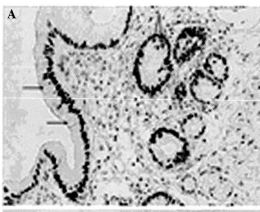

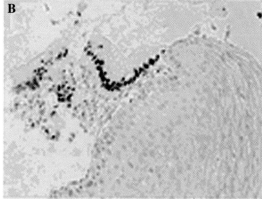

Figure 6. Immunohistochemical staining for CDX2 in biopsies taken from the esophagogastric junction. (A) Positive strong nuclear staining in columnar epithelial cells including cells suspected of being goblet cells (arrows). (B) Strong nuclear staining in columnar cells without any goblet cells or any cells remotely resembling goblet cells. Immunoperoxidase staining with hematoxylin counterstaining, 20× objective. (Microscope condenser removed for better delineation of cell membranes to demonstrate shapes of cells).

ble goblet cells, yet all of these cells are strongly positive for CDX2. Although these cells may very well be "pregoblets" and may, with time, become goblet cells, this is just speculative at the present time. Almost all patients who have esophageal biopsies to rule out BE are symptomatic, and do receive treatment, medical or surgical, for GERD. Therefore, it will be extremely difficult to know the natural history of CDX2 biopsies without goblets, as this will be altered by intervention (medical or surgical), and one would expect that since reflux is thought to be the cause of CDX2 expression, adequate treating of GERD, at least in theory, should reverse CDX2 expression or should prevent the CDX2-positive cells from progressing to a goblet phenotype. "Reversal" of established BE with goblet cells with medical treatment has been reported. In one study, CDX2 expression in biopsies of columnar-lined esophagus without goblet cells was found to predict the finding of goblet cells in a second set of biopsies from the same patients (taken either before or after the CDX2-positive biopsies).[53] In the same study, however, 24% of patients with CDX2-positive biopsies without goblet cells had no goblet cells in a second set of biopsies.[53] Because patients with BE are subjected to life-long surveillance and biopsy, anxiety about their increased chances of getting esophageal cancer, cost, and adverse effects of some modalities to treating or eradicating BE, and increased health and life insurance premiums, and because most follow-up studies so far have shown no significant association between columnar-lined epithelium without goblet cells and esophageal cancer, strong evidence of association between CDX2-positive nongoblet cell CLE and esophageal cancer from large-scale prospective studies is required before labeling these patients as having BE.

11. What is the value of molecular markers (CDX2, MUC2, and CK7/20) for identification of patients predisposed to the development of BE?

Antonio Taddei, Giancarlo Freschi, Maria Novella Ringressi, Duccio Rossi Degli'Innocenti, Francesca Castiglione, and Paolo Bechi
antonio.taddei@unifi.it

Homeobox protein CDX2 is encoded by the *CDX2 gene*. In humans, this protein is a caudal homeobox transcription factor, which is involved in the modulation of complex signaling pathways and transcription processes, important both for embryonic development and the homeostasis of adult tissues. Although CDX2 role in BE is not completely understood, it is noticeable that CDX2 is not expressed in the normal squamous esophageal epithelium, whereas it has been shown to be highly expressed in BE.[54]

Mucins are also widely secreted in the gastrointestinal tract, with distinct composition patterns in the different locations. Among mucins, mucin 2 (MUC2) is prominent in the gut, where it is mainly

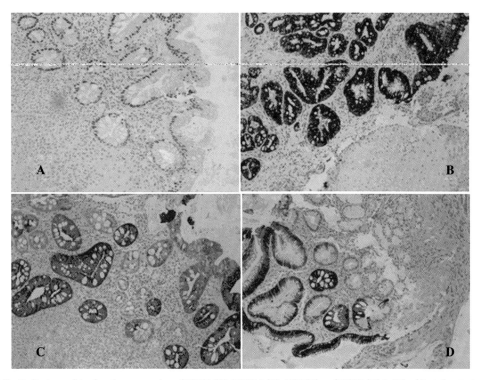

Figure 7. Preliminary data showing expression of CDX2 (A), MUC-2 (B), CK7 (C) and CK20 (D) in BE subjects (see text on p. 12 in question 11).

secreted from goblet cells of the epithelial lining into the lumen of the large intestine.[55]

Cytokeratins (CK) form the building blocks for the intermediate filaments, which contribute to cell cytoskeleton formation. There are variable patterns of expression of cytokeratins in epithelial cells depending on the type, location, and differentiation of epithelium. CK7/20 profiles are considered relevant for the diagnosis of some diseases of the gastrointestinal tract. CK20 is commonly used as a marker of intestinal differentiation. It is widely expressed on the surface and crypt epithelium of the normal colon and small intestine. In the stomach, its expression is limited to the surface foveolar epithelium (no gastric gland/pit expression). In the esophagus, CK7 specific staining is only detectable in the superficial layers of the squamous epithelium, whereas in columnar metaplasia, increased expression is shown more deeply throughout the crypts and the glands.

It has been claimed that a specific staining pattern reliably distinguishes intestinal from the cardial and oxyntic metaplasia.[56] This so-called Barrett's pattern is characterized by CK20 superficial staining and diffuse and strong CK7 staining and has been demonstrated both in long and short segment BE.[56] More recently, the presence of a CK7/20 Barrett's pattern has been confirmed, its presence in ultrashort segment BE has been demonstrated.[57]

We have preliminary data showing indicating that CDX2 was absent in all the patients both of normal epithelium and the esophagitis groups (unpublished data). On the contrary, it was highly expressed in BE: in this group of biopsies a strong nuclear staining was observed (Fig. 7A). MUC2 had exactly the same behavior, it was absent both in normal epithelium and in the esophagitis groups, whereas it was well expressed in BE: in this group of biopsies a strong cytoplasmatic staining was shown (Fig. 7B). CK7 and Ck20 expression showed a distribution that differed from CDX2 and MUC2; their expression (similar for CK7 and CK20) was evident in all three groups patients. However, their expression was significantly ($P = 0.023$) greater in BE than in normal epithelium and esophagitis groups (Fig. 7C & 7D, respectively). It must be stressed that none of the patients in the group with CK7/20 expression developed BE after a five-year follow-up (unpublished data).

In conclusion, although CDX2 and MUC2 are both a definite marker of IM, they cannot be used to identify the patients at risk of BE, since they do not seem to be expressed in any of the patients earlier steps of reflux disease. Moreover, CK7/20 in spite of increased expression in BE than in normal epithelium and esophagitis, do not seem to identify those patients who will develop BE. Therefore, on the basis of this preliminary experience, this panel of immunohystochemical markers, seems certainly useful for BE identification but not to predict its occurrence.

Conflicts of interest

The authors declare no conflicts of interest.

References

1. Wang, K.K. & R.E. Sampliner. 2008. Practice Parameters Committee of the American College of Gastroenterology. Updated guidelines 2008 for the diagnosis, surveillance and therapy of Barrett's oesophagus. *Am. J. Gastroenterol.* **103:** 788–797.
2. Barr, H. & N.A. Shepherd. The management of dysplasia. Guidelines for the diagnosis and management of Barrett's columnar-lined oesophagus: a report of the working Party of the British Society of Gastroenterology August 2005. Available at: http://www.bsg.org.uk.
3. Liu, W., H. Hejin Hahn, R.D. Odze & R.K. Goyal. 2009. Metaplastic esophageal columnar epithelium without goblet cells shows DNA content abnormalities similar to goblet cell containing epithelium. *Am. J. Gastroenterol.* **104:** 816–824.
4. Kelty, C., M. Gough & Q. Van Wyk. 2007. Barrett's oesophagus: intestinal metaplasia is not essential for cancer risk. *Scand. J. Gastroenterol.* **42:** 1271–1274.
5. Gatenby, P.A., J.R. Ramus, C.P. Caygill, *et al.* 2008. Relevance of the detection of intestinal metaplasia in non-dysplastic columnar-lined oesophagus. *Scan. J. Gastroenterol.* **43:** 524–530.
6. Takubo, K., K. Sasa, K. Yamashita, *et al.* 1991. Double muscularis mucosae in Barrett esophagus. *Hum. Pathol.* **22:** 1158–1161.
7. Srivastava, A., R.D. Odze, G.Y. Lauwers, *et al.* 2007. Morphologic features are useful in distinguishing Barrett esophagus from carditis with intestinal metaplasia. *Am. J. Surg. Pathol.* **31:** 1733–1741.
8. Ormsby, A.H., J.R. Goldblum, T.W. Rice, *et al.* 1999. Cytokeratin subsets can reliably distinguish Barrett's esophagus from intestinal metaplasia of the stomach. *Hum. Pathol.* **30:** 288–294.
9. Nurgalieva, Z., A. Lowrey & H.B. El-Serag. 2007. The use of cytokeratin stain to distinguish Barrett's esophagus from contiguous tissues: a systematic review. *Dig. Dis. Sci.* **52:** 1345–1354.
10. Odze, R.D. 2005. Unraveling the mystery of the gastroesophageal junction: a pathologist's perspective. *Am. J. Gastroenterol.* **100:** 1853–1867.

11. Su, Y., X. Chen, M. Klein, *et al.* 2004. Phenotype of columnar-lined esophagus in rats with esophagogastroduodenal anastomosis: similarity to human Barrett's esophagus. *Lab. Invest.* **84:** 753–765.

12. Orlando, R.C. 2006. Mucosal defense in Barrett's esophagus. In *Barrett's Esophagus and Esophageal Adenocarcinoma.* Sharma P. and Sampliner R., pp 60-72. Ed. Blackwell Publishing. Malden.

13. Long, J.D. & R.C. Orlando. 1999. Esophageal submucosal glands: structure and function. *Am. J. Gastroenterol.* **94:** 2818–2824.

14. Li, H., T.N. Walsh, G. O'dowd, *et al.* 1994. Mechanisms of columnar metaplasia and squamous regeneration in experimental Barrett's esophagus. *Surgery* **115:** 176–181.

15. Gillen, P., P. Keeling, P.J. Byrne, *et al.* 1988. Implication of duodenogastric reflux in the pathogenesis of Barrett's oesophagus. *Br. J. Surg.* **75:** 540–543.

16. Vakil, N., S.V. van Zanten, P. Kahrilas, *et al.*; the Global Consensus Group. 2006. The Montreal definition and classification of gastroesophageal reflux disease: a global evidence-based consensus. *Am. J. Gastroenterol.* **101:** 1900–1920.

17. Sharma, P., J. Dent, D. Armstrong, *et al.* 2006. The development and validation of an endoscopic grading system for Barrett's esophagus: the Prague C and M criteria. *Gastroenterology* **131:** 1392–1399.

18. Amano, Y., N. Ishimura, K. Furuta, *et al.* 2006. Which landmark results in a more consistent diagnosis of Barrett's esophagus, the gastric folds or the palisade vessels? *Gastrointest. Endosc.* **64:** 206–211.

19. Riddell, R.H., V. Mann, P. Moayyedi, *et al.* 2006. Targeted esophageal biopsies: what you see is what you get (WYSIWYG)—or not? *Gastroenterology* **130:** A161 (Abstract S1139).

20. De Hertogh, G., P. Van Eyken, N. Ectors, *et al.* 2003. On the existence and location of cardiac mucosa: an autopsy study in embryos, fetuses, and infants. *Gut* **52:** 791–762.

21. Chandrasoma, P. 2005. Controversies of the cardiac mucosa and Barrett's oesophagus. *Histopathology* **46:** 361–73.

22. Peitz, U., M. Vieth, M. Pross, *et al.* 2004. Cardia-type metaplasia arising in the remnant esophagus after cardia resection. *Gastrointest. Endosc.* **59:** 810–817.

23. Hattori, T., K. Mukaisho & K. Miwa. 2005. Pathogenesis of Barrett's esophagus—new findings in the experimental studies of duodenal reflux models. *Nippon Rinsho.* **63:** 1341–1349.

24. Vieth, M. & H. Barr. 2009. Defining a bad Barrett's segment: is it dependent on goblet cells? *Am. J. Gastroenterol.* **104:** 825–874.

25. Liu, W., H. Hahn, R.D. Odze & R.K. Goyal. 2009. Metaplastic esophageal columnar epithelium without goblet cells shows DNA content abnormalities similar to goblet cell-containing epithelium. *Am. J. Gastroenterol.* **104:** 816–824.

26. Stein, H.J., M. Feith & H. Feussner. 2000. The relationship between gastroesophageal reflux, intestinal metaplasia and adenocarcinoma of the esophagus. *Langenbeck's Arch. Surg.* **385:** 309–316.

27. Siewert, J.R., M. Feith, M. Werner & H. Stein. 2000. Adenocarcinoma of the esophagogastric junction: results of surgical therapy based on anantomical/topographic classification in 1,002 consecutive patients. *Ann. Surg.* **232:** 353–361.

28. Gangarosa, L., S. Halter & H. Mertz. 1999. Dysplastic gastroesophageal junction nodules—a precursor to junctional adenocarcinoma. *Am. J. Gastroenterol.* **94:** 835–838.

29. Tytgat, G.N.J., J.W. van Sandick, J.J.B. van Lanschot & H. Obertop. 2003. Role of Surveillance in Intestinal Metaplasia of the Esophagus and Gastroesophageal Junction. *World J. Surg* **27:** 1021–1025.

30. Das, K.M., I. Prasad, S. Garla & P.S. Amenta. 1994. Detection of a shared colon epithelial epitope on Barrett epithelium by a novel monoclonal antibody. *Ann. Intern. Med.* **120:** 753–756.

31. Mirza, Z.K., K.K. Das, R.N. Mapitigama, *et al.* 2003. Gastric intestinal metaplasia as detected by a novel biomarker is highly associated with gastric adenocarcinoma. *Gut* **52:** 807–812.

32. Das, K.M., S. Sakamaki, M. Vecchi & B. Diamond. 1987. The production and characterization of monoclonal antibodies to a human colonic antigen associated with ulcerative colitis: cellular localization of the antigen using the monoclonal antibody. *J. Immunol.* **139:** 77–84.

33. Onuma, E.K., P.S. Amenta, A.F. Jukkola, *et al.* 2001. A phenotypic change of small intestinal epithelium to colonocytes in small intestinal adenomas and adenocarcinomas. *Am. J. Gastroenterol.* **96:** 2480–2485.

34. Glickman, J.N., H. Wang, K.M. Das, *et al.* 2001. Phenotype of Barrett's esophagus and intestinal metaplasia of the distal esophagus and gastroesophageal junction: an immunohistochemical study of cytokeratins 7 and 20, Das-1 and 45 MI. *Am. J. Surg. Pathol.* **25:** 87–94.

35. Fisher, R.S., M.Q. Bromer, R.M. Thomas, *et al.* 2003. Predictors of recurrent specialized intestinal metaplasia after complete laser ablation. *Am. J. Gastroenterol.* **98:** 1945–1951.

36. Bajpai, M., J. Liu, X. Geng, *et al.* 2008. Repeated exposure to acid and bile selectively induces colonic phenotype expression in a heterogeneous Barrett's epithelial cell line. *Lab. Invest.* **88:** 643–651.

37. Das, K.M., Y. Kong, M. Bajpai, *et al.* 2011. Transformation of benign Barrett's epithelium by repeated acid and bile exposure over 65 weeks: a novel in-vitro model. *Int. J. Cancer* **128:** 274–282.

38. Weinstein, W.M. & A.F. Ippoliti. 1996. The diagnosis of Barrett's esophagus: goblets, goblets, goblets. *Gastrointest. Endosc.* **44:** 91–95.

39. Offner, F.A., K.J. Lewin & W.M. Weinstein. 1996. Metaplastic columnar cells in Barrett's esophagus: a common and neglected cell type. *Hum. Pathol.* **27:** 885–889.

40. Chen, Y-Y, H. Wang, D.A. Antonioli, *et al.* 1999. Significance of acid-mucin-positive on goblet columnar cells in the distal esophagus and gastroesophageal junction. *Hum. Pathol.* **30:** 1488–1495.

41. Younes, M., A. Ertan, G. Ergun, *et al.* Goblet cell mimickers in esophageal biopsies are not associated with an increased risk for dysplasia. *Arch. Pathol. Lab. Med.* **131:** 571–575.

42. Paull, A., J.S. Trier, M.C. Dalton, *et al.* 1976. The histologic spectrum of Barrett's esophagus. *N. Engl. J. Med.* **295:** 476–480.

43. Takubo, K., J. Aida, Y. Naomoto, *et al.* 2009. Cardiac rather than intestinal-type bacgkground in endoscopic resection specimens of minute Barrett adenocarcinoma. *Hum. Pathol.* **40:** 65–74.

44. Hahn, H.P., P.L. Blount, K. Ayub, *et al.* 2009. Intestinal differentiation in metaplastic, non-goblet columnar epithelium in the oesophagus. *Am. J. Surg. Pathol.* **33:** 1006–1015.

45. Going, J.J., A.J. Fletcher-Monaghan, L. Neilson, *et al.* 2004. Zoning of mucosal phenotype, dysplasia and telomerase measured by telomerase repeat assay protocol (TRAP) in Barrett's esophagus. *Neoplasia* **6:** 85–92.

46. Abela, Jo-Etienne, James J. Going, John F. Mackenzie, *et al.* 2008. Systematic four-quadrant biopsy detects Barrett's dysplasia in more patients than nonsystematic biopsy. *Am. J. Gastroenterol.* **103:** 850–855.

47. Endo, T., K. Tamaki, Y. Arimura, *et al.* 1998. Expression of sulfated carbohydrate chain and core peptides of mucin detected by monoclonal antibodies in Barrett's esophagus and esophageal adenocarcinoma. *J. Gastroenterol.* **33:** 811–815.

48. Chu, P.G., Z. Jiang & L.M. Weiss. 2003. Hepatocyte antigen as a marker of intestinal metaplasia. *Am. J. Surg. Pathol.* **27:** 952–959.

49. Kumble, S., M.B. Omary, L.F. Fajardo & G. Triadafilopoulos. 1996. Multifocal heterogeneity in villin and Ep-CAM expression in Barrett's esophagus. *Int. J. Cancer* **28:** 48–54.

50. Glickman, J.N., H. Wang, K.M. Das, *et al.* 2001. Phenotype of Barrett's esophagus and intestinal metaplasia of the distal esophagus and gastroesophageal junction: an immunohistochemical study of cytokeratins 7 and 20, Das-1 and 45 MI. *Am. J. Surg. Pathol.* **25:** 87–94.

51. Eda, A., H. Osawa, K. Satoh, *et al.* 2003. Aberrant expression of CDX2 in Barrett's epithelium and inflammatory esophageal mucosa. *J. Gastroenterol.* **38:** 14–22.

52. Kerkhof, M., D.A. Bax, L.M. Moons, *et al.* 2006. Does CDX2 expression predict Barrett's metaplasia in oesophageal columnar epithelium without goblet cells? *Aliment Pharmacol. Ther.* **24:** 1613–1621.

53. Souza, R.F., K. Krishnan & J.S. Spechler, 2008. Acid, Bile, and CDX: the ABCs of making Barrett's metaplasia. *Am. J. Physiol. Gastrointest. Liver Physiol.* **295:** 211–218.

54. Gulmann, C., O.L. Shaqaqi, A. Grace, *et al.* 2004. Cytokeratin 7/20 and MUC1, 2, 5AC, and 6 expression patterns in Barrett's esophagus and intestinal metaplasia of the stomach. *Appl. Immunohistochem. Mol. Morphol.* **12:** 142–147.

55. Ormsby, A.H., J.R. Goldblum & T.W. Rice. 1999. Citokeratyn subset can reliably distinguish Barrett's esophagus from Intestinal Metaplasia of the stomach. *Hum. Pathol.* **30:** 288–294.

56. Couvelard, A., J.M. Cauvin, D. Goldfain, *et al.* 2001. Cytokeratin immunoreactivity of intestinal metaplasia at normal oesophagogastric junction indicates its aetiology. *Gut* **49:** 761–766.

57. Steininger, H., D.A. Pfofe, H. Müller, *et al.* 2005. Expression of CDX2 and MUC2 in Barrett's mucosa. *Pathol. Res. Pract.* **201:** 573–577.

Ann. N.Y. Acad. Sci. ISSN 0077-8923

ANNALS OF THE NEW YORK ACADEMY OF SCIENCES
Issue: *Barrett's Esophagus: The 10th OESO World Congress Proceedings*

Barrett's esophagus: proton pump inhibitors and chemoprevention I

George Triadafilopoulos,[1] Antonio Taddei,[2] Paolo Bechi,[2] Giancarlo Freschi,[2] Maria Novella Ringressi,[2] Duccio Rossi Degli'Innocenti,[2] Francesca Castiglione,[2] Emmanuella Masini,[4] Marek Majewski,[5] Grzegorz Wallner,[5] Jerzy Sarosiek,[6] John F. Dillon,[7] Richard C. McCallum,[7] Katerina Dvorak,[8] Aaron Goldman,[8] Philip Woodland,[9] Daniel Sifrim,[9] Joel E. Richter,[10] Michael Vieth,[11] Helmut Neumann,[12] Cord Langner,[13] Norihisa Ishimura,[14] Yuji Amano,[15] and Valter Nilton Felix[16]

[1]Division of Gastroenterology and Hepatology, Stanford University School of Medicine, Stanford, California. [2]Department of Medical and Surgical Critical Care, Unit of Surgery, University of Florence, Florence, Italy. [3]Department of Medical and Surgical Critical Care, Unit of Human Pathology, University of Florence, Florence, Italy. [4]Department of Pharmacology, University of Florence, Florence, Italy. [5]Medical University of Lublin, 2nd Department of General Surgery, Lublin, Poland. [6]TTUHSC, Paul L. Foster School of Medicine, Department of Medicine, El Paso, Texas. [7]Biomedical Research Institute, University of Dundee, Ninewells Hospital and Medical School Dundee, United Kingdom. [8]Department of Cell Biology and Anatomy, College of Medicine and Arizona Cancer Center, University of Arizona, Tucson, Arizona. [9]Barts and the London School of Medicine and Dentistry, Queen Mary University of London, United Kingdom. [10]Department of Medicine, Temple University, Philadelphia, Pennsylvania. [11]Institute of Pathology, Klinikum Bayreuth, Bayreuth, Germany. [12]Medical Clinic I, University of Erlangen, Erlangen, Germany. [13]Institute of Pathology, Medical University Graz, Graz, Austria. [14]Department of Gastroenterology, Shimane University Hospital, Shimane, Japan. [15]Division of Gastrointestinal Endoscopy, Shimane University Hospital, Shimane, Japan. [16]Department of Gastroenterology, Surgical Division, São Paulo University, São Paulo, Brazil

The following on proton pump inhibitors and chemoprevention in Barrett's esophagus includes commentaries on normalization of esophageal refluxate; the effects of 5-HT$_4$ agonists on EGF secretion and of lubripristone on chloride channels agents; the role of Campylobacter toxin production; the deleterious effects of unconjugated bile acids; the role of baclofen in nonacid reflux; the threshold for adequate esophageal acid exposure; the effects of proton pump inhibitor (PPI) therapy on normalization of esophageal pH and on cell proliferation; the role of the phenotype of cellular proliferation on the effects of PPI therapy; and the value of Symptom Index and Symptom Association Probability in the evaluation of potential response to treatment.

Keywords: Barrett's treatment; omeprazole; duodenogastroesophageal reflux; dysplasia; Symptom Sensitivity Index; Symptom Association Probability; antireflux surgery; PPI; mucin phenotype; pH control; esomeprazole; basal cell layer; hyperplasia; stromal papillae; GABA$_B$ baclofen; lesogaberan; weakly acidic reflux; TLESR; Campylobacter; microbiota; prostone; 5-HT$_4$; TGF-α; GERD; EGF; mucosal protection; CDX2; Barrett's cell lines

Concise summaries

- *In vitro* data in cultured cells suggest that acid and bile exposure is important in Barrett's carcinogenesis. Normalization of esophageal acid exposure—albeit not formally proven in RCT studies—should be beneficial in preventing metaplasia in gastroesophageal reflux disease

(GERD) patients and potentially diminish the likelihood of neoplastic progression.

- Esophageal preepithelial mucosal defense mechanisms in patients with BE are significantly impaired, potentially predisposing metaplastic epithelium to further injury, chronic inflammation and progression to esophageal adenocarcinoma.

doi: 10.1111/j.1749-6632.2011.06047.x

- 5-HT_4 receptor expression significantly increases from the controls to GERD and to BE patients. 5-HT_4 could play a role, involving both EGF and COX-2 pathways, determining PGE2 secretion increase and, consequently, proliferative activity increase, and 5-HT_4 selective antagonists could be the future of GERD therapy and BE chemoprevention.
- The impact of chloride channel stimulators on secretion of protective factors in disease of the esophageal mucosa, especially in patients with Barrett's esophagus (BE) with and without low/high-grade dysplasia (LGD/HGD), remains to be explored.
- Acid suppression therapy with proton pump inhibitors (PPIs) may lead to the bacterial overgrowth and increased reflux of toxic, unconjugated bile acids. This may result in increased cell DNA damage, mutations, and consequently to BE and EAC development. However, the current knowledge about esophageal colonization with Campylobacter species does not justify eradication with antibiotics.
- Most groups currently define adequate acid control in GERD patients as values below normal thresholds for healthy controls, usually a total acid exposure time of less than 4.5–5.5%.
- In patients in whom ongoing symptoms are related to nonacidic reflux events, the reduc-

tion of TLESR frequency $GABA_B$-receptor agonists is a potentially beneficial therapeutic strategy. Baclofen is a reasonable therapeutic add-on in patients under PPIs with persistent symptoms due to nonacid reflux.
- The epithelium of patients with continuous acid exposure is believed to only partially benefit from PPI therapy, whereas the epithelium of patients with pulse acid exposure, leading to more pronounced epithelial changes, might have a greater potential to be positively influenced/cured by PPI therapy.
- For an antisecretory treatment aimed at chemoprevention to be effective, higher PPI dosing, confirmed by pH monitoring, is necessary. PPIs suppress cellular proliferation in BE with the gastric-predominant mucin phenotype, but not in that with the intestinal-predominant mucin phenotype. This finding may partly explain the ongoing controversy effects of acid-suppressive therapy in Barrett's patients.
- Great caution is recommended when using Symptom Sensitivity Index and Symptom Association Probability results to predict a response to PPIs in individual patients, especially in those without classic heartburn or regurgitation.
- There is no significant association between esophageal adenocarcinoma and the use of antisecretory agents *per se.*

---

1. Should the esophageal refluxate be normalized in BE? *In vitro* studies to answer this question

George Triadafilopoulos
vagt@stanford.edu

Two retrospective studies have suggested that controlling esophageal pH may decrease the chances to develop dysplasia. In a VA study, El Serag *et al.*[1] compared the development of dysplasia in patients with BE treated with or without PPI or histamine 2-receptor antagonist (H2RA) over a 20-year time period. They found that the cumulative incidence of dysplasia was significantly lower among patients

who received PPI after BE diagnosis than in those who received no therapy or H2RA. Furthermore, among those on PPIs, a longer duration of use was associated with less frequent occurrence of dysplasia. In the second study,[2] Hillman *et al.* examined whether PPI therapy influences the incidence and progression of dysplasia in patients with BE. They found that ongoing PPI therapy appeared beneficial in the prevention of dysplasia and adenocarcinoma in patients with BE and suggested that all patients with this condition, even those with no esophagitis or symptoms, should be encouraged to continue long term PPI therapy.

Hence, control of the esophageal acid (and bile) exposure by mechanical and pharmacologic means

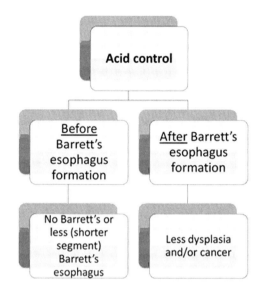

Figure 1. Outline of two scenarios that relate acid control and Barrett's pathogenesis and natural history. Originally published in Ref. 3.

seems quite important in the pathogenesis and natural history of BE. Figure 1 highlights two possible scenarios:[3]

(i) Under the first scenario, acid control before the development of BE may either abort the formation of metaplasia or be associated with shorter segment metaplasia.

(ii) Under the second scenario that occurs after the formation of metaplasia, effective acid control could lead to less dysplasia and cancer, a chemoprevention effect.

Several recent *in vitro* studies have explored the role of the refluxate, such as acid and bile, in affecting BE formation and inducing alterations in the Barrett's cells that would, in turn, favor malignant transformation, but, for brevity, only two recent ones are highlighted herein.

Under the first scenario, Huo *et al.* hypothesized that differences among individuals in molecular pathways activated when esophageal squamous epithelium is exposed to reflux underlie the development of Barrett's metaplasia.[4] They used esophageal squamous cell lines from patients who had GERD with BE and without BE to study the effects of acid and bile salts on expression of the CDX2 gene. They found that both acid and bile salts increased CDX2 messenger RNA (mRNA), protein, and promoter activity in NES-B3T and NES-B10T cells, but not in

NES-G2T or NES-G4T cells. They also found CDX2 mRNA in 7 of 10 esophageal squamous biopsy specimens from patients with BE, but in only 1 of 10 such specimens from patients who had GERD without BE. Since acid and bile salts induce CDX2 mRNA and protein expression in esophageal squamous cells from patients with BE, but not from GERD patients without BE, they speculated that these differences in acid- and bile salt-induced activation of molecular pathways may underlie the development of Barrett's metaplasia.

Hong *et al.* examined whether acid increases methylation of p16 gene promoter and whether NADPH oxidase NOX5-S mediates acid-induced p16 hypermethylation in a Barrett's cell line BAR-T and an EA cell line OE33.[5] Inactivation of the tumor suppressor gene p16 may be important in the malignant transformation of BE. Hypermethylation of p16 gene promoter is an important mechanism inactivating p16. They found that NOX5-S was present in BAR-T and OE33 cells and that acid-induced increase in H_2O_2 production and cell proliferation was significantly reduced by knockdown of NOX5-S (Fig. 2). Exogenous H_2O_2 remarkably increased p16 promoter methylation and cell proliferation. In addition, acid treatment significantly increased p16 promoter methylation and decreased p16 mRNA level. Knockdown of NOX5-S significantly increased p16 mRNA, inhibited acid-induced downregulation of p16 mRNA, and blocked acid-induced increase in p16 methylation and cell proliferation. Conversely, overexpression of NOX5-S significantly decreased p16 mRNA and increased p16 methylation and cell proliferation. The authors postulated that acid reflux may activate NOX5-S and increase production of reactive oxygen species, which, in turn, increase p16 promoter methylation, downregulate p16

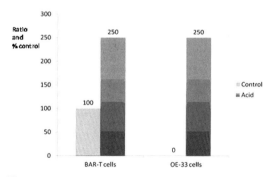

Figure 2. Acid increases methylation levels of p16 gene promoter in BAR-T cells and OE33 cells *in vitro*.

expression, and increase cell proliferation, thereby contributing to malignant progression.

In conclusion, recent *in vitro* data in cultured cells suggest that acid (and bile) exposure is important in Barrett's carcinogenesis. Normalization of esophageal acid exposure—albeit not formally proven in RCT studies—should be beneficial in preventing metaplasia in GERD patients and potentially diminish the likelihood of neoplastic progression of BE.

2. Are esophageal mucosal defense mechanisms different in BE?

Richard W. McCallum and Jerzy Sarosiek
Jerzy.sarosiek@ttuhsc.edu

GERD is defined as the presence of chronic symptoms, predominantly including heartburn/regurgitation with or without mucosal damage produced by an abnormal reflux, i.e., retrograde flow of gastric or mixed duodeno-gastric content into the esophagus and/or mouth. Considering the fact that gastroesophageal refluxate (GER) contains a range of injurious agents, from acid accompanied by seven to eight pepsins and to bile acids mixed with acid/pepsins and pancreatic enzymes, esophageal mucosa has to have in place a plethora of protective factors counteracting these aggressive components, thus preventing injury to the squamous epithelium. Among the esophageal preepithelial protective factors elaborated by salivary or esophageal submucosal mucous glands, buffers and mucins are the leaders, followed by epidermal growth factor (EGF) and transforming growth factor-α (TGF-α), representing a vanguard of mucosal protection in health and disease.[6]

The concept of the role of mucosal protection in health and disease

If protective mechanisms are inadequate or overwhelmed qualitatively or quantitatively by an excessive injurious refluxate, mucosal injury and subsequent repair will take place, thus setting the stage for acute/chronic inflammation.[7,8] It is squamous epithelial repair, in an environment of unabated reflux and dropping pH within the mucosa, that leads highly proliferating mucosal stem cells to replace injured cells, to turn on mucosal differentiation into columnar epithelium, called BE, which is better equipped to cope with the luminal content

of gastroduodenal injurious components.[7] Within 24 h, the composition of GER varies profoundly, from highly and predominantly acidic, especially during the after midnight hours, to highly contaminated with duodeno-gastric reflux during, and shortly after, ingestion of various meals at day time. This continuous variation in the composition of injurious components within GER sets the stage for the final phenotype of Barrett's mucosal cells as incomplete intestinal metaplasia (the mixture of gastric and intestinal cells with some even expressing goblet cell morphology) that is still a subject of injury/repair, as this columnar epithelium exhibits still inadequate mucosal protection.[6–8] This is why highly injurious and proinflammatory stimuli maintain chronic inflammation resulting, in some patients, in the development of complications such as LGD, HGD, and ultimately esophageal adenocarcinoma (AdCa).[6–8]

Although pathophysiology of GERD/BE includes pan-esophageal motility disorder, including defective lower esophageal sphincter (LES), excessive transient LES relaxation (TLESR), and impaired primary and/or secondary esophageal peristalsis and clearance, it is the degree of imbalance between aggressive factors and protective mechanisms that will define absence or presence its final outcome, esophageal adenocarcinoma.[6–8] Setting the stage for potential development of BE, patients with reflux esophagitis have significant impairment in esophageal mucin secretion, as well as esophageal and salivary EGF, which persist even after healing of erosive changes, indicating that this preexisting condition facilitates the development of mucosal injury.[6] Furthermore, esophageal EGF secretion also remains impaired in patients with BE.[9]

Although therapy with PPIs improves the equilibrium between aggressive factors and protective mechanisms by diminishing acidity of GER, some PPIs, such as rabeprazole, may also increase esophageal secretion of protective mucin after healing of erosive mucosal changes.[10] Administration of the serotonin receptor (5-HT$_4$) agonist tegaserod, and potentially other newer agents free of cardiac side effects, results in significant increase in salivary bicarbonate and nonbicarbonate buffers, EGF, and TGF-α, as well as esophageal EGF,[6] promoting further potential restoration of equilibrium. This enhancement of equilibrium can be also promoted further by mastication or chewing sugarless

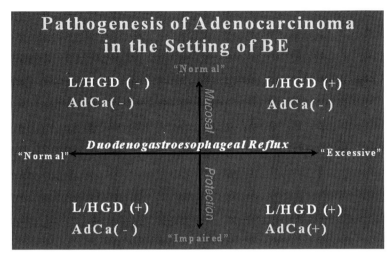

Figure 3. The relationship between disequilibrium between aggressive factors and protective mechanisms in the development of L/HGD and esophageal adenocarcinoma in patients with BE.

chewing gum, which leads to a two- to four-fold increase in salivary buffers, mucin, EGF, and TGF-α.[8] Obviously, administration of GABA$_B$ receptor agonists (baclofen and the newest agents tested in clinical trials) help to prevent GER through inhibition of TLES relaxation.[7] Perhaps in some patients with BE who still exhibit significant GER in spite of BID doses of PPIs, addition of sugarless chewing gum- and/or GABA$_B$ receptor antagonists or 5-HT$_4$ receptor agonist could lead to restoration of equilibrium, thus diminishing profoundly subsequent complications such as LGD, HGD, and adenocarcinoma. This, however, requires confirmation in randomized, placebo-controlled, double-blind clinical trials.

Theoretically, fundoplication, if perfectly performed, should have the greatest potential of inhibition of not only reflux of the acid/pepsins component of GER but also its duodeno-gastric mixture.[7] Its adenocarcinoma preventive potential in patients with BE still remains to be demonstrated. Our illustration (Fig. 3) may help to outline the role of equilibrium between aggressive factors within duodeno-GER and protective factors within salivary and esophageal secretions in maintaining the integrity within the BE mucosa and prevention of the development of esophageal AdCa.

If pharmacological or surgical therapy normalizes the quality and the quantity of duodeno-gastroesophageal reflux and mucosal protective factors remain normal, LGD/HGD should not develop (left upper panel); however, if mucosal protection still remains low (left lower panel), L/HGD may develop but could remain nonprogressive. If pharmacological or surgical therapy diminishes but does not normalize the quality and the quantity of DGER and mucosal protection remains strong or normal, L/GHD could still develop without progression to AdCa (right upper panel); however, if mucosal protection also remains impaired (right lower panel), L/HGD may inevitably develop and exhibit progression to AdCa.

Conclusion

Esophageal preepithelial mucosal defense mechanisms in patients with BE are significantly impaired, potentially predisposing metaplastic epithelium to further injury, chronic inflammation, and progression, through LGD and HGD, to esophageal adenocarcinoma.

3. What is the effect of 5-HT$_4$ agonists on esophageal EGF secretion in patients with GERD and BE?

Antonio Taddei, Paolo Bechi, Giancarlo Freschi, Maria Novella Ringressi, Duccio Rossi Degli'Innocenti, Francesca Castiglione, and Emmanuella Masini
antonio.taddei@unifi.it

Serotonin (5-HT) was discovered in intestinal cells by an Italian researcher, Vittorio Erspamer, in the early 30s. Since then both agonists and antagonists drugs towards 5-HT receptors have been particularly used for gastrointestinal motility disorders, such as constipation, irritable bowel syndrome, nausea, and vomiting.[11,12] There are many 5-HT receptors subtypes and some of them play a mitogenic role throughout their activation.[13] So far, there is no evidence concerning the role of 5-HT$_4$ receptors in GERD and BE patients. It is well known that EGF is very important in the regulation of the tissue integrity and its receptors seem to play a role in cell proliferation as well as in oncogenesis of the gastrointestinal tract.[14] Moreover, these receptors are present throughout all the intestine and are significantly increased in GERD.[15]

Preliminary experience

This preliminary study includes 22 patients, divided in to three groups: controls, GERD, and BE patients. Esophageal samples were taken from each patient and cells were isolated and studied in order to evaluate cell proliferation, Western blotting, and secretion analysis.

5-HT$_4$ receptor expression, although present in all the patients, significantly increases from controls to GERD patients and then to BE patients.

Our preliminary data show that proliferation, evaluated by means of tritiated thymidine incorporation, significantly increases from basal levels in each of the three studied groups after incubation with 5-HT. This effect is more evident after cell preincubation with 5-HT agonists, such as Cisapride, a partial agonist for both 5-HT$_3$ and 5-HT$_4$ receptors, and CJ033466, which is a selective 5-HT$_4$

receptor agonist. On the contrary, preincubation with a selective HT$_4$ antagonist reverses proliferative activity to basal levels.

EGF expression and secretion was also studied, and our findings show that EGF expression increases from controls to BE patients. These data are confirmed by the analysis of the secretion in basal conditions in the three groups. Incubation with Cisapride or selective HT$_4$ agonists significantly increases EGF secretion, and the selective antagonist reduces it to basal levels (Fig. 4). In addition to 5-HT$_4$ receptors, EGF has the same effect on proliferative activity evaluated by means of thymidine incorporation in the three groups. Preincubation with EGF significantly increases proliferative activity in the three groups, on the contrary, preincubation with a selective COX-2 inhibitor, such as Celecoxib, reduces proliferative activity to basal level. Finally, our data show that 5-HT agonists and, mostly, selective HT$_4$ agonists increase PGE2 secretion. Conversely PGE2 is decreased by the selective 5-HT$_4$ antagonist that, therefore, determines the COX-2 activity increase.

In conclusion, in GERD and BE patients, 5-HT$_4$ could play a role that involves both EGF and COX-2 pathways, both determining PGE2 secretion increase, and consequently proliferative activity increase. Our preliminary data suggest that the 5-HT$_4$ receptor involvement may be very important, at an early stage of GERD multistep process, inducing cell proliferation by means of EGF and/or COX-2 increased activity. Therefore, 5-HT$_4$ selective antagonists could be the future of GERD therapy and

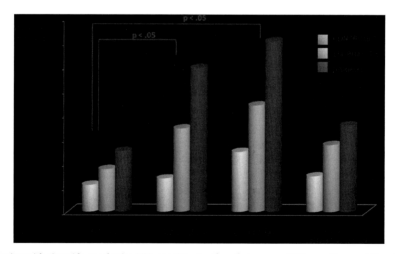

Figure 4. Incubation with cisapride or selective HT$_4$ agonists significantly increases EGF secretion, and the selective antagonist reduces it to basal levels.

BE chemoprevention, but further both experimental and clinical studies in order to support this hypothesis are needed.

4. What is the effect of lubiprostone on chloride channel-2 (ClC-2) driven secretion of protective components of mucus in the human esophagus?

Marek Majewski, Grzegorz Wallner, and Jerzy Sarosiek
Jerzy.sarosiek@ttuhsc.edu

The alimentary tract mucosa is covered by a viscoelastic, approximately 200 micron thick, mucus–buffer layer. The primary role for this layer is to protect the delicate surface epithelium from various chemical and physical aggressive factors and forces, either elaborated endogenously or from exogenous food components, providing also lubrication facilitating propagation and propulsion of nondigestible food solids. There is a close interrelationship between the rate of mucus release from the gastrointestinal mucous cells or from submucosal mucous glands within the esophageal mucosa, and the rate of chloride secretion, setting the optimal conditions for hydration of mucus and formation of its viscoelastic gel layer. Chloride channels type 2 (ClC-2) are widely distributed in tissues through the body and are expressed in many epithelia, especially within the alimentary tract. Lubiprostone, a member of a group of compounds called prostones, within the family of prostanoids, is a locally acting chloride ClC-2 channel activator that enhances a chloride-rich fluid secretion, subsequently resulting in an increase of the alimentary tract secretion, including mucus, driven by stimulation of chloride sodium, thus accelerating transit and alleviating symptoms associated with chronic constipation regardless its etiology. It has been clearly demonstrated that the human esophageal mucosal secretory response is closely related to its luminal exposure to acid and pepsin, thus setting the stage for its role in esophageal mucosal protection during gastroesophageal reflux. This secretory response is augmented by serotonin receptor 5-HT$_4$ agonist. Therefore, administration of lubiprostone may result in increase of secretion of other protective factors within the mucus-buffer layer such as prostaglandins, EGF, transforming growth factor α (TGF-α), thus enhancing the esophagel preepithe-

lial defence mechanisms. Hypothetically, by promoting the quantity and the quality of the mucus barrier along the alimentary tract, lubiprostone could also be of value in mucosal protection during administration of nonsteroidal–antiinflammatory drugs (NSAIDs), well known for their ulcerogenic potential both within the upper and the lower alimentary tract, mediated by an impairment of COX-1-generated prostaglandins and subsequent depletion in mucus production, thus increasing the risk of complications.

The integrity of the alimentary tract mucosa depends upon equilibrium between aggressive factors and defense mechanisms.[16] Since aggressive factors within the alimentary tract always act on the luminal side of the mucosa, preepithelial defense, defined as the mucus-buffers layer with its inherent pH gradient, represents the vanguard of mucosal defense.[17] Mucin, also called mucus glycoprotein, generates the architectural framework or scaffold within the mucus layer supporting contribution of other protective components, including hydrophobic phospholipids and buffers to its ultimate defensive potential.[16,17] Therefore, the rate of synthesis and secretion of mucin is pivotal for the thickness of the mucus-buffers layer and its ability to inhibit hydrogen ion back-diffusion and maintain a pH gradient, from acidic on its luminal perimeter to near neutral at mucus–epithelial cell membrane inter phase.[18] Administration of a conventional NSAID, leading to the development of peptic ulcer disease (PUD), or inducing symptoms of nonulcer dyspepsia (NUD) or chronic constipation, results both in decreased generation of gastroprotective prostaglandins generated by COX-1 and diminished production of gastric mucin.[19]

We have recently demonstrated, in a double-blind, placebo-controlled study protocol where administration conventional NSAID, naproxen, 500 mg bid, resulted in a significant decline of gastric mucus production by 44% ($P < 0.001$) in basal conditions and by 35% ($P < 0.001$) in pentagastrin-stimulated conditions, mimicking the food-stimulated scenario.[19] Furthermore, the rate of secretion of gastric mucin, the major component of mucus, during naproxen administration, declined by 39% in basal conditions ($P < 0.01$) and by 49% in pentagastrin-stimulated conditions ($P < 0.005$).[19] Of note, administration of rabeprazole, one of the most effective PPIs, resulted in significant restorative capacity on naproxen-induced decline of mucus secretion bringing it rate of secretion almost to prenaproxen levels.[19] This decline of mucus and mucin production during administration of naproxen may at least partly explain the propensity of patients receiving NSAIDs for the development of alimentary tract symptoms and complications.

An interrelationship exists in the esophageal mucosa between secretion of mucin and other protective mucus components and chloride through ClC-2 within the alimentary tract.

It is hard to overestimate the value of adequate chloride secretion into the alimentary tract lumen, which is pivotal in regulating optimal rate of hydration of the luminal content, securing adequate fluidity, and promoting its adequate propulsion along the alimentary tract.[20,21] Furthermore, chloride secretion is instrumental in secretion and hydration of gastric mucus and its ability to form gel-like, viscous physical property, instrumental in mucosal protection and lubrication. Recently, a novel agent, the chloride channel activator lubiprostone, has been introduced into our clinical armamentarium, targeting an important pathogenetic link leading to chronic constipation.[20,21] The stimulatory impact of lubiprostone on mucus and mucin production and its viscous, gel-like forming property in asymptomatic volunteers and patients with chronic constipation has recently been explored (unpublished data).

Future implications

The impact of chloride channel stimulators, especially from the family of prostanoids, as well as from the group of prostones on secretion of protective factors such as sodium bicarbonate, mucin, EGF, and TGF-α from salivary and esophageal submucosal mucous glands in the health and disease of the esophageal mucosa, especially in patients with BE with and without LGD/HGD, remains to be explored.

5. In view of the high levels of toxin-producing Campylobacter species found in Barrett's patients, should prophylactic use of antibiotics be considered?

John F. Dillon and Katie Blackett
j.f.dillon@dundee.ac.uk

BE is a premalignant state leading to adenocarcinoma of the esophagus, its close proximity to the stomach raises the obvious question whether bacteria also play a role in disease progression in the esophagus. The GI tract plays host to a large range of bacteria, which helps the physiological process of digestion, while boosting immunity to microbial and other antigens from birth. The immune system requires the presence of commensal bacteria to facilitate its development and maintain its natural immunity to pathogenic microorganisms. The microbiota, and its dysregulation, lead to chronic inflammation, as seen in gastric cancer and possibly colon cancer. In the gastro intestinal tract, these organisms play a major role in immune regulation, and therefore changes in bacterial composition in GERD due to cellular modifications may initiate or maintain neoplastic progression to esophageal carcinoma. So the first step to answering the posed question is what bacteria are present in the esophagus?

The esophagus can be infected with a number of organisms, including *Candida, Cryptococcus*, mycobacteria, and herpes virus. However, studies by Osias *et al.*,[22] Pei *et al.*,[23] and McFarlane *et al.*[24] have demonstrated a biofilm in the esophagus. They have identified many species of bacteria belonging to different genera and phyla. Although the majority of species are of an oral origin, the predominant oral phyla, spirochaetes are not present, providing evidence that not all oral bacteria can colonize these tissues. Studies have been done on the bacterial colonization in patients with reflux esophagitis and BE. Several groups of bacteria have been identified like Streptococci, Staphylococci, Gemella, Veillonella, Neisseria, Prevotella, and Fusobacteria. Although total colony forming units in healthy and BE patients were similar, there is great species diversity.[23–25] More recently, studies have shown the continuation of this colonization of the esophagus by campylobacter into those with esophageal carcinomas. The five bacterial phyla that are commonly identified in all patients at different stages of the reflux–GERD–Barrett's spectrum are: Firmicutes, Actinobacteria, Proteobacteria, Bacteroidetes, and Fusobacteria. The above studies did not reveal any specific organisms that were present in the majority of disease phenotypes that did not occur in any of the healthy controls. Nevertheless, differences in the prevalence of particular bacterial groups, and relative bacterial numbers were observed, with the microbiota becoming increasingly Gram-negative. *Campylobacter* manifested the greatest increase during disease progression. The increased presence of potentially pathogenic nitrate-reducing *Campylobacter* species in disease patients is of concern. The increased prevalence of nitrate-reducing *Campylobacter concisus*, not only in BE patients as found previously but also in those with GERD and ADC, may increase the mutagenic potential of refluxate.

This evidence confirms the presence of these bacteria in association with disease progression, and they have biological effects that could enhance mutagenesis or mitogenesis within the esophagus, but, thus far, there is no evidence of causality. This provides justification for further research but little evidence on which to base therapy upon. Turning again to the question posed, we have to ask if antibiotics are the correct therapy to consider, if we did want to eradicate campylobacter from the esophagus. The paradigm proposed is based directly on experience of *Helicobacter pylori* eradication in the stomach, where there is a very selective niche for colonization and an acid barrier to prevent recolonization. The same conditions do not apply in the esophagus where there is a very diverse microbiota and a ready reservoir of bacterial recolonization from the mouth. This would require continuous use of antibiotics with the attendant problems of resistance and secondary infections.

Therefore, the current knowledge about the microbiota of the esophagus, and in particular it's colonization with *Campylobacter* species, does not justify eradication with antibiotics.

6. What is the link between presence of unconjugated bile acids and the deleterious effect of refluxate in patients taking PPIs?

Katerina Dvorak and Aaron Goldman
kdvorak@email.arizona.edu

In BE, normal esophageal mucosa is replaced by columnar epithelium resembling intestinal tissue. This lesion of distal esophagus is associated with chronic GERD and predisposes patients to develop esophageal adenocarcinoma (EAC). However, the precise mechanism of development of BE and EAC is unclear. The incidence of EAC has been rapidly increasing in the last three decades and, interestingly, this increase correlates with the introduction of PPIs on market.

Epidemiological, animal, and clinical studies suggest that BE is formed in response to stress induced by two major components of refluxate: gastric acid and bile acids. Bile acids in combination with acid induce nitrosative stress, oxidative stress, DNA damage, and alterations in cell signaling. Furthermore, bile acids may induce the expression of proteins associated with phenotypic switch from normal squamous to intestinal phenotype such as Klf-4, villin, and CDX2.

PPIs, since their discovery in the late 1980s, have been largely used for treatment of acid related disorders, including BE. PPIs decrease secretion of gastric acid by inhibiting H^+/K^+ ATPase of parietal cells and alleviate symptoms associated with acid reflux. However, it is not clear if this therapy can completely suppress reflux of duodenal contents. Clinical studies using the Bilitec 2000® probe demonstrated that bile reflux is more common, and concentrations of bile acids are significantly higher in patients with BE than in patients with GERD. Furthermore, during the last five years, concerns have been raised, since long-term treatment with PPIs may produce adverse effects. In this review, we summarize the effects of PPIs on bile acids.

No treatment (pH ~2)

- Unconjugated and glycine-conjugated acids irreversibly precipate at normal stomach pH
- Taurine conjugated bile acids are soluble but they constitute only ~20% of total bile acids
- No bacterial overgrowth; no formation or secondary bile acids
- Bile acids are less concentrated
- Normal gastric emptying
- Normal gastrin levels

PPI (pH >4)

- Unconjugated and glycine-conjugated acids are soluble; they can interact with esophageal mucosa
- PPIs decrease overall stomach secretion and thus bile acids present in the stomach are more concentrated
- Bacterial overgrowth; bacteria induce formation of more toxic unconjugated bile acid
- Delayed gastric emptying
- Hypergasterinemia

Bile acids present in bile are conjugated with glycine or taurine, however there is small fraction of unconjugated bile acids in the normal bile. Glycine-conjugated bile acids represent more than 70% of all bile acid pool while taurine conjugated bile acids represent about 20%. Unconjugated bile acids are known to be more toxic compared to bile acids conjugated with glycine or taurine.

First, the stomach is normally free of bacteria, with the exception of *H. pylori*. PPI treatment is associated with bacterial overgrowth in the upper gastrointestinal tract, since the increase in pH creates environment more permissive for bacterial proliferation.[26,27] A majority of bacterial species residing in the stomach and duodenum may induce the deconjugation and dehydroxylation of primary bile acids to form more toxic, unconjugated, secondary bile acids, such as deoxycholic acid.[26,27] Indeed, studies show bacterial overgrowth and elevated levels of unconjugated bile acids in the gastric juice of patients treated with PPI.[28] The recent study of Yang *et al.* indicates that intestinal metaplasia of the distal esophagus is associated with alterations in the microbiome (a shift from a Gram-positive microbiome in normal esophagus to that of a Gram-negative anaerobic microbiome in inflamed/BE), however it is not clear from this study if patients were treated with PPIs.[28]

Second, the majority of bile acids (glycine conjugated and unconjugated) irreversibly precipitate at normal acidic environment of stomach (pH $\sim$2), thus they cannot cause cell damage or the alterations in cell signaling. In contrast, at higher pH (i.e., pH > 4) glycine conjugated bile acids are soluble, unionized, and thus active since their pKa is about 4. Glycine conjugated bile acids are the most prevalent bile acids in human bile and thus increase of stomach pH by PPIs treatment to pH > 4 may lead to the cellular damage by bile acids. Unconjugated bile acid have pKa $\sim$6.2, and thus they are are most active at this pH. In our studies, we have previously shown that acid, in combination with a bile acid cocktail that reflects the composition of bile acids present in the refluxate, induces oxidative DNA damage *in vitro* in different cell lines and *ex vivo* in esophageal biopsies.[29]

Third, since secretion of gastric acid in the stomach is reduced, then volume of secreted gastric juice is also low. Thus, concentration of bile acids refluxed into stomach and, consequently, to esophagus, is higher compared to the normal stomach where the secretion of gastric juices is high.

Fourth, PPIs may cause hypergastrinemia. Increased gastrin is linked to proliferation and cancer development.[30] Finally, PPIs have been shown to induce delayed gastric emptying, which may compromise the LES and increase the reflux of bile in the esophagus.

In summary, acid suppression therapy with PPIs may lead to the bacterial overgrowth and increased reflux of toxic, unconjugated bile acids. This may result in increased cell DNA damage, mutations, and, consequently, to BE and EAC development.

7. Should baclofen be added to PPIs to address nonacid and bile reflux factors?

Philip Woodland and Daniel Sifrim
d.sifrim@qmul.ac.uk

GERD, which is refractory to PPI therapy, is a frequently encountered clinical problem. This situation is most commonly, although not exclusively, found in patients with nonerosive reflux disease (NERD) in whom the response rate may be as low as 45%. In some cases of PPI refractoriness, the mechanism may be insufficient acid suppression by the PPI. This may be due to patient factors such as poor compliance or improper dosage time (i.e., not taken 30 min before mealtimes), or phamacokinetic/pharmacodynamic factors such as reduced PPI bioavailability, rapid PPI metabolism, or biological resistance to PPIs. These reasons may be best addressed by patient education, rationalization of medication regimes, and use of alternative acid-suppressant agents. However, a proportion of GERD patients have continued reflux-associated symptoms despite adequate efficacy of PPI therapy. These patients often have physiological esophageal acid exposure, yet when tested with 24-h multichannel intraluminal impedance (MII) studies, they have symptoms associated with reflux events that are not acidic, i.e., they may have sensitivity to reflux of other types. The refluxate in these cases may be weakly acidic (pH > 4), and may contain bile components from DGER, or even gas.

Weakly acidic reflux as a cause of GERD symptoms

A study of 60 symptomatic GERD patients taking, and refractory to, PPI revealed that weakly acid

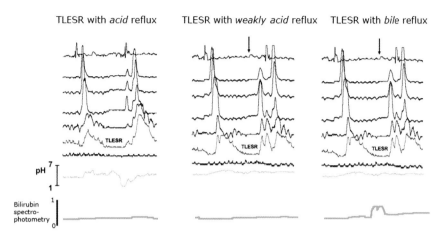

Figure 5. Transient lower esophageal sphincter relaxations can be responsible for acid, weakly acidic, and bile reflux events.

reflux was responsible for persisting regurgitation in 35%, cough in 20%, and heartburn in 7% of cases. Weakly acidic reflux appears to be of particular importance in NERD patients. Emerenziani *et al.* showed that 24% of GERD symptoms in NERD patients were attributed to weakly acidic reflux. There has been recent interest in the role of gaseous reflux symptom generation in GERD. Within their pH-MII study in GERD patients, Emerenziani *et al.* investigated the relationship between gaseous reflux (as measured by MII) and symptoms. They showed that in patients with NERD, the presence of gas with the liquid refluxate was associated with an increased probability of symptom perception. A similar study using pH-MII demonstrated that patients with NERD had an increase in gas-containing reflux episodes compared to controls. DGER is believed to be important in the genesis of a proportion of continuing symptoms despite PPI therapy, although the extent of its role remains controversial. Initial studies by the Leuven group suggested a significant role for DGER in PPI-refractory GERD. When patients with persistent reflux symptoms, despite therapy, were studied PPI, DGER (measured by esophageal bilirubin spectrophotometry) was found to be rather important, being related to 18% of symptomatic episodes versus 7% for acid and 10% for mixed reflux. Conversely, other studies have suggested a less important role for DGER in PPI-refractory GERD. Gasiorowska *et al.* studied a similar group of patients, and found DGER alone to be of a relatively lesser relevance, being related to 9% of symptom events versus 32% for acid and 32% for mixed reflux. Moreover, the amount of DGER

in PPI-refractory patients was similar to that in PPI-responsive patients.

The TLESR as a therapeutic target

If weak acid, DGER, and gas can be responsible for GERD symptoms, it is perhaps not surprising that a proportion of patients remain refractory to PPI therapy. Although PPIs have been shown to reduce both acid and DGER, it would follow that for some patients an alternative therapeutic target to the proton pump should be addressed. The common factor associated with any reflux, be it acid, weak acid, DGER or gas, is the TLESR (Fig. 5). TLESRs are triggered in response to activation of stretch receptors in the stomach and are thought to be mediated by a vago-vagal reflex pathway. Gastroesophageal reflux almost always occurs in the context of a TLESR, and so the suppression of these relaxations is an attractive therapeutic target. This was first shown to be plausible by Mittal *et al.* in 1995 when atropine was shown to reduce both TLESR frequency and the number of reflux events in normal subjects.[31] Subsequently, $GABA_B$ agonists (an example of which is baclofen) have also been shown to reduce the rate of postprandial TLESRs and reflux episodes in humans. $GABA_B$ receptors act at several points along the vagal mechanoreceptor signaling pathway. Vela *et al.* studied nine healthy volunteers and nine symptomatic reflux patients with esophageal pH-impedance after both placebo and a single dose of baclofen. Baclofen was found to cause a significant reduction in both acid and nonacid reflux in all subjects.[32] The potential benefits of baclofen on DGER have also been shown. Koek *et al.* investigated patients with PPI-refractory GERD who showed normal esophageal acid exposure, but who had pathological DGER on Bilitec monitoring. The addition of baclofen 20 mg three times daily to high-dose PPI therapy significantly reduced the number of DGER episodes, esophageal duodenal reflux exposure, and symptoms.[33] A further placebo-controlled study of 16 patients showed that 10 mg baclofen four times daily significantly reduced reflux events and improved symptoms.[34] Although effective at inhibiting TLESRs, the clinical use of baclofen is limited by its side-effect profile, causing troublesome symptoms such as dizziness and nausea. Recently, attention has turned towards new GABA$_B$-receptor agonists that act primarily at peripheral sites and, therefore, have better tolerability. The newly developed, peripherally acting GABA$_B$-receptor agonist lesogaberan has been shown to have a favorable safety and tolerability profile. Furthermore, in a randomized, double-blind, placebo-controlled trial in patients with PPI-refractory symptoms, lesogaberan significantly reduced TLESR frequency and number of reflux episodes compared to placebo.[35]

Summary

PPI-refractory GERD is a commonly encountered clinical problem. Before considering add-on therapy, reversible reasons for PPI failure (e.g., patient compliance) should first be sought. However, a subgroup of patients can be identified in whom ongoing symptoms are related to reflux events that are not acidic. In this group of patients the reduction of TLESR frequency is a potentially beneficial therapeutic strategy. GABA$_B$-receptor agonists have been

shown to be effective in reducing acidic and weakly acidic reflux events, and can reduce DGER. Baclofen is a reasonable therapeutic add-on in those with persistent symptoms due to nonacid reflux in those who can tolerate it. The development of newer drugs with more favorable side-effect profiles is encouraging progress for the management of this difficult-to-treat group of patients. The search for the ideal TLESR-inhibiting drug remains ongoing.

8. In patients on PPI therapy, what is the threshold for adequate suppression of esophageal acid exposure as expected by pH monitoring?

Joel E. Richter
jrichter@temple.edu

The normal esophageal pH values for healthy volunteers are well defined. However, many patients we study today are taking PPIs, and the degree of appropriate acid control on antacid medications has clinical relevance. Unfortunately, the threshold for adequate esophageal acid control on PPI therapy is poorly studied.

The single, widely quoted study addressing this question is from Brad Kuo, MD and Donald Castell, MD at Graduate Hospital, Philadelphia.[36] They studied 19 healthy male volunteers (mean age 25 years) assessing both esophageal and gastric pH in a randomized singled blinded protocol with three dosing arms: 40 mg omeprazole in the morning before breakfast, 40 mg omeprazole in the evening before dinner, and 20 mg twice a day before breakfast and dinner. Before each session, a baseline ambulatory pH study on each patient was done. Each

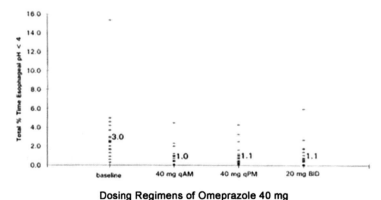

Figure 6. Dosing regimens caused a significant reduction ($P < 0.01$) in distal esophageal acid exposure compared with baseline.

session was carried out over at least five weeks with each dose session separated by at least a one-week washout period. Subjects received seven days of each dosing regimen followed by pH testing.

As shown in Figure 6, all dosing regimens caused a significant reduction ($P < 0.01$) in distal esophageal acid exposure compared with baseline. However, there was no significant difference among these dosing regimens with the range of means very tight at 1.0% to 1.1% for the total acid exposure time. The 95% confidence interval for the upper limit of acid exposure in these 19 volunteers across all studies was 1.6% on omeprazole 40 mg.

Using this threshold value of 1.6%, the same group performed a retrospective analysis of 45 patients with persistent GERD symptoms on omeprazole 20 mg BID.[37] Of this group, 14 (31%) had reflux that was poorly controlled based on the new threshold value of 1.6%. However, this separation did not characterize patients who would respond to increasing the omeprazole dose to 20 mg QID. Of the five patients with typical GER symptoms and pH $>1.6\%$, three responded to the higher omeprazole dose. All three of the responders had a good symptom response on pH testing. In the ten patients (one overlapped with heartburn) with primarily atypical symptoms and pH $>1.6\%$, only one patient with a good symptom correlation improved with QID omeprazole treatment. Thus, only 4 of 11 (36%) patients (three lost to treatment follow up in the atypical group) with pH thresholds $>1.6\%$ and persisted symptoms improved with higher doses of PPIs.

This data gives us little confidence in the proposed pH threshold $<1.6\%$ on PPI therapy and suggest that larger studies and possibly a multicenter study is required to appropriately address this issue. Until this time, our and most other groups, define adequate acid control in GERD patients as values below normal thresholds for healthy controls, usually % total acid exposure time of less than 4.5–5.5%.

9. What are the effects of PPIs on stabilization of basal cell proliferation, reduction of cell cycle abnormalities, and hyperplasia of the basal cell layer?

Michael Vieth, Helmut Neumann, and Cord Langner
Vieth.LKPathol@uni-bayreuth.de

The effects of PPIs on esophageal mucosa are dependent on the type of epithelium present. Physiologically, the esophagus is covered by squamous epithelium. When the squamous epithelium is replaced by columnar epithelium (BE), effects on columnar epithelium can be observed as well.

Squamous epithelium

The esophagus is physiologically lined by nonkeratinized squamous epithelium. Proliferation (regeneration) starts from the basal cell layer. Stromal papillae that extend into the epithelium mainly contain small capillaries. In reflux disease, increased proliferation leads to thickening of the basal cell layer and elongation of stromal papillae (Fig. 7). Capillaries are now located closer to the mucosal surface, and this corresponds to increased redness of the mucosa during endoscopy. At high magnification endoscopy dilated capillary loops may be seen.

The thickness of the basal cell layer and the length of the papillae can be expressed as percentages in relation to the thickness of the entire squamous epithelium. A relationship between these percentages and the severity of disease may be noted: the more severe the reflux disease (according to the Los Angeles classification), the more pronounced the thickness of the basal cell layer and the length of the papillae. After PPI therapy these values drop down markedly. Even if missing or poor controls do not allow a precise definition of what is normal and what is already abnormal, it may be speculated that normal values are very close by to these values induced by PPI therapy (Fig. 8). Since under PPI the length of papillae decreases, capillaries move further away

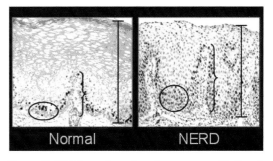

Figure 7. Histology of esophageal squamous epithelium in an individual without pathological changes (left) and an individual with endoscopy negative reflux disease (NERD) (right). Proliferating cells are marked immunohistochemically by Ki67. Circle = basal cell layer; brackets = length of stromal papilla; distance holder = epithelial thickness.

from the lumen leading to a decreased redness of the mucosa up until virtual normalization during endoscopy.[38]

Columnar epithelium

Columnar metaplasia of the distal esophagus (BE) is regarded as a precancerous condition. The risk for malignant transformation is up to 125 times higher than in the normal population. Cancer risk can also be expressed as 0.5% per year for individuals with BE. How to decrease this risk? One option is to remove the esophagus or at least part of it by surgery. This approach would be linked to numerous procedure-related side effects. The question is whether PPI therapy is capable of lowering the risk of malignant transformation, since PPI therapy is known to decrease proliferation, enhance differentiation, and promote epithelial maturation. Not many publications are available on this topic and the study design of the few reports available is limited. It appears, however, that PPI therapy reduces the risk of malignant transformation.[39–42] NSAIDs are thought to cause a trend only, but no significant reduction on its own. Of note, several reports stressed that the effects of PPI therapy may be related to different profiles in acid exposure. Namely there are differences in continuous versus pulse acid exposure. The epithelium of patients with continuous acid exposure is believed to only partially benefit from PPI therapy, whereas the epithelium of patients with pulse acid exposure, leading to more pronounced epithelial changes, might have a greater potential to be positively influenced/cured by PPI therapy.

It needs to be stressed that these data, although corresponding nicely with our expectations, are so far only limited, based upon few (observational) studies with few tested individuals, sometimes biased by poor study design (such as decreased bile reflux under PPI-therapy), or even nonreproducible. Thus, although the mechanisms have not yet been fully understood, at least a trend to risk reduction during PPI-therapy is accepted in the literature.

Length regression of BE has been known for a long time,[43] but to be significant it should exceed 10% of the area covered by columnar epithelium. Especially in short segments this cannot properly be accessed by endoscopy since, for example, 10% of 3 cm would sum up as only 3 mm in length reduction. Again only a trend has been documented so far even if Barrett's will not disappear completely in most cases.

In conclusion, established PPI effects on squamous epithelium are:

1. increase of squamous islands;
2. reduction of cell proliferation;
3. improvement of differentiation;
4. reduction of acid reflux;

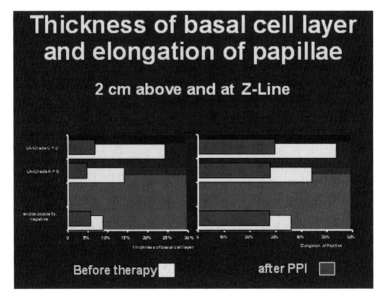

Figure 8. Changes in esophageal squamous epithelium after PPI therapy focusing on length of stromal papillae and thickness of basal cell layer related to severeness of reflux disease assessed by Los Angeles classification (LA Grade). Modified after Vieth *et al.* [38]

5. ERD healing improves detection of neoplasia;
6. adjuvant treatment to ablation therapy; and
7. symptom control.

PPI effects on columnar epithelium are partially based on much weaker evidence:

1. regression of Barrett's length (10% !);
2. reduction of cell proliferation (?);
3. improvement of differentiation (?);
4. decreased COX-2/VEGF expression and PGE2 release;
5. reduction of bile reflux (?);
6. ERD healing improves detection of neoplasia;
7. adjuvant treatment to ablation therapy; and
8. symptom control.

10. Can PPI therapy achieve normalization of esophageal pH in Barrett's patients?

George Triadafilopoulos
vagt@stanford.edu

The use of PPIs is almost universal in patients with BE. These drugs effectively control reflux symptoms; heal mucosal damage; prevent recurrent esophagitis and/or stricture formation; partly regress the metaplastic surface; induce formation of neosquamous islands; reduce DEGR, minimizing the impact of bile on the metaplastic epithelium; facilitate the recognition and regression of dysplasia; and may prevent dysplasia and adenocarcinoma by decreasing cell proliferation, exerting potentially a chomoprevention effect. In this context, maximum esophageal pH control (esophageal pH normalization) is generally considered as essential. PPI therapy is also an important adjuvant treatment to ablation modalities, facilitating neoepitheliazation.[44]

Figure 9A shows an example of "ideal" pH control in BE, where the esophageal pH was normalized to pH < 4.0 for less than 4% using esomeprazole 40 mg bid, and partial suppression of intragastric acidity was accomplished. In contrast, Figure 9B shows "poor" pH control in BE where the esophageal pH remained persistently abnormal despite esomeprazole 40 bid; partial and inadequate suppression of intragastric acidity, particularly at night was noted. In one study, 62% of patients failed to achieve complete esophageal acid suppression (24-h pH < 4.0 for > 5% time) despite esomeprazole 40 mg bid; typically esophageal pH reflects gastric pH, particularly at night (supine position).[45] In another "dose response" study with esomeprazole, 31 patients with BE were noted to accomplish gastric pH >4.0 for 88.4%, 81.4%, and 80.4% of day 5

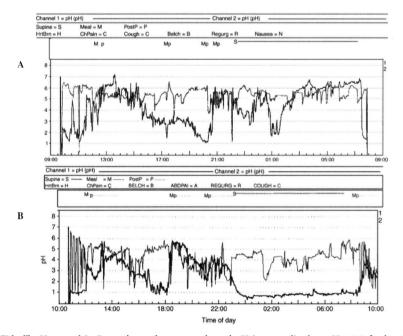

Figure 9. (A) "Ideal" pH control in Barrett's esophagus: esophageal pH is normalized to pH <4.0 for less than 4%; partial suppression of intragastric acidity. (B) "Poor" pH control in Barrett's esophagus. Esophageal pH is persistently abnormal despite esomeprazole 40 bid; partial and inadequate suppression of intragastric acidity (originally published in Ref. 45).

after treatment with esomeprazole 40 mg tid, 40 mg bid, and 20 mg tid, respectively. The esophageal pH remained abnormal in 16%, 23%, and 19% of patients receiving esomeprazole 40 mg tid, 40 mg bid, and 20 mg tid, respectively.[46]

In a crossover trial, there were no significant differences among three PPIs (lansoprazole, omeprazole, and esomeprazole) in controlling esophageal pH. Although all these patients had no GER symptoms, many exhibited persistently abnormal esophageal pH.[47] There are no predictors of normalization of esophageal acid exposure in BE patients. In a cohort study of 46 patients with BE, 25% continued to have abnormal esophageal pH profiles despite bid PPI, and age, BE length, and hiatal hernia size did not predict the persistence of abnormal intraesophageal pH.[48] It appears that acid remains in the esophagus of Barrett's patients because of poor peristalsis of the esophageal body, and most of the reduction in esophageal pH exposure with PPI happens in the upright, not supine position. Similarly, upright—not supine—duodeno-gastro-esophageal (bile) reflux was significantly reduced by PPI in such patients.[49]

In conclusion, a high percentage of patients with BE continue to exhibit pathologic GERD and low gastric pH despite high (bid-tid) doses of PPI and all PPIs have a similar effect. For an antisecretory treatment aimed at chemoprevention to be effective, higher PPI dosing, confirmed by pH monitoring, is necessary.

11. Are different effects of PPI therapy to be expected in relation to the predominant phenotype of cellular proliferation in Barrett's epithelium?

Norihisa Ishimura and Yuji Amano
amano@med.shimane-u.ac.jp

The chemopreventive effect of PPIs for BE has been extensively studied; however, its role remains unclear. Epidemiologic studies suggest a protective effect of PPIs against neoplastic changes and progression in BE; however, the data are contradictory. It is well known that BE consists of two secreted mucin phenotypes, namely gastric and intestinal. The predominant mucin phenotype has been reported to have a more malignant potential. Consistently, we have shown that Barrett's epithelium with intestinal

predominant mucin phenotype showed markedly elevated cellular proliferation and suppressed apoptosis, as compared to that with gastric predominant mucin phenotype.[50,51] Therefore, the controversy regarding the chemopreventive potential of PPI, including the suppression of COX-2 expression and cell proliferation, and the induction of apoptosis, may be the diversity of the mucin phenotype of Barrett's mucosa. The aim of this study[52] was to evaluate the effect of PPIs on cellular proliferation, COX-2 expression, and apoptosis in BE with different mucin phenotypes.

Materials and methods

Four hundred and nineteen consecutive patients with histologically proven BE were enrolled in the study.[52] Patients were divided into two groups, nontreatment patients ($n = 358$), and chronic PPI users ($n = 61$), which were defined when they were continuously administrated from at least two months before endoscopy. Four hundred and sixty-six biopsy samples of BE from 358 nontreatment patients and 81 from 61 chronic PPI users were immunohistochemically examined using anti-COX-2 protein, antiproliferating cell nuclear antigen (PCNA), and antisingle strand DNA (ssDNA) antigens in both mucin phenotypes of BE.

Results

Among nontreatment patients and PPI users, there was no significant difference between the gastric and intestinal predominant mucin phenotype.[52] Prevalence of the COX-2 expression pattern did not significantly differ between the nontreatment and PPI users. In those using PPIs, significant suppression of cellular proliferation assessed by PCNA was found in BE with the gastric predominant mucin phenotype, but not with the intestinal predominant mucin phenotype. Apoptosis indices assessed by ssDNA in chronic PPI users did not significantly differ between the two mucin phenotypes.[52]

Discussion

Acid exposure is considered the main factor not only in the development of BE, but also in the carcinogenesis of Barrett's adenocarcinoma. In this study, we have demonstrated that PPIs showed an inhibitory effect on cellular proliferation only in the gastric predominant mucin phenotype but not in the intestinal predominant mucin phenotype showing more accelerated cellular proliferation activity (Fig. 10).[52]

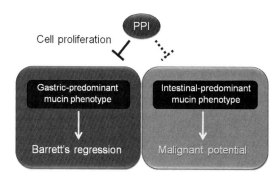

Figure 10. The effect of PPI on cell proliferation in BE.

In BE with the intestinal-predominant mucin phenotype, COX-2 expression and subsequent possible overproduction of prostaglandins is closely related with the acceleration of cellular proliferation and the inhibition of apoptosis. However, the suppressive effect of PPIs for COX-2 expression in BE was not found in this study.

Conclusion
PPIs suppress cellular proliferation in BE with the gastric-predominant mucin phenotype but not in that with the gastric-predominant mucin phenotype. This finding may at least partly explain the ongoing controversy surrounding the notion that all cases of BE respond to acid-suppressive therapy.

12. What are the respective values of the Symptom Index, the Symptom Sensitivity Index, and the Symptom Association Probability for the interpretation of causality of symptoms, and the potential response to medical treatment?

Joel E. Richter
jrichter@temple.edu

The first symptom indices to relate acid reflux by ambulatory pH testing with patients symptoms evolved in the late 1980s.[53] The "symptom index" (SI) is defined as the percentage of symptom episodes that are related to reflux:

Number of reflux related symptom episodes/
Total number of symptom episodes × 100%.

The distribution of SIs in a population of patients with heartburn appears to be bimodal, and the result of receiver operating characteristic analysis indicates that the optimal threshold for SI is 50%. The

major shortcoming of the SI is that this index does not factor in the total number of reflux episodes, hence the higher the frequency of acid reflux, the greater the likelihood that a symptom is associated by chance. For this reason the "symptom sensitivity index" (SSI) was proposed as an additional parameter. SSI is defined as:

Number of symptom associated reflux episodes/
Total number of reflux episodes × 100%.

SSI values of 10% or higher are considered to be positive.[53] It should be noted that these determined thresholds have only been validated for heartburn and regurgitation—not for chest pain or extraesophageal symptoms. Furthermore, these indices have not been validated for nonacid episodes. Both the SI and SSI suffer from the disadvantage that they do not integrate all factors determining the relationship between symptoms and reflux. The "symptom association probability" (SAP) is calculated by dividing 24-h pH data into consecutive two minute windows.[54] For each of these two minute windows, it is determined whether reflux occurred and whether symptoms occurred, giving a 2 × 2 contingency table of S+R+, S–R+, S+R–, S–R–, respectively. Fishers' exact test is used to calculate the probability (p) that the observed distribution could occur by chance alone. SAP is calculated as $(1 - p) \times 100\%$; by statistical convention, SAP ≥ 95% is positive. Limitations of validation outside classical GERD symptoms also apply to the SAP.

Despite the availability of these symptom indices, there is surprisingly little literature assessing their predictive accuracy in a clinical population. To perform this appropriately, a large patient population needs testing with outcomes followed after aggressive PPI therapy or antireflux surgery. The only study to date taking this approach was performed by Taghavi *et al.* from Iran.[55] The authors studied 52 patients with a predominant symptom of heartburn with baseline symptom scores calculated at the first visit. After 24-h pH testing off all PPIs, the symptom reflux indices were calculated. All patients were placed on high dose omeprazole (40 mg AM, 20 mg at night) and symptom scores recorded again one week later. A reduction of >50% in the heartburn score was considered a positive omeprazole test. Overall, the omeprazole test was positive in 23 patients (52%). The concordance of the three symptom indices and the omeprazole test

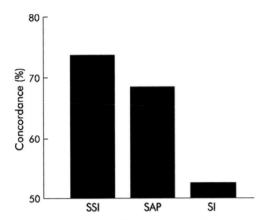

Figure 11. Concordance of the three symptom indices and the omeprazole test.

is shown in Figure 11. All these indices were significantly related to each other ($P < 0.001$). However, only the SAP and SSI had a statistically significant relationship with the omeprazole test ($P < 0.05$ for both). SSI had the highest positive (80.9%) and negative (57.9%) predictive values and sensitivity (73.9%). The specificity of the SSI and SAP (73.3% for both) was lower than the SI (80%). These authors could find no cutoff point at which the results of SI could be related significantly to the omeprazole test results. The authors concluded, "these symptom reflux indices are unable to predict the response of the one most typical symptom of GERD (heartburn) to the one most effective medical treatments available."[55]

No other studies have been reported to date to address this issue in individual patients. However, other studies have shown favorable trend data for both the SAP and SI when assessing the response for heartburn and regurgitation to PPI therapy over several weeks.[56,57] In these studies, those with a positive symptom index and abnormal reflux values performed as a group best, followed by a positive symptom correlation even with a normal pH test, while not surprisingly those with both tests negative did the worst. Based on these limited data, great caution is urged when using these test results to predict a response to PPIs in individual patients, especially those without classic heartburn or regurgitation. Large, possibly multicenter studies need to be performed using strong clinical endpoints such as symptom resolution to prolonged high dose PPI therapy (BID dose for four to eight weeks) or antireflux therapy. Additional studies are also required to

validate the use of these indices with nonacid reflux measured by impedance technology.

13. Can correlation between use of PPI and development of dysplasia be considered?

Valter Nilton Felix
v.felix@terra.com.br

Use of PPIs may be useful to avoid the development of dysplasia if there are not concomitant duodenogastroesophageal reflux (DGER) and other systemic factors interacting, and if it could really normalize esophageal acid exposure.

Reflux symptoms can be controlled in most patients with PPI therapy. Twice a day dosing may be necessary in a subgroup of patients. However there are currently no data that directly support the use of high dose antisecretory therapy to delay or prevent the development of Barrett's esophagus or EAC. Even on higher doses of omeprazole of 40 mg bid, as many as 24% of Barrett's patients were shown to have abnormal total or supine distal esophageal acid exposure values. Limited prospective studies have demonstrated normalization of esophageal pH with q.d. PPI therapy in over 90% of patients with typical reflux symptoms. On the other hand, patients with more severe degrees of erosive esophagitis have significantly greater abnormal esophageal acid exposure in spite of PPI therapy.[58]

Furthermore, adequate acid suppression may mask the detection of nonacid reflux events. PPIs, although effective in controlling the acid component of the refluxate, do not eliminate the reflux of bile, which some believe to be a major contributor to the pathogenesis of Barrett's epithelium. DGER occurs in more than 50% of patients with erosive esophagitis and BE,[59] and the majority of bile reflux events occurred concomitantly with acid reflux. Tack *et al.*[60] have recently published a series of studies suggesting a possible role for DGER in both symptoms and esophagitis in a subset of patients with difficult to manage, symptomatic reflux. Surprisingly, 51% of patients had erosive esophagitis on endoscopy despite the fact that they were on PPI therapy at the time of the study.[60]

Chronic inflammation seems to have a central role in the development of esophageal adenocarcinoma and its precursor lesions. The refluxate contains numerous substances in addition to gastric acid, including bile salts, pancreatic enzymes, and ingested foods and their metabolites, which can cause acute and chronic inflammation of the oesophageal epithelium with resulting oxidative stress.

Abdominal obesity, in addition to promoting gastroesophageal reflux, is also increasingly being recognized as causing a state of low-level systemic inflammation, characterized by increased plasma levels of proinflammatory cytokines and receptors, such as interleukin-6 (IL-6), TNF-α and TNF-α receptor 2, C-reactive protein and leptin.

In addition, cigarette smoking can cause inflammation both systemically and in the esophageal epithelium in response to swallowed smoking products. In turn, a chronic state of systemic and localized inflammation and oxidative stress promotes DNA damage, cellular proliferation and telomere shortening, which can increase the risk of developing clones containing small- and large-scale genomic alterations, eventually leading to widespread chromosomal instability and esophageal adenocarcinoma.

The advisability of prescribing aggressive antireflux therapy for all patients with BE, irrespective of the severity of their underlying GERD, has been debated. One recent study has shown a decrease in development of dysplasia in patients treated with or prescribed PPIs.[61] In multivariate analysis, the use of PPI after BE diagnosis was independently associated with reduced risk of dysplasia, hazards ratio: 0.25 (95% CI 0.13–0.47), $P < 0.0001$. In this same route, a retrospective observational study of 344 patients with BE, PPI treatment after diagnosis of BE was associated with a reduced risk of HGD or cancer.[62]

On the other hand, several uncontrolled, observational studies have found fewer cases of dysplasia and cancer among patients with BE who had antireflux surgery than among those who had received medical treatment, and some even have proposed that antisecretory therapy might predispose to malignancy. However, the limited studies that have addressed this issue directly have not found a significant association between esophageal adenocarcinoma and the use of antisecretory agents *per se.*

Conflicts of interest

The authors declare no conflicts of interest.

References

1. El-Serag, H.B., T.V. Aguirre, S. Davis, *et al.* 2004. Proton pump inhibitors are associated with reduced incidence of dysplasia in Barrett's esophagus. *Am. J. Gastroenterol.* **99:** 1877–1883.

2. Hillman, L.C., L. Chiragakis, B. Shadbolt, *et al.* 2004. Proton-pump inhibitor therapy and the development of dysplasia in patients with Barrett's oesophagus. *Med J Aust.* **180:** 387–391.

3. Triadafilopoulos, G. 2008. Proton pump inhibitors in Barrett's esophagus: Pluripotent but controversial. *Eur. Surg.* **40:** 58–65.

4. Huo, X., H.Y. Zhang, X.I. Zhang, *et al.* 2010. Acid and bile salt-induced CDX2 expression differs in esophageal squamous cells from patients with and without Barrett's esophagus. *Gastroenterology.* **139:** 194–203.

5. Hong, J., M. Resnick, J. Behar, *et al.* 2010. Acid-induced p16 hypermethylation contributes to development of esophageal adenocarcinoma via activation of NADPH oxidase NOX5-S. *Am. J. Physiol. Gastrointest. Liver Physiol.* **299:** G697–G706

6. Majewski, M., T. Jaworski, I. Sarosiek, *et al.* 2007. Significant enhancement of esophageal pre-epithelial defense by tegaserod: Implications for an esophagoprotective effect. *Clin. Gastroenterol. Hepatol.* **5:** 430–438.

7. Oh, D.S. & S.R. DeMeester. 2010. Pathophysiology and treatment of Barrett's esophagus. *World J. Gastroenterol.* **16:** 3762–3772.

8. Sarosiek, J., C.J. Scheurich, M. Marcinkiewicz & RW McCallum. 1996. Enhancement of salivary esophagoprotection: Rationale for a physiological approach to gastroesophageal reflux disease. *Gastroenterology* **110:** 675–681.

9. Sarosiek, J., M.C. Edmunds, Z. Namiot, *et al.* 1994. Secretory profile of Barrett's esophagus: Its significantly modified protective potential. *Gastroenterology* **106:** A173.

10. Sarosiek, I., M. Olyaee, M. Majewski, *et al.* 2009. Significant increase of esophageal mucin secretion in patients with reflux esophagitis after healing with rabeprazole: Its Esophagoprotective potential. *Dig. Dis. Sci.* **54:** 2137–2142.

11. Abdulnour-Nakhoul, S., N.A. Tobey, N.L. Nakhoul, *et al.* 2008. The effect of tegaserod on esophageal submucosal glands bicarbonate and mucin secretion. *Dig. Dis. Sci.* **53:** 2366–2372.

12. Kahrilas, P.J., E.M. Quigley, D.O. Castell, *et al.* 2000. The effects of tegaserod (HTF 919) on oesophageal acid exposure in gastro-oesophageal reflux disease. *Aliment. Pharmacol. Ther.* **14:** 1503–1509.

13. Ataee, R., S. Ajdary, M. Rezayat, *et al.* 2010. Study of 5HT3 and HT4 receptor expression in HT29 cell line and human colon adenocarcinoma tissues. *Arch. Iran. Med.* **13:** 120–125.

14. Lanuti, M., G. Liu, J.M. Goodwin, *et al.* 2008. A functional epidermal growth factor (EGF) polymorphism, EGF serum levels, and esophageal adenocarcinoma risk and outcome. *Clin. Cancer. Res.* **14:** 3216–3222.

15. Marcinkiewicz, M., S.Z. Grabowska & E. Czyzewska. 1998. Role of epidermal growth factor (EGF) in oesophageal mucosal integrity. *Curr. Med. Res. Opin.* **14:** 145–153.

16. Sarosiek, J., B.J. Marshall, D.A. Peura, *et al.* 1991. Gastroduodenal mucus gel thickness in patients with *Helicobacter*

pylori: a method for assessment of biopsy specimens. *Am. J. Gastroenterol.* **86:** 729–734.

17. Namiot, Z., J. Sarosiek, R.M. Rourk, *et al.* 1994. Human esophageal secretion: mucosal response to luminal acid and pepsin. *Gastroenterology* **106:** 973–981.

18. Majewski, M., T. Jaworski, I. Sarosiek, *et al.* 2007. Significant enhancement of esophageal pre-epithelial defense by tegaserod: Implications for an esophagoprotective effect. *Clin. Gastroenterol. Hepatol.* **5:** 430–438.

19. Jaworski, T., I. Sarosiek, S. Sostarich, *et al.* 2005. Restorative impact of rabeprazole on gastric mucus and mucin production impairment during naproxen administration: its potential clinical significance. *Dig. Dis. Sci.* **50:** 357–365.

20. Camilleri, M., A.E. Bharucha, R. Ueno, *et al.* 2006. Effect of a selective chloride channel activator, lubiprostone, on gastrointestinal transit, gastric sensory, and motor functions in healthy volunteers. *Am. J. Physiol. – GI & Liver Physiol.* **290:** G942–G947.

21. McKeage, K., G.L. Plosker & M.A. Siddiqui. 2006. Lubiprostone. *Drugs* **66:** 873–879.

22. Osias, G.L., M.Q. Bromer, R.M. Thomas, *et al.* 2004. Digestive diseases and sciences, **49:** 228–236. Esophageal bacteria and Barrett's esophagus:A Preliminary Report.

23. Zhiheng, Pei, E.J. Bini, L. Yang, *et al.* 2004. Bacterial biota in the human distal esophagus *PNAS* **101:** 4250–4255.

24. Macfarlane, S., E. Furrie, G.T. Macfarlane & J.F. Dillon. 2007. Microbial colonization of the upper gastrointestinal tract in patients with Barrett's esophagus. *Clin. Infect. Dis.* **45:** 29–38.

25. Yang, L., X. Lu, C.W. Nossa, *et al.* 2009. Inflammation and intestinal metaplasia of the distal esophagus are associated with alterations in the microbiome. *Gastroenterology* **137:** 588–597.

26. Laine, L., D. Ahnen, C. McClain, *et al.* 2000. Review article: potential gastrointestinal effects of long-term acid suppression with proton pump inhibitors. *Aliment. Pharmacol. Ther.* **14:** 651–668.

27. Williams, C. 2001. Occurrence and significance of gastric colonization during acid-inhibitory therapy. *Best. Pract. Res. Clin. Gastroenterol.* **15:** 511–521.

28. Yang, L., X. Lu, C.W. Nossa, *et al.* 2009. Inflammation and intestinal metaplasia of the distal esophagus are associated with alterations in the microbiome. *Gastroenterology* **137:** 588–597.

29. Dvorak, K., C.M. Payne, M. Chavarria, *et al.* 2007. Bile acids in combination with low pH induce oxidative stress and oxidative DNA damage: relevance to the pathogenesis of Barrett's oesophagus. *Gut* **56:** 763–771.

30. McCarthy, D.M. 2010. Adverse effects of proton pump inhibitor drugs: clues and conclusions. *Curr. Opin. Gastroenterol.* **26:** 624–631.

31. Mittal, R.K., R. Holloway & J. Dent. 1995. Effect of atropine on the frequency of reflux and transient lower esophageal sphincter relaxation in normal subjects. *Gastroenterology* **109:** 1547–1554.

32. Vela, M.F.,R. Tutuian, P.O. Katz & D.O. Castell. 2003. Baclofen decreases acid and non-acid post-prandial gastro-oesophageal reflux measured by combined multichannel intraluminal impedance and pH. *Aliment. Pharmacol. Ther.* **17:** 243–251.

33. Koek, G.H., D. Sifrim, T. Lerut, *et al.* 2003. Effect of the GABA(B) agonist baclofen in patients with symptoms and duodeno-gastro-oesophageal reflux refractory to proton pump inhibitors. *Gut* **52:** 1397–1402.

34. Ciccaglione, A.F. & L. Marzio. 2003. Effect of acute and chronic administration of the GABA B agonist baclofen on 24 hour pH metry and symptoms in control subjects and in patients with gastro-oesophageal reflux disease. *Gut* **52:** 464–470.

35. Boeckxstaens, G.E., H. Beaumont, V. Mertens, *et al.* 2010. Effects of lesogaberan on reflux and lower esophageal sphincter function in patients with gastroesophageal reflux disease. *Gastroenterology* **139:** 409–417.

36. Kuo, B. & D.O. Castell. 1996. Optimal dosing of omeprazole 40 mg daily. Effects on gastric and esophageal pH and serum gastric in healthy controls. *Am. J. Gastroenterol.* **91:** 1532–1538.

37. Katzka, D.A., V. Paoletti, L. Leite & D.O. Castell. 1996. Prolonged ambulatory pH monitoring in patients with persistent GERD symptoms: testing while on therapy identifies the need for more aggressive anti-reflux treatment. *Am. J. Gastroenterol.* **91:** 2110–2113.

38. Vieth, M., M. Kulig, A. Leodolter, *et al.* 2006. Histological effects of esomeprazole therapy on the squamous epithelium of the distal oesophagus. *Aliment. Pharmacol. Ther.* **23:** 313–319.

39. Nguyen, D.M., H.B. EL-Serag, L. Henderson, *et al.* 2009. Medication usage and the risk of neoplasia in patients with Barrett's esophagus. *Clin. Gastroenterol. Hepatol.* **7:** 1299–1304.

40. El-Serag, H.B., T.V. Aguirre, S. Davis, *et al.* 2004. Proton pump inhibitors are associated with reduced incidence of dysplasia in Barrett's esophagus. *Am. J. Gastroenterol.* **99:** 1877–1883.

41. Cooper, B.T., W. Chapman, C.S. Neumann & J.C. Gearty. 2006. Continuous treatment of Barrett's oesophagus patients with proton pump inhibitors up to 13 years: observations on regression and cancer incidence. *Aliment. Pharmacol. Ther.* **23:** 727–733.

42. Hillman, L.C., L. Chiragakis, B. Shadbolt, *et al.* 2004. Proton-pump inhibitor therapy and the development of dysplasia in patients with Barrett's oesophagus. *Med. J. Aust.* **180:** 387–391.

43. Devière, J., M. Buset, J.M. Dumonceau, *et al.* 1989. Regression of Barrett's epithelium with omeprazole. *N. Engl. J. Med.* **320:** 1497–1498.

44. Yeh, R.W., L.B. Gerson & G. Triadafilopoulos. 2003. Efficacy of esomeprazole in controlling reflux symptoms, intraesophageal, and intragastric pH in patients with Barrett's esophagus. *Dis. Esophagus.* **16:** 193–198.

45. Gerson, L.B., K. Shetler & G. Triadafilopoulos. 2005. Control of intra-oesophageal and intra-gastric pH with proton pump inhibitors in patients with Barrett's oesophagus. *Dig. Liver Dis.* **37:** 651–658.

46. Spechler, S.J., P. Sharma, B. Traxler, *et al.* 2006. Gastric and esophageal pH in patients with Barrett's esophagus treated with three esomeprazole dosages: a randomized, double-blind, crossover trial. *Am. J. Gastroenterol.* **101:** 1964–1971.

47. Gerson, L.B. & G. Triadafilopoulos. 2005. A prospective study of oesophageal 24-h ambulatory pH monitoring in patients with functional dyspepsia. *Dig. Liver. Dis.* **37:** 87–91.

48. Wani, S., R.E. Sampliner, A.P. Weston, *et al.* 2005. Lack of predictors of normalization of oesophageal acid exposure in Barrett's oesophagus. *Aliment. Pharmacol. Ther.* **22:** 627–633.

49. Smythe, A., G.P. Troy, R. Ackroyd & N.C. Bird. 2008. Proton pump inhibitor influence on reflux in Barrett's oesophagus. *Eur. J. Gastroenterol. Hepatol.* **20:** 881–887.

50. Amano, Y., S. Ishihara, Y. Kushiyama, *et al.* 2004. Barrett's oesophagus with predominant intestinal metaplasia correlates with superficial cyclo-oxygenase 2 expression, increased proliferation and reduced apoptosis: changes that are partially reversed by non-steroidal anti-inflammatory drugs usage. *Aliment. Parmacol. Ther.* **20:** 793–802.

51. Amano, Y., Y. Kushiyama, T. Yuki, *et al.* 2007. Predictors for squamous re-epithelialization of Barrett's esophagus after endoscopic biopsy. *J. Gastroenterol.* **22:** 901–907.

52. Amano, Y., D. Chinuki, T. Yuki, *et al.* 2006. Efficacy of proton pump inhibitors for cellular proliferation and apoptosis in Barrett's oesophagus with different mucin phenotypes. *Aliment. Pharmacol. Ther.* **24**(Suppl 4): 41–48.

53. Bredenoord, A.J., Balm Weusten & A.P.J.M. Smout. 2005. Symptom association analysis in ambulatory GERD monitoring. *Gut* **54:** 1810–1817.

54. Weusten, Balm, J.M. Roelofs, L.M. Akkermans, *et al.* 1994. The symptom association probability: an improved method for symptom analysis of 24 hour pH data. *Gastroenterology* **107:** 1741–1745.

55. Taghavi, S.A., M. Ghasedi, M. Saberi-Firooz, *et al.* 2005. Symptom association probability and symptom sensitivity index: preferable but still suboptimal predictors of response to high dose omeprazole. *Gut* **54:** 1067–1071.

56. Aanen, M.C., Balm Weusten, M.E. Numans, *et al.* 2008. Effect of proton-pump inhibitor treatment on symptoms and quality of life in GERD patients depends on the symptom-reflux association. *J. Clin. Gastroenterol.* **42:** 441–447.

57. Watson, R.G.P., T.C.K. Tham, B.T Johnston & N.I. Mcdougall. 1997. Double blind cross-over placebo controlled study of omeprazole in the treatment of patients with reflux symptoms and physiological levels of acid reflux—the "sensitive oesophagus." *Gut* **40:** 587–590.

58. Ours, T.M., W.K. Fackler, J.E. Richter, *et al.* 2003. Nocturnal acid breakthrough: Clinical significance and correlation with esophageal acid exposure. *Am. J. Gastroenterol.* **98:** 545–550.

59. Felix, V.N., R.G. Viebig. Simultaneous bilimetry and pHmetry in GERD and Barrett's patients. *Hepato-Gastroenterol.* **52:** 1453–1455.

60. Tack, J., G. Koek, I. Demedts, *et al.* 2004. Gastroesophageal reflux disease poorly responsive to single-dose proton pump inhibitors in patients without Barrett's esophagus: Acid reflux, bile reflux, or both? *Am. J. Gastroenterol.* **99:** 981–988.

61. El-Serag, H.B., T.V. Aguirre, S. Davis, *et al.* 2004. Proton pump inhibitors are associated with reduced incidence of dysplasia in Barrett's esophagus. *Am. J. Gastroenterol.* **99:** 1877–1883.

62. Nguyen, DM, H.B. El-Serag, L. Henderson, *et al.* 2009. Medication usage and the risk of neoplasia in patients with Barrett's esophagus. *Clin. Gastroenterol. Hepatol.* **7:** 1299.

Ann. N.Y. Acad. Sci. ISSN 0077-8923

Barrett's esophagus: proton pump inhibitors and chemoprevention II

Joel E. Richter,[1] Roberto Penagini,[2] Daniel Pohl,[3] Katerina Dvorak,[4,5] Aaron Goldman,[5]
Edoardo Savarino,[6] Patrizia Zentilin,[6] Vincenzo Savarino,[6] Joshua T. Watson,[7]
Roy K.H. Wong,[7] Fabio Pace,[8,9] Valentina Casini,[8] David A. Peura,[10] Shoshana Joy Herzig,[11]
Takeshi Kamiya,[12] Iva Pelosini,[13] Carmelo Scarpignato,[13] David Armstrong,[14]
Kenneth R. DeVault,[15] Paolo Bechi,[16] Antonio Taddei,[16] Giancarlo Freschi,[16]
Maria Novella Ringressi,[16] Duccio Rossi Degli'Innocenti,[17] Francesca Castiglione,[17]
Emmanuella Masini,[18] and Richard H. Hunt[19]

[1]Department of Medicine, Temple University, Philadelphia, Pennsylvania. [2]Dipartimento di Scienze Mediche, Università degli Studi and Fondazione IRCCS "Ca Granda," Ospedale Maggiore Policlinico, Milan, Italy. [3]Department of Internal Medicine, University Hospital, Zürich, Switzerland. [4]Department of Cell Biology and Anatomy, College of Medicine, Tucson, Arizona. [5]Arizona Cancer Center, The University of Arizona, Tucson, Arizona. [6]Division of Gastroenterology, Department of Internal Medicine, University of Genoa, Genoa, Italy. [7]Department of Medicine, Gastroenterology, Walter Reed Army Medical Center, Washington, District of Columbia. [8]Gastrointestinal Unit "Bolognini" Hospital Seriate (BG), Milan, Italy. [9]University of Milan, Milan, Italy. [10]University of Virginia Medical Center, Charlottesville, Virginia. [11]Division of General Medicine, Beth Israel Deaconess Medical Center, Boston, Massachusetts. [12]Department of Gastroenterology and Metabolism, Nagoya City University Graduate School of Medical Sciences, Nagoya, Japan. [13]Laboratory of Clinical Pharmacology, Division of Gastroenterology, Department of Clinical Sciences, School of Medicine and Dentistry, University of Parma, Parma, Italy. [14]Division of Gastroenterology, McMaster University Medical Centre, Hamilton, Ontario, Canada. [15]Mayo Clinic College of Medicine, Jacksonville, Florida. [16]Department of Medical and Surgical Critical Care, Unit of Surgery, University of Florence, Florence, Italy. [17]Department of Medical and Surgical Critical Care, Unit of Human Pathology, University of Florence, Florence, Italy. [18]Department of Pharmacology, University of Florence, Florence, Italy. [19]Farncombe Family Digestive Disease Research Institute, Department of Gastroenterology, McMaster University Health Science Centre, Hamilton, Ontario, Canada

The following on proton pump inhibitors (PPIs) and chemoprevention in relation to Barrett's esophagus includes commentaries on 48-h pH monitoring, pH-impedence, bile acid testing, dyspepsia, long/short segment Barrett's esophagus, nonerosive reflux disease (NERD), functional heartburn, dual-release delivery PPIs, immediate-release PPIs, long-term PPI use, prokinetic agents, obesity, baclofen, nocturnal acid breakthrough, nonsteroidal anti-inflammatory drugs (NSAIDs), and new PPIs.

Keywords: pH testing; 48-h acid reflux monitoring; ACG guidelines; PPI therapy; Symptom Association Probability; GERD; bile acids; Bilitec probe; functional dyspepsia; functional heartburn; Barrett's esophagus; acid suppression; NERD; ilaprazole; tenatoprazole; CMA omeprazole; rabeprazole; dexlansoprazole; fundic glands polyp; *Clostridium difficile*; erosive esophigitis; pharmacokinetic changes; GABA$_B$; baclofen; TLESR; nocturnal acid breakthrough; COX-2 inhibitors; AspECT trial; STU-Na; API-023

Concise summaries

- In nonerosive reflux disease (NERD) patients, refractory to proton pump inhibitors (PPIs) and undergoing 96-h wireless pH monitoring, off- and on-therapy testing may be useful.
- The performance of the catheter-free wireless pH capsule in measuring esophageal acid exposure has been validated in simultaneous controlled trials. It can be now recommended to perform pH tests on patients with a "low probability" of GERD and persistent symptoms on PPIs "off-therapy" for at least seven days. In this scenario, acid measurement alone is sufficient because nonacid reflux is only relevant during acid suppression.

doi: 10.1111/j.1749-6632.2011.06048.x

- pH-impedance is currently the diagnostic tool of choice in the evaluation of patients with persistent symptoms on PPI therapy.
- The major goal of bile and acid testing should be to evaluate the type of reflux, so that the patients with mixed reflux can be identified and followed more closely, because these patients have a potentially increased risk to develop dysplasia and esophageal adenocarcinoma.
- No therapy has been shown to be highly effective in patients with functional dyspepsia (FD). Patients with an overlap of functional heartburn (FH) and dyspeptic symptoms respond less than patients with NERD and hypersensitive esophagus to antisecretory therapy, and this seems to sustain the fact that patients with functional GI disorders are less likely to respond to antisecretory drugs.
- Given some of the differences that have been found between long-segment BE patients and short-segment BE patients, it seems logical that long-segment BE patients would require a higher dose of PPI to achieve adequate intraesophageal acid suppression, but this is still to be shown. Esophageal pH monitoring is required to determine the appropriate PPI dose.
- The low response rate of NERD to PPIs is probably a feature of true NERD patients, whereas FH patients should not respond at all to these drugs. In patients "refractory" to PPI therapy, the underlying pathogenesis of symptoms needs to be reevaluated, preferably by pH-impedance monitoring, conducted "off" therapy.
- Developing PPIs with longer half-lives or ones that incorporate delivery technologies to prolong their absorption are rational ways to improve their pharmacology and effectiveness. The only one of these newer drugs currently available in the United States, dexlansoprazole-MR, does have more convenient dosing, a longer duration of action, consistent clinical efficacy, and excellent safety and tolerability.
- The clinical implications of long-term use of PPIs can best be understood by calculating numbers-needed-to-harm, using the estimates of relative risk and unexposed incidence rate of the complication, from the major studies in each area.
- Newer PPIs, formulated for delayed release appear to reduce nocturnal intragastric acidity to a greater extent than current delayed release PPIs, when given once-daily. On the other hand, immediate release PPIs have several advantages over enterically-coated PPIs. They have outstanding nocturnal acid control when given twice daily and can provide very good acid support when given at bedtime. An additional advantage is the ability to take the medication independent of food consumption. Prokinetic agents may be considered as a valuable addition to the treatment of Barrett's patients. Taking into account the comorbidities and consequent cotherapies often needed in obese patients, the low propensity for drug-to-drug interactions of rabeprazole makes this PPI particularly suitable for these patients with any acid-related diseases.
- Published studies on baclofen, a GABA$_B$ agonist, relate to its effects on the lower esophageal sphincter (LES) and esophageal reflux in normal and reflux patients. However, although baclofen has been shown to decrease TLESRs specifically in the postprandial state, there are a few studies to suggest that it may be effective in supine reflux and duodenogastroesophageal reflux.
- No trial has definitely shown the efficacy of any kind of chemoprevention in BE. However, relevant but not decisive clinical and experimental data stand for the association aspirin/PPIs to be potentially capable of a synergistic effect.
- In spite of uncertainties, the prospect of truly once-daily antisecretory drugs is now real, and they offer a lack of significant food interaction and an overall consistent acid control with less pulsatile acid exposure and improved control of nighttime acid secretion with fewer episodes of so-called "nocturnal acid breakthrough." The potential benefit of this new generation of antisecretory drugs is to prevent GERD complications, and the progression of Barrett's esophagus (BE).

1. Should 48-h acid reflux monitoring be strongly recommended in patients on PPIs with persistent GERD symptoms?

Joel E. Richter
jrichter@temple.edu

The wireless pH system (Bravo capsule, Given Imaging, Israel) uses a radiotelemetry pH-sensing capsule that is attached to the mucosa of the distal esophagus. It is positioned by endoscopy 6 cm above the squamocolumnar junction or can be placed after traditional manometry 5 cm above the proximal border of the LES. The capsule simultaneously measures pH and transmits data via a radiofrequency signal to a pager-sized receiver clipped to the patient's belt. The performance of the catheter-free wireless pH capsule in measuring esophageal acid exposure has been validated against catheter-based antimony pH electrode systems in simultaneous controlled trials.[1]

The main advantages of the wireless system are the lack of a transnasal catheter and that its position can be fixed. Tolerability is better with the wireless system when compared with catheter-based pH monitoring in both uncontrolled observations and randomized comparison studies.[2] As a result, patients can be more active, eat regularly, sleep better, and attend work or other activities that may other-

wise aggravate their GERD symptoms. Tolerability also allows the study to be done for up to 48 h routinely, and sometimes longer, if the battery is changed. Not surprisingly, longer studies are better for identifying abnormal acid exposure times (AETs) or reflux symptom relationships when compared to the traditional 24-h study.[3,4] However, it must be remembered that the capsule with its antimony pH electrode is only accurate in measuring acid reflux and should be done with the patient off PPIs for one to two weeks.

Many studies have shown that patients with typical or atypical symptoms on PPIs do not have acid reflux. Despite the enthusiasm for nonacid reflux, an average of only 30–40% have increased episodes of nonacid (pH 4–6) reflux, with or without symptom correlation. Thus, 50–60% of patients on PPIs have normal studies, even if impedance testing is performed.[5] In these settings, we are left with the unsettling question of what to do with PPI therapy. Should the PPIs be continued because GERD is controlled and symptoms have another etiology? Or, perhaps the patient never had GERD, and therefore PPIs can be stopped while alternative diagnoses are evaluated? The latter situation is particularly important in patients with atypical GERD symptoms, where the lack of acid reflux allows the gastroenterologist to refer these patients back to ENT, lung,

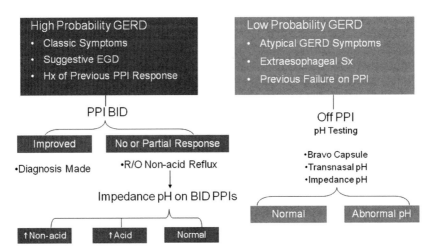

Figure 1. All forms of pH testing can be done, but, clinically, the Bravo capsule is usually preferred because of its tolerability and ease for recording acid reflux for at least 48 h. If pH testing while off PPIs is negative (normal acid exposure time and a negative symptom–reflux association), GERD is very unlikely. Patients with heartburn as a predominant symptom may be labeled as having functional heartburn, whereas those with atypical symptoms will require workup for other etiologies.

or cardiac specialists for evaluation of alternative diagnoses.

As shown in Figure 1, many experts now recommend performing pH tests on patients with a "low probability" of GERD and persistent symptoms while using PPIs "off-therapy" for at least seven days.[5,6] In this scenario, acid measurement alone is sufficient because nonacid reflux is only relevant during acid suppression.

2. Should use of a wireless system with recording of off- and on-therapy testing be recommended for patients with normal endoscopy that do not respond to PPI therapy?

Roberto Penagini and Andrea Tenca
roberto.penagini@unimi.it

The wireless system for pH monitoring has some advantages over the traditional catheter-based system. Owing to the more prolonged period of recording, it has a higher likelihood of detecting symptom/reflux association, especially when infrequent symptoms are present, as well as pathological esophageal AET. In addition, it allows endoscopic and pH monitoring assessment in the same session. Finally, it allows pH monitoring in patients who refuse or do not tolerate the traditional pH or pH + impedance catheter-based testing. These patients represent around 8% of all patients referred for pH testing.

A few studies have investigated if it was feasible to study patients both off and on PPIs during the same test. Calabrese *et al.*[7] assessed 24 patients with NERD responding to PPIs during one day off and three days on PPI, randomizing the patients to omeprazole, 20 mg; pantoprazole, 40 mg; or lansoprazole, 30 mg once daily. They found that by the second day on PPI, AET was normalized in 7/8 patients with each of the three drugs.

Two studies have involved patients refractory to PPIs[8,9]: Hirano *et al.*[8] studied 18 NERD patients during one day off and three days on rabeprazole, 20 mg twice daily. One patient was excluded for premature capsule detachment. On day 1, 9/17 patients had pathological AET and 15/17 had symptoms, four of whom had a positive symptom index (SI). On day 4, one patient only had both pathological AET and positive SI; all the others had normal AET, but 11 still had symptoms. Garrean *et al.*[9] studied

Table 1. Patients with capsule detachment during 96-h wireless pH monitoring (percentage in parentheses)

	≤ Day 2	Day 3	Day 4
Hirano *et al.*[8]	0/18	1/18 (6%)	1/18 (6%)
Scarpulla *et al.*[10]	5/83 (6%)	26/83 (31%)	14/83 (17%)
Calabrese *et al.*[7]	0/24	0/24	0/24
Garrean *et al.*[9]	0/60	4/60 (7%)	5/60 (8%)
Grigolon *et al.*[11]	3/57 (5%)	9/57 (16%)	9/57 (16%)

60 patients, 49 of whom had NERD during two days off and two days on either rabeprazole, 20 mg, or omeprazole/sodium bicarbonate, 40 mg twice daily. Twenty studies were discarded, either because of capsule detachment or loss of data transmission. On day 1 or 2, 14/40 patients had pathological AET, and 36/40 had symptoms; in 18 of them the symptom association probability (SAP) was positive. On day 4, all patients apart from 1 had a normal AET; however, 28 were still symptomatic, and SAP was positive in only four of them. These data confirm that most patients refractory to PPIs either do not have GERD or are not only sensitive to acid.

In conclusion, in NERD patients refractory to PPIs and undergoing 96-h wireless pH monitoring, off- and on-therapy testing may be useful. Clinicians should be aware, however, of two limitations: a considerable number of capsules may detach during day 3 or 4 (Table 1), thus decreasing the power of on-therapy testing; and the role of weakly acidic reflux cannot be assessed.

3. Are there therapeutic implications for impedance testing in patients unresponsive to PPI therapy?

Daniel Pohl
daniel.pohl@usz.ch

GERD is a prevalent clinical condition occurring in 10–30% of the population. The majority of patients respond to PPI therapy. However, community-based studies have shown that approximately 40% of patients supplement their prescription PPI with oral antacids and/or H_2-receptor antagonists, indicating that partial or complete therapy failure may occur in a significant proportion of patients.

The single most important reason for a failing PPI is a wrong diagnosis of GERD. The primary goal, therefore, must be to validate the diagnosis of GERD in a patient presenting with PPI failure. According to the Montreal classification, GERD is diagnosed on the basis of refluxate entering the esophagus, which causes symptoms and/or mucosal damage. In the absence of erosions in the esophagus, which are rarely present in a patient on PPI treatment, an association between patient symptoms and reflux should be documented. Objective parameters, such as an abnormal number of reflux episodes or AET, support the diagnosis of GERD. Because establishing a true diagnosis of GERD is key, the most appropriate diagnostic tools should be used.

Even with perfect acid control, patients may still experience reflux symptoms. Weakly acidic or nonacidic reflux may cause typical (and atypical) symptoms of reflux disease. Up to 70% of heartburn episodes in PPI refractory patients may be associated with weakly acidic reflux, and only esophageal proximal extent has been identified as an important factor in reflux perception.[12] pH-impedance allows the association between weakly acidic/nonacidic reflux and patient symptoms, as well as validation of acid reflux by acid reflux episodes, thereby differentiating reflux disease from functional disorders that should be considered outside the realm of GERD and treated differently.[13]

Few outcome studies are available based on findings from pH-impedance testing. Mainie *et al.* followed 19 patients who were refractory to PPI twice a day that underwent a successful laparoscopic Nissen fundoplication. Before surgery, 18 of the 19 patients were found to have a positive symptom association on MII-pH monitoring (14 with nonacid and 4 with acid reflux). After a mean follow-up of 14 months, 16 of the 18 patients with a positive symptom association were asymptomatic.[14] Becker *et al.* assessed 56 patients with persistent symptoms on a once daily dose of PPI and abnormal MII-pH monitoring results. Most of these patients had a positive symptom association, and later demonstrated a significantly higher response rate to increasing the PPI dose to twice a day compared to patients with normal MII-pH monitoring results.[15] Del Genio *et al.* prospectively assessed the outcomes of laparoscopic Nissen fundoplication in patients who were PPI nonresponsive or noncompliant. All 62 surgically treated patients had a positive MII-pH monitoring result. The overall patient satisfaction rate was 98.3%, and no differences were found in clinical outcomes based on preoperative MII-pH or manometry results.[16]

In conclusion, pH-impedance is currently the diagnostic tool of choice in the evaluation of patients

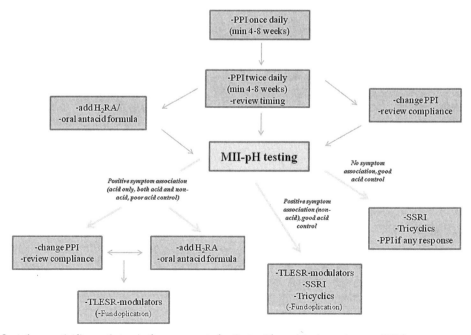

Figure 2. A therapeutic/diagnostic tree in the assessment of patients with persistent symptoms on PPI therapy.

with persistent symptoms on PPI therapy. A therapeutic/diagnostic tree in the assessment of patients with persistent symptoms on PPI therapy is suggested in Figure 2.

4. What can be currently expected from bile and acid reflux testing?

Katerina Dvorak and Aaron Goldman
kdvorak@email.arizona.edu

The major risk factor for BE development is gastroesophageal reflux disease (GERD). Although the importance of gastroesophageal reflux in the pathogenesis of BE is undisputed, it is not yet clear which elements in the refluxate are responsible for metaplastic change to the intestinal epithelium.[17] Hydrophobic bile acids are associated with gastrointestinal cancers, including colon cancer, and they are considered to play also a major role in BE and EAC development.[17] A majority of BE patients and especially those with dysplastic BE have mixed reflux (bile and acid). Importantly, the damaging effects of gastric acid and bile are synergestic. Our recent studies revealed that a combination of bile acids and weak acid induces DNA damage that is significantly higher compared to damage induced by individual agents alone. Therefore, simultaneous bile and acid testing is important.

Pathologic exposure to duodenal refluxate, as measured by Bilitec monitoring, was observed in 22.2% of patients with esophagitis (EE), 54.5% of patients with BE, and 78.6% of patients with EAC, indicating the importance of bile acids in EAC pathogenesis.[18] Duodenoesophageal reflux is mutagenic as shown by *in vivo* experiments using Big Blue rats[19] and Big Blue mice.[20] In agreement with this conclusion, Fein *et al.* also demonstrated that duodenoesophageal reflux induces EAC without exogenous carcinogen. In addition, another study showed that the typical injuries and cellular changes seen in severe reflux EE, that may lead to development of BE, are induced in rats by continuous perfusion with bovine bile treatment for only four weeks. Overall, the evidence indicates that bile acids contribute to the development of BE and EAC. A diet high in fat increases the release of bile acids into the gastrointestinal tract, thus also increasing the concentration of bile acids in the refluxate.

However, currently only pH monitoring and management of acid reflux is the main strategy to evaluate and treat patients with GERD and BE. The probes to measure exposure to acid were successfully developed and they can accurately measure changes in esophageal pH. By contrast, the reflux of bile is not routinely monitored and the studies evaluating actual bile reflux are not common. The major problem is that the methods that are used to study bile reflux are cumbersome and have limitations.

The presence of bile in the esophagus may be detected spectrophotometrically by a miniature fiber optic system (Bilitec probe). This method of measuring bilirubin absorbance can be combined with a pH probe and allows prolonged monitoring of duodenal reflux. Direct aspiration studies of refluxate followed by gas or liquid chromatography are the most precise methods for the detection of the concentration and individual bile acids present in the refluxate. However, these methods are not useful for routine monitoring, because they are demanding and require special instruments.

Impedance is another method that can measure the frequency, duration, and extent of reflux episodes. This method detects gastroesophageal reflux events on the basis of a change in resistance to the flow of an electrical current between pairs of electrodes. When this method is combined with pH monitoring, it is possible to determine acid, weak acid, and alkaline reflux. However, this method cannot determine the composition of refluxate and/or the concentration of bile acids in the esophagus.

Importantly, the activity of bile acids depends on the pH. There are marked differences in the behavior of bile acids depending on the pH of the solution. At low pH in the stomach (pH $\sim$2), the majority of bile acids present in the refluxate irreversibly precipitate. Only taurine-conjugated bile acids are soluble at this pH; however, taurine-conjugated bile acids constitute only $\sim$20% of total bile acids present in the refluxate. At a higher pH ($\sim$4–7) glycine-conjugated and unconjugated bile acids are soluble, unionized, and thus they interact with esophageal mucosa and cause cell damage. This pH zone is considered the most dangerous, because the combined effects of bile acids and acid lead to altered signaling, increased DNA damage, and mutations.

Molecular imprinting using a biosensor specific for bile acid is a promising novel technique that can be developed to detect bile acids present in the esophagus. The principle of this technology involves selection of a polymer that is capable of forming noncovalent interactions with a template molecule such as glycocholic acid.[21] Currently, however, the Bilitec probe in combination with pH monitoring is the only approach to monitor true reflux of bile and acid. There are five major outcomes that can be expected: (1) no reflux, (2) reflux of acid only, (3) reflux of bile only, (4) weak acid and bile reflux, and (5) acid and bile reflux.

In summary, the major goal of bile and acid testing should be to evaluate the type of reflux, so that patients with mixed reflux can be identified and followed more closely; potentially these patients have increased risk of developing dysplasia and esophageal adenocarcinoma.

5. Are patients with dyspepsia less responsive to PPI therapy?

Edoardo Savarino, Patrizia Zentilin, and Vincenzo Savarino
edoardo.savarino@unige.it

FD is a frequent disorder in Western countries.[22] In recent years many definitions of dyspepsia have been attempted and, actually, the last iteration of the Rome III criteria defined FD as the presence of one or more of the following symptoms (epigastric pain, epigastric burning, postprandial fullness, early satiation) thought to originate in the gastroduodenal region, in the absence of any organic, systemic, or metabolic disease that would otherwise likely explain the symptoms.[23]

The pathophysiology of FD is unclear, but it is likely to be multifactorial.[22] Putative mechanisms include overlapping disorders of upper gastrointestinal motor and sensory function. Among them, delayed gastric emptying, impaired fundic accommodation to a meal, altered visceral sensation (e.g., increased gastric hypersensitivity to mechanical distention, and duodenal hypersensitivity), *Helicobacter pylori* induced gastritis, and increased sensitivity to acid infusion have been encountered in many patients with FD. Therefore, the main therapeutic approaches to its management are represented by acid inhibition, prokinetic drugs, and *H. pylori* eradication (Fig. 3).

However, the role of acid suppression is controversial, and randomized controlled trials evaluating the efficacy of antisecretory therapy have given conflicting results.[22,24] A meta-analysis of controlled,

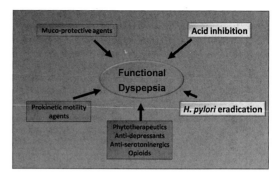

Figure 3. Treatment options for functional dyspepsia.

randomized trials with PPIs in FD reported that this class of agents was superior to placebo with a number needed to treat (NNT) of 7. In particular, four trials compared PPI therapy with placebo and antacids in 2,164 patients with uninvestigated dyspepsia. PPI therapy was more effective (RR, 0.65; 95% confidence interval [CI], 0.55–0.78), with a NNT of 5 (95% CI, 4–7). Eight trials compared PPI therapy with placebo in 3,293 patients with nonulcer dyspepsia. PPI therapy was significantly superior to placebo with a NNT of 9. The lower rate of response compared with that obtained in patients with uninvestigated dyspepsia was due to the exclusion of patients with organic dyspepsia by endoscopy, because these latter ones respond satisfactorily to PPIs. Anyway, there was significant heterogeneity between results, and the major problem with these trials remains potential misclassification bias regarding GERD. In a more recent meta-analysis, Wang *et al.*[25] evaluated a total of seven studies consisting of 3,725 patients analyzed. There was a modest but statistically significant difference in symptom relief in FD patients receiving PPIs (40.3%) compared with those given placebo (32.7%) (RRR, 10.3%; 95% CI, 2.7%–17.3%). The estimated NNT was 14.6 patients (95% CI, 8.7–57.1). This finding was consistent across different doses of PPIs and the patients' status of *H. pylori* infection.

It is relevant to note that a large placebo effect has been documented in many trials aimed at treating FD, which can range from 5% to 85% of patients, with an average value of about 40%.[22,24,25] It has been speculated that this may be due to variance in trial duration, patient selection, recruitment issues, number of subjects included in the study, and other study design factors. Finally, we have recently published a large prospective study,[26] where patients

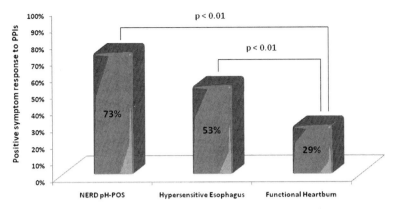

Figure 4. Treatment response to PPIs of patients with nonerosive reflux disease, hypersensitive esophagus, and functional heartburn.

with FH, identified by means of impedance-pH monitoring, had a high association with dyspeptic symptoms, and these results showed them to be less responsive to PPI treatment than patients with pH-POS NERD and hypersensitive esophagus (Fig. 4). This finding seems to confirm the poor response of FD to PPIs.

In conclusion, no therapy has been shown to be highly effective in patients with FD. PPIs seem to be more effective than placebo in several meta-analyses, but this occurs mainly in dyspeptic patients complaining of epigastric pain and burning, even if the degree of treatment response appears to be from mild to moderate. Patients with an overlap of FH and dyspeptic symptoms respond less well than patients with NERD and hypersensitive esophagus to antisecretory therapy, and this seems to sustain the fact that patients with functional GI disorders are less likely to respond to antisecretory drugs. Other treatments have to be adopted.

6. Should the dose of PPI be the same for short- and long-segment Barrett's esophagus?

Joshua T. Watson and Roy K.H. Wong
Joshua.watson5@us.army.mil

BE is a consequence of chronic acid reflux, and many patients with BE are placed on high-dose PPIs indefinitely to adequately control reflux symptoms or to achieve adequate acid suppression. Some gastroenterologists have postulated that achieving adequate acid suppression may be more difficult in long-segment BE patients as opposed to short-segment

BE patients. As such, BE patients are commonly prescribed high dosages of PPIs; however, with the mounting concerns about the potential negative consequences of long-term, high-dose PPIs, such as inhibition of bone resorption, small bowel bacterial overgrowth, enteric infections, bloating, and abdominal pain, gastroenterologists must take another look at their use of PPIs and ask, Are we using too much?

Given some of the differences that have been found between long-segment and short-segment BE patients, it seems logical that long-segment BE patients would require a higher dose of PPI. First, in a study by Loughney *et al.*,[27] they found that long-segment BE patients had weaker LESs and decreased distal esophageal peristaltic contractions compared to short-segment BE patients and controls, which could contribute to a greater reflux diathesis in the long-segment BE patients. They also showed that long-segment BE patients have significantly higher Johnson–DeMeester (JD) scores than patients with short-segment BE or controls. Interestingly, this trend held true even at 0 cm from the LES, where one would think that the groups may have more similar acid reflux exposure. Similar trends were also seen for percent total reflux, percent upright reflux, and percent supine reflux with long-segment BE having a greater degree of both upright and supine reflux than short-segment BE patients. This study and others have thus suggested that long-segment BE patients tend to have weaker LESs, decreased distal esophageal peristaltic contractions, and a greater degree of acid reflux.

Fass *et al.* later showed that there was a direct correlation between intraesophageal acid exposure and the length of Barrett's mucosa.[28] They demonstrated that the greater percentage of total time the esophageal pH is less than 4, the longer the Barrett's segment tends to be. This trend was also seen for percent upright time pH < 4 and percent supine time pH < 4. Thus, they concluded that the duration of esophageal acid exposure is an important contributing factor in determining the length of Barrett's mucosa. Given the correlation between upright and supine reflux, it is also likely that both nocturnal and diurnal esophageal acid exposure are important in determining the length of BE as well. Other studies have also implicated duodenogastroesophageal reflux in the development of BE and have shown that long-segment BE patients tend to have more duodenogastroesophageal reflux than short-segment BE patients.

Overall, existing studies suggest that long-segment BE patients tend to have less competent LESs, longer hiatal hernias, greater esophageal acid exposure, and a greater degree of duodenogastroesophageal reflux. However, what is yet to be determined is if these factors translate clinically into long-segment BE patients requiring higher doses of PPI than short-segment BE patients to achieve adequate intraesophageal acid suppression. Only a few studies have broached this question, most of which have done so indirectly. The fact that achieving symptomatic control in BE patients does not predict normalization of intraesophageal acid has been well established. Outau-Lascar *et al.* performed a study in which BE patients' dose of PPI was escalated until symptom control was achieved; then 24-h ambulatory pH monitoring was performed. They found that the length of Barrett's mucosa did not predict those who were going to have pathologic reflux despite symptom control.[29] As in many studies that have looked at PPI dosing, they based the PPI dose on symptoms, not on Barrett's length or pH monitoring results; so, it is unclear if treating based on normalization of pH would have yielded different results. In another study by Fass *et al.*,[30] BE patients were treated with high-dose PPI (omeprazole, 40 mg twice daily). They found no difference in the rates of failure to achieve acid control between short-segment and long-segment BE patients. However, they only enrolled short-segment BE patients with Barrett's mucosa of at least 2 cm in length and long-segment BE patients with Barrett's mucosa of 6 cm or fewer. Wani *et al.* also placed

BE patients on high-dose PPI therapy and then performed 24-h pH testing.[31] With patients taking rabeprazole, 20 mg twice daily, they noted that the length of Barrett's mucosa was not significantly different between those with normal pH profiles and those with abnormal pH profiles. While these studies suggest that there is no difference between short-segment and long-segment BE patients with regard to the difficulty in achieving adequate acid suppression, no study has directly compared the dose of PPI needed to achieve normal intraesophageal acid exposure in short segment BE patients versus long-segment BE patients.

A study is currently in progress at Walter Reed Army Medical Center that will hopefully provide more insight into this area. Patients with BE and with gastroesophageal junction–specialized intestinal metaplasia are being enrolled and started on, or switched to, omeprazole, 20 mg once daily. After being on this dose for at least one week, patients fill out a symptom questionnaire and undergo an EGD with placement of a Bravo pH monitoring capsule. Day 2 data from the Bravo pH study are used to calculate a JD score and to assess percent time that the esophageal pH is less than 4.2%. If patients have a normal pH study, defined as having an esophageal pH < 4 for less than 4.2% of the time and a normal JD score, they are considered adequately controlled. If, however, they have an abnormal pH study, the dose of omeprazole is increased to 20 mg twice daily. Again, after at least a week on the increased dose, they fill out a symptom questionnaire and undergo a second EGD with Bravo capsule placement. Thus far, we have completed data on 26 patients: 6 with ultrashort segments, 13 with short segments, and 7 with long segments. As with most BE studies, the patients are mostly Caucasian (88%) and male (77%), and prevalence of hiatal hernias is high

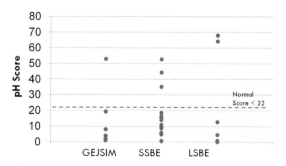

Figure 5. Bravo pH score for omeprazole, 20 mg.

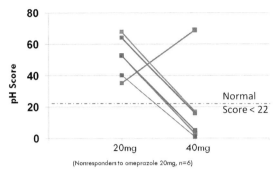

Figure 6. Change in Bravo pH score: single- vs. double-dose PPI.

(85%). No differences between the groups reach statistical significance at this time, but 2/7 (29%) long-segment BE patients have required twice daily dosing compared to 3/13 (23%) short-segment BE patients and 1/6 (17%) ultrashort-segment BE patients. Surprisingly, 20/26 (77%) patients overall have been controlled on once daily dosing (Fig. 5), and only one patient has not been adequately controlled on twice daily dosing (Fig. 6). These early data show that normalization of intraesophageal pH can be achieved in a significant percentage of patients taking omeprazole, 20–40 mg daily, which suggests that BE patients may require lower doses of PPIs than previously thought. Also, despite significant pathophysiologic differences that have been demonstrated between short-segment and long-segment BE patients, there is no evidence so far that long-segment BE patients routinely require higher PPI doses than short-segment BE patients. Larger numbers may be needed to show a difference between the two groups. Finally, our study and several other studies have suggested that esophageal pH monitoring may be required in BE patients to determine the appropriate PPI dose.

7. Is a low response to PPIs a challenge for the treatment of patients with NERD or of those classified as patients with functional heartburn? Should pathogenesis of symptoms be reevaluated in these cases?

Fabio Pace and Valentina Casini
fabio.pace@unimi.it

NERD is at present defined according to the Vevey Working Groups, as follows: "NERD is a subcategory of GERD characterized by troublesome reflux-related symptoms in the absence of esophageal mucosal erosions/breaks at conventional endoscopy and without recent acid-suppressive therapy."[32] The question posed by the title may be split into two more specific ones: do NERD patients respond to PPI similarly to ERD patients? And should NERD nonresponders be further investigated (by pH or pH-impedance monitoring)?

Concerning the first issue, it has been known for many years that NERD patients, for the most part, tend to respond to PPI therapy less effectively; as an example, Dean *et al.* have shown in a systematic review of the literature that the PPI symptomatic response pooled rate was 36.7% in NERD patients and 55.5% in those with erosive EE.[33] The lower response rate in NERD could be due to one of several factors: it is possible that the symptoms in these patients have nothing to do with GERD and are related to other factors. In particular, because NERD is a negatively defined clinical entity, it is possible that a percentage of so-called NERD patients are rather patients affected by FH, which by definition does not respond to PPI therapy.[34]

To overcome the possible influence of an involuntary inclusion of FH patients, we designed a therapeutic study on GERD patients with typical symptoms with and without erosive EE. The study started with a two-week period of high-dose omeprazole, 20 mg twice daily (the so-called omeprazole test). Patients responding to this test period entered an acute phase (3 months) of treatment with any available PPI at a standard dose. In this way we presumably excluded patients not responding to PPI therapy, that is, FH by definition; 577 patients with heartburn were recruited, 306 with EE and 271 without (NERD). Of them, 519 (89.9%) had a positive PPI test, with a greater response in EE patients (96.4%) compared with NERD (82.6%) ($P = 0.011$). Both the percentage of completely asymptomatic patients and the reduction of heartburn intensity at 3 months were significantly higher in the EE compared with NERD patients ($P < 0.01$). The study suggests therefore that "true" NERD may in fact have a genuine lower response to PPIs, that is, not due to misdiagnosis.

Concerning the second question as to whether NERD patients refractory to PPI therapy should be further investigated by esophageal pH monitoring or by esophageal pH impedance (pH-IM), a recent position paper by the ROME 3 Working

Groups has clarified that either examinations can be performed, but necessarily off-therapy. We would like to recall our own experience,[35] conducted on 460 consecutive outpatients referred to our laboratory to undergo pH-IM, largely due to refractoriness to PPI therapy. In this retrospective study we found that pH-IM resulted positively in 45% of patients with a negative pH monitoring (67% of the total), leading to a change in the treatment in about 47% of cases. Thus, pH-IM, and not pH-monitoring alone, was able to substantially increase the diagnostic yield. On the basis of this experience, we recommend that NERD patients refractory to PPI therapy undergo pH impedance, possibly "off" therapy.

To finally answer the initial question, we may conclude that the low response rate of patients with NERD to PPIs is probably a feature of actual NERD patients, whereas FH patients should not respond at all to these drugs. When a NERD patient is "refractory" to PPI therapy, the underlying pathogenesis of symptoms needs to be reevaluated, preferably by investigating the reflux pattern by pH-impedance monitoring, conducted "off" therapy.

8. What is to be expected from the "dual-release delivery" action of newly developed PPIs?

David A. Peura
dap8v@virginia.edu

Pharmacologic treatment for GERD is directed at acid suppression, and PPIs have emerged as the medication class of choice. PPIs irreversibly block the final step of acid secretion by binding to the proton pump, and secretion can only be restored when new pumps are activated or synthesized. In addition, PPIs only inhibit active proton pumps, and activation largely occurs by eating food. Not all pumps are activated during a meal, so later food intake will stimulate dormant pumps. Also new pumps are continually regenerated throughout the day. Because all PPIs share the same mechanism of action and all have short half-lives (approximately one to two h), the potential for subsequent acid secretion exists when dormant or newly regenerated pumps are activated after drug concentrations fall below therapeutic levels. Because food is the primary stimulus for pump activation, PPIs need to be taken at

mealtime (usually 30–60 min before breakfast) to ensure maximum pharmacodynamic (PD) effect. The short half-life and requirement for meal-timed administration are inherent pharmacologic limitations of the PPI class that likely explain compliance and adherence-related persistent or breakthrough symptoms in as many as 40% of regular PPI users.

Strategies to extend the duration of action (and AUC) of PPIs include administering a higher dose of medication, using a more slowly metabolized enantiomer, or dosing medication twice daily. Higher dose medication and more slowly metabolized enantiomers only minimally affect plasma/time drug concentrations and still require meal-timed administration. Twice daily dosing increases cost of treatment, can negatively affect compliance, and is currently not FDA approved, which makes insurance approval more difficult. Developing PPIs with longer half-lives or ones that incorporate delivery technologies to prolong their absorption are more rational ways to improve their pharmacology and effectiveness. Longer half-life drugs include ilaprazole (3.6 h), which is currently marketed in China, and tenatoprazole (8–14 h), which has yet to reach the world market. Chemically metered absorption (CMA) omeprazole (not yet marketed), extended-release rabeprazole (FDA accepted NDA 6/4/10), and dexlansoprazole-MR[36] (available in the United States) are examples of prolonged absorption technologies. The later compound incorporates the more slowly metabolized dextrorotatory isomer of lansoprazole, (R)-lansoprazole, with a pH-dependant dual-delayed release delivery system.

The elimination half-life of dexlansoprazole is about one to two hours, which is similar to other PPIs, but the dual-delayed release formulation extends drug plasma time concentration to 10–12 hours,[37] which in turn enhances its ability to control intragastric pH. PK and PD studies show that dexlansoprazole-MR can be given without regard to food and can be dosed any time of day. Such dosing versatility is especially useful for patients who skip meals (especially breakfast), who find it difficult to dose medication before meal time, or who eat at irregular times.

Clinical studies[38] show that dexlansoprazole-MR, 60 mg, consistently heals all grades of erosive EE during eight weeks of dosing. The 30-mg dose effectively maintained daytime and night symptom control and EE healing during 6 months of treatment. The 30-mg dose also provides full 24-h heartburn relief for patients with symptomatic nonerosive GERD. The safety and tolerability profiles of both 60- and 30-mg doses are similar to lansoprazole.

PPIs have inherent pharmacologic limitations, short half-lives and a requirement for meal-related dosing, which influences their effectiveness and patient compliance. Newer technologies that extend PPI duration of action permit more versatile administration. Whether these newer medications improve compliance, overall effectiveness of acid suppression, and clinical outcomes remains to be seen. The only one of these newer drugs currently available in the United States, dexlansoprazole-MR, has more convenient dosing, a longer duration of action, consistent clinical efficacy, and excellent safety and tolerability. In this regard, it does address some of the unmet needs of the traditional PPIs.

9. How should issues regarding long-term use of PPIs be considered?

Shoshana J. Herzig
sherzig@bidmc.harvard.edu

Since the introduction of omeprazole in 1988, the use of PPIs has climbed rapidly. Although incident use has been relatively stable in the last several years, prevalent use of these drugs continues to increase, reflecting increased numbers of long-term users. Long-term use accounts for a large proportion of use of these medications, if not the majority, depending on the definition used—one study found that 84% of PPI prescriptions are repeat prescriptions. Up to half of initial prescriptions occur during a hospitalization, and 50% are subsequently continued without any evaluation of efficacy/need to continue. Although they are highly effective medications, research has consistently found that a large proportion of PPI prescriptions are not indicated.[39] Given these statistics, reports of risk have important implications. Although PPIs are relatively "safe" medications for the individual patient, even a relatively safe drug, if administered broadly, can become "unsafe" from a public health standpoint.

Fundic gland polyps
The first reports of risk associated with PPIs came in the mid-to-late 1990s when several case reports of fundic gland polyps (FGPs) were published. Since then, several large case-control and cohort studies have been conducted with somewhat conflicting findings. Although most studies find increased odds of FGPs in patients on PPIs, these odds ratios, as well as the unexposed risk estimates, vary widely among the studies, making interpretation difficult. Furthermore, the clinical significance of FGPs is uncertain, as most studies have found an exceedingly low rate of associated dysplasia. Accordingly, the association between PPIs and FGPs, should one exist, does not have obvious clinical implications at the present time. More research is necessary to more conclusively define the association and determine the clinical significance of such an association. Until then, there does not seem to be a role for routine surveillance endoscopy in patients on PPIs, other than that associated with the clinical indication for the medication.

Clostridium difficile *infection*
Studies have found that loss of stomach acidity is associated with colonization of the normally sterile upper gastrointestinal tract. Although *Clostridium difficile* is relatively acid stable, it is possible that survival of *C. difficile* spores may be facilitated by reduced gastric acidity. Given reports of increased risk of other enteric infections in patients on PPIs, several cohort and case-control studies have investigated the association between PPIs and *C. difficile* infection. A systematic review of 12 such studies found an increased risk of taking antisecretory therapy in those infected with *C. difficile* (pooled odds ratio [OR] 1.94; 95% CI, 1.37–2.75).[40]

Community-acquired pneumonia
Increased bacterial colonization of the upper gastrointestinal tract may also predispose one to development of pneumonia, as demonstrated in several studies in ventilated patients.[41] In addition, some studies have demonstrated impaired leukocyte function in patients on PPIs. Given these findings, several authors have investigated the association between PPIs and community-acquired pneumonia, generally finding an association between current use of PPIs and pneumonia, with ORs ranging from 1.02 to 1.9. An interesting finding in several studies is that there seems to be an inverse relationship between the magnitude of the association and the duration of exposure. Thus, patients who have been on long-term PPI therapy may actually be at

Table 2. Risks of long-term PPI therapy

Risk	NNTH[a]	Number exposed annually in the United States	Number harmed
C. difficile	2,400[b]	6 million	2,500
Hip fracture	1,200[c]	6 million	5,000
Pneumonia	226[41]	6 million	26,550
Fundic gland polyps	?[e]		

[a]Number needed to harm.
[b]Extrapolated from Odds ratio = 2.9; unexposed event rate = 22/100,000 persons.
[c]Extrapolated from Ref. 86. Odds ratio = 1.44; unexposed event rate = 1.8/1000 person-years.
[e]Odds ratios, as well as unexposed risk estimates vary widely among the studies, prohibiting NNTH calculation.

less risk for community-acquired pneumonia than patients in whom these medications have been recently initiated.

Hip fractures

The biological plausibility of an association between PPIs and hip fractures has been questioned, as the role of pH in calcium absorption is controversial. One large case-control study found an OR for hip fracture in patients prescribed long-term (>1 year) PPI of 1.44 (95% CI, 1.30–1.59). However, subsequent studies have failed to confirm this association, including one study using the same data set, but slightly different methods. Thus, given the controversial biological plausibility, and conflicting findings, there is insufficient evidence on which to base any clinical recommendations. However, given that vitamin D deficiency and osteoporosis are prevalent in the elderly, all elderly patients, including those on PPIs, should be reminded to assure adequate dietary calcium intake.

Conclusions and implications

The clinical implications of these risks can best be understood by calculating the numbers needed to harm. Using the estimates of relative risk and unexposed incidence rate of the complication from the major studies in each area, we can generate the approximate numbers needed to harm as listed in Table 2. With approximately 2% of the U.S. population on long-term PPIs at any given time, these numbers needed to harm translate to approximately

34,000 patients potentially harmed annually in the United States alone. Thus, although the risks are small at an individual patient level, they are potentially quite large from a population perspective.[42] Although these risks have not been conclusively demonstrated, the fact that such a large proportion of prescriptions are not indicated, coupled with the possibility of risk, should prompt us to reevaluate prescribing practices.

More specifically, the need for long-term PPI therapy should be periodically reevaluated. For those who do require long-term therapy, the lowest effective dose and the lowest effective level of acid suppression should be used.[43] Use of a histamine-2 receptor antagonist should be considered instead of a PPI, and a "step-up" approach should be used. Older adults should be reminded to ensure adequate dietary calcium intake, and consideration should be given to calcium citrate and vitamin D supplementation. Finally, behavioral interventions for nonulcer dyspepsia should be encouraged, such as eating smaller meals, weight loss, smoking cessation, and head-of-bed elevation.

10. Should prokinetic agents, such as dopaminergic antagonists, be considered as a valuable addition to the treatment of Barrett's patients?

Takeshi Kamiya
kamitake@med.nagoya-cu.ac.jp

The answer to this question may be *yes*. GERD is a major risk factor for BE and adenocarcinoma of the esophagus. Patients with GERD, including reflux EE, may develop BE, as the esophagus repeatedly is exposed to acidic gastric contents. Adenocarcinoma may develop from BE, a metaplastic change of the esophageal epithelium from squamous to intestinalized mucosa, which is associated with chronic reflux. Unfortunately, there are no evidences of the efficacy of prokinetic agents in BE. Instead, several reports concerning the role of prokinetics in the treatment of GERD have been reported.

For example, 300 mg of itopride treatment for 30 days showed a significant decrease in the instances of acid reflux.[44] Another report[45] is about the effect of addition of a prokinetic agent to PPI, in which after a 12-week treatment of PPI alone, additional mosapride for 12 weeks showed significant improvement in GERD symptoms. One randomized trial[46] showed that a combination of pantoprazole and mosapride is more effective than pantoprazole alone in patients with erosive GERD. In our study,[47] GERD patients revealed delayed gastric emptying, and mosapride showed efficacy in GERD patients, especially in those with disturbed gastric motility. In healthy volunteers, two weeks' intake of omeprazole resulted in delayed gastric emptying, and concomitant administration of tegaserod prevented delayed gastric emptying induced by omeprazole monotherapy.[48] This effect may be seen in GERD or Barrett's patients being treated with omeprazole or other PPIs.

In conclusion, these data suggest that prokinetic agents may be considered as a valuable addition to the treatment of Barrett's patients.

11. Is there a more effective proton pump inhibitor in the obese patient with GERD?

Iva Pelosini and Carmelo Scarpignato
scarpi@tin.it

Obesity represents a worldwide problem that has reached the status of an epidemic. According to the latest estimates from the World Health Organization, more than 1.5 billion adults worldwide are overweight, and 400 million of these are clinically obese (http://apps.who.int/bmi/index.jsp). Several epidemiological studies have shown an association between a patient's higher body mass index (BMI) and the risk of GERD symptoms and lesions (http://www.medscape.org/viewarticle/560076). There is also evidence to suggest that high BMI is an independent risk factor for the development of erosive EE and is associated with an increased risk of esophageal adenocarcinoma. Data from mechanistic investigations indicate that high BMI may also predispose individuals to pathologic gastroesophageal reflux. Indeed, many of the pathophysiological mechanisms involved in adult GERD are exaggerated in obesity. They include an increased prevalence of hiatus hernia, negatively affecting esophago-gastric junction integrity and function, an increased number of transient LES relaxations, increased intragastric pressure, and impaired esophageal motility.

In spite of the well-documented evidence supporting the association between obesity and GERD,

there is a surprising paucity of information in the literature concerning the impact of overweight/obesity on the efficacy of acid-suppressive therapies, such as histamine$_2$-receptor antagonists (H$_2$RAs) and PPIs. Only recently have demographic data (like BMI) been included in the analysis of the results from clinical studies. The few available data looking at body weight as prognostic indicator provide conflicting results.

Although it is known that obesity does affect drug PKs and PDs (http://www.orthosupersite.com/view.aspx?rid=19166), only few data are available in the literature dealing with the clinical efficacy of acid suppressive therapy (either H$_2$RAs or PPIs) and no one addressing their PK.

McDougall *et al.*[49] first investigated the effect of BMI and other demographic and clinical characteristics on overall prognosis in a long-term (3–4.5 years), prospective study of 77 patients with GERD. Patients requiring daily acid suppression at follow-up had significantly higher mean BMIs than those who did not (26.7 kg/m^2 vs. 23.6 kg/m^2; $P = 0.001$). Logistic regression analysis found that increased age, increased BMI, as well as initial diagnosis of EE were independently associated with an ongoing need for chronic acid-suppressive therapy ($P < 0.01$).[49] At variance with these results, Talley *et al.*[50] in a *post hoc* analysis conducted on patients receiving PPI therapy (omeprazole, 20 mg; esomeprazole, 20 or 40 mg daily) for NERD were unable to find an association between baseline BMI and the probability of patients reporting complete heartburn relief after four weeks of treatment. In this study, however, parameters assessing rapidity of symptom relief were not specifically investigated.

Two studies from the same group[51,52] investigated specifically the influence of BMI on PPI efficacy in patients with erosive EE. In the first study, Sheu *et al.*[3] tried to relate demographic factors, including BMI, to cumulative healing rates of patients with severe EE (grades C and D according to Los Angeles classification) treated with esomeprazole (40 mg daily) during a six-month period. They found that a high BMI (≥ 25 kg/m^2) was an independent risk factor to determine mucosal healing by esomeprazole. Indeed, at the end of treatment, although 98% of patients with a BMI < 25 kg/m^2 were healed, only 60% of those with a BMI ≥ 25 kg/m^2 achieved mucosal healing ($P < 0.001$). Multivariate logistic regression analysis showed a 3.6-fold increase in

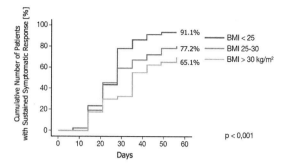

Figure 7. Sustained symptomatic response to esomeprazole in patients with Grade A-B reflux esophagitis, according to their BMI value.

odds of healing for a decrease of BMI > 1.5 kg/m²[51] The second study,[52] performed in patients with mild EE (A and B according to Los Angeles classification), addressed the influence of body weight on the efficacy of maintenance *on demand* therapy. Here again, BMI influenced negatively the symptomatic response to esomeprazole: the higher the patients' BMI, the lower the number of patients with a sustained symptomatic response (Fig. 7). A high BMI also increased the need for medication (measured as number of tablets taken each month) and the failure rate.[52]

A recent *post hoc* analysis[53] was performed to assess the effect of BMI on rabeprazole's clinical efficacy in patients with erosive GERD. The data were derived from a comparative trial assessing mucosal healing and symptom relief of rabeprazole and omeprazole (both given at 20 mg daily) in patients with mild to moderate erosive EE. Although there were no significant differences between treatments for the primary end point (i.e., healing of esophageal lesions), rabeprazole was significantly more effective than omeprazole for several secondary end points, particularly those concerning time to symptom relief. In patients with a BMI ≥ 25 kg/m², the mean time to first day of satisfactory heartburn relief (intensity ≤ 1) with rabeprazole 20 mg (2.6 ± 0.3 days) was significantly shorter versus that observed with omeprazole, 20 mg (3.8 ± 0.4 days, *P* = 0.0113; Fig. 8).

In patients with a BMI < 25 kg/m², there was a numerical trend in favor of rabeprazole compared with omeprazole, but the difference fell short of statistical significance (3.1 ± 0.5 vs. 5.0 ± 0.9 days, respectively; *P* = 0.1996). Similarly, significantly more patients taking rabeprazole in the overweight/obese

BMI category achieved satisfactory heartburn relief in each of the first three treatment days compared with patients who received omeprazole (59.2% vs. 46.6%; *P* = 0.0256). By contrast, in lean patients no differences between rabeprazole and omeprazole were found for this end point (rabeprazole, 52.7%; omeprazole, 48.8%; *P* = 0.6065).

Although it is difficult to compare the results obtained with various PPIs in different studies, due to different patient populations and different experimental design, the opposite behavior (better versus lower efficacy in GERD) of rabeprazole and esomeprazole suggests that the influence of overweight/obesity on drug efficacy is molecule dependent and does not represent a class effect. The reasons underlying the observed difference between these two PPIs are not clear but may reflect unknown PK changes in obesity. Either the volume of distribution (Vd) and/or the hepatic catabolism of PPIs could be altered in the obese patients. Indeed, large variations of Vd of lipophilic drugs (as are PPIs) and impaired cytochrome P450 activity (mainly of the 3A subfamily) have been reported in obesity (http://www.orthosupersite.com/view.aspx?rid =19166). Unfortunately, no PK study has ever been performed in this special patient population and, given the obesity epidemic, this kind of study is nowadays mandatory for all the widely used drugs. Whatever the reason (be it PK or PD) and despite the methodological limitations, this study shows that the clinical efficacy of rabeprazole is maintained in overweight/obese patients with GERD and suggests that this subgroup of patients may derive from rabeprazole even greater benefit than lean patients. Taking into account the comorbidities

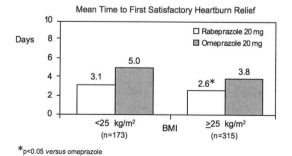

Figure 8. Symptomatic relief with rabeprazole or omeprazole in patients with erosive esophagitis, according to their BMI value (from Ref. 5).

(http://www. biomedcentral.com/1471-2458/9/88) and consequent cotherapies, often needed in these patients, the low propensity for drug-to-drug interactions of rabeprazole makes this PPI particularly suitable for obese patients with any acid-related diseases.

12. What is the role of baclofen, an agent that blocks TLESR, in the treatment of Barrett's esophagus?

Roy K.H. Wong
roykhw@gmail.com

There are no data concerning the treatment of BE with baclofen. Baclofen is a $GABA_B$ agonist, and $GABA_B$ is a major inhibitory neurotransmitter in the central nervous system. $GABA_B$ receptors are located in the enteric nervous system and centrally (brainstem). Baclofen inhibits TLESR through vagal–vagal pathways that transmit impulses from GABA receptors in the proximal stomach to the brainstem in the nucleus tractus solitarius and dorsal vagal nucleus. These impulses are processed, and efferent signals are sent through the vagus nerve to GABA receptors in the LES.

Published studies on baclofen relate to its effects on the LES and esophageal reflux in

Table 3. Effects of acute chronic baclofen therapy: acute $GABA_B$ agonist studies

Author	n	Patients	Dose	PR TLESRs	Reflux episode
Lidums[87]	20	Healthy	Baclofen 40 mg, 90 minutes prior	$5.7 \rightarrow 2.2$	$1 \rightarrow 0.3$ LESP 8.7 $\rightarrow 10.8$
Zhang[88]	20	GERD	Baclofen 40 mg, 90 minutes prior	$15 \rightarrow 9$ (<0.002)	$7 \rightarrow 4, P < 0.02$
Cange[89]	20	GERD	Baclofen 10 mg, BID× 24 hours		$16.5 \rightarrow 7.9, P < 0.0001$ 24 hours
Ciccaglione[90]	15	GERD	Baclofen 40 mg		GERD $149 \rightarrow 73$, $P < 0.003$
	9	Control			Control $42 \rightarrow 18$, $P < 0.007$
Vela[91]	9	GERD	Baclofen 0.5 mg/kg	$7.6 \rightarrow 3.6, P < 0.05$	$15 \rightarrow 6$ acid reflux, $P < 0.004; 4 \rightarrow 2$ nonacid, $P < 0.003$
	9	Control			$7 \rightarrow 1$ acid reflux, $P < 0.02; 2 \rightarrow 0$ nonacid, $P < 0.005$
Omari[92]	30	GERD, children ages 2–17	Baclofen 40 mg, 90 minutes prior		$4.2 \rightarrow 1.7, P < 0.05; 114 \rightarrow 61$, $P < 0.05$ (24 hours)
Boeckxstaens[54]	21	GERD 63% EE continued PPI	Lesogaberan 65 mg PO 1dose Q12× 3 ↑ LESp 28%	$15.5 \rightarrow 11.6$ ($\downarrow 25\%$)	Upright $25 \rightarrow 12$ episodes; supine $4.3 \rightarrow 1$ episode
Gerson[55]	44	GERD 3x/wk 20 Reflux Epi./2 hours	Arbaclofen 10, 20, 40, 60 mg qd, 2 hours before meal		$60.9 \rightarrow 50.5$, (17%). All doses $P < 0.005$, monitored for 12 hours

Table 4. Summary of four semichronic baclofen studies that ranged from two to four weeks

Author	n	Patients	Dose	Duration	Total number reflux episodes	Time pH < 4	Symptom
Koek[93]	16	GERD + Bile Reflux	20 mg QID graded 4 OMP 20 mg BID	14 days	OMP vs. OMP + B 14 → 17 (NS) DGER 17 → 12 (< 0.05)	OM P vs. OMP + B (NS)	Improved $P < 0.01$
Ciccaglione[94]	10		10 mg QID		220 → 52 ($P < 0.003$)	5.8 → 2.7 $P < 0.02$	Improved $P < 0.0007$
Kawai[95]	8	GERD Peds (neurologically impaired)	0.7 mg/ kg/day	7 days	24 hours ($P < 0.01$) PR ($P < 0.049$)	NS	
Cossentino[98]	43	GERD	20 mg PO TID	14 days	69 → 47, $P < 0.045$, PP episodes, $P < 0.04$	Total, $P < 0.003$, upright, $P < 0.016$	Significantly improved

normal patients and those with reflux. Six studies are short-term studies, lasting a few hours during the pre- and postprandial period to 24 hours (Table 3). Two studies concern lesogabaran[54] and arbaclofen (R isomer of baclofen),[55] compounds similar to baclofen. One of the six studies was performed in children (Omari). In five studies, baclofen was administered as a single dose (30–40 mg) 90 minutes before a meal; in one study baclofen, 10 mg twice daily, was administered, and patients were monitored for 24 hours. Lesogaberan, 65 mg, was given every 12 h, three doses, and administered with PPIs. Arbaclofen, 10, 20, 40, and 60 mg, was administered as a dose-ranging study and monitored for reflux for 12 h following the initial dose. Seven of eight studies showed a significant decrease in reflux episodes (except lesogaberan). All four studies that monitored TLESRs showed a decrement in TLESRs, with two being significantly different from controls or placebo.

There have been only four semichronic baclofen studies that ranged from two to four weeks (Table 4). One study was in neurologically impaired children. The doses of baclofen in the four studies ranged from 10 mg, po qid, to 20 mg, po tid to qid. Baclofen was the only antireflux agent in

all studies except for one (Ref. 56) that continued omeprazole use. In the Koek study, duodenogastroesophageal reflux was measured with a Bilitec probe, as these patients were symptomatic in spite of PPI therapy. Four of four studies showed significant decreases in reflux episodes, whereas three of four showed significant improvement in reflux symptoms. The Koek study showed significant improvement in duodenogastroesophageal reflux but not esophageal reflux.

One study by Orr *et al.*[57] looked at baclofen or placebo and was given to reflux patients before sleep at night. Polysomnography was performed over a two-day period. Although there was no difference in acid contact time, the number of reflux events, sleep time, and sleep efficiency was significantly improved in the baclofen-treated patients. This suggests that baclofen may facilitate sleep in GERD patients without increasing acid contact time.

In conclusion, although baclofen has been shown to decrease TLESRs specifically in the postprandial state, there are a few studies to suggest that it may be effective in supine reflux and duodenogastroesophageal reflux. Semichronic studies have shown symptomatic efficacy.

13. What is the comparative effect of proton pump inhibitors on nocturnal acid breakthrough?

David Armstrong
armstro@mcmaster.ca

Acid suppression therapy for patients with erosive EE produces healing rates that are proportional to the degree and duration of acid suppression achieved. PPIs, given once daily, produce marked suppression of gastric acid secretion and gastric acidity that is significantly greater than that produced by histamine H_2-receptor antagonists (H_2-RAs), achieving healing in 80–90% of patients within eight weeks. Despite this, esophageal erosions and reflux symptoms persist in a proportion of patients receiving once-daily PPI therapy. Divided-dose PPI therapy produces greater acid suppression but recurrent or "breakthrough" acid secretion is well documented even in individuals receiving a PPI twice daily.[58]

Nocturnal acid breakthrough (NAB) has been defined, arbitrarily, as the persistence of an intragastric pH below 4, for at least one hour, within 12 h of the intake of a PPI in the evening.[1] The initial report of NAB indicated that acid breakthrough occurred approximately 7.5 h after the evening PPI dose, regardless of whether the subjects received omeprazole or lansoprazole.[58] On the basis of these data, it was proposed that NAB is a class effect, attributable to the PKs of the most common, currently available, delayed-release (DR) PPIs—esomeprazole, lansoprazole, omeprazole, pantoprazole, and rabeprazole—which have a short $t_{\frac{1}{2}}$ (0.5–1.5 h) and a short t_{max} (1.0–3.5 h).[59] As a consequence, there is little PPI prodrug available to inhibit new or newly activated proton pumps once seven to eight hours have elapsed since the last intake of drug.

Although the majority of currently available DR PPIs have similar PK properties, they differ with respect to the duration of acid suppression—defined as an intragastric pH below 4.0—achieved when they are given once daily. In a five-way, cross-over study of once-daily, standard-dose DR PPIs, the time during which intragastric pH remained above 4.0, at steady state, ranged from 10.1 h for pantoprazole, 40 mg daily, to 14.0 h for esomeprazole, 40 mg daily.[60] These differences were also evident in a meta-analysis that included data from 57 studies in an evaluation of the acid suppression produced by the same five DR PPIs at a variety of daily doses (Table 5). The extent of persistent acid suppression, presented as the time during which gastric pH was below 4.0, was dose dependent, ranging from 10.5 h (esomeprazole, 20 mg) to 19.6 h (omeprazole, 10 mg daily) at "half-dose," from 8.5 h (esomeprazole, 40 mg) to 12.3 h (omeprazole, 20 mg daily) at "standard-dose" and from 3.6 h (esomeprazole, 80 mg) to 8.8 h (omeprazole, 40 mg daily) at "double-dose;" the relative potencies of the DR PPIs, compared to omeprazole, were reported as 0.23, 0.90, 1.00, 1.60, and 1.82 for pantoprazole, lansoprazole, omeprazole, esomeprazole, and rabeprazole, respectively.[61] This analysis did not, however, evaluate the effect of twice-daily DR PPI administration, and it is not, therefore, applicable directly to the relative effects of different PPIs on NAB.

The effect of twice-daily dosing on nocturnal acid suppression, in particular, was evaluated in an analysis of 16 PD studies, with 31 arms, of the effects of standard dose DR PPIs administered twice daily on intragastric pH at steady state (i.e., for five to eight days) in healthy subjects. Consistent with the results of previous studies, this analysis (Table 6) reported times (%) with intragastric pH below 4.0 of 15.4% and 19.0% for esomeprazole (40 mg

Table 5. Time (% 24-h period) with gastric pH below 4.0: meta-analysis of gastric pH data at steady state in healthy subjects[61]

PPI	Esomeprazole	Lansoprazole	Omeprazole	Pantoprazole	Rabeprazole
Dose	40 mg	30 mg	20 mg	40 mg	20 mg
Half	43.7	54.1	81.7	57.6	48.8
Standard	35.4	44.9	51.3	46.4	42.3
Double	15.1	35.3	36.8	29.2	29.2

twice daily) and omeprazole (20 mg twice daily), respectively, compared with 35.1% and 36.4% for lansoprazole (30 mg twice daily) and pantoprazole (40 mg twice daily), respectively[62]; no comparative data were available for rabeprazole.

In conclusion, the data available for currently available DR PPIs indicate that gastric acid secretion returns, to an important extent, in a high proportion of individuals receiving standard, once-daily DR PPIs and that this is not abolished by twice-daily administration. Although there are limited data relevant, specifically, to the definition of NAB, the comparative effects of the different DR PPIs, at approved doses, seem to be similar for 24-h acid suppression, nocturnal acid suppression, and nocturnal acid breakthrough; thus, on the basis of the analysis of 24-h intragastric pH for the five DR PPIs,[4] esomeprazole and rabeprazole are similar in potency, and more potent than omeprazole and lansoprazole, which are, themselves, similar in potency and, in turn, more potent than pantoprazole.[4]

Newer PPIs, formulated for delayed release—for example, dexlansoprazole and AGN 201904-Z—or characterized by a longer half life—for example, S-tenatoprazole (STU-Na)—appear to reduce nocturnal intragastric acidity to a greater extent than current DR PPIs, when given once daily.[2] Despite this, nocturnal return of gastric acid secretion is a common phenomenon, regardless of the PPI and administration frequency. A fall in intragastric pH at night may be characterized as nocturnal acid breakthrough; however, because NAB is defined in the context of twice-daily PPI administration, more precise quantification of nocturnal intragastric acidity (e.g., time with gastric pH below 4.0) may yield a better understanding of the effect of newer agents on nocturnal acid secretion and their therapeutic effect in GERD.

14. Compared to PPIs given at bedtime, what are the advantages of the low overnight gastric and esophageal acidity observed with immediate release omeprazole?

Kenneth R. DeVault
devault.kenneth@mayo.edu

Until recently, all PPIs were enteric coated to enable delivery and release of the agent in the proximal

Table 6. Mean time (% 24-h period, % daytime, % night-time) with gastric pH below 4.0: meta-analysis of gastric pH data at steady state (day 5 to day 8) in healthy subjects[62]

Dose	Mean time (%) gastric pH < 4.0 [number of study arms, number of subjects]		
	24-hour period	Daytime	Nighttime
Esomeprazole 40 mg bid	15.2 [2, 55]	19.0 [1, 25]	15.4 [2, 55]
Lansoprazole 30 mg bid	30.5 [2, 22]	7.0 [1, 12]	35.1 [1, 12]
Omeprazole 20 mg bid	19.1 [3, 39]	23.7 [1, 16]	19.0 [3, 38]
Pantoprazole 40 mg bid	29.2 [1, 30]	–	36.4 [1, 30]
Rabeprazole 20 mg bid	10.4 [2, 23]	–	–

small bowel. These agents suppress acid for up to 15 h per day when given once daily and up to 19 h per day when given more than once daily. In addition, most agents take three to five days to reach steady state and are most effective when taken before meals.

A new formulation of nonenterically coated omeprazole combined with sodium bicarbonate has been developed. Sodium bicarbonate is required in this preparation to protect the omeprazole from degradation by stomach acid and also seems to stimulate proton pumps enabling them to be efficiently blocked by the PPI. This combination has been described as immediate-release omeprazole (IR-OME).[63] IR-OME was originally marketed as a powder to be constituted with water but is now also available in capsules containing 20 or 40 mg of omeprazole combined with sodium bicarbonate. The PDs of this combination has been well studied in healthy volunteers where both the maximal concentration of the PPI was higher and occurred earlier after ingestion than the more traditionally formulated PPIs.[64]

A potential advantage of this medication is nocturnal use. IR-OME taken at bedtime has been shown to control 24-h and nighttime gastric acid more completely than pantoprazole taken once or twice daily.[65] On the twice daily dose, the 24-h acid exposure was 12.2% for IR-OME and 43% for pantoprazole, whereas the overnight acid exposure was 8.0% and 63.5%, respectively. Another preliminary study compared nocturnal doses of OME-IR, 40 mg; lansoprazole, 30 mg; and esomeprazole, 40 mg.[66] Although 92% of patients experienced NAB when treated with either lansoprazole or esomeprazole, only 61% of patients experienced NAB when treated with OME-IR. This was mainly related to the lower acid early in the evening (likely due to a combination of neutralization by the bicarbonate and more rapid absorption of the omeprazole). A downside of this medication is the relatively high sodium load (460 mg in each 40 mg omeprazole dose), especially when taken more than once daily.

In summary, IM-OME has several advantages over enterically coated PPIs. It has outstanding nocturnal acid control when given twice daily and can provide very good acid support when given at bedtime. An additional advantage is the option to take the medication independent of food consumption.

15. Is combination of PPIs with antinflammatory drugs (NSAIDs) and aspirin to be considered the future of chemoprevention in BE?

Paolo Bechi, Antonio Taddei, Giancarlo Freschi, Maria Novella Ringressi, Duccio Rossi Degli'Innocenti, Francesca Castiglione, and Emmanuella Masini
antonio.taddei@unifi.it

Many potential agents for esophageal adenocarcinoma chemoprevention in BE have been suggested, but those for which substantial evidence of effectiveness in humans has been shown are PPIs and NSAIDs. The rationale for PPIs in chemoprevention comes first from the well-recognized role of GERD in the multistep process of esophageal adenocarcinogenesis and second from limited observational data that demonstrated an association of PPI use and the reduced incidence of dysplasia in BE.[67] The rationale for aspirin use in chemoprevention comes from its action as a nonselective COX-2 inhibitor, thus preventing COX-2 proinflammatory and carcinogenetic effects exerted through an increase in cell proliferation, inhibition of apoptosis, and activation of angiogenesis. In this respect, selec-

tive COX-2 inhibitors such as the coxib family have been most widely studied and have appeared for a, although the most promising drugs in this particular application. However, some agents in this family seem to be responsible for heavy cardiovascular side effects; thus, their use in this chemopreventive application does not seem any longer justified. Moreover, aspirin has a chemoprevention efficacy for esophageal cancer more than other NSAIDs (efficacy of 40%). Therefore, aspirin has the best risk–benefit ratio, especially for esophageal cancer.[68]

The rationale for the association in chemoprevention of aspirin with PPIs is provided by the symptomatic improvement induced by PPIs in patients with BE suffering from GERD; in other words, most of these patients would take PPI medication anyway, and PPIs reduce the risk of upper gastrointestinal complications due to NSAIDs (from 4% to 1.5% per year for aspirin). The AspECT trial has been devised to answer our question. The aim of the AspECT trial is to verify the efficacy of chemoprevention with PPIs and/or aspirin in BE metaplasia. It is the biggest multicenter controlled trial and has reached its target of 2,500 patients. It is now in its fourth year, and its results, due in 2016 with an interim analysis in 2011 and 2012, are expected to be decisive. Effects of therapy on mortality and conversion rate from Barrett's metaplasia to high-grade dysplasia or adenocarcinoma will be registered. Indications are also expected concerning the best age to begin the treatment, dosage, and duration of therapy. However, so far there is no evidence from long-term randomized controlled studies regarding the use of PPIs and/or aspirin to reduce the risk of esophageal adenocarcinoma. Looking forward to 2016, to support our conclusion regarding chemoprevention with PPIs and aspirin, we do not yet have a long-term randomized controlled study, but only inconclusive epidemiological data;[69] however, very important but indecisive clinical and experimental data are available.[70,71]

Personal, preliminary experience
We studied PPIs and aspirin effects on isolated cells from mucosal biopsies in seven patients with BE metaplasia (unpublished data). Proliferative activity was studied by means of tritiated thymidine incorporation. After the EGF stimulus, which obviously determines a very significant increase in

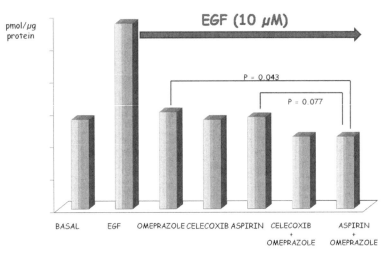

Figure 9. Proliferative activity measured by means of tritiated thymidine incorporation before and after EGF stimuli in BE samples.

proliferative activity, both aspirin and omeprazole, when separately preincubated, were capable of showing a similar decrease in proliferative activity. The incubation with both aspirin and omeprazole at the same time induced a decrease in proliferative activity significantly greater than that induced separately by any of the two drugs. This seems a demonstration of a synergistic effect of the two drugs (unpublished data) (Fig. 9). The same findings were shown by means of the immunohistochemical evaluation. Moreover, pretreatment of the cells with aspirin alone significantly reduced the expression of the receptor of EGF (EGFR); this effect was significantly greater when omeprazole was added, whereas the effects of aspirin on proliferative activity are well known and due to its action as a nonselective COX-2 inhibitor (unpublished data). The effect of omeprazole on proliferative activity could be mediated by the lowering of intracellular pH, of which omeprazole has been shown to be capable in our experiments. Lowering of intracellular pH seems to increase caspase-3 activity, which, in turn, could affect apoptosis and proliferative activity.

In conclusion, looking forward to the AspECT trial, no trial has so far definitely shown the efficacy of any kind of chemoprevention in BE. However, relevant, but indecisive clinical and experimental data support the association of aspirin/PPIs, which on the basis of our experiments seem potentially capable of a synergistic effect.

16. What can be the expected effect from new PPI drugs currently under investigation on prolonged plasma concentration of drug and intake regardless of meal timing?

Richard H. Hunt
huntr@mcmaster.ca

Therapeutic acid suppression in GERD is used to control symptoms, heal erosive EE, and more recently to prevent the evolution and progression of Barrett's metaplasia. It is known that exposure to gastric acid increases cell proliferation in the distal esophagus and that there is a synergistic effect of acid when combined with bile on cell proliferation. Moreover, there is some evidence that pulsatile esophageal acid exposure increases an undifferentiated cell phenotype, although continuous acid exposure does the opposite.[72,73] Some of the effects of acid are summarized in Figure 10A.

One of the many remaining questions is whether pH is important, and, if so, what pH? We know that during standard dosing of current DR PPIs given twice daily in healthy volunteers, there is increased intragastric acidity for up to one-third of the nighttime. After esomeprazole, 40 mg twice daily for five to eight days, results showed that 15% of the nighttime intragastric pH was <4.[74] Moreover, other studies show that ~60–80% of patients have persistent nocturnal acidification despite twice daily

A

	Good Effects	Bad Effects	Flaws
In-vitro	↓ Proliferation	↓ P53 anti-proliferative effect	Cells transformed and unrepresentative
Ex-vivo	↓ MAPK signaling		Explants unreliable
In-vivo models	↓ Acid damage	↑ Adenomas in Min- mouse	Models poorly reflective of human disease
Epidemiology	↓ Reflux damage / strictures	↑ Cancer	Confounding effects with PPI and severity of acid reflux
Phase II/III	↓ Reflux damage / strictures	↑ Gastrin	Short-term surrogates of cancer unvalidated
Phase IV	AspECT trial under way	AspECT trial under way	We will have to wait 8 yr

B

Intragastric suppressing effect of esomeprazole 40mg OM (n=43), by *post hoc* analysis of two of our recent PD studies in healthy volunteers				
Mean % time (95%CI)	24 h (0700-0700)	Day (0700-1900)	Night (1900-0700)	Midnight (0000-0700)
pH ≤4	39.96 (34.60 to 45.33)	21.50 (18.32 to 24.67)	58.07 (49.81 to 66.33)*	69.75 (64.00 to 75.49)
pH ≤3	29.69 (26.58 to 32.79)	13.60 (11.24 to 15.96)	45.47 (40.41 to 50.53)	59.33 (52.70 to 65.97)
pH ≤2	18.72 (15.76 to 21.68)	6.57 (5.08 to 8.06)	30.65 (25.38 to 35.92)	41.67 (34.74 to 48.61)

Figure 10. PPIs and cancer risk in Barrett's esophagus.

PPIs,[75] and ~25% patients with reflux symptoms do not respond to twice daily PPIs given for four to eight weeks.[76] In GERD patients who are refractory to PPIs, pH was abnormal at 30% for once-daily PPIs, and in 25% of patients on twice-daily PPI.[77] Certainly, in healthy volunteers taking esomeprazole, 40 mg once daily 30 min before breakfast, the intragastric pH is < 4 for 75% of the time between midnight and 0700 hours, but of more concern is the fact that pH is <2 for over 40% of that time (2.87 h or 172 min) (Fig. 10B).[78] Thus, there are now a number of new antisecretory drugs under development by the pharmaceutical industry, and these have recently been reviewed by Scarpignato and Hunt (Fig. 11A).[79]

In short, of those drugs recently introduced or likely to be seen in clinical development in the near future, these include new formulations of existing drugs, such as dexlansoprazole; novel chemical entities, such as tenatoprazole or API-023; or the new class of potassium channel blocking drugs. Dexlansoprazole has recently been introduced in both the United States and Canada; results show a modest increase in plasma residence time and AUC in the fed versus fasting state, thus prolonging the antisecretory effect and removing the absolute necessity for giving the drug before food, which offers an important advantage in patients with complex GERD.[80,81] However, it is hard to determine a clinically meaningful difference in mean intragastric 24-h pH. Both API-023, previously known as AGN 201904Z, and the sodium salt of the S-isomer of tenatoprazole, STU-Na, have been shown to predictably and consistently maintain an intragastric pH ≥ 4 throughout the 24-h period (Fig. 11B).[82,83]

The last class of drugs mentioned here includes the potassium-channel acid-blocking drugs or PCABs, which include AZD-0865, which was a short-acting compound with some toxicological

A

New formulations	• Extended-release formulations PPI: ChroNAB technology & AcuFormTM delivery technology for omeprazole **dexlansoprazole (TAK-390MR) for lansoprazole,** extended-release version of rabeprazole • Immediate-release (IR) omeprazole • Vecam: combines PPI with a chemical 'acid pump activator'
Novel PPIs	• **AGN 201904-Z** • **Tenatoprazole, S-isomer of tenatoprazole-Na (STU-Na)**
P-CABs	• Linaprazan (AZD0865), revaprazan, soraprazan, **TAK-438**
PPI-H₂RA combination	• OX-17 (fixed dose combination of a PPI and H$_2$RA), H$_2$RA + tenatoprazole
Looking to the future	• NO-donating antisecretory compounds, NO-PPIs: NMI-826 for lansoprazole

B

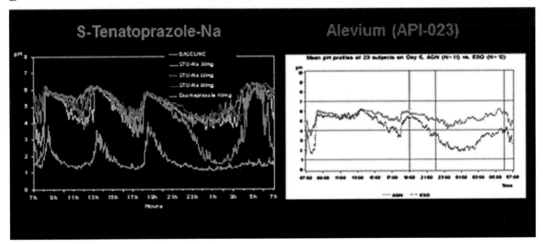

Figure 11. New anti-secretory drugs with long plasma residence time.

problems that resulted in its being withdrawn from development.[84] A current long-acting PCAB is TAK-438, which has an impressive dose-dependent 24-h antisecretory profile and remains in development in Japan.[85]

Thus, the prospect of truly once-daily antisecretory drugs is now real, and they offer a lack of significant food interaction and an overall consistent acid control with less pulsatile acid exposure and improved control of nighttime acid secretion

that avoids the time period of nocturnal acidification with fewer episodes of so-called "nocturnal acid breakthrough." The potential benefit of this new generation of antisecretory drugs is designed to prevent GERD complications, including ulceration and stricture, but particularly in preventing the progression of BE.

Conflicts of interest

The authors declare no conflicts of interest.

References

1. Pandolfino, J.E., M.A. Schreiner, T.J. Lee, *et al.* 2005. Comparison of the Bravo wireless and Digitrapper catheter-based pH monitoring systems for measuring esophageal acid exposure. *Am. J. Gastroenterol.* **100:** 1466–1476.

2. Pandolfino, J.E., J.E. Richter, T. Ours, *et al.* 2003. Ambulatory esophageal pH monitoring using a wireless capsule. *Am. J. Gastroenterol.* **98:** 740–749.

3. Prakash, C. & R.E. Clouse. 2005. Value of extended recording time with wireless pH monitoring in evaluating GERD. *Clin. Gastroenterol. Hepatol.* **3:** 329–334.

4. Prakash, C. & R.E. Clouse. 2006. Wireless pH monitoring in patients with non-cardiac chest pain. *Am. J. Gastroenterol.* **101:** 446–452.

5. Pandolfino, J.E. & M.F. Vela. 2009. Esophageal-reflux monitoring. *GIE* **69:** 917–930.

6. Hirano, I. & J.E. Richter. 2007. ACG practice guidelines: esophageal reflux testing. *Am. J. Gastroenterol.* **102:** 668–685.

7. Calabrese, C., G. Liguori, V. Gabusi, *et al.* 2008. Ninety-six-hour wireless oesophageal pH monitoring following proton pump inhibitor administration in NERD patients. *Aliment Pharmacol. Ther.* **28:** 250–255.

8. Hirano, I., Q. Zhang., J.E. Pandolfino, *et al.* 2005. Four-day Bravo pH capsule monitoring with and without proton pump inhibitor therapy. *Clin. Gastroenterol. Hepatol.* **3:** 1083–1088.

9. Garrean, C.P., Q. Zhang, N. Gonsalves, *et al.* 2008. Acid reflux detection and symptom-reflux association using 4-day wireless pH recording combining 48-hour periods off and on PPI therapy. *Am. J. Gastroenterol.* **103:** 1631–1637.

10. Scarpulla, G., S. Camilleri, P. Galante, *et al.* 2007. The impact of prolonged pH measurements on the diagnosis of gastroesophageal reflux disease: 4-day wireless pH studies. *Am. J. Gastroenterol.* **102:** 2642–2647.

11. Grigolon, A., D. Consonni, I. Bravi, *et al.* 2009. 96 h wireless vs 24 h traditional pH monitoring: an outcome study. *Gut* **58**(Suppl. II): A430.

12. Zerbib, F., A. Duriez, S. Roman, *et al.* 2008. Determinants of gastro-oesophageal reflux perception in patients with persistent symptoms despite proton pump inhibitors. *Gut* **57:** 156–160.

13. Savarino, P. *et al.* 2009. Functional heartburn has more in common with functional dyspepsia than with non-erosive reflux disease. *Gut* **58:** 1185–1191.

14. Mainie, I., R. Tutuian, A. Agrawal, *et al.* 2006. Combined multichannel intraluminal impedance-pH monitoring to select patients with persistent gastro-oesophageal reflux for laparoscopic Nissen fundoplication. *Br. J. Surg.* **93:** 1483–1487.

15. Becker, V., M. Bajbouj, K. Waller, *et al.* 2007. Clinical trial: persistent gastrooesophageal reflux symptoms despite standard therapy with proton pump inhibitors: a follow-up study of intraluminal-impedance guided therapy. *Aliment Pharmacol. Therapeut.* **26:** 1355–1360.

16. del Genio, G., S. Tolone, F. del Genio, *et al.* 2008. Prospective assessment of patient selection for antireflux surgery by combined multichannel intraluminal impedance pH monitoring. *J. Gastrointest. Surg.* **12:** 1491–1496.

17. Nehra, D., P. Howell, C.P. Williams, *et al.* 1999. Toxic bile acids in gastro-oesophageal reflux disease: influence of gastric acidity. *Gut* **44:** 598–602.

18. Stein, H.J., W.K. Kauer, H. Feussner & J.R. Siewert. 1998. Bile reflux in benign and malignant Barrett's esophagus: effect of medical acid suppression and nissen fundoplication. *J. Gastrointest. Surg.* **2:** 333–341.

19. Theisen, J, J.H. Peters, M. Fein, *et al.* 2005. The mutagenic potential of duodenoesophageal reflux. *Ann. Surg.* **241:** 63–68.

20. Fein, M., J.H. Peters, & T.R. Demeester. 2007. Carcinogenesis in reflux disease—in search for bile-specific effects. *Microsurgery* **27:** 647–650.

21. Nehra, D. 2010. Bile in the esophagus-model for a bile acid biosensor. *J Gastrointest. Surg.* **14**(Suppl. 1): S6–S8.

22. Talley, N.J., N. Vakil, & P. Moayyedi. 2005. American Gastroenterological Association technical review on the evaluation of dyspepsia. *Gastroenterology* **129:** 1756–1780.

23. Tack, J., N.J. Talley, M. Camilleri, *et al.* 2006. Functional gastroduodenal disorders. *Gastroenterology* **130:** 1466–1479.

24. Moayyedi, P., B.C. Delaney, N. Vakil, *et al.* 2004. The efficacy of proton pump inhibitors in nonulcer dyspepsia a systematic review and economic analysis. *Gastroenterology* **127:** 1329–1337.

25. Wang, W.H., J.Q. Huang, G.F. Zheng, *et al.* 2007. Effects of proton-pump inhibitors on functional dyspepsia: a meta-analysis of Randomized Placebo-controlled Trials. *Clin. Gastroenterol. Hepatol.* **5:** 178–185.

26. Savarino, E., D. Pohl, P. Zentilin, *et al.* 2009. Functional heartburn has more in common with functional dyspepsia than with non-erosive reflux disease. *Gut* **58:** 1185–1191.

27. Loughney, T., C.L. Maydonovitch, & R.K. Wong. 1998. Esophageal manometry and ambulatory 24-hour pH monitoring in patients with short and long segment Barrett's esophagus. *Am. J. Gastroenterol.* **93:** 916–919.

28. Fass, R., R.W. Hell, H.S. Garewal, *et al.* 2001. Correlation of oesophageal acid exposure with Barrett's oesophagus length. *Gut* **48:** 310–313.

29. Ouatu-Lascar, R. & G. Triadafilopoulos. 1998. Complete elimination of reflux symptoms does not guarantee normalization of intraesophageal acid reflux in patients with Barrett's esophagus. *Am. J. Gastroenterol.* **93:** 711–716.

30. Fass, R., R.E. Sampliner, I.B. Malagon, *et al.* 2000. Failure of oesophageal acid control in candidates for Barrett's oesophagus reversal on a very high dose of proton pump inhibitor. *Aliment Pharmacol. Ther.* **14:** 597–602.

31. Wani, S., R.E. Sampliner, A.P. Weston, *et al.* 2005. Lack of predictors of normalization of oesophageal acid exposure in Barrett's oesophagus. *Aliment Pharmacol. Ther.* **22:** 627–633.

32. Modlin, I.M., R.H. Hunt, P. Malfertheiner, *et al.* 2009. Diagnosis and management of nonerosive reflux disease. *Vevey NERD Consensus Group-Digest.* **80:** 74–88.

33. Dean, B.B., A.D. Gano, Jr., K. Knight, *et al.* 2004. Effectiveness of proton pump inhibitors in nonerosive reflux disease. *Clin. Gastroenterol. Hepatol.* **2:** 656–664.

34. Galmiche, J.P., R.E. Clouse, A. Balint, *et al.* 2006. Functional esophageal disorders. *Gastroenterology* **130:** 1459–1465.

35. Casini, V., F. Pace, S. Pallotta, *et al.* 2008. Usefulness of pH impedance monitoring in a tertiary referral centre. *Gut* **57**(Suppl. II): A37.

36. Metz, D.C., M. Vakily, T. Dixit & D. Mulford. 2009. Review article: dual delayed release formulation of dexlansoprazole MR, a novel approach to overcome the limitations of conventional single release proton pump inhibitor therapy. *Aliment Pharmacol. Ther.* **29:** 928–937.

37. Lee, R.D., D. Mulford, J. Wu & S.N. Atkinson. 2010. The effect of time-of-day dosing on the pharmacokinetics and pharmacodynamics of dexlansoprazole MR: evidence for dosing flexibility with a Dual Delayed Release proton pump inhibitor. *Aliment Pharmacol. Ther.* **31:** 1001–1011.

38. Whittbrodt, E.T., C. Baum & D.A. Peura. 2009. Delayed release dexlansoprazole in the treatment of GERD and erosive esophagitis. *Clin. Exp. Gastroenterol.* **2:** 117–128.

39. Jacobson, B., T. Ferris, T. Shea, *et al.* 2003. Who is using chronic acid suppression therapy and why? *Am. J. Gastroenterol.* **98:** 51–58.

40. Leonard, J., J. Marshall & P. Moayyedi. 2007. Systematic review of the risk of enteric infection in patients taking acid suppression. *Am. J. Gastroenterol.* **102:** 2047–2056.

41. Laheij, R., M. Sturkenboom, R. Hassing, *et al.* 2004. Risk of community-acquired pneumonia and use of gastric acid-suppressive drugs. *JAMA* **292:** 1955–1960.

42. Katz, M. 2010. Failing the acid test: benefits of proton pump inhibitors may not justify the risks for many users. *Arch. Intern. Med.* **170:** 747–748.

43. Raghunath, A., C. Morain & R. McLoughlin. 2005. Review article: the long-term use of proton-pump inhibitors. *Aliment Pharmacol. Ther.* **22:** 55–63.

44. Kim, Y.S. *et al.* 2005. Frequency scale for symptoms of gastroesophageal reflux disease predicts the need for addition of prokinetics to proton pump inhibitor therapy. *World J. Gastroenterol.* **11:** 4210–4214.

45. Miyamoto, M. *et al.* 2007. Comparison of efficacy of pantoprazole alone versus pantoprazole plus mosapride therapy of gastroesophageal reflux disease: a randomized trial. *J. Gastroenterol. Hepatol.* **23:** 746–751.

46. Madan, K. *et al.* 2004. Comparison of efficacy of pantoprazole alone versus pantoprazole plus mosapride in therapy of gastroesophageal reflux disease: a randomized trial. *Dis. Esophagus.* **17:** 274–278.

47. Kamiya, T. *et al.* 2009. Impaired gastric motility and its relationship to reflux symptoms in patients with nonerosive gastroesophageal reflux disease. *J. Gastroenterol.* **44:** 183–189.

48. Tougas, G. *et al.* 2005. Omeprazole delays gastric emptying in healthy volunteers: an effect prevented by tegaserod. *Aliment Pharmacol. Ther.* **22:** 59–65.

49. McDougall, N.I., B.T. Johnston, J.S. Collins, *et al.* 1998. Three- to 4.5-year prospective study of prognostic indicators in gastro-oesophageal reflux disease. *Scand. J. Gastroenterol.* **33:** 1016–1022.

50. Talley, N.J., D. Armstrong, O. Junghard & I. Wiklund. 2006. Predictors of treatment response in patients with non-erosive reflux disease. *Aliment Pharmacol. Ther.* **24:** 371–376.

51. Sheu, B.S., W.L. Chang, H.C. Cheng, *et al.* 2008. Body mass index can determine the healing of reflux esophagitis with Los Angeles Grades C and D by esomeprazole. *Am. J. Gastroenterol.* **103:** 2209–2214.

52. Sheu, B.S., H.C. Cheng, W.L. Chang, *et al.* 2007. The impact of body mass index on the application of on-demand therapy for Los Angeles grades A and B reflux esophagitis. *Am. J. Gastroenterol.* **102:** 2387–2394.

53. Pace, F., B. Coudsy, B. DeLemos, *et al.* 2011. Does body mass index affect clinical efficacy of proton pump inhibitor therapy in GERD? The case for rabeprazole. *Eur. J. Gastroenterol. Hepatol.* In press.

54. Boeckxstaens, G.E., H. Beaumont, V. Mertens, *et al.* 2010. Effects of Lesogaberan on reflux and lower esophageal sphincter function in patients with gastroesophageal reflux disease. *Gastroenterol* **139:** 409–417.

55. Gerson, L.B., F.J. Huff, A. Hila, *et al.* 2010. Arbaclofen Placarbil decreases postprandial reflux in patients with gastroesophageal reflux disease. *Am. J. Gastroenterol.* **105:** 1266–1275.

56. Koek, G.H., D. Sifrim, T. Lerut, *et al.* 2003. Effect of the GABAB agonist baclofen in patients with symptoms and duodeno-gastro-oesophageal reflux refractory to proton pump inhibitors *Gut* **52:** 1397–1402.

57. Orr, W.C., *et al.* 2010. Gastroenterol, M1863 (abstract).

58. Peghini, P.L., P.O. Katz, N.A. Bracy & D.O. Castell. 1998. Nocturnal recovery of gastric acid secretion with twice-daily dosing of proton pump inhibitors. *Am. J. Gastroenterol.* **93:** 763–767.

59. Armstrong, D., & D. Sifrim. 2010. New pharmacologic therapies in gastroesophageal reflux disease. *Gastroenterol. Clin. N. Am.* **39:** 393–418.

60. Miner, P., Katz P.O., Chen Y. & Sostek M. 2003. Gastric acid control with esomeprazole, lansoprazole, omeprazole, pantoprazole, and rabeprazole: a five-way crossover study. *Am. J. Gastroenterol.* **98:** 2616–2620.

61. Kirchheiner, J., S. Glatt, U. Fuhr, *et al.* 2009. Relative potency of proton pump inhibitors—comparison of effects on intragastric pH. *Eur. J. Clin. Pharmacol.* **65:** 19–31.

62. Yuan, Y. & R.H. Hunt. 2008. Intragastric acid suppressing effect of proton pump inhibitors twice daily at steady state in healthy volunteers: evidence of an unmet need? *Am. J. Gastroenterol.* **103**(Suppl. 1): S50 (Abstract #128).

63. Castell, D.O. 2005. Review of immediate-release omeprazole for the treatment of gastric acid related disorders. *Expert Opin. Pharmacother.* **6:** 2501–2510.

64. Vakily, M., W. Zhang, J. Wu, *et al.* 2009. Pharmacokinetics and pharmacodynamics of a known active PPI with a novel dual delayed release technology, dexlansoprazole MR: a combined analysis of randomized controlled clinical trials. *Curr. Med. Res. Opin.* **25:** 627–638.

65. Castell, D.O., R. Bagin, B. Goldlust, *et al.* 2005. Comparison of the effects of immediate-release omeprazole powder for oral suspension and pantoprazole delayed-release tablets on nocturnal gastro-oesophageal reflux disease. *Aliment Pharmacol. Ther.* **21:** 1467–1474.

66. Katz, P.O., D. Ballard, F.K. Koch, *et al.* 2006. Nocturnal gastric acidity after bedtime dosing of proton pump inhibitors in patients with nighttime GERD symptoms. *Gastroenterology* **130:** A175.

67. Shaib, Y., & H.B. El-Serag. 2004. The prevalence and risk factors of functional dyspepsia in a multiethnic population in the United States. *Am. J. Gastroenterol.* **99:** 2210–2216.

68. Jankowski, J. & R. Hunt. 2008. Cyclooxygenase-2 inhibitors in colorectal cancer prevention: counterpoint. *Cancer Epidemiol. Biomarkers Prev.* **17:** 1858–1861.

69. Corley, D.A., K. Kerlikowske, R. Verma, *et al.* 2003. Protective association of aspirin/NSAIDs and esophageal cancer: a systematic review and meta-analysis. *Gastroenterology,* **124:** 47–56.

70. Triadafilopoulos, G., B. Kaur, S. Sood, *et al.* 2006. The effects of esomeprazole combined with aspirin or rofecoxib on prostaglandin E2 production in patients with Barrett's oesophagus. *Aliment Pharmacol. Ther.* **23:** 997–1005.

71. Liu, J.F., G.G. Jamieson, P.A. Drew, *et al.* 2005. Aspirin induces apoptosis in oesophageal cancer cells by inhibiting the pathway of NF-kappaB downstream regulation of cyclooxygenase-2. *ANZ J. Surg.* **75:** 1011–1016.

72. Fitzgerald, R.C. 2005. Barrett's oesophagus and oesophageal adenocarcinoma: how does acid interfere with cell proliferation and differentiation? *Gut* **54**(Suppl. 1): i21–i26.

73. Leedham, S. & J. Jankowski. 2007. The evidence base of proton pump inhibitor chemopreventative agents in Barrett's esophagus—the good, the bad, and the flawed! *Am. J. Gastroenterol.* **102:** 21–99.

74. Yuan, Y. & R.H. Hunt. 2008. Intragastric acid suppressing effect of proton pump inhibitors twice daily at steady state in healthy volunteers: evidence of an unmet need? *Am. J. Gastroenterol.* **103**(Suppl. 1): S50.

75. Richter, J.E. 2006. The patient with refractory gastroesophageal reflux disease. *Dis. Esophagus* **19:** 443–447.

76. Richter, J.E. 2007. How to manage refractory GERD. *Nat. Clin. Pract. Gastroenterol. Hepatol.* **4:** 658–664.

77. Mackalsk, B.A. & A. Ilnyckyj. 2008. Esophageal pH testing in patients refractory to proton pump inhibitor therapy. *Can. J. Gastroenterol.* **22:** 249–252.

78. Wang, C.C., Y. Yuan, Y. Chen & R.H. Hunt. 2008. Night-time pH holding time: what is hidden by the % of time pH $\leq$ 4? *Am. J. Gastroenterol.* **103**(Suppl. 1): S51.

79. Scarpignato, C. & R.H. Hunt. 2008. Proton pump inhibitors: the beginning of the end or the end of the beginning? *Curr. Opin. Pharmacol.* **8:** 677–684.

80. Lee, R.D., D. Mulford, J. Wu & S.N. Atkinson. 2010. The effect of time-of-day dosing on the pharmacokinetics and pharmacodynamics of dexlansoprazole MR: evidence for dosing flexibility with a dual delayed release proton pump inhibitor. *Aliment Pharmacol. Ther.* **31:** 1001–1011.

81. Lee, R.D., M. Vakily, D. Mulford, *et al.* 2009. Clinical trial: the effect and timing of food on the pharmacokinetics and pharmacodynamics of dexlansoprazole MR, a novel dual delayed release formulation of a proton pump inhibitor—evidence for dosing flexibility. *Aliment Pharmacol. Ther.* **29:** 824–833.

82. Hunt, R.H., D. Armstrong, M. Yaghoobi, *et al.* 2008. Predictable prolonged suppression of gastric acidity with a novel proton pump inhibitor, AGN 201904-Z. *Aliment Pharmacol. Ther.* **28:** 187–199.

83. Hunt, R.H., D. Armstrong, M. Yaghoobi & C. James. 2010. The pharmacodynamics and pharmacokinetics of S-tenatoprazole-Na 30 mg, 60 mg and 90 mg vs. esomeprazole 40 mg in healthy male subjects. *Aliment Pharmacol. Ther.* **31:** 648–657.

84. Dent, J., P.J. Kahrilas, J. Hatlebakk, *et al.* 2008. A randomized, comparative trial of a potassium-competitive acid blocker (AZD0865) and esomeprazole for the treatment of patients with nonerosive reflux disease. *Am. J. Gastroenterol.* **103:** 20–26.

85. Hori Y., A. Imanishi, J. Matsukawa, *et al.* 2010. 1-[5-(2-Fluorophenyl)-1-(pyridin-3-ylsulfonyl)-1H-pyrrol-3-yl]-N-methylmethanamine monofumarate (TAK-438), a novel and potent potassium-competitive acid blocker for the treatment of acid- related diseases. *J. Pharmacol. Exp. Ther.* **335:** 231–238.

86. Yang, Y. *et al.* 2006. *JAMA* **296:** 2947–2954.

87. Lidums, I. *et al.* 2000. Control of transient lower esophageal sphincter relaxations and reflux by the GABA$_B$ agonist baclofen in normal subjects. *Gastroenterology* **118:** 7–13.

88. Zhang, Q., A. Lehmann, R. Rigda, J. Dent, R.H. Holloway. 2002. Control of transient lower oesophageal sphincter relaxations and reflux by the GABA$_B$ agonist baclofen in patients with gastro-oesophageal reflux disease. *Gut* **50:** 19–24.

89. Cange, L., E. Johnsson, H. Rydholm, *et al.* 2002. Baclofen-mediated gastro-oesophageal acid reflux control in patients with established reflux disease. *Aliment Pharmacol. Ther.* **16:** 869–873.

90. Ciccaglione, A.F., S. Bartolacci, & L. Marzio. 2002. Effects of one month treatment with GABA agonist baclofen on gastro-esophageal reflux and symptoms in patients with gastro-esophageal reflux disease. *Gastroenterology* **122:** A-196.

91. Vela, M.F., R. Tutuian, P.O. Katz, *et al.* 2003. Baclofen decreases acid and non-acid post-prandial gastro-oesophageal reflux measured by combined multichannel intraluminal impedance and pH. *Aliment Pharmacol. Ther.* **17:** 243–251.

92. Omari, T.I., M.A. Benninga, L. Sansom, *et al.* 2006. Effect of baclofen on esophagogastric motility and gastroesophageal reflux in children with gastroesophageal reflux disease: a randomized controlled trial. *J. Pediatr.* **149:** 436–438.

93. Koek, G.H., D. Sifrim, T. Lerut, *et al.* 2002. Effect of the GABA$_B$ agonist baclofen in patients with symptoms and duodeno-gastro-oesophageal reflux refractory to proton pump inhibitors. *Gut* **52:** 1397–1402.

94. Ciccaglione, A.F. & L. Marzio. 2003. Effect of acute and chronic administration of the GABA$_B$ agonist baclofen on 24 hour pH metry and symptoms in control subjects and in patients with gastro-oesophageal reflux disease. *Gut* **52:** 464–470.

95. Kawai, M., H. Kawahara, S. Hirayama, *et al.* 2004. Effect of baclofen on emesis and 24-hour esophageal pH in neurologically impaired children with gastroesophageal reflux disease. *J. Pediatr. Gastroenterol. Nutr.* **38:** 317–323.

96. Cossentino, M.J., C. Maydonovitch, L. Belle, *et al.* 2003. The effect of baclofen on patients with gastroesophageal reflux disease: A prospective, randomized, double-blinded, placebo-controlled study. *Gastroenterol* **124:** A226.

Ann. N.Y. Acad. Sci. ISSN 0077-8923

ANNALS OF THE NEW YORK ACADEMY OF SCIENCES
Issue: *Barrett's Esophagus: The 10th OESO World Congress Proceedings*

Barrett's esophagus: endoscopic treatments I

Michael D. Saunders,[1] Alejandro Nieponice,[2,3] Katerina Dvorak,[4] Aaron Goldman,[4] Edgardo Diaz-Cervantes,[5] A. De-la-Torre-Bravo,[6] S. Sobrino-Cossio,[7] E. Torres-Durazo,[8] O. Martínez-Carrillo,[5] J. Gamboa-Robles,[9] Melissa Upton,[10] Henry D. Appelman,[11] Luigi Bonavina,[12] Richard I. Rothstein,[13] and Vic Velanovich[14]

[1]Digestive Disease Center, University of Washington Medical Center, Seattle, Washington. [2]University of Pittsburgh, Pittsburgh, Pennsylvania PA. [3]University of Favaloro, Buenos Aires, Argentina. [4]Department of Cell Biology and Anatomy, College of Medicine and Arizona Cancer Center, The University of Arizona, Tucson, Arizona. [5]Saint Joseph's Hospital, Gastroenterology, Endoscopy and Motility Unit, Zacatecas, México. [6]Angeles Metropolitan Hospital, Mexico, Distrito Federal, México. [7]Cancerology's National Institute, México, Distrito Federal, México. [8]Angeles Mocel Hospital, Siglo XXI, México, Distrito Federal, México. [9]General Hospital, Pathology Division, Fresnillo Zacatecas, México. [10]University of Washington Medical Center, Seattle, Washington. [11]Department of Pathology, The University of Michigan Hospitals, Ann Arbor, Michigan MI. [12]Department of Surgery, IRCCS Policlinico San Donato, University of Milano Medical School, Milan, Italy. [13]Section of Gastroenterology, Dartmouth-Hitchcook Medical Center, Lebanon, New Hampshire. [14]Division of General Surgery, Henry Ford Hospital, Detroit, Michigan

The following on endoscopic treatments of Barrett's esophagus includes commentaries on indications for endoscopic treatments; endo-luminal plication procedures; the cellular modifications induced by the endoscopic ablation therapies; eradication by banding without resection; the evaluation of complete ablation; recurrence after ablation; association of antireflux surgery; radiofrequency ablation; and nondysplastic Barrett's esophagus.

Keywords: Barrett's esophagus; esophagectomy; esophageal cancer; radiofrequency ablation; dysplasia; goblet cell; band ligation; banding without-resection; banding without-snare; fundoplication; GERD; antireflux surgery; endolumenal procedures; intramucosal carcinoma

Concise summaries

- There is good evidence supporting the efficacy and safety of endoscopic treatment (photodynamic therapy (PDT), RFA, endoscopic resection (ER)) in early Barrett's cancer. The role of endoscopic treatment for those with no dysplasia or low-grade dysplasia (LGD) is uncertain and cannot be uniformly recommended at this time.

- The current optimal approach for endoscopic management of early Barrett's cancer is ER of visible mucosal lesions followed by eradication of any residual Barrett's mucosa with RFA.

- It is not clear if ablative therapies reduce cancer risk. In susceptible BE patients, they may induce formation of cells with damaged DNA and mutations and thus with higher risk to develop esophageal adenocarcinoma (EAC). Additional markers that have been reported to be abnormal in Barrett's intestinal metaplasia and EAC deserve to be studied.

- The most recent devices launched in the field of endoluminal plication procedures allow for the creation of a valve that resembles a laparoscopic fundoplication with a high-pressure zone and interesting anatomical appearance.

- Argon plasma coagulation (APC), at a power output of 60–90 W, allows a safe ablation of BE and LGD with a high success rate. In most series of patients treated with APC, the newly developed squamous epithelium remains stable at up to five-year follow-up.

- Radiofrequency ablation (RFA) seems optimal for treating flat, nonnodular Barrett's esophagus (BE). Nodular disease may be treated with RFA following the removal of the nodular segments with endoscopic mucosal resection. Proof of true cancer reduction with implementation of

doi: 10.1111/j.1749-6632.2011.06049.x

Ann. N.Y. Acad. Sci. 1232 (2011) 140–155 © 2011 New York Academy of Sciences.

RFA as a treatment strategy in nondysplastic BE is still lacking.

- Banding without-resection (BWR) is a new ablation modality that probably collects the desired criteria for a simple and effective ablative technique for BE. BWR has some advantages and may have fewer risks than EMR and other ablative modalities because it is minimally invasive.

- The factors of recurrence of Barrett's mucosa after ablation cannot be defined yet, but the difference between recurrence and hidden residual Barrett's mucosa has to be defined first.

- It has been shown that the addition of an antireflux operation, most typically a laparoscopic Nissen fundoplication, reduces the rate of recurrent or persistent BE.

---

1. What are the current indications and results of the endoscopic treatments of BE?

Michael D. Saunders

mds@u.washington.edu

The role of endoscopic therapy in BE has evolved. Once considered experimental for high-grade dysplasia (HGD), it is now becoming established as the treatment of choice in that setting. The indications for endoscopic therapy in BE are summarized in Table 1.

Endoscopic therapies available include ER, RFA, photodynamic therapy (PDT), cryotherapy, and other modalities such as APC, multipolar electrocautery, and laser therapy. There is good evidence supporting the efficacy and safety of endoscopic treatment (PDT, RFA, and ER) in early Barrett's cancer. The role of endoscopic treatment for those with no dysplasia or LGD is uncertain and cannot be uniformly recommended at this time.

Endoscopic resection

ER is superior to mucosal biopsies for diagnosis and staging of dysplasia, changing the initial histologic diagnosis and management in about 25% of cases.[1] ER is an excisional therapy, allowing for removal of visible neoplastic mucosal lesions. Negative margins obtained with ER correlate with surgical pathology. Importantly, there is a low rate (<3%) of lymph node metastases with mucosal neoplasia (intramucosal carcinoma).[2] Following ER, metachronous lesions develop in approximately 20% during follow-up.[3]

Ablation

The only modalities studied in controlled fashion for early Barrett's cancer are PDT and RFA (Table 2). Both were superior to medical therapy in eradication of HGD and decreased progression to cancer. Stricture rate was higher with PDT than RFA.

Multimodality therapy

The current optimal approach for endoscopic management of early Barrett's cancer is ER of visible mucosal lesions followed by eradication of any residual Barrett's mucosa, with RFA being the ablative procedure of choice. Table 3 below summarizes the prospective studies evaluating multimodality therapy, highlighting an efficacy of over 90% in eradication of dysplasia and Barrett's mucosa with relatively low complication rates (13–17%).

Recommendations

Endoscopically visible mucosal lesions are removed with ER, allowing for accurate staging and potentially curative excision of the mucosal neoplasia. ER

Table 1. Indications for endoscopic therapy in Barrett's esophagus

Pathology	Endoscopic treatment recommended?
HGD, intramucosal carcinoma (early Barrett's cancer)	Definitely
Nondysplastic Barrett's, indefinite, low-grade dysplasia	Not uniformly
	Consider if other factors present such as family history of esophageal cancer
Localized, invasive cancer in nonsurgical candidate	Individualized
	Considered palliative

Table 2. Summary results for endoluminal plication devices

	PDT ($n = 138$)	RFA ($n = 42$)
Author	Overholt *et al.*[5]	Shaheen *et al.*[6]
Medical therapy	Omeprazole 20 mg BID	Esomeprazole 40 mg BID
Nodular disease	33%, additional 50 J/cm PDT	9%, EMR allowed prior to study entry
Ablation treatments	Mean 2.3	Mean 3.5
Follow-up	24 months	12 months
Eradication of IM	52% vs. 7%	74% vs. 2.3%
Eradication of HGD	77% vs. 39%	81% vs. 19%
Progression to cancer	13% vs. 28%	2.4% vs. 19%
Stricture	36%	6%

Adapted from Wolfsen.[4]

Table 3. Diseases with cancer-prone epithelium and operations designed to reduce cancer risk

Study	n	Modality	Outcome	Follow up	Complications
Pech *et al.*[3]	349	EMR (255) EMR + PDT (11)	Long-term complete response 95% 5-year survival 84%	64 months	17%
Pouw *et al.*[8a]	82	EMR + RFA	CR-N 100%, CR-IM 93%	12 months	13%

[a]Euro II study: interim analysis of ongoing prospective multicenter trial.

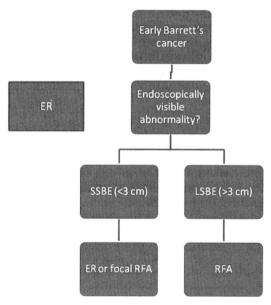

Figure 1. Current optimal approach to endoscopic treatment of early Barrett's cancer.

can be safely performed to semi-circumferential, 2 cm in length areas. ER is repeated until all endoscopically visible abnormalities are removed. The residual Barrett's mucosa should then be eradi-

cated given the risk of developing metachronous lesions.

RFA is the preferred ablation modality in BE following ER of visible mucosal lesions or in flat dysplasia. For long segments of Barrett's mucosa (>3 cm), balloon-based RFA (Halo 360) is preferred initially. For short segments or residual Barrett's following balloon ablation, probe-based RFA (Halo 90) is recommended. Alternatively, ER can be performed exclusively in those with short segments of Barrett's (<3 cm). The recommended approach to endoscopic treatment of early Barrett's cancer is summarized in the following algorithm (Fig. 1).

2. What are the results of the endoluminal plication procedures?

Alejandro Nieponice

Nieponicea@upmc.edu

In the last decade, several endoluminal devices have gained attention as promising tools for treatment of gastresophageal reflux disease (GERD) as an alternative to laparoscopic fundoplication. However, several requirements need to be met for them to prove successful: they need to be safe, effective,

Table 4. Summary results for endoluminal plication devices

Plicator (NDO)	Rothstein	2006	78	3 m	50	23 Plicator
			80			24	15 sham
	Pleskow	2007	29	3 yrs	57	n/a
		2008	33	5 yrs	67	n/a
EndoCinch (Bard)	Abou-Rebyeh	2005	38	1 yr	20	14
	Schiefke	2005	70	1.5 yrs	6	28
EsophyX (EGS)	Cadière – Phase 1	2008	17	1 yr	82	63
		2009	14	2 yrs	79	n/a
	Cadière – Phase 2	2008	79	1 yr	85	37/48
		2009	51	2 yr	71	n/a

user-independent, and economically viable. That strong combination has yet to be seen and has driven several of these devices to failure. As opposed to bulking agents, plication devices have made further achievements by starting with the right concept of recreating the anatomy of a valve at the GE junction. But this concept is far from being a simple task and technical challenges have hampered most of the attempts. The first plication device was Endocinch (BARD, Inc., Murray Hill, NJ, USA), which showed good initial control of symptoms but lack of objective reflux control with PH monitoring. The symptom control failed in the long-term follow-up, plication seemed to be loosened, and this procedure has been abandoned.[8] With similar results but a mild improvement in reflux control the Plicator (NDO Surgical, Inc., Mansfield, MA, USA) has shown a better transmural fixation trying to ensure serosa-to-serosa contact.[9] However, a real valve with a long esophageal segment could not be achieved. This procedure has also been discontinued by most of the surgical community. The most recent device launched to the market is the Esophyx (EndoGastric Solutions) that allows the creation of a valve that resembles a laparoscopic fundoplication with a high-pressure zone and interesting anatomical appearance. Initially reported results were more encouraging than previous competitors and mixed results started to appear as the technique spreads out.[10,11]

A large clinical trial undergoing in the U.S. will probably set faith for this approach. A summary of available results for all these devices is reported in Table 4. In order to accurately understand the results of the endoluminal plication procedures, we need to analyze what the expectations were, what we compared them to, and what the optimal patient population is. Initially the stakes were set too high as everyone thought of this as the perfect alternative to withdraw patients from PPIs without the need of undergoing a laporoscopic surgery and its known side-effects. Comparison with laparoscopic surgery is probably the wrong idea for these devices, as we have learned that hiatal hernias are a big limitation for these procedures. If there is a room for an endoluminal procedure, it will be in a middle-world between chronic medication and the Nissen fundoplication. Therefore, comparisons should be made with medical therapy.

And last but definitely not least, patient selection will turn out to be the key if any endoluminal plication will survive. In a retrospective study, Khajanchee *et al.* showed that patients with lower DeMeester scores, heartburn scores lower than 2, and body mass index lower than 30 had a significantly better outcome when undergoing an endoluminal plication.

This tendency shows that only a highly selected population will benefit from these technologies making the market still available but much less attractive for the companies that need to work on the evolution of these devices. This fact deserves a paragraph on insurance carriers that are ever searching for ways to reduce medical costs, and they are very cautious after the first iteration of endolumenal antireflux procedure and require concrete evidence of efficacy prior to authorizing payment for these novel procedures. George Bernard Shaw said "When I was a young man I observed that nine out of ten things I did were failures. I didn't want to be a failure, so I did ten times more work". This seems to be the case if we want to find a safe, effective and reliable endoscopic method for our patients.

3. May endoscopic ablation therapies induce formation of cells more susceptible to genomic damage?

Katerina Dvorak and Aaron Goldman
kdvorak@email.arizona.edu

BE is a premalignant condition associated with the development of EAC. Patients with this cancer have a poor prognosis with a median survival of less than one year. It is becoming clear that acid suppression therapies alone, using surgery or drugs, have no significant effect on reversing BE. Endoscopic ablation therapies are becoming more popular in recent years, especially for patients with HGD or with intramucosal adenocarcinoma. Endoscopic ablation of abnormal tissue is less invasive and safer compared to esophagectomy that used to be the only routine clinical treatment of HGD and EAC. A number of endoscopic therapies to eradicate esophageal columnar epithelium were developed over recent years including APC, multipolar electrocoagulation, PDT, laser therapy, cryotherapy, and RFA. However, concerns remain regarding incomplete ablation, strictures, and buried glands that are not readily detected and may represent a risk for esophageal cancer development.

In the setting of complete ablation, the neosquamous epithelium is not different from normal squamous epithelium and represents low cancer risk. Garewal *et al.* have shown low expression of Ki67, p53, and low activities of ornithine decarboxylase in new squamous epithelium in completely ablated esophagus.[12] Furthermore, new squamous epithelium exhibits low level of staining for Ki67 and p53 as well as no DNA abnormalities after RFA. Cytokeratin expression (CK-8 and -14) and miRNAs were also similar in postablation neosquamous epithelium and normal squamous epithelium.

However, in the setting of incomplete ablation the data are not so clear. Krishnadath *et al.* reported that three patients who were free of dysplasia after photodynamic therapy developed dysplasia during follow-up and also had increased expression of at least one of the markers associated with increased cancer risk (Ki67, aneuploidy, p53 expression, or p16 promoter hypermethylation).[13] Similarly, Hage *et al.* found that after ablation therapy, residual or recurrent BE glands retain or accumulate abnormalities such as p53 overexpression, increased proliferation, and DNA abnormalities even in the absence of dysplasia.[14] In contrast, a recent biomarker study by Prasad *et al.* shows that DNA abnormalities detected by fluorescence *in situ* hybridization (FISH) were significantly decreased after PTD therapy. However, a subset of patients (19%) without dysplasia had positive FISH results and developed recurrent HGD.[15] Hornick *et al.* reported that buried glands after PDT show reduced crypt proliferation and lower level of DNA abnormalities, and they suggest that these glands have lower neoplastic potential.

The majority of these studies evaluated only biopsies of columnar epithelium from incompletely ablated patients. Only few studies evaluated changes in squamous epithelium after ablative therapies and only few patients were included in these studies. Furthermore, even fewer studies were focused on biomarker alterations at new squamo-columnar junctions that are formed after incomplete ablation. Our group has shown that these new junctions stain positively for several cancer risk associated biomarkers, such as cyclooxygenase 2, Ki67, and p53 in a subset of patients.[16] Importantly, the expression of these biomarkers was low in the preablation BE biopsies.

The major approach to eradicate BE is combination of injury by different ablative techniques and acid suppression. In this environment, intestinal epithelium is healed and replaced primarily with neosquamous epithelium; however, the effect on cancer risk remains unknown, and the question of whether ablation decreases the cancer risk remains unanswered. Wound healing that follows ablation is a complex process that involves different cytokines, enzymes and growth factors, and activation of signaling pathways. This process can be divided into inflammation, proliferation, and maturation phases. After injury, inflammatory cells invade the wound tissue. They produce proteinases, reactive oxygen species, and reactive nitrogen species as a defense against bacteria. Inflammatory cells are also an important source of growth factors and cytokines, which initiate the proliferative phase of wound repair. Wound healing is associated with increased expression of IL-1α, IL-1β, IL-6, TNF-α, or hepatocyte growth factor (HGF) and members of the epidermal growth factor (EFG) family. Importantly, overexpression of these cytokines and growth factors and their receptors is often found in BE and EAC and is likely to have a role in esophageal tumorigenesis. Furthermore, reactive oxygen species produced by inflammatory cells can cause DNA damage resulting in mutations. Most of the genes that orchestrate the wound-healing process are also important regulators of cancer growth and progression. Therefore, epithelium undergoing these changes is possibly more prone to genomic instability and is susceptible to DNA damage in a subset of BE patients especially those, who require repeated ablation. In addition, DNA damage and increased cytokine and growth factor expression may even be elevated if acid and bile reflux is not well controlled. Indeed, both these components of refluxate were shown to induce DNA damage.

In summary, it is not clear if ablative therapies reduce cancer risk. In susceptible BE patients, they may induce formation of cells with damaged DNA and mutations and, thus, with higher risk to develop EAC. Additional markers that have been reported to be abnormal in Barrett's intestinal metaplasia and EAC deserve to be studied to further address this important clinical issue.

4. What can be expected from Banding without-resection for Barrett's esophagus?

Edgardo Diaz-Cervantes
edgardoscopio@hotmail.com

Most of the ablative treatments for Barrett's esophagus are expensive, potentially hazardous, require specialized training, and are not universally available. Furthermore, these ablative techniques may fail to eradicate all of the Barrett's epithelium and often leave remnants of metaplastic mucosa behind in the form of visible islands or in the form of glands buried under a layer of neosquamous epithelium.[17] An effective ablative therapy for BE that is relatively inexpensive, safe, simple, and readily available would be highly desirable. We have been working on BWR from April 2004 to date (seven years); this work has been formerly published in 2007.[18]

BWR is a new ablation modality that probably collects the above desired criteria for an ideal ablative technique. It is *simple*, because there is no need for special skills—you just need an endoscope, a multiband ligator, and some technique; there is no need for an injector, snare, or anything else. BWR is also very *effective*: during the last seven years we have gotten rid of Barrett's in 110 patients, by banding one or two spots of Barrett's epithelium on each session and repeating at three month intervals until the metaplastic epithelium has been completely eradicated. We have obtained 98% of complete resolution of intestinal metaplasia compared to only 2% in our control group consisting of 76 patients (with omeprazol bid for years, only). BWR is a minimally invasive and "easy" procedure for the esophagus because only a very small, superficial

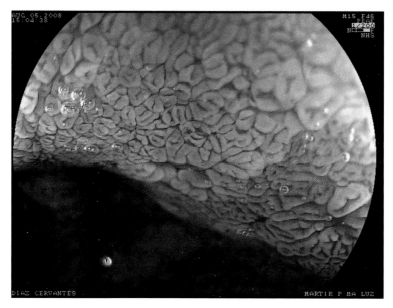

Figure 2. This C1M3 BE was completely ablated in just 2 sessions and 3 rubber bands. The image is enhanced by magnification and acetic acid.

ulceration must heal—the residual scar is thin, small, superficial, and this is probably the main reason for the absence of residual stenosis. BWR is not expensive and is available worldwide. This new Barrett's ablation technique is "low tech" but has "high results."

Number of banding and sessions for complete resolution of BE

How many banding sessions were needed to get complete resolution of BE in the treated group consisting of 101 SSBE and 9 LSBE segment Barrett's? A mean of 2.6 sessions (very similar to other ablation procedures). How many bands were needed for complete resolution of BE in these patients? A mean of 4.7 bands.

Long-lasting changes

One of the big concerns after any ablation procedure is what happens years after ablation and how durable the changes are. In our 110 ablated patients, posteradication changes seems to be durable. The longer follow up in 44 of our 110 patients ranges between 50 and 70 ms with permanent or durable changes. After the last banding procedures, there is no modification at all, on the endoscopic finding even after four to six years (Fig. 3).

Comparison between techniques

A frequent inquiry about BWR is the lack of tissue sampling after ablation; the answer to this is that ablation modalities do not enable tissue sampling after ablation because, except for endoscopicmucosal resection, all of them are *in situ* tissue-destroying techniques. BWR has a deeper penetration mechanism, the same as endoscopic mucosal resection EMR (submucosal), whereas other ablation procedures affect only the mucosal layer. Because of its mechanism of action, this nonresection technique avoids the risk of perforation and bleeding (Fig. 2).

Conclusions

(1) BWR is a new ablation procedure for Barrett's and is very different than EMR.

(2) BWR has the potential to remove HGD because it achieves good depth of ablation.

(3) BWR has many advantages and appears to have fewer risks than EMR and other ablative modalities because it is minimally invasive ("easy" on the esophagus).

(4) In our 110 patients, we found no complications at all (no stricture, bleeding, or perforation), and 98% complete resolution of intestinal metaplasia.

(5) BWR may be the procedure of choice in cirrhotic patients with BE and HGD

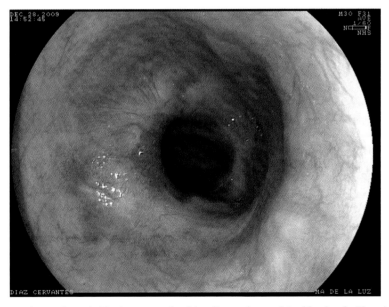

Figure 3. The same patient as shown in Fig. 2 one year after 2 banding sessions and 3 rubber bands. There is no stenosis at all. Four years of follow up has demonstrated no further changes, with apparent BE endoscopically and histologically cleared.

(6) Posteradication changes seem to be durable even after six years of follow-up.

BWR appears to be a safe, effective, simple, and widely available technique for eradicating short-segment and tongued large-segment BE. Nevertheless, further studies are needed.

5. How should *complete* ablation of Barrett's mucosa be defined?

Melissa P. Upton
mupton@u.washington.edu

Before defining "complete ablation of Barrett mucosa," it is essential to acknowledge that there is still no international agreement regarding the definition of Barrett mucosa. What are we trying to ablate?

The original definition by Mr. Norman Barrett was columnar lining of the tubular esophagus, and it dominated the thinking of physicians and scientists for decades. It remains the definition in England and in some other countries, including Japan. According to this definition, esophageal columnar lining can include any type of columnar metaplasia—oxyntic, cardiac, and intestinalized mucosae. This would also include multilayered epithelium, a hybrid epithelium identified more recently and seen in association with chronic reflux. Using this definition, complete ablation would require ablation of *all* columnar lining in the esophagus.

In contrast, the American definition of Barrett's esophagus, adopted in the mid-1990s, requires an endoscopic–histologic correlation. The endoscopist must recognize irregular tongues of pink columnar-appearing epithelium extending into the esophagus proximal to the GE junction, and the pathologist must confirm the histologic finding of specialized columnar epithelium, intestinalized epithelium with goblet cells containing acidic mucins, in biopsies designated as esophageal in location. The American definition came into use following the recognition that the overwhelming majority of cases of EAC and high-grade glandular dysplasia occurred in a setting of columnar metaplasia with goblet cells detected on biopsy. Using the American definition, if the goal is ablation of all Barrett mucosa, we would theoretically ablate the columnar lining of the esophagus only in patients with histologically documented goblet cells.

One problematic issue with the American definition is the challenge of sampling, because goblet cell distribution may be extensive, or focal and patchy. Occasionally, many biopsies may be needed to identify goblet cells, especially in patients with extensive neoplastic alterations. Although the Seattle protocol of biopsy sampling has been recommended as the standard approach, it is clear from a review of practice settings that many gastroenterologists do not use large-jaw biopsy forceps or take the recommended numbers of biopsies at the prescribed distance intervals between biopsies outlined in this protocol. In addition, both in historic mapping series and in more recent studies of endoscopic mucosal resection specimens, cases of adenocarcinoma have been reported in a setting of columnar lined esophagus without histologic documentation of goblet cells. The epithelium adjacent to and in carcinomas may not have identifiable intestinal phenotype. In addition, aneuploidy, and cell cycle abnormalities have been reported in epithelium without histologic features of neoplasia.

It is likely that intestinal metaplasia is simply a histologic marker of risk. Neoplastic changes probably arise in a mutated stem cell population with the capability of differentiating into a neoplastic clone with or without histologically recognizable intestinal phenotype or acidic mucin production. In addition, there may be important contributions to the development of neoplastic risk by stromal components and by populations of the submucosal glands of the esophagus.[19] Ablation limited to the mucosa or superficial epithelium and lamina propria may not be adequate. To confirm if endoscopic ablative techniques can eradicate the risk of future neoplasia, will require longer follow-up intervals, rigorous and careful postablation surveillance biopsies, and additional investigation into the molecular mechanisms of neoplastic development. More work is needed to identify the cells of origin and the permissive microenvironment that favors neoplasia.

In addressing the issue of complete ablation, what are we trying to ablate? Is the goal to ablate neoplastic mucosa? Presumably, the goal is not to simply ablate already detectable neoplastic epithelium, but also to ablate mucosa that is at risk for future neoplastic alterations. Will we refer only patients with documented goblet cells, associated with higher risk for malignancy in the American series? Will we include patients with any columnar lining of the esophagus, given recent EMR data suggesting that neoplasia may develop in cardiac mucosal background?

Some investigators have suggested that all patients with Barrett's esophagus are potentially at risk for neoplasia and should be considered for ablation of the entire columnar lining. But ablation is costly, and patients will require continued surveillance after ablative treatment. Therefore, any decision for mucosal ablation must balance the potential costs and risks of the procedure and continued surveillance with the benefits of ablation. Instead of ablating all patients with Barrett's mucosa, perhaps we should treat only selected groups within the large population of patients with BE, treating only those with histologically proven neoplasia or those who show specific molecular markers for increased risk of progression, such as aneuploidy or increased synthetic fraction when studied by DNA flow cytometry.

Future studies are needed to address whether molecular markers, such as methylation or mutation of p16, can assist in selection of patients at increased risk for neoplasia for whom ablation is clearly indicated. And we must design robust and thorough methods of follow-up for treated patients, both to avoid missing neoplasms that may develop in the postablation period, and also to gain understanding of how the esophagus and its microenvironment (including molecular events) are altered by ablation procedures, and if this alters the risk for future neoplastic changes.

6. Can the factors of recurrence of intestinal metaplasia (Barrett's mucosa) be defined?

Henry D. Appelman
appelman@umich.edu

This can be paraphrased to this question: once Barrett's mucosa is destroyed by any type of ablation, and it recurs, is there an explanation for the recurrence? To answer this question, we need data from a study that begins with Barrett's mucosa, which is then ablated by any technique and replaced by new squamous epithelium. Then the study design has to find a way to prove unequivocally that the Barrett's has been completed destroyed, and that no residual Barrett's mucosa is present beneath the

new squamous mucosa, presumably by biopsy of the entire previous Barrett's segment. The study then must continue with extensive follow-up, and in those cases in which the Barrett's mucosa recurs, the study must identify the reasons for the recurrence. I looked everywhere for this study, and I could not find it. So I looked for published hints.

In one study of 72 patients with 2–6 cm of Barrett's mucosa treated with radio frequency ablation, 92% achieved complete response with no recurrence at five years.[20,21] The definition for complete response was the lack of residual intestinal metaplasia in any biopsy. The biopsy protocol involved four quadrants at every level in one to two centimeter increments, which clearly left a lot of esophageal mucosa not sampled. 8% of these patients did not have a complete response, possibly indicating recurrence in some patients. However, no factors were evaluated in this 8% to help me answer the question above.

In another study on laser ablation in 31 patients, 21 achieved complete response, which was not clearly defined in the study, but presumably it was lack of intestinal metaplasia on any biopsy.[22] Unfortunately, the biopsy protocol was not defined. Eight patients had recurrence of Barrett's from 6 to 44 months after presumably successful ablation, and six of these had a colonic epithelial protein antigen in cardiac-type epithelium without goblet cells, the Das antigen suggesting that this protein is a reasonable predictor of recurrence. However, the antigen was expressed in cardiac-type mucosa, often buried under squamous mucosa, not in goblet cell–containing mucosa. In the British definition of Barrett's mucosa, this cardiac-type mucosa with the Das antigen would have been considered Barrett's mucosa if there were appropriate endoscopic findings.

One likely explanation for recurrent Barrett's mucosa is that this mucosa has become covered by metaplastic squamous epithelium induced by the ablation technique, and this hid residual Barrett's from endoscopic detection and from biopsy. No study can guarantee that this has not happened, because no study followed ablation with biopsy of the entire previous Barrett's segment. Another explanation is that Barrett's recurred, because the new squamous epithelium induced by ablation is subject to the same factors that caused the Barrett's mucosa to occur originally. If we only knew how Barrett's developed in the first place. Unfortunately, we do not.

To summarize, can the factors of recurrence of Barrett's mucosa after ablation be defined? The answer is not yet, but we should keep trying. However, first we have to define the difference between recurrence and hidden residual Barrett's mucosa.

7. Is the combination of APC with antireflux surgery a good means to enhance late results?

Luigi Bonavina
luigi.bonavina@unimi.it

BE is defined as a biopsy-proven change in the distal esophageal epithelium, with normal squamous epithelium being replaced by columnar epithelium containing goblet cells. This condition, also known as intestinal metaplasia, occurs in approximately 10% of patients with gastroesophageal reflux disease.[23] Intestinal metaplasia is a premalignant condition associated with an increased risk of EAC especially when LGD or HGD is found in the biopsies. On the other hand, molecular alterations may even precede the development of intestinal metaplasia in BE.[24]

Retrospective studies have demonstrated that patient survival is improved if an endoscopic surveillance strategy detects cancer at earlier stages compared to a strategy of no surveillance.[25] However, surveillance is a strategy designed to detect cancer, not to prevent cancer. Over the past decade, research efforts have been directed toward endoscopic mucosal ablation to eliminate the risk of cancer and allow regeneration of squamous epithelium following pharmacological or surgical control of reflux.[26] The clinical value of endoscopic ablation of nondysplastic BE combined with acid suppression therapy or antireflux surgery remains controversial.

APC, at a power output of 60–90 Watts, allows a safe ablation of BE and LGD with a high success rate. In our series including 94 patients with nondysplastic BE, the eradication rate was 72.3% with an average of three treatment sessions. Of the 68 eradicated patients, 27 underwent fundoplication and 41 were treated with proton pump inhibitors; the eradication rate was 89.4% and 87.5%, respectively, with a mean follow-up of 26 months.[27] Bright *et al.* recently published the results of a randomized trial of APC versus endoscopic surveillance for BE after antireflux surgery. Regression of BE after fundoplication was more likely, and greater in extent, in patients who underwent prior ablation with APC. Moreover, in most patients treated with APC, the newly developed squamous epithelium remained stable at up to five-years follow-up. The only case of progression to HGD occurred in a patient who was not treated with APC before surgery.[28]

8. Optimizing techniques for RFA to treat BE

Richard I. Rothstein, MD
richard.i.rothstein@hitchcock.org

Attention to radiofrequency device evolution and procedural techniques, along with individualized patient factors, will permit optimization of outcomes from this innovative and beneficial therapy for BE. RFA is optimal for treating flat, nonnodular BE. Individuals with nodular disease may be treated with RFA following the removal of the nodular segments with endoscopic mucosal resection (EMR). A delay of six to eight weeks between the time of EMR to the performance of RFA of Barrett's tissue should provide adequate time for healing of the resected mucosa and is necessary for the best treatment outcomes. RFA is a safe and effective treatment for dysplastic Barrett's as well as intestinal metaplasia with foci of intramucosal carcinoma (staged by endoscopic ultrasound and EMR). Selected nondysplastic Barrett's patients can be safely and effectively treated with RFA and it can be cost-effective for the management of that condition compared to the surveillance strategies in current practice.

The performance of RFA involves the use of specialized devices and a sophisticated control unit (Halo 360 and 90, Barrx Medical). With the Halo RFA system, thermal energy is precisely delivered to the treated tissue to a depth of 500–1000 μm, to remove the mucosal layer and limit damage to the deeper submucosal layer. That effectively reduces the problem of stricture formation, which is a major problem with other ablation treatments such as wide-field EMR and PDT.

The Halo 360 system uses a sizing balloon catheter and variable-sized electrode treatment balloons. The procedure is done following a standard upper endoscopic exam during which the landmarks are recorded for the upper border of the Barrett's segment and the top of the gastric folds as well as the geographic pattern of the intestinal metaplasia. The Barrett's segment is cleaned with a spray of dilute *n*-acetylcysteine to remove surface mucous and a guidewire is left in the distal stomach as the gastroscope is removed. Over this guidewire, the sizing balloon is passed and localized 12 cm proximal to the top of the gastric folds (placed even higher if needed to be above the proximal extent of the Barrett's for ultra-long segment disease). Stepwise inflation and deflation of the balloon as it is moved centimeter-by-centimeter towards the cardia allows the determination (shown on the digital monitor of the control unit) of the size of the esophageal lumen, which is used to determine the effective treatment balloon size. In the situation of multiple balloon sizes recorded along the length of the esophagus, the recommendation is to use the smallest treatment balloon size recommended. However, in the situation of smaller proximal lumen and a consistently larger distal lumen, as may be seen in longer-segment disease, it is appropriate to use a smaller treatment balloon proximally and the larger size distally. In all situations, it is important to view that the selected treatment balloon size permits effective contact of its electrodes to the esophageal wall.

After the sizing steps have been completed, the sizing balloon is removed and the selected treatment balloon is introduced over the guidewire. The gastroscope is introduced alongside the Halo 360 catheter since the RFA treatment is done under direct vision. The proximal part of the electrode segment of the treatment balloon is best placed 1 cm proximal to the top of the Barrett's segment. For Barrett's with dysplasia, the setting for ablation is typically set on the unit at 12 joules/cm^2, whereas for nondysplastic it is recommended to be 10 joules/cm^2. The Barrett's segment is treated proximal to distal with a 5 mm to 1 cm overlap in order to obtain uniform treatment without "skip" areas. Once treated, the endoscope and the balloon with guidewire are all removed from the patient. A soft sort distal cap is placed on the gastroscope, which is reintroduced and used to scrape away all of the treated sloughing mucosa. This step is very important to optimize the ablation outcome, and enough time should be spent to ensure adequate cleaning of the treated segment. The guidewire is replaced

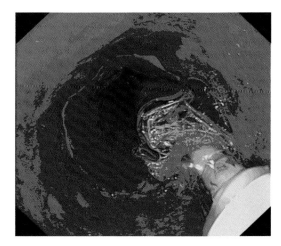

Figure 4. Halo 360 postablation view.

into the stomach and the endoscope removed. The treatment technique of balloon passage and use is repeated as described, with all of the Barrett's segment treated a second time. Following removal of the endoscope, balloon, and guidewire, the patient is recovered, and instructed to continue on bid proton pump inhibitors and to consume a liquid diet for two days and then a soft diet for three to five days before resuming a regular diet. Mild analgesics may be needed, and patients should be given instructions and education about the typical sensations to expect following the RFA treatment (Fig. 4).

In follow-up RFA sessions where there may be residual small areas of Barrett's remaining after the circumferential balloon treatment, the Halo 90 system may be employed. This endoscope-mounted system, with an electrode pattern of 13 × 20 mm, can also be used for primary therapy of short segment disease. After a standard upper endoscopy, the Halo 90 device is mounted on the endoscope which is reintroduced and used in a patchwork fashion with 3 mm overlap onto treated segments to treat all areas of intestinal metaplasia. In contrast to the single application of thermal energy with the circumferential balloon, followed by cleaning of the segment and then retreatment, with the Halo 90 the Barrett's mucosa is treated twice, then scraped clean, and then retreated. Instead of a cap, the mounted RFA device can be used for removal of the sloughed tissue. When treating short segment disease, the device is placed to straddle the top of the gastric folds, and the treatments done by rotating the scope to permit an overlap of a few millimeters and moving around the gastroesophageal junction, usually taking six treatment sites to cover the circumference. Posttreatment recommendations are as for the circumferential treatment described.

As for all new advanced endoscopic procedures, adequate training and mentoring are essential to optimize the clinical outcomes and ensure the best safety for RFA of Barrett's. For references to this section, see Refs 6, 21, 29, 30 and 31.

9. Ablation of nondysplastic Barrett's epithelium: a surgeon's perspective

Vic Velanovich
vvelano1@hfhs.org

Ablation of BE has been shown to be an effective means of eliminating Barrett's epithelium[32] and to decrease the incidence of EAC in patients with HGD.[6] Nevertheless, controversy exists as to whether or not ablating nondysplastic Barrett's epithelium should be done.[22] This paper provides the surgeon's perspective on this issue.

The concept of eliminating cancer-prone epithelium is not new to surgeons. There are several disease processes which have had operations designed specifically to reduce cancer risk (Table 5). Therefore, it is not a conceptual leap for the surgeon to apply ablative techniques to Barrett's epithelium to reduce cancer risk.

Although the risk of EAC in BE is low, prevention is still worthwhile due to the serious consequences of developing adenocarcinoma. EAC is primarily treated with esophagectomy. Esophagectomy carries significant and not easily ignored immediate

Table 5. Diseases with cancer-prone epithelium and operations designed to reduce cancer risk

Disease	Operation
Colonic adenoma	Colonoscopy polypectomy
Ulcerative colitis	Total proctocolectomy
Familial adenomatous polyposis-colon	Total colectomy with rectal mucosal stripping
Familial adenomatous polyposis-duodenum	Pancreas-sparing duodenectomy
Hereditary medullary carcinoma	Total thyroidectomy
BRCA mutations-breast cancer	Bilateral total mastectomy

and long-term adverse events. In the short-term, even in the best of hands, the morbidity rate is over 50%, with a measurable mortality rate. In general practice, the mortality rate can be as high as 10%. Stricture at the anastomosis can occur in 25–50% of patients. This not only leads to dysphagia, but may require multiple dilations. Long-term, even with curative surgery, the quality of life effects of an esophagectomy are substantial. Djarv *et al*.[33] have shown that three years after curative esophagectomy for esophageal cancer, patients have lower quality of life score compared to population norms in several physical functioning domains as well as several constitutional symptoms. Therefore, prevention of an esophagectomy is almost as worthwhile goal as the prevention of adenocarcinoma. In many respects, ablation of Barrett's epithelium can be considered a means of preventing esophagectomy.

BE can recur after ablation. This is prevented by a strict regimen of acid-suppression therapy. However, the development of Barrett's is promoted most aggressively by the combination of acid and bile reflux. Although proton pump inhibitor therapy is effective in reducing acid reflux, it does nothing for bile reflux. We have previously shown that the addition of an antireflux operation, most typically a laparoscopic Nissen fundoplication, reduces the rate of recurrent or persistent BE.[34] Clearly, a randomized trial is needed to confirm these findings.

10. RFA for nondysplastic BE: the gastroenterologist's perspective

Srinadh Komanduri
koman1973@gmail.com

Perhaps the most intriguing aspect of endotherapy for BE is its application in nondysplastic disease. Although offering therapy for patients with dysplastic BE is a cost-effective strategy, the same is not so evident for nondysplastic disease. However, treating only patients with dysplasia will likely limit our ability to reach the ultimate goal of eradication of EAC.

RFA offers an effective, safe, and durable treatment for patients with BE. Most recently, five years data from the AIM II trial demonstrated 92% complete eradication of BE (CR-IM). This is extremely exciting data and encourages to expand our indications for endotherapy in BE. Although RFA in nondysplastic BE appears to be cost-effective if surveillance can be discontinued, it remains to be seen where this fits in the management paradigm when surveillance is continued.

Currently, there is insufficient data to recommend cessation of surveillance after endotherapy despite achieving CR-IM. A potential solution is to risk-stratify our patients with BE for consideration for RFA. Although many biomarkers are under investigation, we are still far from a simple blood test to define risk in nondysplastic BE. That being said, we currently have a safe therapy that can eliminate not only disease, but any of these molecular changes that may drive stem cell differentiation. In addition, we must consider quality of life (QOL) in this cohort. It is considered standard of care to eliminate all pre-cancerous lesions in the body (e.g., colon polyps, breast lumps, and actinic keratosis). This paradigm creates a dilemma when we tell our patients that we will not remove their precancerous BE. It is difficult for patients to consider the small rate of progression to cancer in these circumstances. Therefore, we must consider how this would affect a patient's quality of life when making treatment decisions. Previous data have shown incremental improvement in QOL with successful eradication of BE. Ultimately, it would be ideal to have data that demonstrates a true cancer reduction with implementation of RFA as a treatment strategy in nondysplastic BE. However, given the progression rate, this will likely not be feasible any time soon. Despite the lack of this data, the durability of RFA and a recent meta-analysis clearly suggests that implementation of RFA would decrease the incidence of EAC.

Currently, RFA should be considered in select patients who fully understand the limitations of currently available data. These may include patients who are young (age <50), those with long segment disease, and patients with family history of BE-dysplasia or EAC. Regardless of this choice, it is imperative to have an extensive discussion with these patients and discuss the current data to allow them to make an educated decision about their disease. [For references to this section, see Refs 35–38]

11. What is the mechanism of regression of Barrett's esophagus after BWR?

Edgardo Diaz-Cervantes, A. De-la-Torre-Bravo, S. Sobrino-Cossio, E. Torres-Durazo, O. Martínez-Carrillo, and J. Gamboa-Robles
edgardoscopio@hotmail.com

Because Barrett's epithelium has a thickness of only 0.5 to 0.6 mm,[39] banding might be expected to result in its complete eradication. Indeed, an event in our endoscopy unit revealed an ablative technique for Barrett's esophagus (BE) that could fulfill a number of the ideal criteria for an ablative alternative. During an endoscopic variceal ligation in a patient who had bleeding esophageal varices, we placed a band on a varix that had an overlying tongue of BE. Proton pump inhibitors were prescribed. To our surprise the BE was no longer visible on a follow-up endoscopic examination one month later; this observation suggested that banding had eradicated the BE.[18]

METHOD	CR-IM	SCAR THICKNESS	STENOSIS %	PERFORATION %	BLEEDING %	BURIED BARRETT'S %
CRYO	21					0 - 18
MPEC	67		1		0 - 14	
APC	55 - 76		0 - 15	0 - 3	0 - 4	
RFA	54 - 89			0.03	- 1	0.6
PDT	52		23 - 35	0 - 1	0 - 14	6 - 60
BWR	98%	THIN	0	0	0	0.8
MBL-EMR		GROSS	10 - 70	0 – 9	0 – 10	?

Figure 5. Methods of ablation.

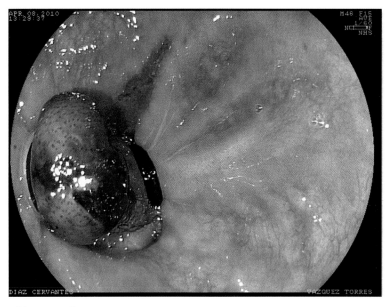

Figure 6. Banding without-resection.

Banding without-resection (BWR) is a novel method of ablation for BE, consisting on the creation of a pseudopolyp by using a multib and ligation device. Its main feature resides in a non-resection technique of the created pseudo-polyp, leaving it just ligated until it spontaneously sloughs off (Fig. 5), leaving a small ulceration that heals with neosquamous epithelium.

Mechanism of regression

1. Ischemia: the band obliterates the blood flow, and 5 to 10 days later the ischemic tissue sloughs off, leaving a small ulceration that heals with the replacement of neosquamous mucosa when acid reflux is controlled by the administration of PPI.
2. The defect of the banded mucosa is replaced by surrounding mucosa. This means that the smaller mucosal defect leads to smaller residual ulcer, resulting into a small, thin, and superficial scar.
2. By BWR, we don't snare, cut, heat; we neither infiltrate nor inject; we just apply suction, band, wait, and follow-up...so simple...so "easy" on the esophagus.

One drawback of BWR is that there is no tissue for histological evaluation; but this is a drawback shared by all ablative *in situ*-destroying procedures for BE, except for EMR (Fig. 6).

Depth of ablation

Because BWR depends on the creation of a pseudopolyp, and the same principle rules for endoscopic mucosal resection (EMR): then, both procedures may have similar depth of ablation. Endoscopic banding has an excellent track record of safety, even in high risk patients with cirrhosis. There are many substantial advantages on BWR when compared to resection, such as:

1. Banding without-resection is *per se* preventive for bleeding and perforation.
2. No need for submucosal injection before banding.
3. The risk of stricture after banding without-resection is minimal or absent. As a result of BWR we obtain only a thin, small and superficial scar, instead of big mucosal defects with long and gross scars that are usually obtained after resection.

Conflicts of interest

The authors declare no conflicts of interest.

References

1. Larghi, A. *et al.* 2005. EUS followed by EMR for staging of high-grade dysplasia and early cancer in Barrett's esophagus. *Gastrointest. Endosc.* **62:** 16.
2. Prasad, G.A. *et al.* 2007. Long-term survival following endoscopic and surgical treatment of high-grade

dysplasia in Barrett's esophagus. *Gastroenterology* **132:** 1226–1233.

3. Pech, O. *et al.* 2008. Long-term results and risk factor analysis for recurrence after curative endoscopic therapy in 349 patients with high grade intraepithelial neoplasia and mucosal adenocarcinoma in Barrett's Oesophagus. *Gut* **57:** 1200.

4. Wolfsen, D. 2009. Endoscopic ablation therapy: imaging and advanced technology in action. *Gastroenterology* **137:** 1225.

5. Overholt, B.F. *et al.* 1995. Barrett's esophagus: photodynamic therapy for ablation of dysplasia, reduction of specialized mucosa and treatment of superficial esophageal cancer. *Gastrointest. Endosc.* **42:** 64–69.

6. Shaheen, N.J. *et al.* 2009. Radiofrequency ablation in Barrett's esophagus with dysplasia. *N. Engl. J. Med.* **360:** 2277–2288.

7. Pouw, R.E. *et al.* 2010. Safety outcomes of Balloon-based RFA after focal endoscopic resection of early Barrett's neoplasia in 118 patients: results of an ongoing European multicenter study. *Gastrointest. Endosc.* **71:** AB126.

8. Schiefke, I. *et al.* 2005. Long term failure of endoscopic gastroplication (EndoCinch). *Gut* **54:** 752–758.

9. Pleskow, D. *et al.* 2004. Endoscopic full-thickness plication for the treatment of GERD: a multicenter trial. *Gastrointest. Endosc.* **59:** 163–171.

10. CadiEre, G.B. *et al.* 2008. Endoluminal fundoplication by a transoral device for the treatment of GERD: a feasibility study. *Surg. Endosc.* **22:** 333–342.

11. CadiEre, G.B. *et al.* 2008. Antireflux transoral incisionless fundoplication using EsophyX: 12-month results of a prospective multicenter study. *World J. Surg.* **32:** 1676–1788.

12. Garewal, H., L. Ramsey, P. Sharma, *et al.* 1999. Biomarker studies in reversed Barrett's esophagus. *Am. J. Gastroenterol.* **94:** 2829–2833.

13. Krishnadath, K.K., K.K. Wang, K. Taniguchi, *et al.* 2000. Persistent genetic abnormalities in Barrett's esophagus after photodynamic therapy. *Gastroenterology* **119:** 624–630.

14. Hage, M., P.D. Siersema, K.J. Vissers, *et al.* 2005. Molecular evaluation of ablative therapy of Barrett's oesophagus. *J. Pathol.* **205:** 57–64.

15. Prasad, G.A., K.K. Wang, K.C. Halling, *et al.* 2008. Correlation of histology with biomarker status after photodynamic therapy in Barrett esophagus. *Cancer* **113:** 470–476.

16. Dvorak, K., L. Ramsey, C.M. Payne, *et al.* 2006. Abnormal expression of biomarkers in incompletely ablated Barrett's esophagus. *Ann. Surg.* **244:** 1031–1036.

17. Urosevic, P. & G.K. Kiroff. 2002. Ablation of Barrett's epithelium: the promise and the problems diseases of the esophagus **15:** 30–38.

18. Diaz-Cervantes, E., A. De-la-Torre-Bravo, S.J. Spechler, *et al.* 2007. Banding without resection(endoscopic mucosal ligation) as a novel approach for the ablation of short-segment Barrett's epithelium: results of a pilot study. *Am. J. Gastroenterol.* **102:** 1640–1645.

19. Saadi, A., N.B. Shannon, P. Lao-Sirieix, *et al.* 2010. Stromal genes discriminate preinvasive from invasive disease, predict outcome, and highlight inflammatory pathways in digestive cancers. *PNAS* **107:** 2177–2182.

20. Fleischer, D.E., B.F. Overholt, V.K. Sharma, *et al.* 2008. Endoscopic ablation of Barrett's esophagus: a multicenter study with 2.5-year follow-up. *Gastrointest. Endosc.* **68:** 867–876.

21. Fleischer, D.E., R. Odze, B.F. Overholt, *et al.* 2010. The case for endoscopic treatment of non-dysplastic and low-grade dysplastic Barrett's esophagus. *Dig. Dis. Sci.* **55:** 1918–1931.

22. Fisher, R.S., M.Q. Bromer, R.M. Thomas, *et al.* 2003. Predictors of recurrent specialized intestinal metaplasia after complete laser ablation. *Am. J. Gastroenterol.* **98:** 1945–1951.

23. Spechler, S.J. 2002. Barrett's esophagus. *N. Engl. J. Med.* **346:** 836–842.

24. Romagnoli S., M. Roncalli, D. Graziani, *et al.* 2001. Molecular alterations of Barrett's esophagus on microdissected endoscopic biopsies. *Lab. Invest.* **81:** 241–247.

25. Incarbone R., L. Bonavina, G. Saino, *et al.* 2002. Outcome of esophageal adenocarcinoma detected during endoscopic biopsy surveillance for Barrett's esophagus. *Surg. Endosc.* **16:** 263–266.

26. Bonavina L., C. Ceriani, A. Carazzone, *et al.* 1999. Endoscopic laser ablation of nondysplastic Barrett's epithelium: is it worthwhile? *J. Gastrointest. Surg.* **3:** 194–199.

27. Pagani M., P. Granelli, B. Chella, *et al.* 2003. Barrett's esophagus: combined treatment using argon plasma coagulation and laparoscopic antireflux surgery. *Dis. Esoph.* **16:** 279–283.

28. Bright T., D.I. Watson, W. Tam, *et al.* 2007. Randomized trial of argon plasma coagulation versus endoscopic surveillance for Barrett's esophagus after anti-reflux surgery: late results. *Ann. Surg.* **246:** 1016–1020.

29. Lyday W.D., F.S. Corbett, D.A. Kuperman, *et al.* 2010. Radiofrequency ablation of Barrett's esophagus: outcomes of 429 patients from a multicenter community practice registry. *Endoscopy* **42:** 272–278.

30. Fleischer, D.E., B.F. Overholt, V.K. Sharma, *et al.* 2010. Endoscopic radiofrequency ablation for Barrett's esophagus: 5-year outcomes from a prospective multicenter trial. *Endoscopy* **42:** 781–789.

31. Vassiliou, M.C., D. von Renteln, D.C. Wiener, *et al.* 2010. Treatment of ultralong segment Barrett's using focal and balloon-based radiofrequency ablation. *Surg. Endosc.* **24:** 786–791.

32. Velanovich, V. 2009. Endoscopic endoluminal radiofrequency ablation of Barrett's esophagus: initial results and lessons learned. *Surg. Endosc.* **23:** 2175–2180.

33. Djarv, T., J. Lagergren, J.M. Blazeby & P. Lagergren. 2008. Long-term health-related quality of life following surgery for oesphageal cancer. *Br. J. Surg.* **95:** 1121–1126.

34. O'Connell, K. & V. Velanovich. 2010. Effects of Nissen fundoplication on endoscopic endoluminal radiofrequency ablation of Barrett's esophagus. *Surg. Endosc.*

35. Wani, S. *et al.* 2009. Esophageal adenocarcinoma in Barrett's esophagus after endoscopic ablative therapy: a meta-analysis and systematic review. *Am. J. Gastroenterol.* **104:** 502–513 [Review].

36. Fleischer, D. *et al.* 2010. AIM II: 5 year durability data. *DDW Plenary.*

37. Wang, J.S., M. Guo, E.A. Montgomery, *et al.* 2009. DNA promoter hypermethylation of p16 and APC predicts neoplastic progression in Barrett's esophagus. *Am. J. Gastroenterol.* **104:** 2153–2160 [Epub 2009 Jul 7].

38. Shaheen, N.J., A.F. Peery, R.H. Hawes, *et al.* 2010. AIM Dysplasia Trial Investigators. Quality of life following radiofrequency ablation of dysplastic Barrett's esophagus. *Endoscopy* **42s:** 790–799 [Epub 2010 Sep 30].

39. Ackroyd, R., N.J. Brown, T.J. Stephenson, C.J. Stoddard, & M.W.R. Reed. 1999. Ablation therapy for Barrett oesophagus: what depth of tissue destruction is needed? *J. Clin. Pathol.* **52:** 509–512.

Ann. N.Y. Acad. Sci. ISSN 0077-8923

ANNALS OF THE NEW YORK ACADEMY OF SCIENCES

Issue: *Barrett's Esophagus: The 10th OESO World Congress Proceedings*

Barrett's esophagus: endoscopic treatments II

Bruce D. Greenwald,[1] Charles J. Lightdale,[2] Julian A. Abrams,[3] John D. Horwhat,[4] Ram Chuttani,[5] Srinadh Komanduri,[6] Melissa P. Upton,[7] Henry D. Appelman,[8] Helen M. Shields,[9] Nicholas J. Shaheen,[10] and Stephen J. Sontag[11]

[1]Division of Gastroenterology and Hepatology, Department of Medicine and Marlene and Stewart Greenebaum Cancer Center, University of Maryland School of Medicine, Baltimore, Maryland. [2]Gastroenterology-Gastrointestinal Endoscopy, Columbia-Presbyterian Medical Center, New York, New York. [3]Division of Digestive and Liver Diseases, Columbia-Presbyterian Medical Center, New York, New York. [4]Walter Reed Army Medical Center, Washington, DC. [5]Beth Israel Deaconess Medical Center, Boston, Massachusetts. [6]Feinberg School of Medicine, Division of Gastroenterology/Hepatology Northwestern University, Chicago, Illinois. [7]University of Washington Medical Center, Seattle, Washington. [8]Department of Pathology, University of Michigan, Ann Arbor, Michigan. [9]Gastroenterology Division, Harvard Medical School and Beth Israel Deaconess Medical Center, Boston, Massachusetts. [10]Center for Esophageal Diseases and Swallowing, University of North Carolina School of Medicine, Chapel Hill, Chapel Hill, North Carolina. [11]Veterans Administration Hospital, Hines, Illinois

The following on endoscopic treatments of Barrett's esophagus includes commentaries on animal experiments on cryotherapy; indications for cryotherapy, choice of dosimetry, number of sessions, and role in Barrett's esophagus and adenocarcinoma; recent technical developments of RFA technology and long-term effects; the comparative effects of diverse ablation procedures and the rate of recurrence following treatment; and the indications for treatment of dysplasia and the role of radiofrequency ablation.

Keywords: cryosurgery; esophageal neoplasms; Barrett's esophagus; dysplasia; adenocarcinoma; specialized intestinal metaplasia; subsquamous glandular mucosa; buried glands; radiofrequency ablation; argon plasma coagulation; multipolar electrocautery; PDT; Halo[90]; Halo[180]; Halo[360]; balloon sizing; carcinoma; subsquamous glands; proton pump inhibitor therapy; AspECT trial; multifocal disease; neosquamous epithelium

Concise summaries

- Spray (noncontact) cryotherapy delivered to the esophagus via standard upper endoscope induces necrosis extending into the submucosa and inflammation into the muscularis propria at doses currently being used clinically. For Barrett's high-grade dysplasia, the lifetime risk of developing adenocarcinoma is high, and cryoablation therapy is one of several modalities that may prevent the development of cancer.

- The clinical experience to date seems to suggest that 10–15 sec freeze times may be adequate for short-term efficacy in ablation of Barrett's esophagus (BE), but the optimum number of freeze-thaw cycles for tissue ablation is still unclear. However, recent work presented at the 2010 OESO World Congress suggests an ability to accomplish this with less than three treatments, on average, and this may reflect advantages gained by the shift toward a dosimetry of 2×20 sec, yielding a more robust treatment response than 4×10 sec sprays.

- There are very limited data available to compare the two cryotherapy methods, but high efficacy in elimination of early neoplasia in BE and excellent safety profiles appear similar at this time.

- Cryotherapy is probably no better than other ablation modalities for palliation of bulky esophageal cancers, but experience is limited. It appears to cause tumor regression for extended periods even if eradication is not possible.

- When sizing and ablation catheter selection are performed according to instructions, circumferential ablation using radiofrequency ablation (RFA) technology is a safe, effective

doi: 10.1111/j.1749-6632.2011.06050.x

procedure with a <0.02% perforation rate and no patient deaths. The possibility of even larger devices, and "one-size fits all" balloon devices that unfurl or unroll to accommodate individual esophageal sizes and shapes, are also in the development pipeline, and these would obviate the need for balloon staging.

- With both RFA and cryotherapy, the strictures that have been reported have for the most part been responsive to single balloon dilation. Overall, the safety profile with RFA and cryotherapy is significantly improved over PDT with RFA currently with the most data in support of its safety profile.
- Endoscopic ablation appears to achieve excellent rates of ablation of Barrett epithelium and Barrett-associated neoplasia; however, longer follow-up is needed to identify risk factors for persistence and recurrence, using regular and careful biopsy surveillance strategies.
- Much remains unknown regarding the utility of ablative therapy in Barrett's. Although preliminary data suggest that in both dysplastic and nondysplastic Barrett's, the neosquamous epithelium is durable in mid-term results, further work will define the long-term durability of the neosquamous reversion. The cancer risk in treated subjects requires further definition.
- There is some variability in recommendations for dealing with low-grade dysplasia (LGD). These recommendations vary from continuing endoscopic biopsy surveillance every six months for LGD for an indefinite period of time, to antireflux therapy followed by endoscopic surveillance every one to three years.
- Concerning the progression of BE to HGD and adenocarcinoma, the role of acid in increasing or decreasing proliferation is still controversial and uncertain. The results of the 10-year prospective controlled trial Aspirin Esomeprazole Chemoprevention Trial (AspECT), to be reported in 2014, will be of great importance to making decisions concerning the use of proton pump inhibitors (PPIs) on a continuous basis to specifically decrease the risk of high-grade dysplasia (HGD) and adenocarcinoma in Barrett's patients.

---

1. What are the results of cryotherapy in animal models?

Bruce D. Greenwald

bgreenwa@medicine.umaryland.edu

This discussion focuses on spray (noncontact) cryotherapy delivered to the esophagus via standard upper endoscope. Two cryotherapy devices are currently available in the United States—a low-pressure liquid nitrogen device (CryoSpray Ablation System, CSA Medical, Inc., Baltimore, MD, USA) and a high-pressure system using CO_2 (Polar Wand, GI Supply, Camp Hill, PA, USA). This device generates cold by the Joule–Thomson effect, whereby rapid expansion of gas at the catheter tip produces a significant decrease in temperature. In both techniques, tissue is repeatedly frozen then allowed to thaw. These freeze-thaw cycles induce tissue necrosis by direct freezing (protein denaturation, extracellular, and intracellular ice formation, and cell membrane disruption), tissue necrosis (vascular stasis, platelet aggregation, and thrombosis), and cryotherapy-induced apoptosis. The procedures are performed using standard endoscopic sedation and techniques in the outpatient setting. To vent gas during the procedure, a modified orogastric tube (cryo-decompression tube) is placed prior to spraying and removed after treatment for the liquid nitrogen system, and a suction catheter is attached to the tip of the endoscope in the CO_2 system. Endoscopic treatment sessions are repeated every four to six weeks as needed.

Animal models were developed to test whether these devices could successfully freeze esophageal tissue and to develop appropriate dosimetry. Initial studies using a prototype of the liquid nitrogen device involved 20 swine, with freeze time varying between 10 and 60 sec.[1] Follow-up endoscopy with biopsy was performed on days 2, 7, 14, 21, and 28 to assess cryotherapy effects and healing. Animals were sacrificed after complete healing was documented, and full-thickness samples of the treated area were evaluated. Cryotherapy produced mucosal freezing in all animals within 30 sec, and tissue thawed within one min after cessation of the spray. Follow-up endoscopy demonstrated varying degrees of injury from superficial erosions to severe mucosal blistering. Histologically, biopsies showed mild superficial inflammation extending to the lamina propria in mild cases but severe acute esophagitis extending to the submucosa with separation of the squamous epithelium in severe cases. Three swine developed esophageal strictures, and histology showed transmural acute inflammation from treatment in these cases.

In initial studies of a prototype CO_2 system, mucosa was frozen in two dogs by spraying until a white frost was seen.[2] Superficial necrosis and acute inflammation was seen on day 1 without submucosal involvement. Re-epithelialization began by day 4 with complete healing by week 3. A later study using the commercial CO_2 device evaluated eight swine treated with varying duration of spray (15, 30, 45, 60, 120 sec) followed by necropsy two days later.[3] Depth of necrosis and injury correlated with spray duration, with necrosis of the mucosa/submucosa at 15–30 sec, muscularis propria at 45–60 sec, and adventitia (transmural) at 120 sec.

A human depth of injury study is ongoing at the University of Miami, Miami, Florida.[4] The liquid nitrogen device is being tested on normal esophageal tissue seven days prior to planned cancer-related esophagectomy, with assessment of inflammation, hemorrhage, and necrosis. Dosimetries used are 10 sec freeze followed by thaw for four cycles and 20 sec freeze then thaw for two cycles. Preliminary results in three patients indicate that inflammation extends to the submucosa/muscularis propria and necrosis to the mucosa/submucosa in the 10 sec group, with inflammation to the muscularis propria and necrosis to the submucosa in the patient treated for 20 sec.

In summary, the following has been learned through the study of cryotherapy in animal and human models:

- spray cryotherapy can induce necrosis extending through the esophageal wall;
- depth of injury is determined by duration of the cryotherapy spray and number of freeze-thaw cycles; and
- in humans, spray cryotherapy induces necrosis extending into the submucosa and inflamma-

tion into the muscularis propria at doses currently being used clinically.

2. What is the difference between liquid nitrogen and carbon dioxide cryotherapy systems with respect to efficacy and to side effects?

Charles J. Lightdale, MD
cjl18@columbia.edu

Liquid nitrogen cryotherapy

This method uses a low-pressure spray of liquid nitrogen to freeze tissue at a very cold $-196\,^\circ$ C.[5] The special plastic catheter carrying the liquid nitrogen gets very cold, as does the endoscope itself, and the catheter routinely becomes unmovable in the biopsy channel. There is a warm air pump to unfreeze the system more rapidly. As the liquid nitrogen spray freezes tissue, it warms to nitrogen gas, which expands and must be evacuated from the upper GI tract. For this purpose, a special oral-gastric suction tube with both active and passive suction is utilized. This tube can sometimes be a technical obstacle. Abdominal massage is also required during treatment to help evacuate gas through the tube and through the mouth. A clear plastic cap on the tip of the endoscope can help decrease the lens fogging associated with the freezing spray.

Carbon dioxide cryotherapy

This method uses compressed carbon dioxide gas spray through a catheter with a tiny opening at the tip (0.005 inch diameter). The rapid expansion of the room temperature carbon dioxide gas causes cooling (Joule–Thomson effect) to $-78\,^\circ$ C, freezing the targeted tissue.[6] For gas evacuation, a cap-like suction device is fixed to the endoscope tip with a connecting flat suction tube along the side of the endoscope. The suction cap can make endoscope passage into the esophagus more difficult in some. The endoscope and catheter do not freeze, and abdominal massage is not required. The compressed carbon dioxide gas reservoir is more stable than liquid nitrogen, and the carbon dioxide system is less expensive. Lens fogging during the treatment is also a problem with this system.

Comparison of efficacy and side effects

Liquid nitrogen. In a series of 17 patients with HGD in BE, the complete response (CR) for HGD was 94%, for all dysplasia (D) 88%, and for intestinal metaplasia (IM) 53%.[5] In a larger series of 60 patients with HGD, CR for HGD was 97%, D was 87%, and IM was 57%.[7] In 49 patients who completed cryotherapy for stage T1 esophageal cancer, the CR was 75%.[8] Reported side effects in these series include variable chest pain and dysphagia, stricture rate 3–13%, mostly related to prior therapies, and one gastric perforation in a patient with Marfan's syndrome.

Carbon dioxide. In 44 patients, the CR for HGD was 86%, D was 84%, and IM was 50%.[9] Side effects were minimal chest discomfort, and no serious adverse events.

Conclusions

There are very limited data available to compare the two cryotherapy methods, but high efficacy in elimination of early neoplasia in BE and excellent safety profiles appear similar at this time. Further studies are also needed to compare cryotherapy to other ablative methods.

3. What is the recommended dosimetry for cryotherapy?

Julian A. Abrams
ja660@columbia.edu

Cryotherapy is a means of tissue destruction that can be used for the successful ablation of BE with or without dysplasia. Short-term data suggest that this treatment modality is both effective and safe. However, there are limited dosimetry data for cryotherapy in BE. Cryotherapy results in two processes, the freeze and the thaw, that both result in tissue damage and destruction. During the freeze, there is direct tissue injury via intra- and extra cellular ice crystal formation. This in turn can lead to both rapid cell death as well as delayed apoptosis several days after treatment. Both faster rates of cooling and longer duration of freeze increase the amount of ice crystal formation. During the thaw period, there is recrystallization and growth of ice crystals, which lead to shear injury. Additionally, thrombosis of small blood vessels occurs, leading to tissue hypoxia and cell death. It is unclear whether the freeze or thaw period is more important, or whether the number of freeze-thaw cycles is the most important factor in determining treatment effect.

Only a few dosimetry studies have been performed with cryotherapy in the esophagus.[3,10,11] Johnston *et al.* used liquid nitrogen spray to treat the esophagus of 20 pigs, with freeze times ranging from 10 to 60 sec.[10] Observed tissue injury ranged from superficial inflammation to coagulative necrosis on the submucosa. The degree of injury did not appear to correlate with freeze time. In a pig model study using cooled carbon dioxide, tissue damage was limited to the submucosa for freeze durations of 15 and 30 sec, but affected deeper layers with longer durations.[3] The clinical relevance of tissue injury and necrosis to deeper layers of the esophagus is unclear, as cryotherapy can result in preservation of the extracellular matrix despite surrounding cell death.

Clinical experience with various doses of cryotherapy has demonstrated seemingly consistent efficacy with a good safety profile. The initial dosing regimen for liquid nitrogen spray in studies of BE with HGD or adenocarcinoma was 20 sec times three cycles. After a case of a patient with Marfan's syndrome who developed a gastric perforation due to overdistention, the dosing protocol was changed to 10 sec times four cycles. Both of these studies demonstrated that liquid nitrogen cryotherapy was efficacious and safe,[7,8] although analyses comparing efficacy in the patients who received (20 sec × 3) versus (10 sec × 4) were not performed. There is an ongoing study of CO_2 cryotherapy, although dosimetry, efficacy, and safety data are not yet available.

In summary, cryotherapy produces a variable depth of tissue injury based on duration of freeze, the number of freeze-thaw cycles, and the distance from the spray origin. The clinical experience to date seems to suggest that 10–15 sec freeze times may be adequate for short-term efficacy in ablation of BE. The optimum number of freeze-thaw cycles for tissue ablation is still unclear. Palliative treatment of esophageal tumors is less clear. Longer freeze times may be more effective in this population; this may be accompanied by a theoretical increased risk of perforation, although this has not been observed clinically. Studies that compare various freeze durations and numbers of freeze-thaw cycles with clinical outcomes are lacking.

4. What are the criteria that determine the mean number of cryotherapy sessions and total length of treatment—is PPI therapy concomitant to cryotherapy mandatory?

John D. Horwhat
john.david.horwhat@us.army.mil

As with any endoscopic technique, ideal application will be influenced by factors that relate to the patient, the procedure and the physician. Presently, cryotherapy remains a largely fledgling technology that is only slowly finding a niche with endoscopists that ablate BE. All (nonabstract) published data relating to cryotherapy and BE have been with the CSA^TM Medical device, and there is no published consensus on dosimetry.[7,8,12]

With respect to patient-related factors, the major determinants are the length of the segment being treated and the goal of therapy. The aim of each treatment cycle is to keep an area of mucosa "painted" with a uniform white cryofrost for 20 sec in the treatment of dysplasia and 30 sec for cancer. Two cycles are typically given for a total treatment dose of 40 sec (dysplasia) and 60 sec (cancer) respectively. If one attempts to treat too large of a segment, there is the risk that the distal mucosa could begin to thaw as the scope is moved proximally, thus diminishing the uniformity of effect. In order to both maintain direct visualization and to ensure that the spray is applied for uniform freezing effect, a 3–4 cm length is the largest segment that should be targeted with each cycle. Whether one chooses to treat in a hemicircumferential or fully circumferential manner depends on the operators experience and ability to maneuver around the decompression tube.

Another patient factor is the goal of therapy. If the goal is regression from HGD to nondysplastic BE, one may not need as many sessions as when the goal is complete re-epithelialization to squamous mucosa. Just as small islands of columnar appearing tissue can remain after the application of RFA or PDT that require addition HALO90^TM or spot treatment with APC, the same can occur with CSA^TM and result in the need for an additional treatment session.

Procedural factors relate to dosimetry, the ability to maintain visualization and to ventilate the volume of gas that is instilled. During the earliest work with CSA^TM, dosimetry required either four 10-sec freeze-thaw cycles or two 20-sec cycles per segment treated. As experience developed and refinements in the dual-lumen decompression tube (CDT^TM) were made, most now use the 2×20 sec dosimetry as this is quicker, easier to perform and

Table 1. Number of treatment sessions required for nondysplastic and dysplastic Barrett's esophagus and esophageal cancer

Cohort	N	Population	Segment length (cm)	Number of treatments/ patient	Dosimetry used
NNMC cohort (includes Johnston GIE)	335	Nondysplastic and LGD/HGD	3.9(1–11)	3	10 @ 2×20 sec hemicircumferential, 25 @ $4 \times$ 10 sec circumferential
WRAMC cohort (unpublished data)	119	Nondysplastic and LGD	2.9(1–10)	4	14 @ 4×10 sec, 5 @ 2×20 sec
Shaheen (GIE)	998	HGD	5.3(1–13)	3.4	Mixture of 4×10 and 2×20 sec
Greenwald (GIE)	779	Cancer	4(1–15) tumor length	3	3×20 sec
Sreenarasimhaiah (OESO)	223	LGD, HGD, and ImCA	5.84	2.25	4×10 and 2×20

NNMC, National Naval Medical Center; WRAMC, Walter Reed Army Medical Center; LGD, low-grade dysplasia; HGD, high-grade dysplasia; GIE, gastrointestinal endoscopy; OESO, 10th World Congress, World Organization for Specialized Studies on Diseases of the Esophagus; sec, seconds.

appears to give a more robust response than the 10-sec freeze-thaw cycles. Visualization and venting are interrelated in that one may encounter some fogging of the lumen after 12–15 sec of freezing. This can be ameliorated by temporarily stopping the flow of gas and allowing decompression to catch up. Recall that liquid nitrogen expands nearly 700 times in volume when changing from a liquid to gas with rewarming, and it is imperative that the decompression tube ventilates this volume to reduce the risk of barotrauma. Since the inception of the CDT[TM], overdistention, and resultant barotrauma have been all but eliminated.

Recent work performed by Ribiero *et al.* has contributed greatly to our knowledge of dosimetry.[13] Patients scheduled for esophagectomy had a 2×2 cm^2 area of mucosa targeted for cryospray with either 4×10 sec or 2×20 sec. Seven days later at esophagectomy the treated area was analyzed histologically. The areas treated with 2×20 sec sprays consistently achieved a depth of necrosis to the level of the superficial or deep submucosa. This evidence adds support to the basis for a dosimetry of 2×20 sec in patients with dysplasia and further work in this area is ongoing by these investigators.

Table 1 shows data from several centers as it relates to dosimetry and includes nondysplastic Barrett's, dysplasia, and cancer. Abstract data presented at OESO 2010 are included. The data from Dumot *et al.* from the Cleveland Clinic are not shown as the prototype devices and dosimetry changed multiple times over the course of his study as the technology evolved, and the data are too heterogeneous to display. Even allowing for the evolution from hemicircumferential spraying to circumferential spraying then from 4×10 sec sprays to 2×20 sec sprays, there is a striking consistency among the various centers for a number of treatment sessions that ranges from 3 to 4. Regarding the issue of whether acid control is necessary during the application of cryotherapy, the only data relating to CSA[TM] ablation come from the original pilot study with CSA[TM] from Johnston *et al.*[12] All patients that entered into the trial that had reversal of their Barrett's to normal squamous had complete acid control demonstrated by 24 h-pH analysis upon entry to the study. Doses of medication were escalated for patients without acid control and repeat testing done at higher dose to ensure an anacid intraesophageal lumen was present during the treatment and healing phases of the study. Sim-

ilarly, work with RFA from the Stanford group has shown a statistically significant ($P < 0.05$) relationship between acid control and treatment response, emphasizing the need for acid control in patients undergoing ablation.[14]

Summary

The current literature demonstrates the ability to accomplish eradication of HGD and intramucosal esophageal cancer with three to four applications of CSA[TM] therapy. Recent work presented at the 2010 OESO World Congress suggests an ability to accomplish this with less than three treatments, on average, and this may reflect advantages gained by the shift toward a dosimetry of 2×20 sec yielding a more robust treatment response than 4×10 sec sprays. Certainly, we await the full results from Ribiero *et al.*[13] as they study more patients undergoing esophagectomy in an effort to confirm whether 2×20 sec dosimetry will continue to consistently demonstrate full thickness mucosal necrosis. If proven in subsequent patients, this full thickness histology would confirm that which we see endoscopically and solidify our ability to embrace this as our standard noncancer dosimetry. And with regard to acid control, we should aim to control acid exposure in all patients undergoing any ablation procedure—whether radiofrequency, resectional procedures, or cryotherapy—to ensure the greatest opportunity for healing with a neosquamous epithelium.

5. Endoscopic spray cryotherapy for esophageal cancer: cure or palliation?

Bruce D. Greenwald
bgreenwa@medicine.umaryland.edu

This review discusses the use of low-pressure endoscopic spray cryotherapy with liquid nitrogen (CryoSpray Ablation System) for the treatment of esophageal cancer. With this technique, esophageal tissue is frozen with liquid nitrogen delivered in a noncontact method via a catheter passed through the working channel of a standard upper endoscope. In cancer, tissue is typically frozen for 20 sec, allowed to thaw completely (approximately one min) then refrozen repeatedly, typically in at least three freeze-thaw cycles. These cycles induce tissue necrosis by direct freezing (protein denaturation, extracellular and intracellular ice formation, cell membrane disruption), tissue necrosis (vascular stasis, platelet aggregation, and thrombosis), and cryotherapy-induced apoptosis. The procedure is performed using standard endoscopic sedation and techniques in the outpatient setting. To vent nitrogen gas formed by evaporation during the procedure, a modified orogastric tube (cryodecompression tube) is placed prior to spraying and removed after treatment. Endoscopic treatment sessions are repeated every four to six weeks as needed.

The first case of endoscopic spray cryotherapy in esophageal cancer was reported by Cash *et al.* in 2007.[15] A 73-year-old man with previous T2N1 tonsillar cancer seven years prior and T4N0 esophageal squamous cell carcinoma three years prior, both treated with concurrent chemotherapy and external beam radiotherapy, presented with a T2N0 esophageal squamous cell carcinoma outside the field of the previous esophageal cancer. He was treated with two sessions of cryotherapy and remained disease free for over two years. He developed an esophageal stricture from treatment that required dilation and placement of a temporary esophageal stent.

The largest reported study on the use of endoscopic spray cryotherapy in esophageal cancer was published earlier this year.[8] In this retrospective study, 79 patients from 10 sites around the U.S. were treated. These patients failed, refused, or were not candidates for standard therapy, including chemotherapy, radiation therapy, or esophagectomy. In this cohort, 74 (94%) had adenocarcinoma, 5 (6%) had squamous cell cancer, and 64 (81%) were male. Median age was 76 (range 51–93) years, and tumor stage at enrollment was T1: 60 (T1a: 33, T1b: 23, not specified: 4; T2: 16, T3/4: 3. Many participants were treated with previous therapy including endoscopic mucosal resection: 27 (42%), concurrent chemotherapy/external beam radiotherapy: 12 (19%), photodynamic therapy (PDT): 11 (17%), external beam radiotherapy alone: 7 (11%), concurrent chemotherapy and external beam radiotherapy then esophagectomy: 2 (3%), argon plasma coagulation (APC): 2 (3%), and one each for chemotherapy alone, esophageal stent, and RFA.

An efficacy cohort of 49 participants completed treatment, either through endoscopic and biopsy-confirmed tumor eradication (CR) or because of tumor progression, patient preference to stop therapy, or comorbid condition precluding further therapy (treatment failure). In this group, tumor stage was T1: 36 (T1a: 24, T1b: 10, not specified: 2); T2: 10, T3/4: 3. Overall CR was 61.2%, including 72.2% for T1 tumors (T1a: 75%, T1b: 60%). Mean follow-up was 10.6 months for all and 11.5 months in the T1a group. The median number of cryotherapy sessions needed to produce a CR was three. Concurrent treatments at the time of cryotherapy included endoscopic resection: 9, external beam radiotherapy: 2, argon plasma coagulation: 3, RFA: 2, and esophagectomy: 4. In a number of patients, cryotherapy was not able to eradicate the tumor but was able to slow or halt tumor progression for extended periods of time, over one year in some cases. In a safety analysis including 332 treatments for the 79 participants, no serious adverse events were reported. Esophageal stricture developed in 10 (13%), with 9/10 noted to have esophageal narrowing due to previous treatment prior to initiation of cryotherapy.

An earlier study of spray cryotherapy included five patients with intramucosal carcinoma.[16] Three of five responded to the treatment, downgrading histology to IM without HGD or carcinoma. Another study, primarily assessing safety and tolerability of spray cryotherapy in 77 patients, included treatment data on seven patients with intramucosal or mucosal carcinoma.[5] Cancer was eliminated in all patients and IM was eliminated in 5/7 (although follow-up was limited).

Limited data are available on the use of spray cryotherapy for debulking of advanced esophageal neoplasms. Treatment in this setting is technically challenging due to luminal stenosis and the presence of the cryodecompression tube, which may make scope manipulation difficult.

In summary, liquid nitrogen spray cryotherapy:

- eradicates T1a (mucosal) esophageal adenocarcinoma in 75% of cases;
- can be used in T1b (submucosal) disease, but risk of lymph node metastasis must be considered;
- is probably no better than other ablation modalities for palliation of bulky esophageal cancers, but experience is limited; and
- appears to cause tumor regression for extended periods even if eradication is not possible.

Disclosures

The author has received research funding from and serves as a consultant and medical advisory board

Table 2. In multiple studies, RFA has resulted in no subsquamous glandular mucosa

	N	FU	CR-IM	CR-D	CR-HGD	Buried glands	Stricture rate
AIM-II trial[25]	61	30 months	98.4%			None	0%
	50	60 months	92%			None	0%
AIM-LGD[96]	10	24 months	90%	100%		None	0%
HGD Registry	92	12 months	54%	80%	90%	None	0.4%
AMC-I[30]	11	14 months	100%	100%		None	0%
AMC-II[31]	12	14 months	100%	100%		None	0%
Comm Registry[68]	429	20 months	77%	100%		None	1.1%
EURO-I[69]	24	15 months	90%	100%		None	4.0%
EURO-II[32]	118	12+ months	96%	100%			
Emory[70]	27	<12 months	100%	100%		None	0%
Dartmouth[71]	25	20 months	78				
Henry Ford[33]	66	Varied	93%			None	6.0%
Mayo[34]	63	24 months	79%	89%		None	0%
LGD[72]	39	24 months	87%	95%		None	0%
HGD[36]	24	23 months	67%	79%		None	0%
AIM RCT (primary)[27]	127 (RFA84)	12 months	77% (83%)	86% (92%)		5.1%	6.0%
Long-term FU[73]	106	24 months	93%	95%		3.8%	7.6%
EMR vs. RFARCT[38]	22	24 months	96%	96%		None	14%

member for CSA Medical, Inc., the manufacturer of the CryoSpray Ablation system.

6. Compared to other thermal ablation modalities, what is the rate of development of subsquamous glandular mucosa following RFA?

Ram Chuttani
rchuttan@bidmc.harvard.edu

Key issues
- Incomplete ablation by any method may result in the glandular mucosa getting "buried" under regenerating neosquamous epithelium.
- This subsquamous glandular mucosa may not be visible endoscopically.
- Inadequate endoscopic surveillance may lead to development of undetected malignancy.

Argon plasma coagulation
In several series, incidence of subsquamous glandular mucosa after APC ablation varies between 4–44%.[17–21] The key factors predicting lower incidence with APC are higher power settings, higher PPI dose, and shorter Barrett's segment.

Photo dynamic therapy ablation and multipolar electro coagulation
Three series compared APC versus PDT; PDT had between 4% and 24% incidence of subsquamous glandular mucosa.[18–20] In addition, the PHOBAR Trial compared PDT with porfimer sodium combined with acid suppression (PHOPDT) to acid suppression alone (OM) in patients with HGD. At baseline, 5.8% of patients in the PHOPDT group, and 2.9% of patients in the OM group had SSIM. After treatment, the percentage of patients with squamous overgrowth increased, but there was no significant difference between the two groups: PHOPDT (30%) and OM (33%) groups ($P = 0.63$).[21]

The data on the incidence of subsquamous glandular mucosa after MPEC therapy are limited. Sharma *et al.* reported SSIM in 27% of NDBE/LGD patients (3/11) who had undergone MPEC and achieved endoscopic and histologic cure (mean follow-up of 24 months after endoscopic reversal of Barrett's).[22]

Other key factors

- Adequate biopsy specimen must be obtained—large capacity forceps are essential to sample lamina propria.
- All of these thermal methods have an unacceptably high incidence of subsquamous "buried" glandular mucosa.
- There are reports of undetected subsquamous adenocarcinoma developing after APC and PDT.[19,23,24]

Radiofrequency ablation

In multiple studies, RFA has resulted in no subsquamous glandular mucosa (Table 2). AIM Trial at 2.5 years showed no subsquamous glandular epithelium in nearly 4,000 total biopsy specimens.[25] AIM-II 5-year durability trial had 1,473 biopsy specimens with no buried glands. A total of 85% of the specimens included lamina propria or deeper tissue.[26] The highest published post-RFA subsquamous glandular mucosa rate to date is 5% of patients in the AIM Dysplasia Trial, a randomized control trial that evaluated RFA versus control (biopsy surveillance and high-dose PPI acid suppression) in LGD and HGD patients. At baseline, 25% of patients had subsquamous glandular mucosa. At the 12-month primary endpoint, this decreased to 5% in the RFA arm and increased to 40% in the control arm.[34] Overall, in the published RFA literature, which includes over 900 patients, there have been six patients with post-RFA biopsy proven subsquamous glandular mucosa (one subsquamous glandular mucosa containing fragment per patient).[27–29] This translates to less than 0.7% of patients having subsquamous glandular mucosa post-RFA.[28–39]

7. What is expected from future technical developments of the RFA technology (automated process) to optimally size the ablation balloon?

Charles J. Lightdale
cjl18@columbia.edu

Current sizing balloon and procedure

In choosing the Halo[360] ablation catheter for circumferential RFA, a sizing balloon is used to select the appropriate catheter, which is made in five inner diameter (ID) sizes: 18 mm, 22 mm, 25 mm, 28 mm, and 31 mm.[40] Sizing is performed at 1 cm intervals beginning at 12 cm above the esophagogastric junction measured as the top of the gastric folds. At every sizing location, the Halo generator provides a measure of the esophageal ID and recommends the ablation catheter size. Data are recorded on a sizing worksheet, and the smallest recommended ablation catheter is selected. Generally 5–7 sizing steps are required, which adds 5–10 min to the procedure.[41] The sizing procedure is generally safe, although it can cause some intraprocedural discomfort and small amounts of bleeding associated with breaks in the mucosa.[26,42,43] When sizing and ablation catheter selection are performed according to instructions, circumferential ablation is a safe, effective procedure with a < 0.02% perforation rate and no patient deaths.

Recent sizing balloon modification

A recent improvement in the sizing balloon involves a change in the balloon material from polyethylene terephthalate (PET) to the softer polyurethane (PU). The earlier PET balloon could measure esophageal ID to ≤ 33.7 mm, while the new PU sizing balloons can measure esophageal ID to ≤ 45 mm. This allows better differentiation between the esophagus and cardia.

Sizing balloon modifications under review

The current inflation pressure of the sizing balloon is 4 pounds/square inch (PSI). A new modification is being considered that will decrease the sizing balloon pressure to 3 PSI. The advantage of a lower-pressure sizing balloon (25% less force applied to esophageal wall) would be to make it less prone to migration within the esophagus and also to further decrease the risk of mucosal tears and bleeding. Using this method, the smallest size ablation catheter should theoretically be used with less stricture formation, although this risk is already low (0–6%). If this modification results in more residual islands of Barrett's mucosa, these are still easily treated using the Halo[90] focal RFA device.

Circumferential use of larger focal ablation device

Another way to improve the sizing balloon step would be to avoid it altogether by using the Halo[90] focal RFA device in a circumferential manner. The Halo[90] has a 13 mm × 20 mm footprint compared to the new Halo Ultra[90] that has a 13 mm × 40 mm footprint, allowing faster ablation of larger Barrett's areas.

Future concepts

The possibility of even larger Halo[180] devices and "one size fits all" balloon devices that unfurl or unroll to accommodate individual esophageal sizes and shapes are also in the development pipeline, and these would obviate the need for balloon staging.

8. What are the comparative adverse effects of the diverse ablation procedures?

Srinadh Komanduri
koman1973@gmail.com

There has been an evolution in strategies for endoscopic ablation of dysplastic Barrett's epithelium and early intramucosal adenocarcinoma. The advances in endoscopic mucosal resection have limited ablative strategies to flat dysplastic disease. Prior ablative strategies including multipolar electrocoagulation (MPEC) and APC have fallen out of favor due to lack of predictability as to depth of ablation. PDT was the mainstay of ablative strategies for many years. PDT has been very effective for treatment of HGD, but it has carried a stricture rate up to 30%, side effects of photosensitivity, nausea, and dehydration.[44] Furthermore, the risk of buried glandular disease, which was reported frequently with PDT, appears too extremely rare with newer technology such as RFA. RFA has the most thoroughly investigated safety profile and safety reporting via the ongoing registry.

Current overall complication rates are <0.25% with stricture rate <1%, nearly nonexistent buried glandular disease despite specifically sampling for this, and minimal bleeding or perforation risk (0.02%).[26] Perforation really has not been a significant issue with any of the therapies but can occur and generally is operator and technique dependent. Finally, the newest therapy for ablation has been cryotherapy. While data have been limited, a recently published study evaluating safety and efficacy of cryotherapy[7] in HGD demonstrated strictures in 3% of patients, buried glands in 3% and one minor case of bleeding. With both RFA and cryotherapy, the strictures that have been reported have for the most part been responsive to single balloon dilation. Overall, the safety profile with RFA and cryotherapy

is significantly improved over PDT with RFA; currently with the most data in support of its safety profile with RFA, cryotherapy is significantly improved over PDT, and RFA currently with the most data in support of its safety profile.

9. Is the potential rate of recurrence of Barrett's epithelium following ablation currently known? What are the reasons for variability in published results?

Melissa P. Upton
mupton@u.washington.edu

"Recurrence" or persistence?

Some papers use the term "recurrence," but there is currently no data to show if Barrett's mucosa or Barrett's-associated neoplasia detected after ablation represents recurrence or persistence. The more precise term, incomplete response (IR), is recommended, when findings such as Barrett's epithelium or neoplastic alterations are seen within a defined interval after ablation.

Table 3. The results of radiofrequency ablation are promising, but long-term follow-up is not yet available

Results of radiofrequency ablation (RFA)			
	Follow-up duration		
Trial	1 year	2.5 years	5 years
AIM trial RFA[27] N = 60	CR-IM 70%	CR IM 98%	CR-IM 92% N = 50
US Multicenter RFA	CR-LGD 90.5% CR-HGD 81% CR-IM 77.4%		
Velanovitch *et al.* N = 60	CR-IM 93%		
US Multicenter for HGD	CR-HGD 90.2% CR-D 80.4% CR-IM 54.3%		
Sharma *et al.*[22] (eight centers) N = 70	CR-IM 70%		
Roorda *et al.*[14]	CR-IM 46% CR-D 71%		

(CR, complete response; IM, intestinal metaplasia; LDG, low-grade dysplasia; HGD, high-grade dysplasia; D, cysplasia).

The results of radiofrequency ablation are promising, but long-term follow-up is not yet available. Table 3 summarizes some of the recent papers in this area.

A recent Cochrane review of a number of ablative techniques summarized the results of 16 studies, including 1,074 patients, with a mean number of 49 patients per study (range 8–108).[45] Studies using PDT had a mean eradication rate of 52% for BE and eradication rates of dysplasia ranging between 56% and 100%. Factors that affected PDT efficacy included variations in drug, light source, and dose of light. Results reported for RFA included a mean 82% eradication rate of BE and a 94% eradication rate of dysplasia.[45]

Factors that may affect detection of Barrett's mucosa following ablation include limitations of endoscopic identification, variations in biopsy strategy and sampling, extent of ablation or incomplete ablation, and buried Barrett's glands that may remain below squamous re-epithelialization. There are limits to standard white light endoscopy, which can only identify luminal contour and luminal lining, visualizing columnar tongues, but lack the resolution to differentiate subtypes of columnar epithelium.

After squamous re-epithelialization, buried glands cannot be seen without specialized endoscopic techniques, such as optical coherence tomography (OCT). Follow-up biopsy strategy must employ careful surveillance such as the Seattle protocol, which includes four-quadrant large-jaw biopsies at each 2 cm of esophagus previously documented to have columnar metaplasia and at each 1 cm of esophagus in patients with history of neoplastic changes. Biopsies must be deep enough to sample subsquamous lamina propria to rule out buried Barrett's glands or neoplasia, and it appears that the rate of buried glands is similar comparing postablation biopsies with sham/PPI biopsies.[46]

Investigators in the AIM Dysplasia Trial reported that 80% of biopsies post-RFA were deep enough to evaluate for subsquamous glands; however, they considered biopsies adequate if they included lamina propria, muscularis mucosae, or submucosa. Squamous mucosa was most apt to provide limited or superficial biopsies. Subepithelial sampling was present in only 78.5% of squamous-only samples, compared to 98.8% of columnar mucosa samples ($P < 0.001$). The investigators stated that "a biopsy that included LP papillae was categorized as LP." Their figure 1F shows a tangentially oriented biopsy of squamous mucosa that does not include subsquamous tissue.[46] If this figure is representative of a portion of the samples that were deemed adequate, more studies and longer follow-up are needed to determine the rate and biologic potential of buried glands post-RFA. It is also worth emphasizing that these results are from experienced investigators using standardized procedures. We do not yet know whether the excellent ablation results reported so far can be achieved in other sites of practice and whether they will be lasting results.

What factors have been associated with "recurrence" (persistence)?

A total of 75% of "recurrences" after cryotherapy or RFA were in cardia.[47] This raises the question of whether the GEJ may be harder to treat, or more difficult to biopsy and screen, than tubular esophagus. Molecular signature may also be associated with difficulty in eradicating disease with RFA. Investigators performed microdissection of mucosal biopsies and studied a panel of 16 allelic imbalances in 21 patients with LGD and BE. If more than 75% of cells carried mutations, the patients were more resistant to RFA treatment, and additional treatment sessions were needed to eradicate mucosa with mutations.[48] Other reported associations with IR include longer lengths of the Barrett's segments, older age of the patients, multifocality of dysplasia, obesity, location of IM at the top of the gastric folds, and longer duration of dysplasia prior to treatment. In one study including pH control, adequate pH was achieved in fewer than 50% of patients undergoing RFA, and ablation efficacy was lower in patients with inadequate pH control.[14]

In conclusion, endoscopic ablation appears to achieve excellent rates of ablation of Barrett's epithelium and Barrett's-associated neoplasia, however, longer follow-up is needed to identify risk factors for persistence and recurrence, using regular and careful biopsy surveillance strategies. Additional investigation and clinical research is needed to optimize control of esophageal pH, and to identify patients at risk for IR or "recurrence," including those with longer segments and increased mutation rates. Better strategies are also needed for surveillance of GEJ and cardia.

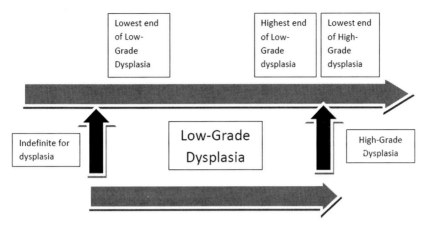

Figure 1. The low-grade dysplasia spectrum: not all things given the diagnosis of low-grade dysplasia are the same.

10. Given the low risk for cancer development, should LGD be treated?

Henry D. Appelman
appelman@umich.edu

Actually, a more appropriate question is, "given the low risk of cancer development, should LGD even require more stringent surveillance?" In order to answer this question, we need a clear definition of LGD. The textbooks offer various definitions that are filled with words like "slightly," "reduced," "larger," "minimal," "more atypical," "mild," "irregular," and "inconspicuous" that are used to define LGD, yet these words have no clear meanings. Therefore, definitions of LGD currently in print are only marginally useful at best.

Regardless of these definitional problems, is it still possible that, in practice, the diagnosis of LGD by different pathologists is good enough for clinicians to use in determining patient management? To begin with, clinicians and pathologists have to recognize that LGD is not a single entity but a group of epithelial changes that look worse than normal, but they do not look as bad as HGD. We know that the histologic diagnosis of LGD has poor agreement even among experienced pathologists.[49] Presumably, LGD has a lowest end and a highest end, and the highest end is next to the lowest end of HGD. (Fig. 1)

This leads to other questions. Is the cancer risk the same at both ends of the low-grade dysplastic spectrum? Is the cancer risk for highest LGD like that for the lowest HGD or is it more like the lowest LGD? Clearly we don't have answers to these questions, because no study has separated LGD into the two groups of highest and lowest ends and evaluated cancer risk for each groups separately. The reason why this has not been done is that no pathologist or groups of pathologists know the criteria for epithelia at both ends of the LGD spectrum. What is obvious is that the diagnosis of LGD is not very dependable, and so clinicians have to decide if they really want to make patient care decisions based upon such an undependable diagnosis.

Presumably, this has lead to the variability in recommendations for dealing with LGD. These recommendations vary from continuing endoscopic biopsy surveillance every six months for LGD for an indefinite period of time to antireflux therapy followed by endoscopic surveillance every one to three years. The Practice Parameters Committee of the American College of Gastroenterology suggests that LGD requires expert pathologist confirmation with follow-up endoscopy at six months and yearly endoscopy until there is no dysplasia on two consecutive yearly endoscopies.[50.] To emphasize the problems in histologic diagnosis of LGD, there is a recent study from the Netherlands of 147 patients who had a diagnosis of LGD from six community hospitals. The biopsies were reviewed by two "expert" pathologists, who downgraded the diagnosis to negative or indefinite for dysplasia in 85% of the cases.[51] They only agreed with the diagnosis of LGD in 15% of these patients. In these 15%, there was an 85% cumulative risk of progression to HGD or carcinoma in 109 months compared to only a 5% risk at 107 months for those cases that were downgraded to negative or indefinite. In another study from four U.S. centers of 618 patients, 147 cases were diagnosed as LGD, but there was no central pathologist review.[52] In this study, it was concluded that the progression to carcinoma from LGD is not significantly different from that of the entire group, most of whom did not have dysplasia. This suggested that LGD patients might have been managed similarly to nondysplastic Barrett's patients in terms of surveillance.

To conclude, based upon this information, more frequent follow-up is clearly indicated for cases of LGD that have been verified by the two expert Dutch pathologists, because there is a high risk of progression to HGD and carcinoma. However, regular follow-up might be recommended for cases of LGD from the four U.S. centers as long as they were not reviewed by the Dutch pathologists, because of their low-risk of progression.

11. What is the effect of *continuous* therapy with PPIs compared to *intermittent* prescription on the rate of progression of BE to HGD and adenocarcinoma?

Helen M. Shields
hshields@caregroup.harvard.edu

The data supporting a chemopreventative effect of acid suppression in BE leading to a reduction of the risk of HGD and esophageal cancer are conflicting. In 1996, using organ culture of endoscopic biopsies of BE, Fitzgerald *et al.* showed that continuous acid exposure resulted in increased villin expression, indicating differentiation because villin is one of the first cytoskeletal proteins to be localized to the apical membrane in development and is widely used as a marker of cell differentiation.[53] They also showed reduced cell proliferation as indicated by proliferating cell nuclear antigen expression (PCNA), suggesting a differentiated phenotype.[53]

In contrast, short acid-pulses dramatically increased cell PCNA expression and proliferation. These authors concluded that variations in acid exposure may contribute to the heterogeneity seen both molecularly and structurally in Barrett's patients. They postulated that acid suppression would need to be effective enough to inhibit acid pulses and cell proliferation. However, Lao-Sirieix *et al.* found that long-term acid suppression reduces proliferation in BE biopsy samples, but it had no advantageous effect on c-myc, apoptosis, or COX-2.[54]

Lao-Sirieix noted that the AspECT trial is important because it will evaluate aspirin and esomeprazole for their effect on the risk of HGD and/or esophageal cancer in a prospective, randomized manner.[54]

Additional controversial results of the effect of acid on proliferation were published in 2007 by Feagins *et al.*, who treated Barrett's cells with short exposures to acid.[55] Acid exposure significantly decreased total cell numbers and resulted in cell cycle prolongation that was associated with greater expression of p53.[55] The authors concluded that acid has p53-mediated, antiproliferative effects in non-neoplastic Barrett's epithelial cells.[55] They speculated that antisecretory medication in dosages beyond that necessary to heal esophagitis may be detrimental rather than helpful. They called for prospective clinical trials to determine the optimal level of acid suppression in BE.[55]

In 2006, Cooper *et al.* reported that BE patients who were continuously treated with PPIs had a low incidence of adenocarcinoma (0.31%) compared to previously published reports.[56] However, de Jonge recently published the largest reported nationwide cohort of unselected patients from the Netherlands with BE and found a 0.4% annual risk of cancer in histologically proven BE patients, which is lower than the frequently quoted 0.5% annual incidence of cancer in Barrett's patients.[57] Male gender, older age (greater than 75 years), and the diagnosis of low-grade dysplasia are independent predictors of malignant progression.[57]

In summary, the role of acid in increasing or decreasing proliferation is still controversial and uncertain. Physicians must balance the safety of the long-term use of PPIs in patients with BE and their possible, but not proven, potential for decreasing the risk of neoplasia over the long term. The annual incidence of esophageal cancer in patients with BE is lower than previously thought making comparisons to older and higher estimates of the risk not useful for decision making. The results of the 10-year 2,513 patient prospective controlled trial AspECT to be reported in 2014 will be of great importance to making decisions concerning the use of PPIs on a continuous basis to specifically decrease the risk of HGD and adenocarcinoma in Barrett's patients.

12. Can the role of RFA in ablating dysplasia be evaluated? What are the late results?

Nicholas J. Shaheen
nshaheen@med.unc.edu

Endoscopic ablative therapy for BE is a rapidly evolving field featuring potentially landscape-shifting technology for the care of these patients. The prospect of improving care in BE is especially enticing given that our practices have been largely unchanged over the last 20 years, during which time the incidence of esophageal adenocarcinoma, the disease to which BE predisposes, has risen dramatically.[59] Because the technology to perform ablation has evolved and become more accessible, and because the morbidity associated with these procedures is generally low, these therapies have gained in popularity. However, considerable questions persist about when in the course of BE these techniques should be used, and which of the several available techniques should be preferred.

It appears that ablation can change the natural history of BE, at least in the short and midterm. Multiple modalities have been demonstrated to effectively cause reversion of IM to neosquamous epithelium.[59–62] Importantly, high-dose acid suppression with PPIs must be given in conjunction with the treatments to induce this change.

Two modalities have been subjected to comparison with intensive endoscopic surveillance in randomized controlled trials, PDT and RFA. Overholt *et al.*[63] randomized 208 subjects with BE and HGD in a 2:1 ratio to either treatment with a PPI, or treatment with PDT plus PPI therapy. The primary outcome was eradication of all HGD at any time during follow-up. Secondary outcomes included complete eradication of IM, cancer incidence, and safety profile. Subjects were assessed with upper endoscopy with biopsies every six months. The mean follow-up in the PDT group was 24 months, and in the PPI group, 19 months. Seventy-seven percent of subjects in the PDT + PPI arm achieved the primary outcome, compared to 39% in the PPI group. Of treated subjects, 52% had complete eradication of IM at some time during follow-up. Cancer incidence was 13% in the PDT + PPI group, compared to 28% in the PPI group, with all differences between groups statistically significant. Esophageal strictures occurred in 12% of subjects

undergoing one PDT treatment, and 38% after two treatments. The authors concluded that PDT was effective in eradication of HGD, and decreased cancer incidence.

A second study compared RFA to intensive endoscopic surveillance.[42] One hundred and twenty-seven subjects with either low-grade ($n = 64$) or high-grade ($n = 63$) dysplasia were randomized in a 2:1 ratio to either RFA + PPI or PPI alone. The primary outcomes were complete eradication of dysplasia and IM at 12 months. Secondary outcomes included cancer incidence and safety profile. Subjects were assessed by upper endoscopy with biopsies every three months (HGD) or every six months (low-grade dysplasia). In the treatment groups, 81% (HGD) and 91% (LGD) achieved eradication of dysplasia, and 77% achieved eradication of IM. In contrast, 21% of controls achieved eradication of dysplasia, and 2% achieved eradication of IM. The cancer risk at one year was 9.3% in controls and 1.2% in treated patients ($P < 0.05$ for all).

A recent study assessing the ability of cryotherapy with liquid nitrogen also presented promising results. Of 98 patients with BE and HGD treated at 10 U.S. sites, 97% were able to be made free of HGD, 86% were free of all dysplasia, and 57% were free of all IM. The side effect profile of the treatment was favorable, with no perforations, three strictures, and two subjects with chest pain managed with narcotics. For ease of use, efficacy, and cost, current data suggest that RFA is a logical choice for ablative therapy in BE. It has a side effect profile superior to that of PDT, with fewer strictures. Efficacy data from rigorous studies demonstrate efficacy as good, or better, than other forms of ablation, and the balloon-based device allows treatment of even long segments of disease in a time-effective manner compared to other devices.

But which patients deserve consideration as candidates for ablation? Is the only good BE burned BE, even if it was nondysplastic before combusted? Both cost-effectiveness analysis data,[64] as well as the data from trials reviewed above, suggest that subjects with HGD are reasonable candidates. While cancer risk is substantially lower in subjects with low-grade dysplasia, certain subgroups of LGD subjects may also deserve consideration. Multifocal disease, dysplasia confirmed by multiple pathologists, and longer segment disease have all been suggested as potential risk factors for progression in LGD.

Interestingly, even among subjects with nondysplastic disease, cost-effectiveness data suggest that ablative therapy may confer a survival advantage at a reasonable cost.[64] The treatment of nondysplastic patients faces an especially high bar, because the vast majority of these subjects will never develop cancer.[65] Therefore, any treatment directed at this subgroup needs to be safe, reasonably priced, and effective. Although this appears to be a formidable task, ablation may in fact turn out to be preferable to our current strategy of endoscopic surveillance,[66] because of the high costs associated with endoscopic surveillance, as well as the extremely high costs and mortality associated with the development of esophageal adenocarcinoma. This is especially true if endoscopic surveillance intervals can be altered after successful ablation. However, to date, vitally needed outcomes data regarding the efficacy of ablation in less severe forms of Barrett's make it impossible to draw firm conclusions about the role of these therapies in subjects with nondysplastic Barrett's and those with LGD.

Much remains unknown regarding the utility of ablative therapy in Barrett's. Although preliminary data suggest that in both dysplastic and nondysplastic Barrett's, the neosquamous epithelium is durable in mid-term results,[26,67] further work will define the long-term durability of the neosquamous reversion. The cancer risk in treated subjects requires further definition. As noted above, further work will be necessary to optimize candidate selection. Until these issues are settled, the use of ablative technologies in BE will continue to be an evolving picture.

13. What are the current indications for cryo-ablative therapy in patients with Barrett's esophagus?

Stephen Sontag
sontagsjs@aol.com

In the past five years a number of institutions have utilized cryo-ablative therapies to destroy unwanted malignant tissues. In general, there are five reports that contain the bulk of the information that is so often referred to when discussing the use of cryo-ablation. These reports are as follows:

- Greenwald *et al.*[8] (10 centers, 79 pts with LGD, HGD, adenocarcinoma—curable but inoperable)
  - Endoscopic spray cryo-therapy for esophageal cancer   safety and efficacy. GIE 2010
- Greenwald *et al.*[5] (4 centers, 77 patients with adenocarcinoma/SCC T1, T2, T3—inoperable)
  - Safety, tolerability and efficacy of endoscopic low-pressure liquid nitrogen spray cryotherapy in the esophagus. Diseases of the Esophagus 2010
- Shaheen *et al.*[7] (9 centers, 98 pts with HGD—curable)
  - Safety & efficacy of endoscopic spray Cryotherapy for BE with HGD. GIE 2010
- Dumot *et al.*[16] (1 center, 30 pts with HGD, Adenocarcinoma—curable but inoperable)
  - CSA for Barrett's esophagus with HGD and early esophageal carcinoma in high risk patients. GIE 2009
- Johnston *et al.*[12] (1 center, 11 pts with BE with or without dysplasia—eradicatable)
  - Cryo-ablation of Barrett's esophagus: a pilot study. GIE 2005

All together, these five reports provide 230 patients with some type of "bad" esophageal disease. The company itself, C.S.A. Medical of Baltimore Maryland provides a "cryo-therapy ablation kit" pamphlet that contains the indications, contraindications and warnings as well as instructions on the use of cryo-therapy. The stated indications for use are contained in a simple generalizable sentence: "The CSA System is intended to be used as a cryosurgical tool for the destruction of unwanted tissue in the field of general surgery, specifically endoscopic applications."

The stated contraindications are somewhat lengthier (Table 4). Of interest is the way a large insurance company looks at use of newer therapies such as cryo-ablation. Aetna Insurance Company in their Clinical Policy Bulletin for Barrett's esophagus surgery states the following:

1. Aetna considers any of the following interventions *medically necessary* for the treatment of members with Barrett's esophagus who have HGD when medical therapy (e.g., PPI's, H-2 RA's, or prokinetic agents) has failed:

a. esophagectomy
b. fundoplication
c. photodynamic therapy
d. endoscopic mucosal resection
e. radiofrequency ablation

2. Aetna considers any of the following ablative interventions *experimental and investigational* for the treatment of members with Barrett's esophagus because their effectiveness for this indication has not been established:

a. Argon plasma coagulation
b. cryo-therapy
c. Laser therapy
d. Multi-polar electro-coagulation
e. Ultrasonic therapy

The wisdom and basis of these decisions is beyond the scope of this paper. Indeed, a conference of endoscopic investigators charged with determining

Table 4.

Category	Contraindication
General	• During pregnancy • Where food is identified in the stomach or proximal duodenum at the time of the procedure and cannot be removed. • In any application in which use of the active suction module is inappropriate.
Compromised Tissue	• Where significant esophageal ulceration or mucosal break is present
Anatomical Volume/ Compliance (Gas Evacuation)	• Where any procedure or anatomy has significantly reduced or restricted the volume of the stomach, including, but not limited to, gastric bypass, stomach stapling and gastrojejunostomy • Where any disease state has significantly reduced the elasticity in the GI tract (e.g. Marfan's Syndrome).

which therapies should and should not be approved would likely make for a very entertaining weekend.

Discussion

Large-scale studies on the benefits of cryo-ablation therapy (or any ablative therapies) are unlikely to be performed soon, and even more unlikely to be funded. In all likelihood, the role of ablative therapies, including cryo-ablation, will be defined by a large number of individual experiences, most important of which would be the safety of the method. Until that time, individual and group experience will be the source upon which we depend. With the knowledge that some therapies considered safe today may have unrecognized long-term deleterious effects, I offer some morsels of food for thought:

Our everyday beloved sun provides us with light and warmth.
But, our treasured sun also provides a high energy assault on our human tissues.
The modalities we use to destroy the evil Barrett's. . .
–MPEC, heat, APC, laser, PDT, radiofrequency, freezing–
Also provide a high energy assault on our human tissues.
And
Skin cancer is linked not so much to chronic exposure,
But rather to a single severe sun burn from years earlier. . .
perhaps to that one really bad burn—when you were a teen.

Conclusion

Without evidence for or against the long-term benefit of ablation of Barrett's dysplasia, I offer the following, which is important to recognize is based only on feelings and opinion. In cryo-ablation (or any ablation) of Barrett's Esophagus, the risks must not outweigh the potential benefits:

1. For Barrett's adenocarcinoma: each patient must be considered individually; the decision to use cryotherapy is a matter between patient and physician.
2. For Barrett's high-grade dysplasia: the lifetime risk of developing AdCa is high; cryoablation therapy is one of several modalities that may prevent the development of cancer.

3. For Barrett's low-grade dysplasia or less: The lifetime risk of developing adenocarcinoma is low; aside from selected cases, routine cryo-ablation therapy cannot be justified.

Conflicts of interest

The authors declare no conflicts of interest.

References

1. Johnston, M.H, P. Schoenfeld, J.V. Mysore & A. Dubois. 1999. Endoscopic spray cryotherapy: a new technique for mucosal ablation in the esophagus. *Gastrointest. Endosc.* **50:** 86–92.
2. Pasricha, P.J, S., Hill., Wadwa, *et al.* 1999. Endoscopic cryotherapy: experimental results and first clinical use. *Gastrointest. Endosc.* **49:** 627–631.
3. Raju G.S., I. Ahmed, S.Y. Xiao, *et al.* 2005. Graded esophageal mucosal ablation with cryotherapy, and the protective effects of submucosal saline. *Endoscopy* **37:** 523–526.
4. Unpublished data, kindly provided by Afonso Ribeiro, MD, University of Miami, Miami, FL.
5. Greenwald, B.D., J.A. Dumot, J.D. Horwhat, *et al.* 2010. Safety, tolerability, and efficacy of endoscopic low-pressure liquid nitrogen spray cryotherapy in the esophagus. *Dis. Esoph* **23:** 13–19.
6. Chen, A.M, P.J. Pasricha. 2011. Cryotherapy for Barrett's esophagus: who, how, and why? *Gastrointest. Endosc. Clin. North Am.* **21:** 111–118.
7. Shaheen, N.J., B.D. Greenwald, A.F. Peery, *et al.* 2010. Safety and efficacy of endoscopic spray cryotherapy for Barrett's esophagus with high-grade dysplasia. *Gastrointest. Endosc.* **71:** 680–685.
8. Greenwald, B.D., J.A. Dumot, J.A. Abrams, *et al.* 2010. Endoscopic spray cryotherapy for esophageal cancer: safety and efficacy. *Gastrointest. Endosc.* **71:** 686–693.
9. Canto, M.I., E.C. Gorospe, E.J. Shin, *et al.* 2009. Carbon dioxide (CO_2) cryotherapy is a safe and effective treatment of Barrett's esophagus (BE) with HGD/intramucosal carcinoma.(Abstract). *Gastrointest. Endosc.* **69:** AB341.
10. Johnston, C. M., L. P. Schoenfeld, J.V. Mysore, Dubois A. 1999. Endoscopic spray cryotherapy: a new technique for mucosal ablation in the esophagus. *Gastrointest. Endosc.* **50:** 86–92.
11. Pasricha, P.J., S. Hill, K.S. Wadwa, *et al.* 1999. Endoscopic cryotherapy: experimental results and first clinical use. *Gastrointest. Endosc.* **49:** 627–631.
12. Johnston, M.H., J.A. Eastone, J.D. Horwhat, *et al.* 2005. Cryoablation of Barrett's esophagus: a pilot study. *Gastrointest. Endosc.* **62:** 842–848.
13. Ribiero A.C. 2010. Poster Session Presented at the 10th World Congress, OESO, Boston, MA.
14. Roorda, A.K., S.N. Marcus, G. Triadafilopoulos, *et al.* 2007 Early experience with radiofrequency energy ablation therapy for Barrett's esophagus with and without dysplasia. *Dis. Esoph.* **20:** 516–520.
15. Cash, B.D., L.R. Johnston, M.H. Johnston, *et al.* 2007. Cryospray ablation (CSA) in the palliative treatment of squamous cell carcinoma of the esophagus. *World J. Surg. Oncol.* **5:** 34.
16. Dumot, J.A., J.J. Vargo, 2nd, G.W. Falk. *et al.* 2009. An open-label, prospective trial of cryospray ablation for Barrett's esophagus high-grade dysplasia and early esophageal cancer in high-risk patients. *Gastrointest. Endosc.* **70:** 635–644.
17. Basu, K.K., B. Pick, R. Bale, *et al.* 2002. Efficacy and one year follow up of argon plasma coagulation therapy for ablation of Barrett's oesophagus: factors determining persistence and recurrence of Barrett's epithelium. *Gut* **51:** 776–780.
18. Kelty, C.J., R. Ackroyd, N.J. Brown, *et al.* 2004. Endoscopic ablation of Barrett's oesophagus: a randomized-controlled trial of photodynamic therapy vs. argon plasma coagulation. *Aliment Pharmacol. Ther.* **20:** 1289–1296.
19. Ragunath, K., N. Krasner, V.S. Raman, *et al.* 2005. Endoscopic ablation of dysplastic Barrett'soesophagus comparing argon plasma coagulation and photodynamic therapy: a randomized prospective trial assessing efficacy and cost-effectiveness. *Scand. J. Gastroenterol.* **40:** 750–758.
20. Hage, M., P.D. Siersema, H. van Dekken, *et al.* 2004. 5-aminolevulinic acid photodynamic therapy versus argon plasma coagulation for ablation of Barrett's oesophagus: a randomised trial. *Gut* **53:** 785–790.
21. Bronner, M.P., B.F. Overholt, S.L. Taylor, *et al.* 2009. Squamous overgrowth is not a safety concern for photodynamic therapy for Barrett's esophagus with high-grade dysplasia. *Gastroenterology* **136:** 56–64.
22. Sharma, P., A. Bhattacharyya, H.S. Garewal. *et al.* 1999. Durability of new squamous epithelium after endoscopic reversal of Barrett's esophagus. *Gastrointest. Endosc.* **50:** 159–164.
23. van Laethem, J.L., M.O. Peny, I. Salmon, *et al.* 2000. Intramucosal adenocarcinoma arising under squamous re-epithelialisation of Barrett's oesophagus. *Gut* **46:** 574–577.
24. Mino-Kenudson, M., S. Ban, M. Ohana, *et al.* 2007. Buried dysplasia and early adenocarcinoma arising in barrett esophagus after porfimer-photodynamic therapy. *Am. J. Surg. Pathol.* **31:** 403–409.
25. Fleischer D.E., B.F. Overholt, V.K. Sharma, *et al.* 2008. Endoscopic ablation of Barrett's esophagus: a multicenter study with 2.5-year follow-up. *Gastrointest. Endosc.* **68:** 867–876.
26. Fleischer, D.E., B.F. Overholt, V.K. Sharma, *et al.* 2010. Endoscopic radiofrequency ablation for Barrett's esophagus: 5-year outcomes from a prospective multicenter trial. *Endoscopy* **42:** 781–789.
27. Shaheen, N.J., P. Sharma, B.F. Overholt. *et al.* 2009. Radiofrequency ablation in Barrett's esophagus with dysplasia. *N. Engl. J. Med.* **360:** 2277–2288.
28. Hernandez, J.C., S. Reicher, D. Chung, *et al.* 2008. Pilot series of radiofrequency ablation of Barrett's esophagus with or without neoplasia. *Endoscopy* **40:** 388–392.
29. Pouw, R.E., J.J. Gondrie, C.M. Sondermeijer, *et al.* 2008. Eradication of Barrett esophagus with early neoplasia by radiofrequency ablation, with or without endoscopic resection. *J. Gastrointest. Surg.* **12:** 1627–1636.

30. Sharma, V.K., H.J. Kim, A. Das, *et al.* 2008. A prospective pilot trial of ablation of Barrett's esophagus with low-grade dysplasia using stepwise circumferential and focal ablation (HALO system). *Endoscopy* **40:** 380–387.

31. Ganz, R.A., B.F. Overholt, V.K. Sharma, *et al.* 2008. Circumferential ablation of Barrett's esophagus that contains high-grade dysplasia: a U.S. multicenter registry. *Gastrointest. Endosc.* **68:** 35–40.

32. Lyday, W.D., F.S. Corbett, D.A. Kuperman, *et al.* 2010. Radiofrequency ablation of Barrett's esophagus: outcomes of 429 patients from a multicenter community practice registry. *Endoscopy* **42:** 272–278.

33. Eldaif S.M., E. Lin, K.A. Singh, *et al.* 2009. Radiofrequency ablation of Barrett's esophagus: short-term results. *Ann. Thorac. Surg.* **87:** 405–410.

34. Vassiliou, M.C., D. von Renteln, D.C. Wiener, *et al.* 2010. Treatment of ultralong-segment Barrett's using focal and balloon-based radiofrequency ablation. *Surg. Endosc.* **24:** 786–791.

35. O'Connell, K., V. Velanovich. 2010. Effects of Nissen fundoplication on endoscopic endoluminal radiofrequency ablation of Barrett's esophagus. *Surg. Endosc.* [Epub ahead of print].

36. Sharma, V.K., H.J. Kim, A. Das, *et al.* 2009. Circumferential and focal ablation of Barrett's esophagus containing dysplasia. *Am. J. Gastroenterol.* **104:** 310–317.

37. Herrero, L.A., F.G. van Vilsteren, R.E. Pouw, *et al.* 2011. Endoscopic radiofrequency ablation combined with endoscopic resection for early neoplasia in Barrett's esophagus longer than 10 cm. *Gastrointest. Endosc.* [Epub ahead of print].

38. Van Vilsteren, F.G., R.E. Pouw, S. Seewald, *et al.* 2011. Stepwise radical endoscopic resection versus radiofrequency ablation for Barrett's oesophagus with high-grade dysplasia or early cancer: a multicentre randomised trial. *Gut* **60:** 765–773.

39. Zehetner J, S.R. Demeester, J.A. Hagen, *et al.* 2011. Endoscopic resection and ablation versus esophagectomy for high-grade dysplasia and intramucosal adenocarcinoma. *J. Thorac. Cardiovasc. Surg.* **141:** 39–47.

40. Ganz, R.A., D.S. Utley, R.A. Stern, *et al.* 2004. Complete ablation of esophageal epithelium with a balloon-based bipolar electrode: a phased evalulation in the procine and in the humanesophagus. *Gastrointest. Endosc.* **60:** 1002–1010.

41. Sharma, V.K., K.K. Wang, B.F. Overholt, *et al.* 2007. Balloon-based, circumferential, endoscopic radiofrequency ablation of Barrett's esophagus: 1-year follow-up of 100 patients. *Gastrointest. Endosc.* **65:** 185–195.

42. Shaheen, N.J., P. Sharma, B.F. Overholt, *et al.* 2009. Radiofrequency ablation in Barrett's esophagus with dysplasia. *N. Engl. J. Med.* **360:** 2277–2288.

43. Van Vilsteren, F.G.I, J.G.H.M. Bergman. 2010. Endoscopic therapy using radiofrequency ablation for esophageal dysplasia and carcinoma in Barrett's esophagus. *Gastrointest. Endoscopy. Clin. North Am.* **20:** 55–74.

44. Overholt, B.F., K.K. Wang, J.S. Burdick, *et al.* 2007. Five-year efficacy and safety of photodynamic therapy with Photofrin in Barrett's high-grade dysplasia. *Gastrointest. Endosc.* **66:** 460–468.

45. Rees JRE, P. Lao-Sirieix, A. Wong. *et al.* 2010. Treatment for Barrett's oesophagus. *Cochrane Data Base Systemic.* Review.

46. Shaheen, N.J., A.F. Peery, B.F. Overholt, *et al.* 2010.AIM Dysplasia Investigators. 2010. Biopsy depth after radiofrequency ablation of dysplastic Barrett's esophagus. *Gastrointest. Endosc.* **72:** 490–496.

47. Halsey K.D., J.W. Chang, B.D. Greenwald, *et al.* Recurrent disease following endoscopic ablation of Barrett's neoplasia. *Gastroenterology* **138:** S-16.

48. Finkelstein, S.D., W.D. Lyday. 2008. The molecular pathology of radiofrequency mucosal ablation of Barrett's esophagus. *Gastroenterology* **134:** A436.

49. Montgomery, E., M.P. Bronner, J.R. Goldblum, *et al.* 2001. Reproducibility of the diagnosis of dysplasia in Barrett esophagus: a reaffirmation. *Hum. Pathol.* **32:** 368–378.

50. Wang K.K., R.E. Sampliner. 2008. Updated guidelines. 2008. for the diagnosis, surveillance and therapy of Barrett's esophagus. *Am. J. Gastroenterol.* **103:** 788–797.

51. Curvers, W.L., F.J. ten Kate, K.K. Krishnadath, *et al.* 2010. Low-grade dysplasia in Barrett's esophagus: overdiagnosed and underestimated. *Am. J. Gastroenterol.* **105:** 1523–1530.

52. Sharma, P., G.W. Falk, AP. Weston, *et al.* 2006. Dysplasia and cancer in a large multicenter cohort of patients with Barrett's esophagus. *Clin. Gastroenterol. Hepatol.* **4:** 566–572.

53. Fitzgerald, R. C., M. B. Omary, G. Triadafilopoulos. 1996. Dynamic effects of acid on Barrett's esophagus. An ex vivo proliferation and differentiation model. *J. Clin. Invest.* **98:** 2120–2128.

54. Feagins, L. A., H.-Y. Zhang, K. Hormi-Carver, *et al.* 2007. Acid has antiproliferative effects in nonneoplastic Barrett's epithelial cells. *Am. J. Gastroenterol.* **102:** 10–20.

55. Lao-Sirieix, P., A. Roy, C. Worrall. *et al.*2006. Effect of acid suppression on molecular predictors for esophageal cancer. *Cancer Epidemiol. Biomarkers Prev.* **15:** 288–293.

56. Cooper, B.T., W. Chapman, C.S. Neumann, *et al.* 2006. Continuous treatment of Barrett's oesophagus patients with proton pump inhibitors up to 13 years: observations on regression and cancer incidence. *Aliment Pharmacol. Ther.* **23:** 727–733.

57. DeJonge, P.F., M. van Blankenstein, C.W.N. Looman, *et al.* 2010. Risk of malignant progression in patients with Barrett's oesophagus: a Dutch nationwide cohort study. *Gut* **59:** 1030–1036.

58. Pohl, H., H.G. Welch. 2005. The role of overdiagnosis and reclassification in the marked increase of esophageal adenocarcinoma incidence. *J. Natl. Cancer Inst.* **97:** 142–146.

59. Dulai, G.S., D.M. Jensen, G. Cortina, *et al.* 2005. Randomized trial of argon plasma coagulation vs. multipolar electrocoagulation for ablation of Barrett's esophagus. *Gastrointest. Endosc.* **61:** 232–240.

60. Sampliner, R.E., B. Fennerty, H.S. Garewal. *et al.* 1996. (Reversal of Barrett's esophagus with acid suppression and multipolar electrocoagulation: preliminary results. *Gastrointest. Endosc.* **44:** 532–535.

61. Overholt, B.F., M. Panjehpour, J.M. Haydek, *et al.* 1999. Photodynamic therapy for Barrett's esophagus: follow-up in 100 patients. [see the comments]. *Gastrointest. Endos.* **49:** 1–7.

62. Sharma, V.K., K.K. Wang, B.F. Overholt, *et al.* 2007. Balloon-based, circumferential, endoscopic radiofrequency ablation of Barrett's esophagus: 1-year follow-up of 100 patients. *Gastrointest. Endosc.* **65:** 185–195.

63. Overholt, B.F., C.J. Lightdale, K.K. Wang. *et al.* 2005. Photodynamic therapy with porfimer sodium for ablation of high-grade dysplasia in Barrett's esophagus: international, partially blinded, randomized phase III trial. *Gastrointest. Endosc.* **62:** 488–498.

64. Inadomi, J.M., M. Somsouk, R.D. Madanick, *et al.* 2009. A cost-utility analysis of ablative therapy for Barrett's esophagus. *Gastroenterology* **136:** 613–623.

65. Schnell, T.G., S.J. Sontag, G. Chejfec *et al.* 2001. Long-term nonsurgical management of Barrett's esophagus with high-grade dysplasia. *Gastroenterology* **120:** 1607–1619.

66. Wang, K.K., R.E. Sampliner 2008. Updated Guidelines 2008 for the Diagnosis, Surveillance and Therapy of Barrett's esophagus. *Am. J. Gastroenterol.* **103:** 788–797.

67. Shaheen, N.J., D.E. Fleischer, G.M. Eisen, *et al.* 2010. Durability of epithelial reversion after radiofrequency ablation: follow-up of the AIM dysplasia trial. *Gastroenterology* **138** (Suppl. 1): 92. Ref Type: Abstract

68. Gondrie, J.J., R.E. Pouw, C.M. Sondermeijer, *et al.* 2008. Stepwise circumferential and focal ablation of Barrett's esophagus with high–grade dysplasia: results of the first prospective series of 11 patients. *Endoscopy* **40:** 359–369.

69. Gondrie, J.J., R.E. Pouw, C.M. Sondermeijer, *et al.* 2008. Effective treatment of early Barrett's neoplasia with stepwise circumferential and focal ablation using the HALO system. *Endoscopy* **40:** 370–379.

70. Pouw, R.E., K. Wirths, P. Eisendrath, *et al.* 2010. Efficacy of radiofrequency ablation combined with endoscopic resection for Barrett's esophagus with early neoplasia. *Clin Gastroenterol Hepatol* **8:** 23–29.

71. Pouw, R.E., R. Bisschops, O. Pech, *et al.* 2010. Safety Outcomes of Balloon-Based Circumferential Radiofrequency Ablation after Focal Endoscopic Resection of Early Barrett's Neoplasia in 118 Patients: Results of an Ongoing European Multicenter Study. *Gastrointest Endosc* **71:** AB126.

72. Velanovich, V. 2009. Endoscopic endoluminal radiofrequency ablation of Barrett's esophagus: initial results and lessons learned. *Surg Endosc* **23:** 2175–2180.

73. Shaheen, N.J., B.F. Overholt, S.E. Sampliner, *et al.* 2011. Durability of Radiofrequency Ablation in Barrett's Esophagus with Dysplasia. *Gastroenterology* May 6. [Epub ahead of print].

Ann. N.Y. Acad. Sci. ISSN 0077-8923

ANNALS OF THE NEW YORK ACADEMY OF SCIENCES
Issue: *Barrett's Esophagus: The 10th OESO World Congress Proceedings*

Barrett's esophagus: surgical treatments

Paolo Parise,[1] Riccardo Rosati,[2] Edoardo Savarino,[3] Andrea Locatelli,[2] Martina Ceolin,[2] Kulwinder S. Dua,[4] Roger P. Tatum,[5] Italo Braghetto,[6] C. Prakash Gyawali,[7] Reza A. Hejazi,[8] Richard W. McCallum,[8] Irene Sarosiek,[9] Luigi Bonavina,[10] Eelco B. Wassenaar,[11] Carlos A. Pellegrini,[11] Brian C. Jacobson,[12] Cheri L. Canon,[13] Adolfo Badaloni,[14] and Gianmattia del Genio[15]

[1]Department of General Surgery IV, Regional Referal Center for Esophageal Pathology, Pisa, Italy. [2]General and Minimally Invasive Surgery, Istituto Clinico Humanitas IRCCS and Department of Surgery, University of Milan, Milan, Italy. [3]Gastroenterology Unit, Istituto Clinico Humanitas IRCCS, University of Milan, Milan, Italy. [4]Department of Medicine, Division of Gastroenterology and Hepatology, Medical College of Wisconsin, Milwaukee, Wisconsin. [5]University of Washington, VA Puget Sound Health Care System, Seattle, Washington. [6]Department of Surgery, University Clinical Hospital Jose Joaquin Aguirre, Santiago, Chile. [7]Division of Gastroenterology, Washington University School of Medicine, St. Louis, Missouri. [8]Department of Internal Medicine, Texas Tech University Health Sciences Center, El Paso, Texas. [9]Department of Internal Medicine, Texas Tech University, Paul L. Foster School of Medicine, El Paso, Texas. [10]Department of Surgery, IRCCS Policlinico San Donato, University of Milano Medical School, Milan, Italy. [11]Department of Surgery, Health Sciences Center, University of Washington School of Medicine, Seattle, Washington. [12]Section of Gastroenterology, Boston University Medical Center, Boston, Massachusetts. [13]Department of Radiology, University of Alabama at Birmingham, Birmingham, Alabama. [14]Clinica San Camilo, University of Favaloro, Buenos Aires, Argentina. [15]Center of Esophago-gastric and Obesity Surgery, Second University of Naples, Naples, Italy

The following on surgical treatments for Barrett's esophagus includes commentaries on the indications for antireflux surgery after medical treatment; the effects of the various procedures on the lower esophageal sphincter; the role of impaired esophageal motility and delayed gastric emptying in the choice of the surgical procedure; indications for associated highly selective vagotomy, duodenal switch, and gastric electrical stimulation; therapeutic strategies for detection and treatment of shortened esophagus; the role of antireflux surgery on the regression of metaplastic mucosa and the risk of malignant progression; the detection of asymptomatic reflux brfore bariatric surgery; the role of non-GERD symptoms on the results of surgery; and the indications of Collis gastroplasty and choice of the type of fundoplication.

Keywords: antireflux surgery; metaplastic epithelium; dysplasia; LES pressure; manometry; esophageal motility; peristalsis; Nissen wrap; dysphagia; highly selective vagotomy; truncal vagotomy; duodenal switch; preoperative HRM; LES; achalasia; esophageal body; spastic disorders; gastric emptying; TLESR; post-vagotomy gastroparesis; gastric electrical stimulation; gastric emptying test; gastrostomy; jejunostomy; bariatric surgery; asymptomatic reflux; preoperative endoscopy; short esophagus; slipped wrap; Collis gastroplasty; impedance

Concise summaries

- A laparoscopic antireflux procedure could be proposed to all patients affected by Barrett's esophagus (BE) as an effective and safe therapeutic alternative, balancing risks and benefits for each patient.
- Surgery should also be offered to patients with poor control of symptoms by medical treatment or with progression to low-grade dysplasia or with pathologic functional studies under medical treatment.

- Numerous studies have shown that the surgical procedures lead to a significant postoperative improvement of manometric parameters of lower esophageal sphincter (LES), mainly in patients with severe gastroesophageal reflux disease (GERD) (erosive disease or BE). Nissen repairs produce a higher LES pressure in comparison to posterior repairs, although the difference is not statistically significant.
- Preoperative knowledge of the baseline esophageal motility will be useful in the

doi: 10.1111/j.1749-6632.2011.06051.x

evaluation of those patients who develop symptoms after antireflux (AR) surgery.

- Addition of highly selective vagotomy (HSV) to antireflux procedures in an attempt to produce both acid suppression, as well as a reflux barrier, does not significantly reduce postoperative GERD recurrence. Duodenal switch appears to be a good solution for the control of the pathophysiological mechanisms participating in the genesis of BE. However, this technique failed to resolve completely the complications of BE due to persistence of acid reflux.

- High-resolution manometry (HRM) in the preoperative setting may identify absolute and relative contraindications to the antireflux surgical procedure. It defines extremes of LES and esophageal body motor abnormalities with high sensitivity. In addition, it may identify esophageal motor features that may have value in preoperative counseling and tailoring of the procedure.

- Gastric emptying time should be routinely obtained preoperatively so that postoperative dyspepsia, gas-bloating, and possible vagal nerve damage can be interpreted. Gastro-electrical stimulation provides a significant reduction of symptoms and nutritional status in patients with postvagotomy gastroparesis related to Nissen fundoplication (NF).

- Twenty-four hour esophageal pH monitoring of proton pump inhibitors (PPIs) therapy remains a reliable test for the diagnosis of recurrent reflux after fundoplication.

- Antireflux surgery seems to reduce the risk of progression to high-grade dysplasia and adenocarcinoma more than medical treatment, but does not eliminate the risk.

- Preoperative identification of a shortened esophagus is paramount for successful fundoplication surgery. Short esophagus can be diagnosed radiographically, so that the surgeons can plan accordingly and incorporate esophageal lengthening procedure, if appropriate.

- Collis gastroplasty with fundoplication allows a tension-free fundoplication in shortened esophagus. Patients refer improvement of symptoms, but have the disadvantage of losing distal esophageal motility and having a secreting gastric mucosa in the neoesophagus that requires chronic PPI use and long-term follow-up. Its indication should be limited to shortened esophagus without large ulcers, peptic stricture, Barrett and only after failure to achieve extensive mediastinal mobilization.

- The role of preoperative endoscopy before lap band has been studied, and it seems reasonable to consider endoscopy for anyone undergoing bariatric surgery, although data are lacking to definitively prove its utility among asymptomatic patients.

- An objective measurement of the influence of the total wrap on the bolus transit may be helpful in refining the optimal antireflux wrap type, and the impact of fundoplication on esophageal physiology can be evaluated by combined multichannel intraluminal impedance and HRM.

---

1. How long should medical treatment be continued before antireflux surgery?

Paolo Parise

p.parise@ao-pisa.toscana.it

There are three goals in the treatment of patients affected by BE: (1) stop reflux, (2) promote the regression of dysplastic or metaplastic epithelium, and (3) stop the progression to dysplasia or adenocarcinoma.

Stop reflux

Most patients are treated with a PPI, but many of them have few or no reflux symptoms, probably as a consequence of altered sensitivity in the metaplastic epithelium. Consequently, symptoms cannot be used as an index of "good" therapy,[1] and patients should be tested while receiving acid-suppression therapy with 24-hour pH-metry, as suggested by Peghini *et al.*[2] Moreover, patients with BE often have larger hiatal hernias, incompetent LESs, and ineffective motility of the distal esophagus; so they need aggressive medical therapy with a high-dose PPI, sometimes associated with an evening dose of the H_2 receptor antagonist, because of the presence of nocturnal breakthrough.[3] Even more, it has been observed that high-dose PPI (lansoprazole 60 mg/day) failed to normalize the 24-hour pH test in more than one-third of patients with BE.[4] Todd *et al.*, in a study of 25 patients with BE treated with omeprazole 40–60 mg/day, observed an 80% normalization of 24-hour pH-metry, but in 60% of cases the esophageal exposure to bile was still abnormal with the Bilitec 2000.[5] Several studies have instead demonstrated that antireflux surgery is able to normalize not only the esophageal exposure to acid in about 90% of patients, but also the exposure to duodenogastric refluxate, with a very low morbidity rate using a laparoscopic approach.[6,7]

Stop progression and promote regression

Weston *et al.* prospectively followed 108 patients affected by BE with or without any-grade dysplasia and treated with PPI for a mean period of 40 months. Among the nondysplastic patients, none regressed to nonmetaplastic epithelium, and 28.7% progressed to low-grade dysplasia but with a subsequent regression rate of 78.2%. In the low-grade dysplasia group, 65% of patients regressed to no dysplasia, but 20% progressed to high-grade dysplasia, subsequently developing cancer or multifocal high-grade dysplasia in 50% cases and nondysplastic BE in the remaining 50% cases. Patients presenting with high-grade dysplasia developed cancer or multifocal high-grade dysplasia in 62.5% of cases and regressed to low-grade or no dysplasia in the other cases.[8]

In a retrospective study from the Netherlands, 105 patients affected by long-segment BE without high-grade dysplasia or cancer at first endoscopy were followed for a mean period of 12.7 years. Low-grade dysplasia was present in 11 patients at entry endoscopy. At the end of follow-up, 6% of patients had developed adenocarcinoma, which equals one cancer case per 221 patient years, or 0.45% per year. High-grade dysplasia was diagnosed in 5% of patients, which equals one cancer case per 266 patient years, or 0.38% per year. Regression from low-grade dysplasia to nondysplastic Barrett's epithelium was observed in 50% of cases.[9]

Antireflux surgery seems to be able to gain better results. In a study of 77 patients treated with antireflux surgery versus 14 patients treated with PPI,[10] complete regression of the metaplastic epithelium was observed in 36.4% of surgical patients versus 7.1% of medical patients ($P < 0.03$). In a more recent paper on 125 patients with short-segment BE treated with laparoscopic NF, duodenal switch, or duodenal diversion, regression to nonmetaplastic mucosa was observed in 61% patients of the Nissen group, and 64% and 65%, respectively, in the other two groups.[7] Regression was observed only in short-segment BE.

A randomized study, published in 2003, compared medical and surgical treatment of BE. In the medical group, 2 of 3 patients regressed from low-grade dysplasia to no dysplasia, and in the surgical group 5 of 5, but in the medical arm, dysplasia *de novo* appeared in 8/40 patients (20%); two of these developed high-grade dysplasia. In the surgical arm, 3 of 53 patients (6%) developed dysplasia *de novo*, and two of these subsequently progressed to high-grade dysplasia, but these two showed a recurrence of gastroesophageal reflux (GER) in functional studies. However, if the patients with pH-metric failure were excluded, dysplasia *de novo* appeared in only 2% of patients, and the surgical group showed a statistically significant difference in the medical group ($P < 0.05$). The rate of malignancy was 0.8% per year in the medical group and 0.5% in the surgical group.[6]

Very interesting data were obtained via a large literature metanalysis. In a recent review, Chang *et al.* included 1,696 patients affected by BE, 700 medically treated and 996 surgically treated. Surgically treated patients demonstrated a higher incidence of disease regression (15.4%) compared with medically treated patients (1.9%). Even when controlled studies only were analyzed, the probability of regression was greater for surgically treated patients (6.5% vs. 0.5% $P = 0.024$); the largest difference between surgical and medical therapy was demonstrated in the probability of regression from nondysplastic Barrett's epithelium to normal squamous epithelium (17% vs. 0.4%).[11] Unfortunately, with regard to progression to adenocarcinoma, when differences in study design are ignored, results suggest that antireflux surgery is associated with a significantly reduced incidence rate of cancer; however, analyzing only randomized controlled trials and cohort studies, a significant difference cannot be demonstrated:[11,12] 4.8 cases per 1,000 patient years in the surgical group versus 6.5 cases per 1,000 patient years in the medical group ($P = 0.32$).

Conclusion

It is not easy to describe how long medical treatment should be continued in patients with BE, but in light of the previously exposed data, it is easier to determine when an antireflux procedure should be proposed. A laparoscopic antireflux procedure could be proposed for all patients affected by BE, as an effective and safe therapeutic alternative, balancing risks and benefits for each patient. Surgery should also be offered to patients with poor control of symptoms, with progression to low-grade dysplasia, or with pathologic functional studies under medical treatment.

2. What is the effect of the various AR procedures on the LES?

Riccardo Rosati, Edoardo Savarino, Andrea Locatelli, and Martina Ceolin
riccardo.rosati@humanitas.it

The main mechanisms involved in the pathogenesis of GERD provoked a defection of the normal antireflux barrier (His angle, LES) continence, esophageal clearance, thorax abdomen pressure gradient). In particular, the majority of patients with severe GERD have a permanent defect of the LES, as demonstrated by physiologic studies; this alteration is more pronounced in the most severe form of reflux disease: patients with BE or severe erosive disease have significantly lower LES resting pressures than patients with nonerosive reflux disease (NERD) or mild erosive disease.[13]

A defective LES is generally defined as a sphincter with a resting pressure of less than 8 mm Hg, an overall length of less than 2 cm, or an intraabdominal length of less than 1 cm. The presence of a mechanically defective sphincter became a criterion for surgery: it has been clearly demonstrated that both total and partial fundoplication procedures restore normal function and length in the structurally defective LES. The degree of increasing pressure increase after fundoplication is usually dependent on the type of plasty:[14] Nissen repairs produce a higher LES pressure in comparison to posterior repairs, although the difference is not statistically significant. The results after anterior repair (Watson) in terms of LES resting and residual pressure and in terms of transient relaxations are similar to Nissen repair and unrelated to body position and gastric distension.[15,16]

The good results with laparoscopic antireflux procedures increased the demand for surgery in patients with NERD who often have normal LES characteristics at rest.[17] In patients with manometrically intact LES, several other mechanisms have been proposed

to explain the impaired competence of the LES: increased frequency and duration of transient LES relaxations (tLESRs), which are both restored by antireflux surgery;[15] impaired esophageal peristalsis; impaired gastric emptying; increased intragastric or intraabdominal pressure; and increased BMI.[18]

However, GERD does not always mean the presence of an incompetent LES (permanent or transient), but there is also a group of patients with hypertensive lower esophageal sphincter (HLES) and GERD. HLES is defined as a pressure of LES above 35 mm Hg, with normal relaxation and no esophageal body motility disorder. The etiology and pathophysiology of HLES is unknown; it has been postulated that it could be secondary to the presence of abnormal esophageal acid exposure, being a sort of defensive mechanism. Some of these patients can benefit from surgery. Varga *et al.* reported a series of patients with HLES, who were submitted to a floppy NF: mean LES pressure changed six weeks after surgery from 50.5 mm Hg to 24.7 mm Hg, and 15.7 mm Hg at late follow-up, and no cases of postsurgery dysphagia were reported in this group of patients.[19]

Besides, abnormality of the LES pressure profile after fundoplication can be determined by an anatomical failure of the wrap (e.g., intrathoracic migration): for example, the recognition of a dual high-pressure zone (HPZ) at HRM correlates with recurrent hiatal hernia.[20]

In conclusion, numerous studies have shown that surgical procedures lead to a significant postoperative improvement of manometric parameters of LES, mainly in patients with severe GERD (erosive disease or BE); further studies may help to predict the outcome of surgical treatment in patients with NERD.

3. What are the consequences of an impaired esophageal motility on the choice of surgical technique?

Kulwinder S. Dua
kdua@mcw.edu

Esophageal manometry is useful in identifying those occasional patients who may have reflux-like symptoms but have achalasia and in whom antireflux surgery is contraindicated. Similarly, antireflux surgery may have adverse consequences in those with severe dysmotility in the form of aperistalsis, as seen in those with scleroderma. However, the vast majority of patients undergoing antireflux surgery have either normal or impaired, but not absent, esophageal motility. Impaired esophageal motility leading to ineffective esophageal peristalsis (IEP), and poor bolus clearance is defined as mean amplitude of the peristaltic waves in the distal 10 cm of the esophagus being less than 25–30 mm Hg.[21] Since a 360° full wrap (FW) results in a higher increase in the esophagogastric junction pressure and also a higher postswallow residual relaxation pressure, as compared to a partial wrap (PW), the customary wisdom and approach has been to use PW in those with IEP and FW in those with normal motility. This tailored approach to antireflux surgery is based on two assumptions: first, in the presence of IEP, FW may result in a higher postoperative dysphagia rate, and second, PW is not as effective as a FW in controlling GER, and hence FW should be the procedure of choice unless there are reasons not to do so. In patients with IEP, Lund *et al.* reported dysphagia in 44% with FW (Nissen) compared to 9% with PW (Toupet).[22] On the other hand, Baigrie *et al.* performed FW (Nissen) in 31 patients with IEP, and the postoperative dysphagia score at one-year follow-up was 6%, which was similar to the score of patients who underwent a Nissen wrap and had normal motility.[23] Similar controversial data exist regarding the efficacy of reflux control with PW as compared to a FW. Several studies in the 1990s have shown inferior control of GER with PW, especially in those with severe reflux disease. However, on a prospective study of 107 patients, 54 patients were randomized to a Nissen wrap and 53 to a partial 180° anterior wrap. Both groups were comparable in preoperative severity of reflux disease and esophageal dysmotility. At the 10-year follow-up, there was no significant difference between the two groups with regard to reflux control, dysphagia, and overall satisfaction.[24] Similar results were found in a well-designed prospective randomized study that was initially published in 2001 and recently updated with a longer follow-up period.[25] Two hundred patients were randomized, as shown in Figure 1.

At two-year follow-up, postoperative dysphagia was more common in the Nissen group, and preoperative motility did not correlate with postoperative dysphagia in either group. Six of 50 patients with normal motility and 13 of 50 with dysmotil-

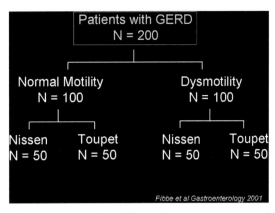

Figure 1. No significant difference between Nissen wrap and a partial 180° anterior wrap with regard to reflux control, dysphagia, and overall satisfaction. Adpated from Ref. 25.

ity in the Nissen group had dysphagia, compared to 3 of 50 (normal motility) and 5 of 50 (dysmotility) in the Toupet group. Toupet proved to be as good as the Nissen procedure in controlling reflux symptoms.

Based on the above conflicting results from the literature, no firm recommendations can be made on the choice of surgery in patients with impaired esophageal motility. Prospective randomized studies are challenging the concept of tailoring surgery on the basis of preoperative esophageal motility testing. There are several reasons that can potentially explain these discrepancies. First, several studies appear to be retrospective reviews of prospectively collected data and we need more prospective randomized studies. Second, the techniques of motility testing used may not have been sensitive enough to accurately assess bolus transit. It will be interesting to see the impact of tailoring surgery based on the recently introduced multiple channel HRM and concurrent impedance testing (reflecting bolus transit). Third, esophageal dysmotility is usually secondary to GERD, and studies have shown reversal of dysmotility after antireflux surgery. This may have confounded the results; currently, there are no tests that can preoperatively predict this reversal.

So, is esophageal motility evaluation before antireflux surgery required? Abnormal esophageal motility does not diagnose reflux disease, but esophageal manometry can diagnose achalasia presenting with reflux-like symptoms or aperistalsis of scleroderma. Knowledge on the baseline preoperative esophageal motility will be useful in the evaluation of those patients who develop symptoms after an antireflux surgery.

4. Should HSV be added to antireflux surgery?

Roger P. Tatum

rtatum@u.washington.edu

Although antireflux surgery is commonly employed as a treatment for more severe and refractory GERD and overall results of most studies reveal a patient satisfaction rate of 90% or greater with the procedure, recurrence of GERD symptoms, with or without esophagitis, is observed in approximately 10–25% of patients after long-term follow-up.[26–29] One recently published randomized trial of laparoscopic antireflux surgery (LARS) versus PPI treatment with 12-year follow-up reported an overall recurrence rate of 47% for surgical therapy.[30] Therefore, in an effort to reduce the recurrence rate of esophageal acid reflux and its symptoms, some authors have, throughout the history of antireflux surgery, suggested the addition of HSV in order to simultaneously reduce gastric acid production.

Specifically, parietal cell vagotomy (or HSV) was first reported as an adjunct to NF for the control of reflux by Bahadorzadeh and colleagues in 1975.[31] None of the 14 patients undergoing this combined procedure were found to have recurrent reflux with a mean 20 months of follow-up. However, a later series of 158 patients by the same group revealed an overall surgical failure rate, defined as the recurrence of moderate to severe symptoms of 17.5% at a mean six-year follow-up.[32] Notably, the addition of a posterior gastropexy to the procedure, in addition to HSV and open NF, resulted in a failure rate of only 9.3%. The authors concluded by recommending that NF with HSV and posterior gastropexy be reserved for those patients who presented with GERD in combination with peptic ulcer disease. In a series of 32 patients undergoing open NF with HSV by Garcia-Rinaldi *et al.*, with a mean 14-month follow-up, three patients (9%) were found to have esophagitis on postoperative endoscopy.[33] In a study of 97 patients who completed postoperative pH testing within six months of open NF with HSV, Bohmer *et al.* reported that 82.5% had normal pH studies, with slightly better overall

symptom control.[34] Therefore, as these data collectively indicate, both objective and subjective results of HSV combined with antireflux surgery are not strikingly different from those of the published series of fundoplication alone.

It is worth mentioning that in the modern era of PPI therapy, HSV is rarely practiced as a procedure for the management of peptic ulcer disease, for which it has traditionally been indicated. Treatment with PPI medications, such as omeprazole, is capable of reducing gastric acidity by 97% and results in an increase in 24-hour serum gastrin levels equivalent to those observed after HSV.[35] Therefore, a particular advantage to HSV in the management of GERD is difficult to argue.

Disadvantages and risks to the performance of HSV in the context of antireflux procedures have been noted by other authors. Stein *et al.*, reporting on a series of patients who presented with recurrent symptoms after failed antireflux procedures, including 12 who had undergone HSV in association with fundoplication, noted that there was a particularly high incidence of slippage of the fundoplication in the HSV patients.[36] Therefore, they specifically advocated against the addition of HSV to fundoplication. Kennedy *et al.* reported four cases of necrosis of the lesser curvature of the stomach in patients who had undergone this combined procedure and cautioned against its use.[37] Delayed gastric emptying (DGE) was demonstrated in patients who had undergone HSV and fundoplication, compared to those after fundoplication alone by Jamieson *et al.*, although there were no differences between the two groups in terms of symptomatic outcome.[38] These specific risks, in combination with the additional time and skill required to perform HSV, argue against the combination of HSV with antireflux surgery.

Notably, truncal vagotomy (unilateral or bilateral), in combination with fundoplication and without an accompanying gastric emptying procedure, has been shown to be safe and is associated with minimal to no side effects (particularly in the case of unilateral vagotomy) in a series by Oelschlager *et al.*[39] As this technique results in a relative increase in the length of esophageal mobilization, up to approximately 3 cm, it has been proposed as a deliberate maneuver to deal with the phenomenon of the short esophagus. Therefore, by inference the recurrence of reflux may be influenced by truncal vagotomy, although this may have as much or more to do with the potential to reduce the incidence of recurrent hiatus hernia in such patients as it does with acid suppression resultant from the vagotomy itself. This was not demonstrated in this series, however, in which approximately 40% of those patients returning for routine postoperative pH testing were found to have abnormal DeMeester scores.

In conclusion, though long-term recurrence rates for antireflux surgery may be in excess of 20%, published data indicate that the addition of HSV to these procedures, in an attempt to produce both acid suppression as well as a reflux barrier, does not significantly reduce GERD recurrence postoperatively. The degree of acid suppression provided by HSV is in some ways comparable, and in others not as complete, as that provided by PPI therapy. Further, disadvantages of this combined approach, beyond the additional time and skill involved in the performance of the procedure, include risks of fundoplication slippage, gastric necrosis, and DGE. In select cases in which adequate length of the esophagus below the hiatus is difficult to achieve, unilateral truncal vagotomy may be considered in order to obtain 3 cm of esophagus below the hiatal closure, although the ultimate effect that this technique has on reflux recurrence has yet to be determined. Overall, the evidence does not support the addition of HSV to antireflux surgical procedures as they are practiced in the current era.

5. What are the indications for duodenal switch in patients with BE?

Italo Braghetto and Attila Csendes
ibraghet@redclinicauchile.cl

BE is defined as the presence of intestinal metaplasia at the distal esophagus as a consequence of chronic and severe reflux.[40,41] The main pathophysiologic factors are an incompetent LES with an increased perimeter of the cardia (dilatation of the esophagogastric junction); severe, abnormal acid reflux; duodenogastroesophageal reflux; and motor alterations of the thoracic esophagus.

Table 1 shows the differences between patients with short-segment BE and long-segment BE with regard to the pathophysiological factors involved.

Table 2 shows the Bilitec 2000 results in controls subjects: patients with GER, erosive esophagitis, and BE.[42–44] Patients with BE have more severe acid and biliary reflux, secondary to defective LES, and anatomic abnormalities, such as very dilated cardia or presence of hiatal hernia.

Currently, different types of clinical and endoscopic manifestations are accepted, which also are treated in different ways; the discussion among gastroenterologists and surgeons persists concerning the best option for treatment for short-segment, long-segment, or complicated BE. Most gastroenterologists until the present were reluctant to indicate surgery in patients with GERD, but now surgeons discuss the different surgical modalities for treatment of BE.[45,46] On the basis of these pathophysiological factors, surgical treatment for patients with BE must increase LESP, suppress acid secretion, or abolish duodenal reflux.

Therefore, there are goals for surgical treatment in BE. (1) Clinical goals: control of symptoms, cessation of acid and duodenal reflux, healing of the esophagitis, and avoidance of complications (ulcer, stricture, dysplasia). (2) Histologic goals are prevention of increase in length of intestinal metaplasia, regression of intestinal metaplasia to cardiac mucosa, prevention of dysplasia, regression of dysplasia, and prevention of progression to adenocarcinoma. The surgical options are fundoplication and gastropexy alone, fundoplication and vagotomy-antrectomy and Roux-en-Y gastrojejunostomy, or fundoplication and HSV and duodenal switch.

Table 1. Clinical results after fundoplication + highly selective vagotomy + duodenal switch in patients with Barrett's esophagus

	Non-complicated ($n = 45$) (%)	Complicated ($n = 21$) (%)	*P* value
Morbidity	6 (13.3)	3 (14.2)	0.78
Post-operative mortality	–	–	
Follow-up Visick I-II	43 (95.5)	13 (61.9)	0.0014
Recurrence	1 (2.2)*	8 (38.1)+	0.00035

Table 2. Clinical results at long term follow up in patients with Barrett's esophagus having undergone duodenal switch compared to acid truncal vagotomy, partial gastrectomy, and Roux-en-Y gastrojejunostomy

Clinical results	Duodenal switch procedure $n = 75$	Truncal vagotomy partial gastrectomy Roux-en-Y anastomosis $n = 245$
Operative mortality	0	2 (0.8%)
Follow up (%)	95%	92%
Months follow-up	55	68
Visick I and II	71%	91%
Visick III and IV	29%	9%
Development of dysplasia	0	0
Development of adenocarcinoma	0	0
Regression of low-grade dysplasia	8/13	15/24

For short-segment BE, there is consensus for performing a fundoplication with very satisfactory long-term results. However, for the long segment there is controversy concerning the long-term results of fundoplication or more complete physiologic procedures.[47,48] Postoperative anatomic failures after fundoplication are more frequent in patients with long-segment BE (5% vs. 12–25%). Farrell reported three times more postoperative anatomic failure in patients with BE compared to non-Barrett's patients.[49–51]

Csendes and others have published very disappointing long-term results in long-segment BE patients and propose to perform other procedures that accomplish all the purposes of surgery, such as fundoplication with addition of acid suppression duodenal diversion procedures.[52] Consequently, fundoplication and HSV and duodenal switch was presented as a physiological procedure for BE, as it prevents pathological duodenogastric reflux, improves LES competence, and decreases gastric acid secretion.[53,54]

Results
We studied the postoperative results of this procedure in patients with short-segment noncompli-

cated and long-segment complicated BE.[55] In complicated long-segment BE, the results regarding the presence of erosive esophagitis were worse, and the persistence of peptic ulcer and stricture were almost 38% and 10%, respectively. Incompetent LES was present in 57% of patients with complicated BE, and positive acid reflux and positive Bilitec 2000 were higher in patients with complicated BE compared to non-complicated BE. At long-term follow-up, recurrence and Visick IV grading were also more frequent in this group of patients (Table 1). More recently, Csendes *et al.*[56] published late results comparing duodenal switch and acid suppression duodenal diversion procedure with antrectomy and Roux-en-Y gastrojejunostomy (Table 2). Better results were observed in patients submitted to the latter procedure.

Conclusions
1. This technique appears to be the ideal solution for the control of all pathophysiological mechanisms participating in the genesis of BE. However, the technique failed to resolve completely the complications of BE, owing to persistence of acid reflux.
2. These results demonstrate that antireflux surgery associated with HSV and duodenal switch gives excellent results in patients with noncomplicated BE; however, in patients with esophageal ulcer or strictures, the results are unsatisfactory with a high recurrence rate.
3. There are two possible explanations for this failure. First, surgery failed to improve LES competence and the inability to control gastric acid secretion. HSV was insufficient for complete abolition of gastric acid secretion.
4. For short-segment BE, duodenal switch is not justified because fundoplication gives very good results at long-term follow-up.[56–59]
5. For patients with long segment, duodenal switch in association with HSV and antireflux surgery should not be the operation of choice in patients with complicated BE.
6. Indications for duodenal switch are currently restricted to selected patients having had previous surgical procedures, such as gastric pull-up after esophagectomy.

6. What information can be expected from preoperative HRM for the choice between various antireflux techniques?

C. Prakash Gyawali

cprakash@wustl.edu

HRM allows detailed interrogation of esophageal motor phenomena with the use of multiple circumferential high-fidelity solid state sensors on an esophageal manometry catheter, dedicated software for filling in data points between recording sites with best fit data, and computerized topographic contour plots wherein preassigned colors reflect contraction amplitudes and pressure phenomena in the esophagus. The entire esophagus can be simultaneously interrogated with the creation of vivid images that are now termed *Clouse plots*, in honor of Ray Clouse, who conceived HRM in the 1990s. For patients undergoing foregut surgery, preoperative HRM can provide useful information in the following areas: anatomic information, LES abnormalities, and esophageal body contraction abnormalities.

Anatomic information

The classic HRM image of esophageal peristalsis is anchored by the two sphincters, the upper esophageal sphincter (UES) and the LES. Therefore, esophageal length can be determined as the distance between the two sphincters, and a shortened esophagus can be quickly identified—this may have an impact on the foregut surgical procedure as an esophageal lengthening procedure may be needed (Fig. 2). Further, components of the LES HPZ, that is, the LES and the diaphragmatic crura, can be individually identified. Hence, a separation between the LES and diaphragmatic crura can be measured to define a hiatus hernia (Fig. 2). The motility catheter may not traverse the diaphragmatic hiatus despite straddling the LES in the presence of a sizable axial hiatus hernia.

LES abnormalities

One of the most frequent findings on preoperative HRM is a hypotensive LES, indicating disrupted sphincteric barrier function—this improves with antireflux surgery, and higher LES basal pressures are typically recorded following fundoplication, reflecting reduced compliance of the gastroesophageal junction HPZ. On the contrary, the finding of an error of LES relaxation may indicate a missed achalasia or achalasia-like disorder and necessitates altering the surgical procedure to include LES

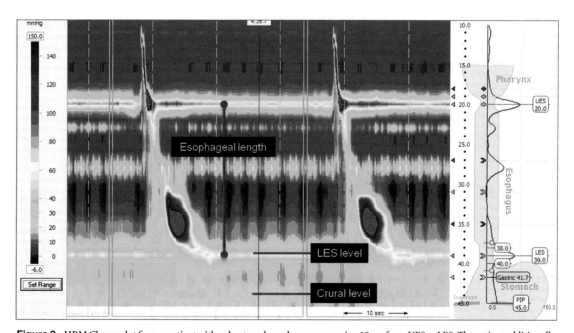

Figure 2. HRM Clouse plot from a patient with a shortened esophagus measuring 19 cm from UES to LES. The patient additionally has a 5 cm hiatus hernia, as depicted by the separation of the LES from the diaphragmatic crural contraction. HRM allows quick assessment of esophageal length and can provide information regarding anatomic relationship between the LES and diaphragmatic crura.

Table 3. Classification of weak peristalsis and implication for antireflux surgery

	Percent failed sequences	Amplitude of transmitted sequences	Implication for antireflux surgery
Normal	Up to 30%	>30 mm Hg	
Mild hypomotility	>30 to ≤50%	<30 mm Hg	Probably none, unless dysphagia
Moderate hypomotility	>50% to ≤80%	<30 mm Hg	
Severe hypomotility	≥80%	Any	Caution for standard surgery

Adapted from reference 61.

myotomy. HRM has particularly high sensitivity and positive predictive value for the diagnosis of LES relaxation errors, with very low false-positive rates.[60] The likelihood of diagnosing achalasia on preoperative HRM before LARS in a large cohort of over 1,000 patients was 1.0%, and an additional 2.5% had significant errors of LES relaxation.[61]

Esophageal body contraction abnormalities

Integrity of esophageal body peristalsis can be assessed by the use of isobaric contour tools. Using a combination of the proportion of failed sequences and peristaltic contraction amplitudes, patients with esophageal body aperistalsis or severe hypomotility (≥80% peristaltic failure with wet swallows) can be identified (Table 3). As many as 3.2% of patients undergoing preoperative HRM testing had aperistalsis, and another 1.3% had severe esophageal body hypomotility in a cohort of over 1,000 patients preoperatively.[61] In patients with severe hypomotility or aperistalsis, a partial (≤270°) fundoplication may reduce the likelihood of postoperative transit symptoms when compared to a 360° NF, but outcome data are limited. With lesser degrees of hypomotility, postoperative transit symptoms are inconsistent except when patients report preoperative dysphagia.[62]

Multiple rapid swallows (MRS) can be potentially used to assess peristaltic reserve in patients undergoing preoperative HRM.[63] When five swallows are administered two to three seconds apart, esophageal body peristalsis is inhibited with profound LES relaxation during the swallows, followed by a robust esophageal body contraction sequence and LES aftercontraction in normal individuals. A normal appearing response has been noted after MRS in as many as 48% of subjects with low distal esophageal body contraction amplitudes (ineffective esophageal motility) after MRS.[63] This may

prove to be a useful tool in predicting postoperative improvement in postoperative manometric function, but outcome data are not available yet and research is ongoing.

A hypermotile or spastic pattern can also be quickly identified by visual inspection as well as with the use of specialized tools, including the pressure volume tool, wherein the distal contractile integral (DCI) can be measured in mm Hg/cm/sec. Normal ranges have been established, and values >5,000 mm Hg/cm/sec are considered abnormal. Other spastic features in the esophageal body include the presence of ≥15% double peaked waves, any triple peaked waves, mean wave duration ≥ 5.7 seconds, simultaneous contractions ≥20%, and mean contraction amplitudes >180 mm Hg. Spastic disorders have been shown to be associated with increased esophageal symptom reporting, and esophageal pain sensitivity to balloon distension correlates well with esophageal body contraction amplitudes. Therefore, spastic disorders reflect esophageal hypersensitivity to noxious and pressure phenomena and can predict a higher likelihood of residual symptoms despite successful antireflux surgery.[64] As many as 23–44% of patients undergoing preoperative HRM may have spastic features.[61]

In summary, HRM in the preoperative setting identifies absolute and relative contraindications to the antireflux surgical procedure in as many as 7% of patients. HRM defines extremes of LES and esophageal body motor abnormalities with high sensitivity. In addition, HRM provides reliable anatomic data that may benefit the foregut surgeon and may identify esophageal motor features that may have value in preoperative counseling and tailoring of the procedure. Use of the MRS procedure may provide assessment of esophageal peristaltic reserve in the presence of weak peristalsis that may further augment the value of preoperative HRM before esophageal foregut surgery.

7. Should gastric emptying be routinely assessed before considering a NF?

Reza A. Hejazi, Irene Sarosiek, and
Richard W. McCallum
richard.mccallum@ttuhsc.edu
reza.abbaszdehhejazi@ttuhs.edu
irene.sariosiek@ttuhsc.edu

Nissen fundoplication (NF) is the most popular and effective antireflux procedure for patients who are refractory to medical treatment and referred for surgical treatment of GERD. However, GERD is often only part of a spectrum of gastrointestinal tract dysfunction. Approximately 20–40% of patients with GERD have associated symptoms, such as early satiety and bloating, suggestive of delayed gastric emptying (DGE).[65] The proposed mechanisms are: the role of gastric distention in increasing the TLESRs; and the role of antral dysmotility and slow gastric emptying in increasing transient LES relaxations.

DGE primarily has not been associated with erosive esophagitis and GERD in recent pediatric literature.[66,67] Recent reports in adult patients did show that DGE does not affect outcomes of GERD following NF. Nevertheless, the patients with DGE have more postoperative gas, bloating and/or nausea compared with patients with normal gastric emptying. This observation may lead to the possible addition of a pyloroplasty to the fundoplication. In our experience of 21 adult patients with GERD where NFs were performed, there was no significant difference in the preoperative versus postoperative gastric emptying times. In 9 (43%) of these patients with prefundoplication DGE, 7 patients also had DGE postfundoplication (Fig. 3). The severity of early satiety increased from an average severity score 9 to 21 (max 28 points), while the severity of heartburn and regurgitation markedly decreased.[68] There are also scattered reports that indicate acceleration of gastric emptying post-fudoplication.[69]

Conclusions

1. Dyspepsia symptoms are very common in GERD patients, both pre- and post-Nissen.
2. GET should be routinely obtained preoperatively to allow for adequate interpretation of dyspepsia symptoms with gas bloating and possible vagal nerve damage in post-op period.
3. NF appears to have no or minimal effect on GET.
4. Slow GET is not necessarily accelerated by Nissen.
5. Delayed GET is not a contraindication to Nissen, but a loose wrap (60 French) is recommended.

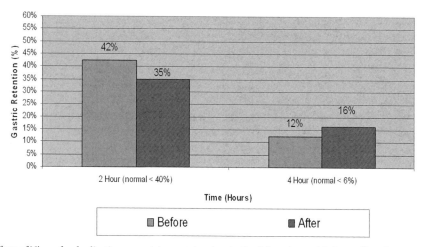

Figure 3. Effects of Nissen fundoplication on gastric emptying time in 21 adult patients with GERD.[68] With permission from John Wiley & Sons.

8. What can be expected from gastric electrical stimulation in the treatment of postvagotomy gastroparesis occurring after NF?

Irene Sarosiek and Richard W. McCallum

irene.sarosiek@ttuhsc.edu

Postsurgical gastroparesis (PSG) develops in up to 10% of patients undergoing intentional or inadvertent vagotomy and in up to 50% of patients undergoing surgery for gastric outlet obstruction. Although gastroparesis in a setting of postabdominal surgery is less frequently diagnosed (13%) when compared with diabetic (29%) or idiopathic (36%) origin, it is identified as a chronic form of gastric atonia from disruption of the normal mechanisms that direct gastric motility. NF is the major surgery associated with PSG symptoms and could be attributed to "accidental" vagal nerve injury during surgery.[70,71] Resection of distal esophagus and gastroesophageal anastomosis in BE complicated by dysphagia or cancer could potentially also lead to PSG. Many therapeutic methods have been used to treat gastroparesis, including diet modification, pharmacological agents (prokinetics and antiemetic), endoscopic techniques (injections of botulinum toxin), psychological counseling, or even surgical placement of feeding tubes.

Gastric electrical stimulation (GES) represents a major advancement for symptom control in a set-

Table 4. The results of GES therapy in post-NF gastroparetics. Interestingly, there was a significant improvement of GET results after pyloroplasty was performed in our P-V gastroparetic patients

Means ± SE (N = 18)	Baseline	Follow-up
TTS (severity: 0–28)	19.1 ± 3.4	10.9 ± 7.6*
Vomiting (severity: 0–4)	2.6 ± 05	10 ± 0.5*
Nausea (severity: 0–4)	3.4102	1.8 ± 0.2*
G and/or J-tubes	4	0
TPN	1	0
Gastric retention (%) four hours	48	40

ting of medically refractory gastroparesis (Fig. 4). GES therapy was approved in 2000 as the Enterra System and has shown a significant and sustained improvement of the GP condition, with 75–80% reduction in major symptoms.[70] The gastric emptying test (GET) assessed with the nuclear medicine 4-hour scintigraphy is an objective measurement of dysmotility, although initial clinical studies have shown mixed results regarding acceleration of GET with GES.[72]

On the basis of already published data,[70] GES is recognized as a treatment option in all drug refractory groups, including the post-vagotomy (P-V) etiology of gastroparesis. Further studies were designed to investigate the clinical outcome of an addition of pyloroplasty (PP) in a subgroup of the P-V patients with GES therapy. Thirty-one patients (mean age 48 [20–70]; F 87%; mean GP duration three years [1–33]) with severe GI P-V symptoms were implanted with the Enterra System. Eighteen of these P-V patients underwent NF before being diagnosed with GP. Also, four of these 18 P-V patients received PP at the time of GES implantation. Tests and evaluations obtained at baseline and after at least 12-month and up to 85-month follow-up visits were as follows: total GP symptoms score (TSS), including nausea (N), vomiting (V), early satiety (ES), postprandial fullness (PF), abdominal bloating (AB), pain (AP), and epigastric burning (EB) (max TSS = 28), gastric emptying test (normal retention at 4 hours <10% of the solid meal), and nutritional status with TPN and G/J tubes presence (Table 4).

We concluded that GES-Enterra Therapy provides a significant reduction of GP symptoms and

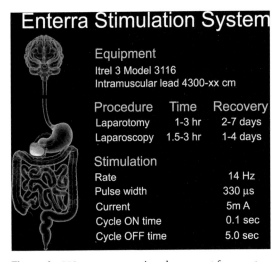

Figure 4. GES represents a major advancement for symptom control in a setting of medically refractory gastroparesis.

nutritional status in patients with P-V gastroparesis related to NF. Pyloroplasty combined with GES maintained this reduction in symptoms but also accelerated gastric emptying in patients with P-V GP refractory to pharmacotherapy. If these gains in GET as well as the reduction in symptoms are confirmed in a larger study population, then pyloroplasty accompanying GES will be an important medical advance and could be regarded as a possible "cure" for this P-V etiology of gastroparesis.

9. Can complete regression of BE after successful antireflux surgery be assessed?

Luigi Bonavina
luigi.bonavina@unimi.it

There is an ongoing debate between gastroenterologists and surgeons as to the optimal treatment of GER in the context of BE. LARS has been shown to effectively control both acid and nonacid reflux. In addition, there is evidence that antireflux surgery can eliminate intestinalization at the cardia in a two-year interval[73] and can heal some patients with a short-segment BE.[74] There also appears to be some protection against the development of dysplasia and adenocarcinoma after an effective fundoplication, whereas evidence for pharmacological therapy having the same benefit is less compelling. Parrilla *et al.*,[45] in the only randomized clinical trial, reported that patients with a well-functioning fundoplication had a significantly reduced incidence of dysplasia compared to medically treated patients.

The concept that elimination of reflux should promote a quiescent state in the BE is supported by studies showing, after fundoplication, a reduced or normalized expression of genes involved in the progression to cancer.[75] To further enhance cancer protection, endoscopic mucosal ablation, performed either before or after a fundoplication, could be incorporated in the therapeutic strategy of patients with BE, but long-term results are still lacking.[76,77]

Zehetner *et al.*[78] recently published the results of antireflux surgery in 75 patients with a minimum follow-up of five years (median 8.9 years, range 5–18 years). Regression of BE was documented in 31% of the patients. Progression occurred in 8%,

and the incidence of a failed fundoplication was significantly greater in these patients (67% vs. 16%). The reported rate of progression from nondysplastic Barrett's to high-grade dysplasia or cancer was 0.8% per patient year. Not surprisingly, the prevalence of progression was significantly increased (sevenfold) in patients with a failed fundoplication.

Yearly endoscopic follow-up with multiple-level biopsies is recommended in patients who underwent antireflux surgery with a diagnosis of BE. It seems reasonable to use the same biopsy protocol that is usually adopted for surveillance. During endoscopy, the fundoplication should be assessed in the retroflexed view and scored according to the Hill classification. Twenty-four hour esophageal pH monitoring of PPI therapy remains a reliable test for the diagnosis of recurrent reflux after fundoplication. Special attention should be given to patients with recurrent reflux symptoms and/or abnormal pH studies, since progression is more likely to happen after a failed antireflux procedure.

10. Can antireflux surgery be considered as reducing or potentially eliminating the risk of malignant progression?

Eelco B. Wassenaar and Carlos A. Pellegrini
pellegri@u.washington.edu

BE is a risk factor for the development of esophageal cancer. The natural history of Barrett's consists of progression of disease due to exposure to gastric contents from GERD from Barrett's metaplasia to dysplasia to esophageal adenocarcinoma (EAC). Dysplasia can regress back to metaplasia, though, and even to normal mucosa.

Treatment of BE has mostly focused on control of reflux. It is still unclear what the effect of treatment (medical, endoscopic, or surgical) is on the natural course of BE. Every patient will have a different response to treatment, and the consequence of failure of treatment to control reflux has to be taken into account. Medical treatment has been shown to reduce the chance of progression to EAC in multiple studies. Nguyen *et al.* recently reported a risk of developing HGD or EAC of 7.4% after a follow-up of eight years. This risk almost doubled in patients not taking PPIs.[79]

Surgical treatment through antireflux surgery has also been shown to reduce progression to EAC.

Multiple case series with up to 90 patients who have BE and undergo antireflux surgery (ARS) have been published with a maximum follow-up of five years. Development of EAC in these series is generally low (0–4%). In a recent review of these case series, the progression was found to be 0.7%.[80] Control of reflux after ARS seems to be key in preventing progression of disease. Patients that progress to adenocarcinoma after ARS are often found to have a failed fundoplication.[81]

When comparing medical treatment with surgical treatment, two studies (an RCT by Parrilla *et al.*[45] and a cohort study by Gatenby *et al.*[82]) have shown decreased progression rates to HGD or EAC of patients after ARS, compared with treatment with PPIs. Several factors influence the interpretation of these results. First of all progression of BE to HGD and EAC is rare and therefore hard to study. Most studies are case series with limited follow-up in a disease that can take decades to develop. When comparing medical versus surgical treatment, one has to take into account that surgical candidates will probably have worse disease than medical treated patients. On the other hand, the complications due to the operation (nor due to medical treatment) are included in the analysis of the results.

Conclusions that can be drawn from this analysis are that ARS seems to reduce the risk of progression of BE to HGD or EAC, especially when surgery is successful. ARS seems to reduce the risk more than medical treatment but does not eliminate the risk.

11. Should systematic preoperative endoscopy be performed in all patients undergoing bariatric surgery to detect asymptomatic reflux lesions that could affect the type of surgery performed?

Brian C. Jacobson
brian.jacobson@bmc.org

Let's first establish what asymptomatic reflux lesions are. These would include BE, minor strictures, asymptomatic esophagitis, and early cancer. One could also classify hiatal hernia as an asymptomatic lesion that is reflux related, though not a lesion resulting from reflux. The role of endoscopy may also depend on the type of surgery being planned. These surgeries can be categorized as restrictive versus malabsorptive. The vertical-banded gastroplasty, sleeve gastrectomy, and laparoscopic adjustable gastric band (lap band) are all restrictive bariatric surgeries, while the biliopancreatic diversion with duodenal switch is malabsorptive. The commonly used Roux-en-Y gastric bypass (RYGBP) has both restrictive and malabsorptive properties. All surgeries leave the gastroesophageal junction intact, although with the RYGBP, only a small upper gastric pouch easily accessible by standard endoscopy. Thus, regardless of procedure chosen, the esophagus and cardia can still be visualized endoscopically after bariatric surgery should the need arise.

What then is the possible role of endoscopy before surgery? First, it may offer the surgeon information that might change the type of operation chosen. For example, if a large hiatal hernia or severe esophagitis is encountered, the surgeon may opt to repair the crural diaphragm during the bariatric procedure. Obviously if early cancer is encountered, the operation of choice may be esophagectomy, but this scenario is likely an exceedingly rare occurrence. Second, a finding such as severe esophagitis or peptic ulcer may postpone the operation to enable appropriate medical management. Third, in the setting of a RYGBP, there may be a desire to visualize the distal stomach before making its access difficult. However, an important distinction should be made between asymptomatic lesions and symptomatic lesions. It seems hard to argue with investigating symptoms before surgery. So the question posed is, What is the role in asymptomatic patients? There are some data, as well as societal guidelines, to help inform this decision.

Several authors have examined the role of preoperative endoscopy before lap band. Some have found a greater risk of subsequent band slippage in the setting of hiatal hernia, with decreased risk of slippage if a crural repair is performed.[83] In one large study of 145 consecutive patients undergoing endoscopy before bariatric surgery, only 10% had clinically relevant findings (mostly hiatal hernias and esophagitis).[84] Symptomatic patients were much more likely to have important findings (62% vs. 2%), leading the authors to suggest a selective use of endoscopy in these patients. However, another series with 190 consecutive patients found that 40% had hiatal hernias resulting in crural repair at the time of surgery.[85] Five percent had esophagitis severe enough to postpone surgery, and 3% had BE. Only roughly

30% of the patients in this series had symptoms, suggesting that endoscopy may be beneficial even among asymptomatic patients.

The European Association for Endoscopic Surgery recommends endoscopy or an upper GI series before all bariatric procedures.[86] The American Society for Gastrointestinal Endoscopy recommends endoscopy for all symptomatic patients and suggests consideration of endoscopy for all patients scheduled to under RYGBP or lap band.[87] Therefore, it seems reasonable to consider endoscopy for anyone undergoing bariatric surgery, although data are lacking to definitively prove its utility among asymptomatic patients.

12. Are there radiographic findings that ascertain the existence of a shortened esophagus, and what is the consequence on the surgical strategy?

Cheri L. Canon
ccanon@uabmc.edu

Preoperative identification of a shortened esophagus is paramount for successful fundoplication surgery. If unrecognized, consequences could include misplaced (low) fundoplication, often also referred to as "slipped wrap," recurrent hernia secondary to crural disruption, and actual wrap disruption.[88] Short esophagus has multiple definitions in the surgical and radiologic literature, further complicating the sometimes contentious topic. Many define it as an esophagus in which a tension-free fundoplication cannot be performed. Because of variability in its definition, its reported incidence covers a broad range from 0% to 60%. Horvath *et al.* estimate its incidence at 10%.[88]

Esophageal shortening can be predicted radiographically, with many reported findings. Some consider a nonreducing hernia 5 cm or longer,[89,90] while others use the finding of a large paraesophageal hernia, stricture, BE, or loss of the angle of His to suggest a short esophagus. However, when these predictors are used, the overall sensitivity is low. Mittall *et al.* reported a sensitivity of 66%, with a positive predictive value of 37% for the diagnosis of short esophagus.[91] However, the esophagram faired better than manometry, which had a reported sensitivity of 43%, with a positive predictive value of 25%. In another study, the posi-

tive predictive value of the esophagram was 50% for the diagnosis of short esophagus.[88]

In addition to the multiple definitions and radiographic findings suggesting short esophagus, the diagnosis is further complicated by occasional difficulty in accurate identification of the gastroesophageal junction, best seen at the termination of the gastric rugal folds. A large ampulla can be confused with a non-reducing hiatal hernia, thus suggesting a short esophagus. In Horvath's article, three categories of short esophagus (10%) were described: true, nonreducible short esophagus (3%); true but reducible (with mediastinal dissection) short esophagus (7%); and an apparent short esophagus.[88] True, nonreducible short esophagus went on to esophageal lengthening procedure, Collis gastroplasty. Apparent short esophagus occurs when patients have a large hernia or paraesophageal hernia but have adequate esophageal redundancy allowing mobilization below the diaphragm.

In a prospective study of 180 patients, intraoperative measurement between the gastroesophageal junction and the angle of His was obtained before and after extensive mediastinal dissection.[92] An esophagus was considered short if the junction was less than 1.5 cm below the angle of His or above the angle. Before dissection, 37.7% of patients had an apparent short esophagus. After extensive mediastinal dissection, with an average increase of 6 cm in esophageal length, 18.8% had persistent short esophagus. This study determined that esophagography and severity and duration of symptoms were the best predictors of a true short esophagus.

There is ongoing debate as to the definition and, therefore, the prevalence of short esophagus. More confusing, there is no agreement on its management, and some surgeons do not even agree on its existence. What we do know is that the esophagram is noninvasive, readily available, and inexpensive. It is the best test for anatomy, hernia reducibility, and stricture. It is probably a good screen for shortened esophagus, although there needs to be appropriate emphasis on technique. Some feel that the "single most important aspect of radiographic examination is to identify the short esophagus."[89] So, to answer the question, short esophagus can be diagnosed radiographically so that the surgeons can plan accordingly and incorporate an esophageal lengthening procedure, if appropriate.

13. What are the indications and long-term outcome of the Collis modification of fundoplication?

Adolfo E. Badaloni
badaloni@arnet.com.ar

The existence of a shortened esophagus, its diagnosis, and therapy have been a topic of controversy for many years. The best accepted definition is when 2.5 cm of a tension-free abdominal esophageal segment cannot be obtained despite extensive mediastinal dissection. The incidence of a shortened esophagus ranges from 2% to 10% of patients undergoing a fundoplication, with important variability among different series.[93,94] Overseeing a short esophageal segment may lead to failure of antireflux surgery that can be seen as a misplaced fundoplication, crural disruption, and herniation of the wrap into the mediastinum.

Once confirmed, the surgeon must choose among a few options. (1) extensive mediastinal dissection (type II).[94] This solves the problem in the majority of patients and should be always attempted before doing another procedure; (2) total duodenal diver-

Table 5. Postoperative function following Collis gastroplasty with fundoplication

(*n* = 15)	(Collis–Nissen *n* = 12)	(Collis–Toupet *n* = 3)	(Late Follow-up *n* = 14 months)
Intact and properly positioned fundoplication			14/14
Recurrent peptic stricture–requiring dilatation			1/14
Biopsy neoesophagus with oxyntic mucosa			11/11
Average LES resting pressure			16 mm Hg
Distal esophageal body function was absent			6/14
Abnormal results in 24-hour pH study			7/14
No dysplactic progression in BE			

Table 6. Disparity between symptomatic and physiological outcomes following esophageal lengthening procedures for antireflux surgery

(1996–2002)	(ARS 1579)	(Collis–Nissen 68–4.3%)
Symptoms significant improvement (*n* = 58)	Chest pain	90%
	Dysphagia	89%
	Heartburn	86%
	Regurgitation	91%
Objective physiologic testing (*n* = 25)	Abnormal pH test or severe esophagitis	80%
	Wrap herniation	16%
	New Barrett's epithelium	8%

Mean follow-up period: 30 ± 4 months.

sion.[95] The classical Roux-en-Y gastrojejunostomy entails transection of the duodenum, resection of all the antrum, and a vagotomy. The blind duodenal limb is anastomosed to the side of the Roux loop, 45–60 cm distal to the gastrojejunal anastomosis. This is the ideal operation for patients with shortened esophagus associated with other morbidity factors, such as multiple interventions, alkaline reflux, peptic strictures, Barrett's or scleroderma. It should be indicated in highly selected patients, as side effects (gastric atony, delayed emptying, altered bowel peristalsis) are not neglectible. (3) Collis gastroplasty:[96] this is the only procedure that creates a tension-free intraabdominal segment of neoesophagus for fundoplication when type II dissection fails. Disadvantages of this method include creation of a distal segment with altered motility, with the ability of secreting acidic content and the risk of leaks through the suture. According to Horvath *et al.*, of 10% of patients undergoing antireflux surgery with a shortened esophagus, 7% can be appropriately managed with extensive mediastinal mobilization of the esophagus, and the remaining 3% require an aggressive surgical approach, including the use of gastroplasty procedures.[94]

In our experience, from 1996 to 2010, with more than 600 antireflux procedures, we have diagnosed 28 cases of shortened esophagus, with only two of them requiring a Collis–Nissen procedure. Seventeen cases were solved with a type II dissection, and six patients underwent a total duodenal diversion.

Three patients required a total esophagectomy, one of them being a failed Collis with a severe nonhealing ulcer. Jobe *et al.*[96] analyzed the outcomes of 15 patients with Collis gastroplasty with fundoplication, observing that anatomical and symptomatic control was excellent, while the physiological and pathological responses were not adequate (Table 5). In another study, Edward Lin *et al.*[97] higlighted the discrepancies between the symptom control and the objective physiological outcomes (Table 6). So in reality, what are we achieving with a Collis procedure? A patient who does not complain while he develops his esophagitis or Barrett's epithelium?

In conclusion, the Collis gastroplasty with fundoplication allows a tension-free fundoplication in shortened esophagus. Patients prefer improvement of symptoms, but have the disadvantage of losing distal esophageal motility and having a secreting gastric mucosa in the neoesophagus that requires chronic PPI use and long-term follow-up. Its indication should be limited to shortened esophagus without large ulcers, peptic stricture, or Barrett's, and only after failure to achieve extensive mediastinal mobilization.

14. Should the choice of the type of fundoplication still be the matter of discussion?

Gianmattia del Genio, Alberto del Genio, Salvatore Tolone, Federica del Genio, and Ludovico Docimo
gdg@doctor.com

Laparoscopic total fundoplication is currently accepted as the most effective procedure in controlling GERD. However, in the recent past many authors favored the use of a partial wrap especially for patients

Table 7. Pre- and postoperative esophageal bolus transit patterns detected at combined impedance and manometry

	Preoperative (N = 15)	Postoperative (N = 15)	P
Liquid swallows			
Complete transit (%)	68.8 ± 23.1	75.5 ± 21.8	N.S.
Incomplete transit (%)	31.1 ± 23.1	23.3 ± 22.9	N.S.
Viscous swallows			
Complete transit (%)	64.4 ± 25.0	86.6 ± 15.8	<0.05
Incomplete transit (%)	35.5 ± 25.0	13.3 ± 15.8	<0.05

with defective peristalsis, as the result of a balanced option between the potential risk of postoperative dysphagia and the benefit of reflux control. Later on, partial antireflux procedures reported less favorable outcomes in assuring a good protection from reflux at long-term follow-up. We undertook the current study to evaluate by means of combined multichannel intraluminal impedance and high-resolution manometry manometry (HrM-MII) the impact of fundoplication on esophageal physiology. An objective measurement of the influence of the total wrap on the bolus transit may be helpful in refining the optimal antireflux wrap type (e.g., partial versus total; Fig. 5).[98]

Methods

In this study, 15 consecutive patients who underwent laparoscopic Nissen–Rossetti fundoplication had HRM-MII and combined 24-hour pH and multichannel intraluminal impedance (MII-pH) before and after the surgical procedure. All patients completed a pre- and postoperative symptom questionnaire. The following were calculated for liquid and viscous deglutition: lower esophageal sphincter pressure (LESP) and relaxation (LESR), the distal esophageal amplitude (DEA), the number of complete esophageal bolus transit (CBT), and the mean total bolus transit time (BTT). The acid and nonacid GER episodes were calculated by MII-pH, with the patient in both upright and recumbent positions.

Results

The postoperative HRM-MII showed an increased LESP ($P < 0.05$), while LESR, DEA did not change after surgery ($P =$ N.S.). CBT and BTT did not change for liquid swallows ($P =$ N.S.) but became faster for viscous after surgery ($P < 0.05$). The

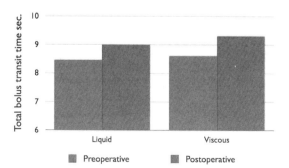

Figure 5. An objective measurement of the influence of the total wrap on the bolus transit may be helpful in refining the optimal antireflux wrap type (e.g., partial versus total).

24-hour pH monitoring confirmed the postoperative reduction of both acid and nonacid reflux ($P < 0.05$) (Table 7).

Discussion

Since the early 1970s, our group sustained the idea that a correctly fashioned total fundoplication does not increase the risk of postoperative dysphagia. The technique included an extensive transhiatal esophageal mobilization to restore the LES to the abdomen; preservation of the lesser omentum and short gastric vessels as important mechanisms of preventing intrathoracic migration, telescopage, or rotation of the wrap; and routine use of intraoperative manometry and endoscopy to control the function (i.e., calibration, length) and anatomy of the wrap (passage through, height in respect of the cardias, and correct geometry around the probe in reverse vision).[99] This feature in controlling reflux without increasing dysphagia occurs because of the elastic feature of the anterior gastric wall (Nissen–Rossetti), which is able to dilate when the bolus passes through the wrap or to increase the pressure for Laplace's law when the gastric fundus is distended, preventing reflux after a meal. A practical confirmation can be found in achalasic patients after extended myotomy, suggesting that the total fundoplication itself creates an adequate barrier without impairing the bolus, also when peristalsis is absent and a myotomy has abolished the LES pressure.[100]

Because the total fundoplication is largely recognized to be superior in controlling GERD,[101,102] this demonstration of an unchanged transit progression of the bolus after total fundoplication, associated with previous observations of good outcomes upon long follow-up in patients with normal, defective, or absent peristalsis,[103] supports the choice of adopting total fundoplication as a unique antireflux technique that is based on intention to treat choice. Appropriate preoperative investigation and a correct surgical technique are mandatory in securing these results.

Conflicts of interest

The authors declare no conflicts of interest.

References

1. Katzka, D.A. & D.O. Castell. 1994. Successful elimination of reflux symptoms does not insure adequate control of acid reflux in patients with Barrett's esophagus. *Am. J. Gastroenterol.* **89:** 989–991.

2. Peghini, P.L., P.O. Katz, *et al.* 1998. Nocturnal recovery of gastric acid secretion with twicw-daily dosing of proton pump inhibitors. *Am. J. Gastroenterol.* **93:** 763–767.

3. DeMeester, S.R. & T.R. DeMeester. 2000. Columnar mucosa and intestinal metaplasia of the esophagus. Fifty year of controversy. *Ann. Surg.* **231:** 303–321.

4. Sampliner, R.E. 1994. Effect of up to 3 years of high-dose lanisoprazole on Barrett's esophagus. *Am. J. Gastroenterol.* **89:** 1844–1848.

5. Todd, J.A., K.K. Basu, *et al.* 2005. Normalisation of oesophageal pH does not guatantee control of duodenogastroesophageal reflux in Barrett's esophagus. *Aliment. Pharmacol. Ther.* **21:** 969–975.

6. Parrilla, P., L.F. Martinez de Haro, *et al.* 2003. Long-term results of a randomized prospective study comparing medical and surgical treatment of Barrett's esophagus. *Ann. Surg.* **237:** 291–298.

7. Csendes, A., I. Braghetto, *et al.* 2009. Late results of surgical treaments of 125 patients with short- segment barrett esophagus. *Arch. Surg.* **144:** 921–927.

8. Weston, A.P., A.S. Badr, *et al.* 1999. Prospective multivariate analysis of clinical, endoscopic, and histological factors predictive of the development of Barrett's multifocal high-grade dysplasia or adenocarcinoma. *Am. J. Gastroenterol.* **94:** 3413–3419.

9. Hage, M., D. Siersema, *et al.* 2004. Oesophageal cancer incidence and mortality in patients with long- segment Barrett's oesophagus after a mean follow-up of 12,7 years. *Scand. J. Gastroenterol.* **12:** 1175–1179.

10. Gurski, R., J.H. Peters, *et al.* 2003. Barrett's esophagus can and does regress after antireflux surgery: a study of prevalence and predictive features. *J. Am. Coll. Surg.* **196:** 706–712.

11. Chang, E.Y., C.D. Morris, *et al.* 2007. The effect of antireflux surgery on esophageal carcinogenesis in patients with Barrett's esophagus. *Ann. Surg.* **246:** 11–21.

12. Corey, K.E., S.M. Schmitz, *et al.* 2003. Does a surgical antireflux procedure decrease the incidence of esophageas adenocarcinoma in Barrett's esophagus? A Meta-Analysis. *Am. J. Gastroenterol.* **98:** 2390–2394.

13. Lord, R.V.N., S.R. DeMeester, J.H. Peters, *et al.* 2009. Lower esophageal sphincter incompetence, and effectivness of nissen fundoplication in the spectrum of gastroesophageal reflux disease. *J. Gastrointestinal. Surg.* **13:** 602–610.

14. Herbella, F.A.M., P. Tedesco, I. Nipomnick, *et al.* 2007. Effect of partial and total laparoscopic fundoplication on esophageal body motility. *Surg. Endosc.* **21:** 285–288.

15. Chrysos, E., E. Athanasakis, G. Pechlivanides, *et al.* 2004. The effect of total and anterior partial fundoplication on antireflux mechanisms of the gastroesophageal junction. *Am. J. Surg.* **188:** 39–44.

16. Wykypiel, H., B. Hugl, M. Gadenstaetter, *et al.* 2008. Laparoscopic partial posterior (Toupet) fundoplication improves esophageal bolus propagation on scintigraphy. *Surg. Endosc.* **22:** 1845–1851.

17. Ritter, M.P., J.H. Peters, T.R. DeMeester, *et al.* 1998. Outcome after laparoscopic fundoplication is not dependent on a structurally defective lower esophageal sphincter. *J. Gastrointest. Surg.* **2:** 567–572.

18. Riedl, O., M. Gadenstaetter, W. Lechner, *et al.* 2009. Preoperative lower esophageal impact manifestations of GERD

nor outcome after laparoscopic Nissen fundoplication. *J. Gastrointest. Surg.* **13:** 1189–1197.

19. Varga, G., A. Kiraly, L. Cseke, *et al.* 2008. Effect of laparoscopic fundoplication on hypertensive lower esophageal sphincter associated with gastroesophageal reflux. *J. Gastrointest. Surg.* **12:** 304–307.

20. Tatum, R.P., R.V. Soares, E. Figueredo, *et al.* 2010. High-resolution manometry in evaluation of factors responsible for fundoplication failure. *J. Am. Coll. Surg.* **210:** 611–619.

21. Kahrilas, P.J., W.J. Dodds & W.J. Hogan. 1988. Effect of peristaltic dysfunction on esophageal volume clearance. *Gastroenterology* **94:** 74–80.

22. Lund, R., G. Wetcher, F. Raiser, *et al.* 1997. Laparoscopic Toupet fundoplication for gastroesophageal reflux disease with poor esophageal body motility. *J. Gastrointest. Surg.* **1:** 301–308.

23. Baigrie, R.J., D.I. Watson, J.C. Myers, & G.G. Jamieson. 1997. Outcome of laparoscopic Nissen fundoplication in patients with disordered preoperative peristalsis. *Gut* **40:** 381–385.

24. Cai, W., D.I. Watson, C.J. Lally, *et al.* 2008. Ten-year clinical outcome of a prospective randomized clinical trial of laparoscopic Nissen versus anterior 180° partial fundoplication. *Br. J. Surg.* **95:** 1501–1505.

25. Strate, U., A. Emmermann, C. Fibbe, *et al.* 2008. Laparoscopic fundoplication: Nissen versus Toupet two-year outcome of a prospective randomized study of 200 patients regarding preoperative esophageal motility. *Surg. Endosc.* **22:** 21–30.

26. Zaninotto, G., G. Portale, M. Costantini, *et al.* 2007. Long-term results (6–10 years) of laparoscopic fundoplication. *J. Gastrointest. Surg.* **11:** 1138–1145.

27. Broeders, J.A., H.G. Rijnhart-de Jong, W.A. Draaisma, *et al.* 2009. Ten-year outcome of laparoscopic and conventional nissen fundoplication: randomized clinical trial. *Ann. Surg.* **250:** 698–706.

28. Braghetto, I, A. Csendes, P. Burdiles, *et al.* 2002. Results of surgical treatment for recurrent postoperative gastroesophageal reflux. *Dis. Esophagus.* **15:** 315–322.

29. Broeders, J.A., W.A. Draaisma, A.J. Bredenoord, *et al.* Long-term outcome of Nissen fundoplication in non-erosive and erosive gastro-oesophageal reflux disease. *Br. J. Surg.* **97:** 845–852.

30. Lundell, L., P. Miettinen, H.E. Myrvold, *et al.* 2009. Comparison of outcomes twelve years after antireflux surgery or omeprazole maintenance therapy for reflux esophagitis. *Clin. Gastroenterol. Hepatol.* **7:** 1292–1298; quiz 1260.

31. Bahadorzadeh, K. & P.H. Jr. Jordan. 1975. Evaluation of the Nissen fundoplication for treatment of hiatal hernia: use of parietal cell vagotomy without drainage as an adjunctive procedure. *Ann. Surg.* **181:** 402–408.

32. Jordan, P.H., Jr. & J. Thornby. 1997. Parietal cell vagotomy performed with fundoplication for esophageal reflux. *Am. J. Surg.* **173:** 264–269.

33. Garcia-Rinaldi, R. & F. Lanza. 1984. Hiatal hernia with severe reflux esophagitis: treatment by superselective vagotomy and Nissen fundoplication. *South Med. J.* **77:** 418–422.

34. Bohmer, R.D., R.H. Roberts, & R.J. Utley. 2000. Open Nissen fundoplication and highly selective vagotomy as a treatment for gastro-oesophageal reflux disease. *Aust. N. Z. J. Surg.* **70:** 22–25.

35. Olbe, L., C. Cederberg, T. Lind, & M. Olausson. 1989. Effect of omeprazole on gastric acid secretion and plasma gastrin. *J. Gastroenterol. Hepatol.* **4**(Suppl 2): 19–25.

36. Stein, H.J., H. Feussner & J.R. Siewert. 1996. Failure of antireflux surgery: causes and management strategies. *Am. J. Surg.* **171:** 36–9; discussion 39–40.

37. Kennedy, T., P. Magill, G.W. Johnston, & T.G. Parks. 1979. Proximal gastric vagotomy, fundoplication, and lesser-curve necrosis. *Br. Med. J.* **1:** 1455–1456.

38. Jamieson, G.G., G.J. Maddern & J.C. Myers. 1991. Gastric emptying after fundoplication with and without proximal gastric vagotomy. *Arch. Surg.* **126:** 1414–1417.

39. Oelschlager, B.K., K. Yamamoto, T. Woltman, & C. Pellegrini. 2008. Vagotomy during hiatal hernia repair: a benign esophageal lengthening procedure. *J. Gastrointest. Surg.* **12:** 1155–1162.

40. DeMeester, S.R., J.H. Peters & T.R. DeMeester, 2001. Barrett's esophagus. *Curr. Probl. Surg.* **38:** 549–640.

41. Falk, G.N. 2002. Barrett's esophagus. *Gastroenterology* **122:** 1569–1579.

42. Eisen, G.M., R.S. Sandler, S. Murray, & M. Gottfried. 1997. The relationship between gastroesophageal reflux disease and its complications with Barrett's esophagus. *Am. J. Gastroenterol.* **92:** 27–31.

43. Csendes, A., G. Smok & J. Quiroz. 2002. Clinical, endoscopic, and functional studies in n408 patients with Barrett's esophagus compared to 174 cases of intestinal metaplasia of the cardia. *Am. J. Gastroent.* **97:** 554–560.

44. Korn, O., A. Csendes, P. Burdiles, *et al.* 2004. Anatomic dilatation of the cardia and competence of the lower esophageal sphuincter: a clinical and experimental study. *J. Gastrointest. Surg.* **4:** 398–406.

45. Parrilla, P., L.F. de Martinez Haro, A. Ortiz, *et al.* 2003. Long-term results of a randomized prospective study comparing medical and surgical treatment of Barrett esophagus. *Ann. Surg.* **237:** 291–298.

46. Peters, J.H. & K.K. Wang. 2004. How should Barrett's ulceration be treated? *Surg. Endosc.* **18:** 338–344.

47. Bowers, S.P., S.G. Mattar, C.D. Smith, *et al.* 2002. Clinical and histologic outcome after antireflux surgery in Barrett's esophagus. *J. Gastrointest. Surg.* **6:** 532–539.

48. Gurski, R.R., J.H. Peters, J.A. Hagen, *et al.* 2003. Barrett's esophagus can and does regress following antireflux surgery; a study of prevalence and predictive features. *J. Am. Coll. Surg.* **196:** 706–713.

49. Desai, K.M., N.J. Soper, M.M. Frisella, *et al.* 2003. Efficacy of laparoscopic antireflux surgery in patients with Barrett's esophagus. *Am. J. Surg.* **186:** 652–659.

50. Horgan, S., D. Pohl, D. Bogetti, *et al.* 1999. Failed antireflux surgery: what have we learned from reoperations? *Arch. Surg.* **134:** 809–815, discussion 815–817.

51. Farrell, T.M., C.D. Smith, R.E. Metreveli, *et al.* 1999. Fundoplication provides effective and durable symptom relief in patients with Barrett's esophagus. *Am. J. Surg.* **178:** 18–21.

52. Csendes, A. 2004. Surgical treatment of Barrett's esophagus: 1980–2003. *World J. Surg.* **28:** 225–231.

53. DeMeester, T.R., K.H. Fuchs, C.S. Ball, *et al.* 1987. Experimental and clinical results with proximal end to end duodenojejunostomy for pathologic duodeno gastric reflux. *Am. Surg.* **206:** 414–426.

54. Csendes, A., I. Braghetto, P. Burdiles, *et al.* 1997. A new physiological approach for the surgical treatment of patients with Barrett's esophagus. Technical considerations and results in 65 cases. *Ann. Surg.* **226:** 123–143.

55. Braghetto, I., A. Csendes, P. Burdiles & O. Korn. 2000. Antireflux surgery, highly selective vagotomy and duodenal switch procedure: post-operative evaluation in patients with complicated and non-complicated Barrett';s esophagus. *Dis. Esophagus* **13:** 12–17.

56. Csendes, A., I. Braghetto, P. Burdiles, *et al.* 2009. Late results of the surgical treatment of 125 patients with short-segment Barrett';s esophagus. *Arch. Surg.* **144:** 921–927.

57. Biertho, L., B. Dallemagne & L. dewandre. 2007. Laparoscopic treatment of Barrett's esophagus: long term results. *Surg. Endosc.* **21:** 11–15.

58. Zaninotto, G., M. Cassaro, G. Pennelli, *et al.* 2005. Barrett's epithelium after antireflux surgery. *J. Gastrointest. Surg.* **9:** 1253–1261.

59. Oeschlager, B.K., M. Barreca & L. Chang, *et al.* 2003. Oleinikov D., Pellegrini CA. Clinical and pathologic response of Barrett's esophagus to laparoscopic antireflux surgery. *Ann. Surg.* **238:** 458–556.

60. Ghosh, S.K., J.E. Pandolfino, J. Rice, *et al.* 2007. Impaired deglutitive EGJ relaxation in clinical esophageal manometry: a quantitative analysis of 400 patients and 75 controls. *Am. J. Physiol.* **293:** G878.

61. Chan, W.W., L.R. Haroian, C.P. Gyawali. 2011. Value of preoperative esophageal function studies before laparoscopic antireflux surgery. *Surg Endosc*; March 18 [epub ahead of print].

62. Montenovo, M., R.P. Tatum, E. Figueredo, *et al.* 2009. Does combined multichannel intraluminal esophageal impedance and manometry predict postoperative dysphagia after laparoscopic Nissen fundoplication? *Dis. Esophagus* **22:** 656–663.

63. Fornari, F., I. Bravi, R. Penagini, *et al.* 2009. Multiple rapid swallowing: a complementary test during standard oesophageal manometry. *Neurogastroenterol. Motil.* **21:** 718–725.

64. Winslow, E.R., R.E. Clouse, K.M. Desai, *et al.* 2003. Influence of spastic motor disorders of the esophageal body on outcomes from laparoscopic antireflux surgery. *Surg. Endosc.* **17:** 738–745.

65. Khajanchee, Y.S., C.M. Dunst & L.L. Swanstrom. 2009. Outcomes of Nissen fundoplication in patients with gastroesophageal reflux disease and delayed gastric emptying. *Arch. Surg.* **144:** 823–828.

66. Struijs, M.C., D. Lasko, S. Somme, & P. Chiu. 2010. Gastric emptying scans: unnecessary preoperative testing for fundoplications? *J. Pediatr. Surg.* **45:** 350–354; discussion 354.

67. Machado, R.S., E. Yamamoto, F.R. da Silva Patricio, *et al.* 2010. Gastric emptying evaluation in children with erosive gastroesophageal reflux disease. *Pediatr. Surg. Int.* **26:** 473–478.

68. Hejazi, R.A., S. Reddymasu, M. Moncure & R.W. McCallum. Delayed gastric emptying in reflux disease patients is not a contraindication to Nissen fundoplication. *Gastroenterology*, **136**(Suppl 1): A-297.

69. Vu, M.K., J.W. Straathof, P.J. Schaar, *et al.* 1999. Motor and sensory function of the proximal stomach in reflux disease and after laparoscopic Nissen fundoplication. *Am. J. Gastroenterol.* **94:** 1481–1489.

70. McCallum, R., Z. Lin, P. Wetzel, *et al.* 2005. Clinical response to gastric electrical stimulation in patients with postsurgical gastroparesis. *Clin. Gastroenterol. Hepatol.* **3:** 49–54.

71. Shafi, M.A. & P.J. Pasricha. 2007. Post-surgical and obstructive gastroparesis. *Curr. Gastroenterol. Rep.* **9:** 280–285.

72. Oubre, B., J. Luo, A. Al-Juburi, *et al.* 2005. Pilot study on gastric electrical stimulation on surgery- associated gastroparesis: long-term outcome. *South Med. J.* **98:** 693–697.

73. DeMeester, T., G. Campos, S. DeMeester, *et al.* 1998. The impact of an antireflux procedure on intestinal metaplasia of the cardia. *Ann. Surg.* **228:** 547–556.

74. Gurski, R., J. Peters, J. Hagen, *et al.* 2003. Barrett's esophagus can and does regress after antireflux surgery: a study on prevalence and predictive features. *J. Am. Coll. Surg.* **196:** 706–712.

75. Oh, D., T. DeMeester, D. Vallbohmer, *et al.* 2007. Reduction of interleukin 8 gene expression in reflux esophagitis and Barrett's esophagus with antireflux surgery. *Arch. Surg.* **142:** 554–559.

76. Bonavina, L., C. Ceriani, A. Carazzone, *et al.* 1999. Endoscopic laser ablation of nondysplastic Barrett's epithelium: is it worthwhile? *J. Gastrointest. Surg.* **3:** 194–199.

77. Fleischer, D., R. Odze, B. Overholt, *et al.* 2010. The case for endoscopic treatment of non-dysplastic and low-grade dysplastic Barrett's esophagus. *Dig. Dis. Sci.* **55:** 1918–1931.

78. ZEhetner, J., S.R. DeMeester, S. Ayazi, *et al.* 2010. Long-term follow-up after anti-reflux surgery in patients with Barrett's esophagus. *J. Gastrointest. Surg.* **14:** 1483–1491.

79. Nguyen, D.M., H.B. El-Serag, L. Henderson, *et al.* 2009. Medication usage and the risk of neoplasia in patients with Barrett's esophagus. *Clin. Gastroenterol. Hepatol.* **7:** 1299–1304.

80. Wassenaar, E.B. & B.K. Oelschlager. 2010. Effect of medical and surgical treatment of Barrett's metaplasia. *World J. Gastroenterol.* **16:** 3773–3779.

81. O'Riordan, J.M., P.J. Byrne, N. Ravi, *et al.* 2004. Long-term clinical and pathologic response of Barrett's esophagus after antireflux surgery. *Am. J. Surg.* **188:** 27–33.

82. Gatenby, P.A., J.R. Ramus, C.P. Caygill, *et al.* 2009. Treatment modality and risk of development of dysplasia and adenocarcinoma in columnar-lined esophagus. *Dis. Esophagus* **22:** 133–142.

83. Dolan, K., R. Finch & G. Fielding. 2003. Laparoscopic gastric banding and crural repair in the obese patient with a hiatal hernia. *Obes Surg.* **13:** 772–775.

84. Korenkov, M. *et al.* 2006. Is routine preoperative upper endoscopy in gastric banding patients really necessary? *Obes. Surg.* **16:** 45–47.

85. Sharaf, R.N. *et al.* 2004. Endoscopy plays an important pre-operative role in bariatric surgery. *Obes. Surg.* **14:** 1367–1372.

86. Sauerland, S. *et al.* 2005. Obesity surgery: evidence-based guidelines of the European Association for Endoscopic Surgery (EAES). *Surg. Endosc.* **19:** 200–221.

87. Anderson, M.A. *et al.* 2008. Role of endoscopy in the bariatric surgery patient. *Gastrointest. Endosc.* **68:** 1–10.

88. Horvath, K.D., L.L. Swanstrom, B.A. Jobe. 2000. The short esophagus: pathophysiology, incidence, presentation, and treatment in the era of laparoscopic antireflux surgery. *Ann. Surg.* **232:** 630–640.

89. Baker, M.E., D.M. Einstein, B.R. Herts, *et al.* 2007. Gastroe-sophageal reflux disease: integrating barium esophagram before and after antireflux surgery. *Radiology* **243:** 329–239.

90. Gastal, O.L., J.A. Hagen, J.H. Peters, *et al.* 1999. Short esoph-agus. Analysis of predictors and clinical implications. *Arch. Surg.* **134:** 633–638.

91. Mittal, S.K., Z.T. Awad, M. Tasset, *et al.* 2000. The preoper-ative predictability of the short esophagus in patients with stricture or paraesophageal hernia. *Surg. Endosc.* **14:** 464–468.

92. Mattioli, S., M.L. Lugaresi, M. Constantini, *et al.* 2008. The short esophagus: intraoperative asssessment of esophageal length. *J. Thorac. Cardiovasc. Surg.* **136:** 834–841.

93. Urbach, D.R. *et al.* 2001. Preoperative determinants o fan esophageal-lengthening procedure in laparoscopic antire-flux surgery. *Surg. Endosc.* **15:** 1408–1412.

94. Horvath, K.D., L.L. Swanstrom & B.A. Jobe. 2000. The short esophagus. Pathophysiology, incidence, presentation and treatment in the era of laparoscopic antireflux surgery. *Ann. Surg.* **232:** 630–640.

95. Peters, J.H. 1998. What are the main drawbacks of diversion of duodenal contents via Roux-en-Y gastrojejunostomy? The esophagogastric junction. In R. Giuli, J.P. Galmiche, G.G. Jamieson, C. Scarpignato, Eds.: 837–842. John Libbey – Eu-rotext. Paris.

96. Jobe, B.A., K.D. Horvath & L.L. Swanstrom. 1998. Postoper-ative function following laparoscopic Collis gastroplasty for shortened esophagus. *Arch. Surg.* **133:** 867–874.

97. Lin, E., R.N. Vickie Swafford, R. Chadalavada, *et al.* 2004. Disparity between symptomatic and physiologic outcomes following esophageal lengthening procedures for antireflux surgery. *J. Gastrointest. Surg.* **8:** 31–39.

98. del Genio, G., S. Tolone, A. D'Alessandro, *et al.* 2011. The impact of total fundoplication on esophageal transit. Analy-sis by combined multichannel intraluminal impedance and manometry. *J Clin Gastroenterol, in press.*

99. del Genio, G., G. Rossetti, L. Brusciano, *et al.* 2007. La-paroscopic Nissen-Rossetti fundoplication with routine use of intraoperative endoscopy and manometry: technical as-pects of a standardized technique. *World J. Surg.* **31:** 1099–1106.

100. del Genio, G., S. Tolone, A. del Geniodel, G Genio, *et al.* 2010. A closure without a closure: impedance pH monitor-ing expanding the indications for antireflux surgery. Replay. *Gastroenterology* **138:** 392.

101. del Genio, G., S. Tolone, F. del Genio, G del Genio, *et al.* 2008. Total fundoplication controls acid and nonacid reflux: evaluation by pre- and postoperative 24-h pH-multichannel intraluminal impedance. *Surg. Endosc.* **22:** 2518–2523.

102. del Genio, G., S. Tolone, F. del Genio, *et al.* 2008. Prospec-tive assessment of patient selection for antireflux surgery by combined multichannel intraluminal impedance pH moni-toring. *J. Gastrointest. Surg.* **12:** 1491–1496.

103. Rossetti, G., L. Brusciano, G. Amato, *et al.* 2005. A total fundoplication is not an obstacle to esophageal emptying after heller myotomy for achalasia: results of a long-term follow up. *Ann. Surg.* **241:** 614–621.

Ann. N.Y. Acad. Sci. ISSN 0077-8923

ANNALS OF THE NEW YORK ACADEMY OF SCIENCES

Issue: *Barrett's Esophagus: The 10th OESO World Congress Proceedings*

Barrett's esophagus: surveillance and reversal

Christine P.J. Caygill,[1] Katerina Dvorak,[2,3] George Triadafilopoulos,[4] Valter Nilton Felix,[5] John D. Horwhat,[6] Joo Ha Hwang,[7] Melissa P. Upton,[8] Xingde Li,[9] Sanjay Nandurkar,[10] Lauren B. Gerson,[11] and Gary W. Falk[12]

[1]UK Barrett's Oesophagus Registry, UCL, Division of Surgery and Interventional Science, Royal Free and University College Medical School, London, United Kingdom. [2]Department of Cell Biology and Anatomy, College of Medicine and [3]Arizona Cancer Center, The University of Arizona, Tucson, Arizona. [4]Division of Gastroenterology and Hepatology, Stanford University School of Medicine, Stanford, California. [5]Department of Gastroenterology, Surgical Division, São Paulo University, São Paulo, Brazil. [6]Gastroenterology Service, Walter Reed Army Medical Center, Washington, DC. [7]Division of Gastroenterology, Department of Medicine and [8]Department of Pathology, University of Washington, Seattle, Washington. [9]Department of Bioengineering, Johns Hopkins University, Baltimore, Maryland. [10]Department of Gastroenterology, Box Hill Hospital, Box Hill, Australia. [11]Division of Gastroenterology, Stanford University School of Medicine, Stanford, California. [12]Division of Gastroenterology, Hospital of the University of Pennsylvania, Philadelphia, Pennsylvania

The following on surveillance and reversal of Barrett's esophagus (BE) includes commentaries on criteria for surveillance even when squamous epithelium stains normally with a variety of biomarkers; the long-term follow-up of surgery versus endoscopic ablation of BE; the recommended surveillance intervals in patients without dysplasia; the sampling problems related to anatomic changes following fundoplication; the value of tissue spectroscopy and optical coherence tomography; the cost-effectiveness of biopsy protocols for surveillance; the quality of life of Barrett's patients; and risk stratification and surveillance strategies.

Keywords: Barrett's esophagus; endoscopy; presence IM; absence IM; incomplete ablation; DNA damage; surveillance guidelines; radiofrequency ablation; PPI; antireflux surgery; dysplasia; esomeprazole; cancer incidence; fundoplication; Collis gastroplasty; postsurgical endoscopy; optical coherence tomography; time trade-off technique

Concise summaries

- There has been increasing recognition that progression to cancer is not inevitable, and that the process can stop at any of the stages along its course. There is also evidence that low grade dysplasia, or even high-grade dysplasia, may regress. In addition, not all patients are observed to progress through each step.

- Endoscopic surveillance of Barrett's esophagus (BE), as currently practiced, has numerous shortcomings. Dysplasia and early adenocarcinoma are endoscopically indistinguishable from intestinal metaplasia without dysplasia. There are considerable interobserver variability and quality control problems in the interpretation of dysplasia in both the community and academic settings. Survey data indicate that while surveillance is widely practiced, there is marked variability in the technique and interval of surveillance as practice guidelines are not widely followed.

- According to potential sampling errors, if the decision to offer surveillance were to be based on the presence or absence of IM at diagnosis, a significant proportion of patients would be lost to follow up.

- For surveillance of these patients, the most frequently used biomarkers include proliferation marker Ki67, p53, cyclooxygenase 2, and DNA abnormalities (such as aneuploidy, chromosome loss, or amplification). The panel of various biomarkers should be recommended to identify patients with an increased risk to develop cancer.

- Concerning the long-term follow-up of Barrett patients following surgery versus radiofrequency ablation, although both regression and

doi: 10.1111/j.1749-6632.2011.06052.x

progression have been noted, surgery does not completely or substantially eliminate metaplasia. Esophago-gastric cancer still develops after 15 years of ARS.

- Radiofrequency ablation (RFA) is effective and durable, but no data on cancer incidence are (yet) available.
- However, no literature exists that has directly addressed the issue of Barrett's surveillance following fundoplication in a direct manner. It should be kept in mind that anatomic changes following fundoplication may have the potential to interfere with the ability to distend and visualize the distal esophagus, especially in patients with short-segment BE.
- The further development and testing of a balloon-based optical coherence tomography imaging catheter will allow the endoscopist to perform systematic surveillance of the esophagus following ablation to detect subsquamous Barrett's epithelium. The development of this technology may improve methods for ablation and patient outcomes.
- Limiting surveillance to high-risk individuals may decrease the endoscopic and financial burden and make surveillance more worthwhile. However, in its current state, surveillance does not appear to be a cost effective strategy.
- The decrement in health related quality of life from symptoms appears to be equivalent in patients with gastroesophageal reflux disease (GERD) and BE. However, there appears to be an additional decrement in quality of life associated with the cancer risk perception and anxiety associated with the diagnosis despite lack of evidence that life expectancy changes after BE diagnosis.

---

1. Should a decision of surveillance be based upon the presence of an intestinal metaplasia at endoscopy, also taking into consideration potential sampling errors?

Christine P.J. Caygill, P.A.C. Gatenby, and A. Watson
c.caygill@ucl.ac.uk

In the United States, detection of intestinal metaplasia (IM) has been a prerequisite for the diagnosis of columnar-lined (Barrett's) esophagus (CLO), and the American College of Gastroenterology guidelines recommend surveillance only of those patients in whom IM is detected.[1] This differs from the the British Society of Gastroenterology guidelines, as UK pathological opinion is that IM can always be identified if sufficient biopsies are taken over time.[2] This poses the question, "If CLO is diagnosed but IM is not detected at index endoscopy, what is the risk of malignant transformation and should those patients undergo surveillance?"

We therefore undertook a large cohort study to examine the time sequence of IM detection in CLO patients and the relationship between the presence of IM at index endoscopy and malignant transformation. We followed up 322 CLO patients with no IM (CLO$^-$) at diagnostic biopsy up to 10 years.[3] The proportion of patients developing IM (CLOIM) in CLO$^-$ over time was analyzed using the Kaplan–Meier survival analysis, and the probability of the finding of IM dependent on gender, patient age at biopsy, metaplastic segment length, and number of samples taken was analyzed using logistic regression. In addition, the CLO$^-$ patients were compared to 612 CLOIM patients for a number of other criteria.

Median follow-up was three and a half years; 34% of CLO patients did not have IM detected at index endoscopy. Survival analysis demonstrated that, overall, 54.8% of patients with CLO$^-$ had developed IM or dysplasia at five years from follow-up; at 10 years, the proportion was 90.8%. The finding of IM is more common in males than females and increases with segment length and number of biopsy samples taken. It also increases with increasing age, but this was not statistically significant. Progression of CLO to esophageal adenocarcinoma (EAC) in the 322 CLO$^-$ patients was compared to that in 612 CLO patients with IM at diagnosis. The results are shown in Table 1. There was a trend for an increased risk of adenocarcinoma in the patients with CLOIM over CLO$^-$, but this was not statistically significant.

Table 1. Adenocarcinoma development

Diagnostic histology	N	N (%) developing EAC
CLO$^-$	322	10 (3.1)
CLOIM	612	20 (3.2)

This study demonstrates that the finding of IM is more common in males and increases with segment length and number of biopsy samples taken. The finding of goblet cells increases with increasing duration of follow-up, and over 50% of patients who originally did not have IM were found to have IM at five years and over 90% at 10 years. This is most likely to be due to sampling errors, though an actual progression from CLO$^-$ to CLOIM cannot be ruled out in some cases. If sufficient biopsy samples are taken over time, the vast majority of patients will demonstrate IM.

There was a trend for an increased risk of EAC in the patients with CLOIM over CLO$^-$, which may represent a lead-time bias in CLO$^-$ patients, but there was no statistically significant difference in EAC development. If the decision to offer surveillance were to be based on the presence or absence of IM at diagnosis, 34% of patients would be excluded. Not all centers adopt a four-quadrant biopsy technique with biopsies every 2 cm. A survey in 2006[4] among gastroenterologists in the United Kingdom revealed that 22 of 30 claimed to do so, although this figure may have risen since. The probability is that IM would have been found more frequently at the diagnostic biopsy had it been searched for more rigorously.

Goyal's group has shown in a small series that CLO patients who progress to EAC development have similar DNA abnormalities irrespective of the detection of IM at index endoscopy.[5] This raises the hypothesis that the DNA profile is more reliable than histological subtype (presence of IM) in determining malignant potential, which is to be tested in a large collaborative study between UKBOR and Harvard.

Conclusion

If the decision to offer surveillance were to be based on the presence or absence of IM at diagnosis, a significant proportion of patients would be lost to follow-up.

2. What should be the right follow-up of treated patients in whom squamous epithelium stains normally with a variety of biomarkers, thus witnessing complete ablation of the Barrett's mucosa?

Katerina Dvorak

kdvorak@email.arizona.edu

Endoscopic ablation therapy using different approaches (radiofrequency therapy, cryotherapy, photodynamic therapy, multipolar electrocoagulation, argon plasma coagulation) is the treatment modality that can completely eradicate Barrett's esophagus in the majority of BE patients. A new squamous epithelium replaces the columnar epithelium as a consequence of injury induced by endoscopic ablation. Several studies demonstrated that if the ablation is complete, the neosquamous epithelium is undistinguishable from normal squamous epithelium and represents minimal cancer risk.[6] However, these studies evaluated only a limited number of biomarkers, and only a few patients were included in these studies.

First, in my opinion, before we answer the question of what should be the right follow-up of patients with normal expression of biomarkers, we need to clarify exactly what biomarkers should be used and if these biomarkers can be routinely used in clinical practice. Most frequently used biomarkers include proliferation marker Ki67, p53, cyclooxygenase 2, and DNA abnormalities (such as aneuploidy or chromosome loss or amplification). The panel of various biomarkers should be recommended to identify patients with an increased risk of developing cancer. Furthermore, much larger studies evaluating cancer risk-associated biomarkers need to be done to confirm that a new squamous epithelium truly does not represent cancer risk.

Second, the primary goal is to achieve complete ablation of BE. This is very important since residual BE glands persisting underneath the neosquamous epithelium may progress to esophageal adenocarcinoma. Indeed, these cases have been reported.[7] Therefore, the esophageal mucosa should be examined with white light and also with narrow band imaging to identify any residual metaplastic lesions. The patients should return for a repeat endoscopy every six to eight weeks until all the islands of intestinal mucosa have been eradicated. The optimal frequency of endoscopic surveillance was not yet determined; however, it has been proposed that an endoscopy should be performed every four months for one year after the esophagus has been cleared, then every six months for another year, and then once a year for five years until more studies are completed. Ideally, a combination of biomarker expression and genetic tests can be used in the future to stratify for surveillance those patients at high risk for developing esophageal adenocarcinoma.

Third, ablated patients should be treated to reduce and eliminate gastroesophageal reflux to stop the damage to the esophageal lining. The majority of the patients that undergo ablation are the patients with high-grade dysplasia or intramucosal adenocarcinoma. These patients have increased reflux of gastric acid and bile acids compared to control patients or patients with uncomplicated GERD.[8] The standard therapy includes proton pump inhibitors (PPIs); however, new emerging drugs that reduce transient lower esophagus sphincter relaxation (TLESR) may be more beneficial in these patients. These drug classes include the $GABA_B$ receptor agonists (including lesogaberan and arbaclofen placarbil).[9] Because of different mechanisms of action, in contrast to PPIs, these drugs reduce not only reflux of gastric acid but also the bile acid reflux. Especially lesogaberan, a $GABA_B$ receptor agonist, is very promising, since this drug does not have serious CNS side effects.[10]

Fourth, recommendations should include also a change of diet and lifestyle. Patients should eat a diet low in fat and stay away from any food that they know triggers their heartburn symptoms, such as tomato sauce, orange juice, and carbonated sodas. Modest weight loss and eating a diet high in fruits and vegetables should be recommended to patients after ablation therapy. Finally, chemoprevention should be considered. There is epidemiologic and experimental evidence to suggest that chemoprevention using nonsteroidal anti-inflammatory drugs, such as aspirin, may reduce the risk of cancer in BE patients.

In summary, more clinical studies using a broad variety of biomarkers are needed to answer these questions: Do patients with complete ablation need surveillance? What is the risk that BE will regrow? And does residual BE represent the same risk as BE?

3. What is the long-term follow-up to surgery in Barrett's esophagus with no dysplasia versus radiofrequency ablation?

George Triadafilopoulos
vagt@stanford.edu

Radiofrequency (RFA) and surgery (fundoplication) are not directly comparable. The former has no impact on symptoms of GERD, while the latter is intended to control such symptoms. Nevertheless, both approaches may have an impact on disease progression and/or regression in the long term, and this is the focus of this comparison.

Another important distinction also needs to be made. Whereas PPIs are only able to decrease acid content in the stomach (and thus change the pH of the refluxate), surgery has the ability to prevent any type of reflux (i.e., bile). RFA is typically combined with PPI therapy that, at least to a major degree, suppresses acid reflux.[11] Fundoplication does not alter the length of Barrett's esophagus, whereas, by contrast, RFA ablates Barrett's metaplasia, and, used together with PPI therapy that suppresses acid reflux, leads to squamous re-epitheliazation.

When comparing RFA to surgery, some definitions are important to bear in mind; *progression* is a change from either intestinal metaplasia to any form of dysplasia or an increase in grade of dysplasia or development of adenocarcinoma. By contrast, *regression* is a change from high-grade dysplasia (HGD) to low-grade dysplasia (LGD) or no dysplasia, change from LGD to metaplasia or loss of metaplasia, and change from IM to squamous

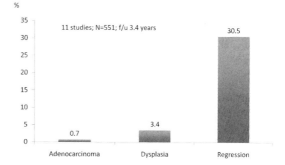

Figure 1. Long-term outcomes of fundoplication in Barrett's esophagus cohorts 11 studies; N = 551; f/u 3.4 years. Originally printed in Ref. 11.

Table 2. Medical therapy versus surgery for Barrett's esophagus n (%)

Publication	Treatments	PPI	Nissen	Progression PPI	Progression Nissen	Regression PPI	Regression Nissen	Study type
Gatenby et al.[3]	PPI vs. Nissen	646	41	154 (24)	4 (10)	NA	NA	Cohort
Parrilla et al.[54]	H2RA/PPI vs. Nissen	43	58	10 (23)	5 (9)	2 (5)	5 (9)	RCT
Rossi et al.[53]	PPI vs. successful Nissen	19	16	NA	NA	12 (63)	16 (100)	Case comparison
Total		708	115	164 (23.8)	9 (9.1)	14 (22.6)	21 (28.4)	

PPI, proton pump inhibitor; H2RA, H2 receptor antagonist; RCT, randomized controlled trial; NA, not applicable. Table adapted from Ref. 12.

epithelium. Shortening of the segment or development of squamous cell islands, although considered by some as regression, usually is not accurately measured and reported.[12]

How good is fundoplication in patients with Barrett's esophagus?

The LOTUS trial involved 554 patients with GERD of whom 60 had Barrett's esophagus. Of these, 28 were randomized to esomeprazole and 32 to laparoscopic antireflux surgery (LARS). Four of 60 patients with Barrett's esophagus on either treatment strategy experienced treatment failure during the three-year follow-up (Fig. 1). The esophageal pH in Barrett's esophagus patients was significantly better controlled after surgical treatment than after esomeprazole, while quality of life (QoL) scores were similar for the two therapies at baseline and at three years. Operative difficulty was slightly greater in patients with BE than those without. There was no difference in postoperative complications or level of symptomatic reflux control.

Figure 1 shows the long-term outcomes of fundoplication in Barrett's esophagus cohorts from 11 studies (551 patients, mean f/u of 3.4 years). Cancer was noted in 0.7% of cases, dysplasia in 3.4%, while regression was noted in 30.5%.[12] Pooled results from three studies involving 708 Barrett's esophagus patients on PPI versus 115 patients post-LARS showed progression in 24% of PPI users versus 9% of LARS patients; regression was seen in 23% and 28%, respectively (Table 2; not significant).[12] A recent 15-year-long population study shows that anti-reflux surgery does not decrease esophageal or cardiac cancer risk.[14]

A multicenter, randomized, sham-controlled study of RFA in patients with dysplastic Barrett's esophagus achieved complete eradication of metaplasia.[15] Complete eradication of HGD occurred in 81% of those treated versus 19% of sham-treated controls; of LGD in 90.5% versus 22.7% of controls, and of intestinal metaplasia in 77.4% versus 2.3% of controls. In terms of disease progression, any progression of disease occurred in 3.6% of those treated versus 16.3% of sham-treated controls; any progression to cancer occurred in 1.2% versus 9.3% of controls; HGD progression to cancer in 2.4% versus 19%; and LGD to HGD in 4.8% versus 13.6%—all quite significant.

Fleischer *et al.* recently reported long-term efficacy data in 50 patients with Barrett's esophagus who had previously completed eradication of metaplasia and then were followed for five years. No strictures or mucosal lesions were found, and many biopsies (mean = 31 per patient) were taken. Forty-six of 50 patients (92%) had complete, long-lasting, clearance of metaplasia, while 4 (8%) had IM (6 of 126 specimens). In all these patients, a single-session focal RFA cleared the residual metaplasia.[16]

In conclusion, although both regression and progression have been noted, surgery does not completely or substantially eliminate metaplasia. Esophagogastric cancer still develops after 15 years of ARS. RFA is effective and durable, but no data on cancer incidence are (yet) available.

4. Using various proposed guidelines, what surveillance interval should be recommended in Barrett's patients with no evidence of dysplasia?

Valter Nilton Felix

v.felix@terra.com.br

The degree of dysplasia is currently used as a marker for risk of progression to cancer, though there is increasing evidence that biomarkers and level of genetic instability may provide better predictive measures. In patients with BE with no evidence of dysplasia on initial endoscopy, a repeat endoscopy should be performed within the next year. If no dysplasia is confirmed, these patients are considered to be at low risk to have their condition progress and/or develop cancer. Therefore, the interval for additional surveillance has been recommended to be every three years, but, on the basis of decision analysis models, the more appropriate interval may be five years.

Recommendations for surveillance of low-grade dysplasia and specialized intestinal metaplasia without dysplasia are largely opinion statements not well supported by objective data. Although cancers identified by surveillance are at earlier stages than those diagnosed without prior endoscopic evaluation, surveillance failures are common. Recommendations for screening and surveillance are not evidence based. Current recommendations are limited by inconsistent endoscopic findings and sampling errors, inconsistent histological diagnoses of Barrett esophagus and dysplasia, and our poor understanding of the natural history of various histological lesions. Future directions include validation of methods that reduce these inconsistencies by *in vivo* detection of abnormalities and by objective diagnostic markers besides grades of dysplasia, such DNA content analysis and molecular markers, and improved understanding of the disease progression.

BE does not produce any symptoms or health impairment other than its associated condition of GERD. However, it is a premalignant condition that may progress to esophageal adenocarcinoma (EAC);[17] Therefore, its diagnosis and management are focused around prevention, early recognition, and early treatment of EAC.[18] The goal of surveillance is to diagnose early stages of cancer in patients with known BE and to intervene so as to prevent progression to fatal cancer.

Surveillance is structured follow-up testing of BE to detect progressive dysplastic changes in the mucosa that herald development of carcinoma. The surveillance program for BE has evolved over the years owing to several factors, including the realization of association of BE with EAC, slow progression of BE to carcinoma through escalating grades of histological dysplasia, dismal outcome of EAC, a rapidly rising incidence of EAC, and most importantly the awareness of the lay public regarding heartburn being complicated by BE and EAC.

Prevalence of cancer is high with low-grade dysplasia (LGD), and even higher with high-grade dysplasia (HGD). It is thought that histological disease in BE progresses sequentially from no dysplasia to LGD, then to HGD, and eventually to EAC, but it now appears that not all cases progress to cancer in a predictable sequence of worsening dysplasia. Moreover, there has been increasing recognition that progression to cancer is not inevitable, and the process can halt itself at any of the stages along its course. There is also evidence that LGD or even HGD may regress. Additionally, not all patients are observed to progress through each step.[19,20]

Since the rate of progression of LGD to cancer is not much different from that of BE without dysplasia, surveillance intervals of only one year for LGD do appear to be justified. This program is continued until the examination shows that LGD has changed when the follow-up plan is also changed accordingly. When the lesion reverts to BE without dysplasia, surveillance is decreased to three-year intervals. If the LGD does not change, yearly surveillance is continued throughout the patient's life. An invasive carcinoma should not occur in patients in the surveillance program. If this happens, it indicates failure of the program.

In patients with BE with no evidence of dysplasia on initial endoscopy, a repeat endoscopy should be performed within the next year. If no dysplasia is confirmed, these patients are considered to be at low risk for having their condition progress and/or develop cancer. Therefore, the interval for additional surveillance has been recommended to be every three years. However, on the basis of decision analysis models, the more appropriate interval may be five years.[21]

5. Can anatomic changes following fundoplication hinder appropriate esophageal sampling during surveillance endoscopy?

John D. Horwhat
john.david.horwhat@us.army.mil

A lack of agreement still exists regarding best surveillance practices for patients with Barrett's esophagus, with controversy remaining related to appropriate time intervals between exams and which equipment to use for optimal detection of dysplasia. Given the growing volume of patients that have undergone antireflux surgery since the advent of laparoscopic techniques, it is surprising to find that no literature exists that has directly addressed the issue of Barrett's surveillance following fundoplication in a direct manner. A review of endoscopy following hiatal hernia repair published in 2000 warned of the possibility of difficulty visualizing short-segment Barrett's after fundoplication, but no references are offered for this statement.[22]

To understand changes with postsurgical endoscopy and to avoid misidentifying the location of the Barrett's segment, it is of paramount importance to know exactly what the anatomic landmarks look like in the native state. When a patient is being surveyed for Barrett's esophagus and the squamocolumnar junction has moved proximally, we need to know where the normal anatomic landmarks are located in order to then determine if the wrap has in any way compromised our ability to distend the area and see the tissue.

Unfortunately, we already have evidence in the literature describing the difficulty that exists when trying to reliably define landmarks in a patient with Barrett's. While experts from the international working group were able to distinguish the anatomic landmarks of the diaphragmatic hiatus and proximal margin of the gastric folds with almost perfect reliability, we have also seen that the ability to use the palisading vessels had a far poorer reliability.[23] So low, in fact, that it should not be used to determine the end of the true esophagus in a patient with Barrett's esophagus. If, then, we are using the margin of the gastric folds as our landmark for performing surveillance, we must be cautious that a tight or long fundoplication could compromise the ability to see this area well.

Fortunately, a question answered during the 1994 OESO World Congress addressing the causes for a failed Nissen fundoplication reported that the problem with wraps being made too tight or too long had, in 1994, become rarely seen because of changes in surgical technique (circa 1983)—when the practice of performing better fundic mobilization and then making a shorter, looser wrap over a 60-Fr bougie became standard. It deserves mention, though, that there is no clear consensus on what type of antireflux surgery should be performed in patients with Barrett's. The USC group has advocated for either liberal use of a Collis gastroplasty to lengthen the esophagus or the use of a transthoracic approach to better mobilize the esophagus when a short esophagus is anticipated.[24] Others have published that the short esophagus is actually a myth, does not exist, and is more a function of having not properly mobilized the fundus. In a series from the University of Tennessee at Memphis, there were no lengthening procedures required in over 628 fundoplication surgeries over a 10-year period.[25] Finally, there are those that advocate that the best type of surgical approach in patients with Barrett's may not even be a fundoplication. After reviewing 25 articles that evaluated surgical treatment of Barrett's esophagus from 1980 to 2003, Csendes *et al.* offered that the best alternative may be acid suppression with a PPI and a duodenal diversion procedure.[26] Clearly, these patients would not have any interference with complete esophageal mucosal visualization at subsequent surveillance endoscopy.

Despite reports of regression and reversal of metaplasia following antireflux surgery, there are counterbalancing reports of patients that have progressed to cancer as well. This argues for the ongoing need to perform surveillance in Barrett's patients that have had antireflux surgery. While improvements in surgical technique may have decreased the potential for intestinal metaplasia to become pulled into a tight/long wrap and consequently become difficult to visualize, we realize that not all patients will experience an ideal surgical outcome, and we must be prepared to address this group of patients with innovative endoscopic techniques. The best means to improve visualization and surveillance in these patients is with the use of a clear plastic cap on the tip of the endoscope (dedicated Olympus distal viewing cap or reprocessed band ligation cap).

This allows one to achieve better distension of the lumen for confirmation of the anatomic landmarks and targeted biopsies as needed.

In summary, anatomic changes following fundoplication may have the potential to interfere with the ability to distend and visualize the distal esophagus, especially in patients with short-segment Barrett's esophagus. This should almost be viewed as a complication of surgery, however, as refinements in technique have largely eliminated the problem of the tight/long fundoplication. We must be cognizant of the normal landmarks of the esophagus and the location of the proximal gastric folds to confidently identify the location of the Barrett's esophagus; this also holds true for the postfundoplication patient. In the event that a patient's distal esophagus is difficult to distend, ensure that your endoscopy lab has clear plastic caps to affix to the end of the endoscope to improve your ability to visualize this tissue and target biopsies.

6. What is the value of optical coherence tomography in the surveillance of patients with Barrett's esophagus?

Joo Ha Hwang, Melissa P. Upton, and Xingde Li
jooha@u.washington.edu

The use of ablative therapies for treatment of Barrett's esophagus is increasing. Ablative therapies include balloon-based RFA, photodynamic therapy (PDT), endoscopic mucosal resection, argon plasma coagulation, and cryotherapy. The previous paradigm for treatment of Barrett's with endoscopic ablative therapies was to treat patients with high-grade dysplasia (HGD) who were not considered to be operative candidates or who refused surgery. However, recent data suggest that endoscopic ablative therapy for Barrett's is both safe and effective. Therefore, endoscopic ablative therapies are being used increasingly in patients who will require long-term surveillance. In addition, ablation of nondysplastic Barrett's is also being evaluated, since Barrett's is perceived as a premalignant condition.[27]

Following ablation of Barrett's mucosa, residual Barrett's epithelium may persist below the neosquamous epithelium as subsquamous Barrett's epithelium. Unfortunately, current optical imaging methods cannot identify subsquamous Barrett's epithelium. The true incidence of subsqua-mous Barrett's epithelium following ablation is currently unknown. In a prospective, multicenter, sham-controlled trial of patients with dysplastic Barrett's esophagus treated with either RFA or a sham procedure demonstrated that subsquamous Barrett's epithelium was identified in 5.1% of patients at 12-month follow-up.[28] The true incidence of subsquamous Barrett's esophagus following ablation is likely to be higher, since the current method of surveillance with random biopsies is subject to sampling error. Furthermore, the incidence of subsquamous Barrett's following PDT is reported to be up to 25%.[29] Therefore, it is logical to assume that the occurrence of subsquamous Barrett's is likely to be higher in RFA compared to PDT, since PDT achieves a deeper ablation compared to current RFA methods.

Although the natural history and significance of subsquamous Barrett's epithelium is not well characterized, most believe that subsquamous Barrett's epithelium remains at risk for malignant transformation.[30] Since subsquamous Barrett's epithelium is thought to have some risk of future malignant transformation, a method to detect subsquamous Barrett's on surveillance endoscopy in patients who have undergone ablative therapy for Barrett's esophagus is needed. Theoretically, a technology that could reliably detect subsquamous Barrett's epithelium would allow endoscopists to improve ablative therapy methods for Barrett's esophagus. In addition, if subsquamous Barrett's epithelium could be completely excluded by systematic imaging, then future surveillance endoscopy may not be necessary, which could make ablative therapy of nondysplastic Barrett's cost-effective. One possible imaging technology that has the ability to do this is optical coherence tomography (OCT).

OCT is an optical method that allows for high-resolution, cross-sectional imaging of tissue microanatomy below the tissue surface. OCT is the optical analog to ultrasound using near infrared low coherence light instead of sound. OCT imaging can be performed in real time with an imaging depth of up to three mm with an axial resolution of up to one μm, depending on the light source. OCT imaging of the esophagus can be performed through a fiberoptic imaging probe that can be passed through the accessory channel of an endoscope.

Ex vivo imaging of human esophagectomy specimens using an ultrahigh resolution OCT imaging

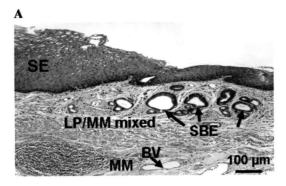

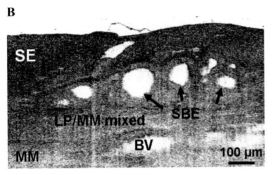

Figure 2. (A) OCT image of subsquamous Barrett's epithelium (SBE) obtained from an *ex vivo* human esophagectomy specimen. Abbreviations: MM, muscularis mucosa; LP, lamina propria; BV, blood vessel; SE, squamous epithelium. (B) Corresponding histology of demonstrating SBE (H&E, 100× magnification). Abbreviations: MM, muscularis mucosa; LP, lamina propria; BV, blood vessel; SE, squamous epithelium. Reprinted from Cobb *et al.*[31] with permission.

system has demonstrated the ability to detect subsquamous Barrett's epithelium (Fig. 2).[31] Although this imaging was performed on *ex vivo* tissue using a laboratory OCT imaging system, it demonstrates the capability of OCT to perform cross-sectional imaging of the esophagus to imaging the microanatomy at depths that are sufficient to detect subsquamous Barrett's epithelium.

Initially, OCT imaging of the esophagus required placement of the catheter tip directly on the esophageal mucosa, which limited its ability to image large areas of the esophageal mucosa. However, the development of balloon-based OCT imaging catheters now allow for rapid imaging of large areas of the esophagus. The imaging catheter is positioned in the center of the balloon catheter and rotated and withdrawn, resulting in a spiral scanning pattern. The further development and testing of a balloon-based OCT imaging catheter will allow the endoscopist to perform systematic surveillance

of the esophagus following ablation to detect subsquamous Barrett's epithelium. The development of this technology may improve methods for ablation and patient outcomes.

7. Considering the variability of data concerning cancer incidence in patients with Barrett's esophagus, and as most cases of adenocarcinoma are diagnosed at entry, should cost-effectiveness of intensive biopsy protocols to assess the degree of dysplasia be questioned?

Sanjay Nandurkar
sanjay.nandurkar@monash.edu

Patients with Barrett's esophagus undergo periodic endoscopic surveillance to improve early detection of dysplasia and or adenocarcinoma. Although Barrett's esophagus would appear an ideal model for surveillance, the cost-effectiveness of this practice has been questioned.[32] Indeed, there are two aspects that need to be evaluated in this context: first, whether a surveillance program is effective (regardless of its cost), and second regarding the cost to run such a program in order to save a life.

The published literature had shown that the majority of the cancers within Barrett's are detected at index endoscopy or within a few years; very few cancers are detected subsequently. In the vast majority of individuals, Barrett's is often identified for the first time with coexisting dysplasia or cancer. Hence, we do not often have a lead time with the majority of the cancers associated with Barrett's esophagus, as they are not regarded as surveillance cancers. Thus, the true impact of surveillance on reducing adenocarcinoma-related mortality is small. Hence, after removal of all prevalent cancers detected within the first year of index endoscopy, if 1,000 patients with Barrett's without dysplasia were to be entered into a surveillance program, we would expect that only four patients would develop adenocarcinoma per year.[33] Furthermore, the majority of the patients entering the surveillance program are old and often have coexisting morbidity. Thus, it is expected that a subset of patients would die from other causes and many others may become too frail to continue surveillance.[34] Thus, from a broader health perspective, it remains questionable whether the money spent is worth the potential gain. Moreover, even if surveillance were to be successful in detecting the cancers at an earlier stage, amenable to be effectively treated, the impact of such a surveillance program on reducing the overall cancer-related mortality in Barrett's esophagus would be low. Hence, even perfect surveillance programs would have minimal impact on reducing the burden of disease.

Unfortunately, there are no randomized control trials that have evaluated the efficacy of surveillance and or surgical intervention. Such trials would require large numbers of patients and a duration of more than 10 years to complete, which is highly expensive and logistically difficult. Thus, most studies that have grappled with this question have employed Markov models on which to base their predictions. In the absence of real data these models are essentially hypothetical scenarios based on a lot of assumptions. There is an inherent elasticity applicable to the input variables deemed as sensitivity analysis. For example, the risk of developing cancer can vary from 0.4% to 1% per year, and the cost associated with endocopy and esophagectomy would vary significantly, depending upon where it is performed. Although, objective parameters are easier to measure and input into the model, subjective variables such as pain and suffering after surgery are difficult to gauge. Models incorrectly assume 100% uptake and retention in a surveillance program. Also, models fail to account for the impact on quality of life from being in a surveillance program.

U.S. researchers reported that with a cancer risk of 0.4% per year, a surveillance interval of less than five years did not show benefit in quality of life.[35] Recently, a British study using a PENTAG Markov model developed to assess cost utility reported that endoscopic surveillance of nondysplastic Barrett's at three-year intervals, low-grade dysplasia at yearly intervals, and high-grade dysplasia at three monthly intervals did more harm than good when compared to no surveillance.[36] Furthermore, surveillance was projected to result in fewer quality of life years gained versus no surveillance.

Studies have suggested that male gender and Caucasian race are more likely to develop cancers, whereas absence of aneuploidy at index endoscopy is a negative predictor. Limiting surveillance to high-risk individuals may decrease the endoscopic and financial burden and make surveillance more worthwhile. However, in its current state, surveillance does not appear to be a cost-effective strategy.

8. Quality of life of Barrett's patients

Lauren B. Gerson
lgerson@stanford.edu

Health-related quality of life (HRQOL) is defined as: *the capacity of an individual to perform social and domestic roles so as to meet the challenges of everyday living without emotional distress or physical disability*.[37] For patients with Barrett's esophagus (BE), the decrement in health-related quality of life from chronic heartburn symptoms may be as important as the decrement associated with the potential cancer risk.[38] Decrements from a disease on HRQOL can have important future impact regarding subsequent ethical, financial, and policy health-care decisions.

A large number of instruments are available to measure HRQOL, including generic, disease-specific, and health-state utility preference assessments. The SF-36, a widely used generic instrument, asks patients 36 questions regarding overall physical and emotional functioning, bodily pain and role limitations, social function, mental health, and general health perception.[39] Patients with GERD have demonstrated lower SF-36 scores compared to the general population and equivalent scores to other chronic conditions, including diabetes and depression.[40] However, SF-36 scores have not been demonstrated to be lower in patients with GERD and BE compared to patients with GERD alone.[38,41] Disease-specific instruments ask targeted questions regarding the impact of a particular disease or symptom, such as heartburn, on quality of life. For example, the Quality of Life in Reflux and Dyspepsia (QOLRAD) assesses five domains for patients with GERD and dyspeptic symptoms, including emotions, vitality, sleep, eating/drinking, and physical/social functioning.[42] Questions are graded from 1 (symptom present all of the time) to 7 (absence of symptoms). Prior studies have not shown important differences in subscale scores on the QOLRAD between patients with GERD and those with GERD and BE. Again, the scores were significantly lower compared to a control population without GERD and improved with PPI therapy.[43]

Patient-derived health state utility assessments are designed to provide numerical indications of health-related quality of life on a scale of 0 to 1, where 0 represents death or a state equivalent to death and 1 represents ideal health. In the standard gamble technique, patients are asked to compare life in a particular health state, such as GERD, to a gamble with a probability P, where existence without GERD is the outcome and $1- P$ is immediate death. The probability P is varied until the preference for the perfect health is equal to the preference for the gamble.[44] In patients with GERD and BE, the mean standard gamble scores did not differ significantly compared to a cohort with GERD alone, (mean values of 0.95 versus 0.94), but SG scores were lower for both cohorts when assessed off of PPI therapy (0.93 for GERD and 0.94 for BE compared to 0.94 and 0.95 respectively on PPI therapy).[38]

In the time trade-off technique, patients are asked to trade-off years or months of life in a state of disease or less-than-perfect health like GERD for a shorter life span in a state of perfect health.[45] The patient's life expectancy is calculated from available U.S. Life Tables and the preference value calculated as 1 (number of years traded/years remaining). As patients are often more willing to trade away time rather than take a risk of death, values using the TTO technique are often lower compared to SG values. For example, the mean values for GERD patients off PPI were 0.90 for TTO, compared to 0.94 using SG ($P = 0.003$) and did not change statistically for the cohort with GERD and BE. In a subsequent study when patients were ask to trade away the potential risk of dysplasia and/or esophageal adenocarcinoma compared to heartburn symptoms, mean TTO values did not differ between GERD and BE cohorts, but the TTO values decreased significantly as the grade of dysplasia increased. For a scenario of esophageal carcinoma, the mean TTO value was 0.67.[46] There was poor correlation between SF-36 scores and utility values in both of the utility studies comparing GERD patients to GERD with BE.

In summary, the decrement in HRQOL from symptoms appears to be equivalent in patients with GERD and BE. However, there appears to be an additional decrement in HRQOL associated with the cancer risk perception and anxiety associated with the diagnosis despite lack of evidence that life expectancy changes after BE diagnosis. Other studies have also demonstrated that repeated endoscopic examinations may increase HRQOL decrements in this patient population.[47] Future research should focus on physician education regarding HRQOL decrements from GERD symptoms, and providing accurate information to both patients and physicians regarding risks of dysplasia and cancer associated with BE.

9. What is a safe method of surveillance in Barrett's esophagus?

Gary W. Falk
gary.falk@uphs.upenn.edu

The goal of endoscopic surveillance of Barrett's esophagus is to detect dysplasia or cancer at an early and potentially curable stage. Current practice guidelines recommend endoscopic surveillance of patients with Barrett's esophagus. This is supported by observational studies that uniformly show that Barrett's esophagus patients in whom adenocarcinoma was detected in a surveillance program have their cancers detected at an earlier stage, with markedly improved five-year survival compared to similar patients not undergoing routine endoscopic surveillance.

Candidates for endoscopic surveillance

Only patients with documented Barrett's esophagus are candidates for surveillance. Before entering into a surveillance program, patients should be advised about risks and benefits, including the limitations of surveillance endoscopy as well as the importance of adhering to appropriate surveillance intervals.[48] Other considerations include age, likelihood of survival over the next five years, and ability to tolerate either endoscopic or surgical interventions for early esophageal adenocarcinoma.

Surveillance techniques

At the time of endoscopy, landmarks should be carefully identified, including the diaphragmatic pinch, the gastroesophageal junction, as best defined by the proximal margin of the gastric folds and level of the squamocolumnar junction. The new Prague classification scheme, which describes the circumferential extent (C value) and maximum extent (M value) of columnar mucosa above the proximal margin of the gastric folds, should be used because of its excellent reliability coefficients for segments >1 cm in length. Current guidelines suggest obtaining systematic four quadrant biopsies at 2 cm intervals along the entire length of the Barrett's segment once inflammation related to GERD is controlled with antisecretory therapy.[48] Active inflammation makes it more difficult to distinguish dysplasia from reparative changes and thus the presence of ongoing erosive esophagitis is a contraindication to performing surveillance biopsies. Before commencing biopsies, meticulous high-resolution white light endoscopy is crucial in an effort to detect any mucosal abnormalities no matter how subtle for targeted biopsies or endoscopic resection. A variety of new optical imaging enhancements have been developed to allow for detailed inspection of the mucosal and vascular surface patterns, but these do not necessarily lead to enhanced detection of early neoplasia compared to high-resolution white light endoscopy.

A systematic biopsy protocol clearly detects more dysplasia and early cancer compared to ad hoc random biopsies.[49] Subtle mucosal abnormalities, no matter how trivial, such as ulceration, erosion, plaque, nodule, stricture, or other luminal irregularity in the Barrett's segment, should also be extensively biopsied, as there is an association of such lesions with underlying cancer. Current guidelines now recommend that mucosal abnormalities, especially in the setting of high-grade dysplasia, should undergo endoscopic mucosal resection.[48] Furthermore, EMR will change the diagnosis in approximately 50% of patients when compared to endoscopic biopsies, given the larger tissue sample available for review by the pathologist. The safety of systematic endoscopic biopsy protocols has been demonstrated.[50] Current evidence does not support the routine use of jumbo biopsy forceps. A new large capacity forceps that can be passed through standard diameter endoscopes provides larger samples than standard large capacity forceps and may increase the yield of dysplasia.[51] However, the extensive use of endoscopic mucosal resection has changed biopsy sampling considerably and makes much of this debate of historical interest only.

Surveillance intervals

Surveillance intervals, determined by the presence and grade of dysplasia, are based on our limited understanding of the biology of esophageal adenocarcinoma. Surveillance every three years is recommended by the American College of Gastroenterology as adequate in patients without dysplasia after two negative examinations.[48] If low-grade dysplasia is found, the diagnosis should first be confirmed by an expert gastrointestinal pathologist owing to the marked interobserver variabil-

ity in interpretation of these biopsies. Data suggest that if there is a consensus diagnosis by two or three expert GI pathologists, the risk of progression is greater than if there is no such agreement. These patients should receive aggressive antisecretory therapy to decrease the changes of regeneration that make pathologic interpretation of this category so difficult. A repeat endoscopy should then be performed within six months of the initial diagnosis. If low-grade dysplasia is confirmed, annual surveillance is recommended when low-grade dysplasia is present until two examinations in a row are negative. There is no agreement on the biopsy protocol to use, although a protocol of four quadrant biopsies at 1 cm intervals, as would be used for high-grade dysplasia, makes sense. Endoscopic mucosal resection should be performed if any mucosal abnormality is present in these patients. If high-grade dysplasia is found, the diagnosis should first be confirmed by an experienced gastrointestinal pathologist as well. If the segment is flat and without any mucosal abnormalities, the endoscopic biopsy protocol should then be repeated within three months to exclude an unsuspected carcinoma, using careful inspection with high-quality white light endoscopy. The presence of any mucosal abnormality warrants endoscopic mucosal resection in an effort to maximize staging accuracy. Management options for these patients include continued surveillance, endoscopic therapy, or esophagectomy.

Limitations of surveillance

Endoscopic surveillance of Barrett's esophagus, as currently practiced, has numerous shortcomings. Dysplasia and early adenocarcinoma are endoscopically indistinguishable from intestinal metaplasia without dysplasia. The distribution of dysplasia and cancer is highly variable, and even the most thorough biopsy surveillance program has the potential for sampling error. There are considerable interobserver variability and quality control problems in the interpretation of dysplasia in both the community and academic settings. Current surveillance programs are expensive and time consuming. Survey data indicate that while surveillance is widely practiced, there is marked variability in the technique and interval of surveillance, as practice guidelines are not widely followed. Recent work by Abrams *et al.* found that adherence to guidelines was seen in only 51% of cases, and the longer the segment length, the worse the adherence encountered.[52] However, education programs can enhance compliance with guidelines.

Conflicts of interest

The authors declare no conflicts of interest.

References

1. Wang, K.K. & R.E. Sampliner. 2008. The Practice Parameters Committee of the American College of Gastroenterology. Updated guide-lines 2008 for the diagnosis, surveillance and therapy of Barrett's esophagus. *Am. J. Gastroenterol.* **103:** 788–797.

2. Watson, A., R.C. Heading & N.A. Shepherd. 2005. Guidelines for the diagnosis and management of Barrett's columnar-lined oesophagus: a report of the working party of the british society of gastroenterology, *BSG Guidelines Gastroenterol.* 1–42.

3. Gatenby, P.A.C., J.R. Ramus, C.P.J. Caygill, *et al.* 2008. The relevance of the detection of intestinal metaplasia in non-dysplastic columnar-lined oesophagus. *Scand. J. Gastro.* **43:** 524–530.

4. Ramus, J.R., C.P.J. Caygill, P.A.C. Gatenby & A. Watson.2008. Current uk practice in the diagnosis and management of columnar-lined oesophagus; results of the uk national barrett's oesophagus registry (ukbor) endoscopist questionnaire. *Eur. J. Cancer. Prev.* **17:** 422–425.

5. Liu, W., H. Hahn, R.D. Odze & R.K. Goyal. 2009. Metaplastic esophageal columnar epithelium without goblet cells shows DNA content abnormalities similar to goblet cell-containing epithelium. *Am. J. Gastroenterol.* **104:** 816–824.

6. Garewal, H., L. Ramsey, P. Sharma, *et al.* 1999. Biomarker studies in reversed Barrett's esophagus. *Am. J. Gastroenterol.* **94:** 2829–2833.

7. Van Laethem, J.L., M.O. Peny, I. Salmon, *et al.* 2000. Intramucosal adenocarcinoma arising under squamous re-epithelialisation of Barrett's oesophagus. *Gut.* **46:** 574–577.

8. Vaezi, M.F. & J.E. Richter. 1996. Role of acid and duodenogastroesophageal reflux in gastroesophageal reflux disease. *Gastroenterology* **111:** 1192–1199.

9. Koek, G.H., D. Sifrim, T. Lerut, *et al.* 2003. Effect of the GABA(B) agonist baclofen in patients with symptoms and duodeno-gastro-oesophageal reflux refractory to proton pump inhibitors. *Gut.* **52:** 1397–1402.

10. Boeckxstaens, G.E., H. Beaumont, V. Mertens, *et al.* Effects of lesogaberan on reflux and lower esophageal sphincter function in patients with gastroesophageal reflux disease. *Gastroenterology* **139:** 409–417.

11. Arora, G., S. Basra, A.K. Roorda & G. Triadafilopoulos.2009. Radiofrequency ablation of Barrett's esophagus. *Eur. Surg.* **41:** 19–25.

12. Wassenaar, E.B. & B.K. Oelschlager. 2010. Effect of medical and surgical treatment of Barrett's metaplasia. *World J. Gastroenterol.* **16:** 3773–3779.

13. Attwood, S.E., L. Lundell, J.G. Hatlebakk, *et al.* 2008. Medical or surgical management of GERD patients with Barrett's

esophagus: the LOTUS trial 3-year experience. *J. Gastrointest. Surg.* **12:** 1646–1654.

14. Lagergren, J., W. Ye, P. Lagergren & Y. Lu. 2010. The risk of esophageal adenocarcinoma after antireflux surgery. *Gastroenterology.* **138:** 1297–1301.

15. Shaheen, N.J., P. Sharma, B.F. Overholt, *et al.* 2009. Radiofrequency ablation in Barrett's esophagus with dysplasia. *N. Engl. J. Med.* **360:** 2277–2288.

16. Fleischer, D. *et al.* 2010. "Endoscopic radiofrequency ablation for Barrett's esophagus: five-year durability outcomes from a prospective multi-center trial" *DDW* (Abstract 358).

17. Sharma, P. & R.E. Sampliner. 2001. *Barrett's Esophagus and Esophageal Adenocarcinoma.* Blackwell. Malden, MA.

18. Spechler, S.J. 2002.Barrett's esophagus. *N. Engl. J Med.* **346:** 836–842.

19. Felix, V.N. 2008.GERD to cancer: what is involved? In *Annals of Diagnostic & Therapeutic Approaches for GI Malignancies: Past, Present & Future.* pp. 32–36. Athens.

20. Wood, R.K. & Y.X. Yang. 2008. Barrett's esophagus in 2008: an update. *Keio. J. Med.* **57:** 132–138.

21. Hirota, W.K., M.J. Zuckerman, D.G. Adler, *et al.* 2006. The role of endoscopy in the surveillance of premalignant conditions of the upper GI tract. *Gastrointest. Endosc.* **63:** 570–580.

22. Johnson, D.A., Z. Younes & W.J. Hogan. 2000. Endoscopic assessment of hiatal hernia repair. *Gastrointest. Endosc.* **52:** 650–659.

23. Sharma, P., J. Dent, D. Armstrong, *et al.* 2006. The development and validation of an endoscopic grading system for barrett's esophagus: the prague c & m criteria. *Gastroenterology* **131:** 1392–1399.

24. Jackson, C.C. & S.R. Demeester. 2005. Surgical therapy for Barrett's esophagus. *Thorac. Surg. Clin.* **15:** 429–436.

25. Madan, A.K., C.T. Frantzides & K.L. Patsavas. 2004. The myth of the short esophagus. *Surg. Endosc.* **18:** 31–34.

26. CSENDES, A. 2004. Surgical treatment of Barrett's esophagus: 1980–2003. *World J. Surg.* 225–231. [Epub 2004 Feb 17].

27. Fleischer, D.E., B.F. Overholt, V.K. Sharma, *et al.* 2010. Endoscopic radiofrequency ablation for Barrett's esophagus: 5-year outcomes from a prospective multicenter trial. *Endoscopy* **42:** 781–789.

28. Shaheen, N.J., P. Sharma, B.F. Overholt, *et al.* 2009. Radiofrequency ablation in Barrett's esophagus with dysplasia. *N. Engl. J. Med.* **360:** 2277–2288.

29. Mino-Kenudson, M., S. Ban, M. Ohana, *et al.* 2007. Buried dysplasia and early adenocarcinoma arising in Barrett esophagus after porfimer-photodynamic therapy. *Am. J. Surg. Pathol.* **31:** 403–409.

30. Van Laethem J.L., M.O. Peny, I. Salmon, *et al.* 2000. Intramucosal adenocarcinoma arising under squamous re-epithelialisation of Barrett's oesophagus. *Gut.* **46:** 574–577.

31. Cobb, M.J., J.H. Hwang, M.P. Upton, *et al.* 2010. Imaging of subsquamous Barrett's epithelium with ultrahigh-resolution optical coherence tomography: a histologic correlation study. *Gastrointest Endosc.* **71:** 223–230.

32. Nandurkar, S. & N.J. Talley. 1998. Surveillance in Barrett's oesophagus: a need for reassessment? *J. Gastroenterol. Hepatol.* **13:** 990–996.

33. De Jonge, P.J., M. Van Blankenstein, C.W.N. Looman, *et al.* 2010. Risk of malignant progression in patients with

Barrett's oesophagus: a Dutch nationwide cohort study. *Gut.* **59:** 1030–1036.

34. Macdonald, CE., A.C. Wicks & R.J. Playford. 2000. Final results from ten year cohort of patients undergoing surveillance for Barrett's oesophagus: observational study. *BMJ.* **321:** 1252–1255.

35. Provenzale, D., C. Schmitt & J.B. Wong. 1999. Barrett's esophagus: a new look at surveillance based on emerging estimates of cancer risk. *Am. J. Gastroenterol.* **94:** 2043–2053.

36. Garside, R., M. Pitt, M. Somerville, *et al.* 2006. Surveillance of Barrett's oesophagus: exploring the uncertainty through systematic review, expert workshop and economic modeling. *Health Technol. Assess.* **10:** 1–142, iii-iv.

37. Tarter, R.E., J. Switala, A. Arria, *et al.* 1991. Quality of life before and after orthotopic hepatic transplantation. *Arch. Intern. Med.* **151:** 1521–1526.

38. Gerson, L.B., N. Ullah, T. Hastie, *et al.* 2005. Patient-derived health state utilities for gastroesophageal reflux disease. *Am. J. Gastroenterol.* **100:** 524–533.

39. Stewart, A.L., S. Greenfield, R.D. Hays, *et al.* 1989. Functional status and well-being of patients with chronic conditions. Results from the Medical Outcomes Study. *JAMA* **262:** 907–913.

40. Revicki, D.A., M. Wood, P.N. Maton, *et al.* 1998. The impact of gastroesophageal reflux disease on health-related quality of life. *Am. J. Med.* **104:** 252–258.

41. Eloubeidi, M.A. & D. Provenzale. 2000. Health-related quality of life and severity of symptoms in patients with Barrett's esophagus and gastroesophageal reflux disease patients without Barrett's esophagus. *Am. J. Gastroenterol.* **95:** 1881–1887.

42. Wiklund, I.K., O. Junghard, E. Grace, *et al.* 1998. Quality of Life in Reflux and Dyspepsia patients. Psychometric documentation of a new disease-specific questionnaire (QOLRAD). *Eur. J. Surg. Suppl.* 41–49.

43. Kulig, M., A. Leodolter, M. Vieth, *et al.* 2003. Quality of life in relation to symptoms in patients with gastro-oesophageal reflux disease– an analysis based on the ProGERD initiative. *Aliment. Pharmacol. Ther.* **18:** 767–776.

44. Llewellyn-Thomas, H., H.J. Sutherland, R. Tibshirani, *et al.* 1982. The measurement of patients' values in medicine. *Med. Decis. Making* **2:** 449–462.

45. Torrance G.W. 1986. Measurement of health state utilities for economic appraisal. *J. Health. Econ.* **5:** 1–30.

46. Gerson, L.B., N. Ullah, T. Hastie, *et al.* 2007. Does cancer risk affect health-related quality of life in patients with Barrett's esophagus? *Gastrointest. Endosc.* **65:** 16–25.

47. Kruijshaar, M.E., M. Kerkhof, P.D. Siersema, *et al.* 2006. The burden of upper gastrointestinal endoscopy in patients with Barrett's esophagus. *Endoscopy* **38:** 873–878.

48. Wang, K.K. & R.E. Sampliner. 2008. Practice Parameters Committee of the American College of Gastroenterology. Updated guidelines 2008 for the diagnosis, surveillance and therapy of Barrett's esophagus. *Am. J. Gastroenterol.* **103:** 788–797.

49. Abela, J.E., J.J. Going, J.F. Mackenzie, *et al.* 2008. Systematic four-quadrant biopsy detects Barrett's dysplasia in more patients than nonsystematic biopsy. *Am. J. Gastroenterol.* **103:** 850–855.

50. Levine, D.S., P.L. Blount, R.E. Rudolph, B.J. Reid. 2000. Safety of a systematic endoscopic biopsy protocol in patients with Barrett's esophagus. *Am. J. Gastroenterol.* **95:** 1152–1157.

51. Komanduri, S., G. Swanson, L. Keefer, S. Jakate. 2009. Use of a new jumbo forceps improves tissue acquisition of Barrett's esophagus surveillance biopsies. *Gastrointest. Endosc.* **70:** 1072–1078.

52. Abrams, J.A., R.C. Kapel, G.M. Lindberg, *et al.* 2009. Adherence to biopsy guidelines for Barrett's esophagus surveillance in the community setting in the United States. *Clin. Gastroenterol. Hepatol.* **7:** 736–742.

53. Rossi, M., M. Barreca, N. de Bortoli, *et al.* 2006. Efficacy of Nissen fundoplication versus medical therapy in the regression of low-grade dysplasia in patients with Barrett esophagus: a prospective study. *Ann. Surg.* **243:** 58–63.

54. Parrilla, P., L.F. Martinez de Haro, *et al.* 2003. Long-term results of a randomized prospective study comparing medical and surgical treatment of Barrett's esophagus. *Ann. Surg.* **237:** 291–298.

Ann. N.Y. Acad. Sci. ISSN 0077-8923

Barrett's esophagus: progression to adenocarcinoma and markers

Dianchun Fang,[1] Kiron M. Das,[2] Weibiao Cao,[3] Usha Malhotra,[4] George Triadafilopoulos,[5] Robert M. Najarian,[6] Laura J. Hardie,[7] Charles J. Lightdale,[8] Ian L.P. Beales,[9] Valter Nilton Felix,[10] Paul M. Schneider,[11] and Andrew M. Bellizzi[12]

[1]South West Hospital, Third Military Medical University, Chongqing, China. [2]UMDNJ Robert Wood Johnson Medical School, New Brunswick, New Jersey. [3]Department of Medicine, Rhode Island Hospital and Warren Alpert Medical School, Brown Medical School and Rhode Island Hospital, Providence, Rhode Island. [4]Division of Hematology/Oncology, University of Pittsburgh Department of Medicine, Pittsburgh, Pennsylvania. [5]Division of Gastroenterology and Hepatology, Stanford University School of Medicine, Stanford, California. [6]Department of Pathology, Section of Gastrointestinal and Hepatobiliary Pathology, Beth Israel Deaconess Medical Center and Harvard Medical School, Boston, Massachusetts. [7]Molecular Epidemiology Unit, Centre for Epidemiology and Biostatistics, University of Leeds, Leeds, United Kingdom. [8]Gastroenterology-Gastrointestinal Endoscopy, Columbia-Presbyterian Medical Center, New York, New York. [9]Norfolk and Norwich University Hospital, University of East Anglia, Norwich, United Kingdom. [10]Department of Gastroenterology, Surgical Division, São Paolo University, São Paolo, Brazil. [11]Department of Visceral and Transplantation Surgery, University Hospital Zurich, Zurich, Switzerland. [12]Department of Pathology, Brigham and Women's Hospital, Harvard Medical School, Boston, Massachusetts

The following on progression to adenocarcinoma and markers of Barrett's esophagus includes commentariess on the expression of claudin 4 in Barrett's adenocarcinoma; the role of acid and bile salts; the role of insulin-like growth factor; the value of reactive oxygen species; the importance of abnormal methylation; genetic alterations in stromal cells and genomic changes in the epithelial cells; the value of confocal laser endomicroscopy for the subsurface analysis of the mucosa; indications for statins as adjuvant chemotherapeutic agent; the sequence of molecular events in malignant progression in Barrett's mucosa; and the value of the macroscopic markers and of p53 mutations.

Keywords: claudin 4; squamous epithelium; GERD; acid exposure; bile exposure; carcinoma; *in vitro* transformation; phenotype changes; morphological changes; Cdx2 mRNA expression; p53 protein; NOX5; COX2; PGE$_2$; p16; Barrett's esophagus; aneuploidy; tetraploidy; confocal laser endomicroscopy; eCLE; pCLE; hydroxymethyl-CoA reductase inhibitors; cyclooxygenase-2 inhibitors; protein farnesyltransferase; neoplastic progression

Concise summaries

- Although several molecular events associated with the progression from metaplastic to cancer tissue have been identified in recent years, little is known about the molecular changes that occur in the beginning of the disease. Conversion of squamous mucosa to columnar mucosa is perhaps the most critical one, and

- The study on mRNA expression of claudin 4 reconfirmed that claudin 4 expression is significantly correlated with exposure of the distal esophagus to acid reflux, suggesting alteration of claudin 4 expression to be one of the specific changes in the earliest stage of gastresophageal reflux disease (GERD).

- The molecular mechanism for the transition from Barrett's esophagus (BE) to cancer is still unclear. Repeated exposure to acid and bile selectively induces a colonic phenotype expression in BAR-T cells, and, when repeated over 65 weeks, causes transformation of benign Barrett's epithelial cells to neoplastic phenotype.

- The transformed cells have increased Cdx2 mRNA expression, increased proliferation and reduced apoptosis, and it is possible that the activated DNA damage response machinery

doi: 10.1111/j.1749-6632.2011.06053.x

might play an important role in tumorigenesis in BE.

- Upregulation of COX2 and downregulation of *p16* increase cell proliferation and decrease apoptosis in these cells. Persistent acid reflux present in BE patients may cause changes including high levels of reactive oxygen species (ROS), increased cell proliferation, and decreased apoptosis, which may lead to DNA damage and increased mutations and thereby contribute to the progression from metaplasia to dysplasia and to EA.

- Hypermethylation leads to silencing of p16 tumor suppressor gene. This event appears to be an early event in BE, and its frequency increases on progression from dysplasia to adenocarcinoma.

- A number of genes that have been shown to have altered expression due epigenetic changes in adenocarcinoma on BE are currently being studied. Based on available data, there has been a lot of interest in this field, and the utility of combining these panels with clinical variables is also being explored.

- The genome-wide assessment provided by current DNA microarrays reveals many candidate genes and patterns not previously identified. Stromal gene expression in BE and adenocarcinoma is similar, indicating that these changes precede malignant transformation. There is a distinct stage-specific stromal signature in Barrett's carcinogenesis, with predominance of inflammation- and TGF-β–related genes.

- Despite strong evidence for the predictive value of biomarkers used in panels and in concert with evaluation of a mucosal biopsy, there are several limitations to the use of individual biomarkers alone to evaluate a given patient's risk for BE-associated neoplasia. The role played by environmentally induced damage from acid reflux and ingested irritants in the development of carcinoma is poorly understood, although may explain why molecular abnormalities are neither specific to, nor sufficient for the development of adenocarcinoma.

- Genetic variation in the insulin-like growth factor (IGF) axis has also been shown to modify risk of esophageal adenocarcinoma (EAC) development, and disruption to this axis may provide a mechanistic link between obesity and adenocarcinoma.

- There have been several new developments in the endoscopic detection of early neoplastic lesions in Barrett's patients. Today, magnification endoscopy, which enhances mucosal detailing, is generally used in combination with chromoscopy. The mucosal details as seen with magnification endoscopy can be further increased by using narrow band imaging without the use of dyes.

- Confocal laser endomicroscopy (CLE), allowing sub-surface analysis of the mucosa, is a reliable tool for detection of BE-associated neoplasia, with the potential to decrease the number of biopsies taken, allowing for immediate guidance of endoscopic therapy and making surveillance more cost-effective.

- Statins alter intracellular signaling pathways to induce apoptosis and inhibit proliferation. They would be expected to have a beneficial effect on the excess circulatory mortality associated with BE. They seem to offer exciting potential as chemo-preventative agents in BE.

- Despite the enthusiasm triggered by various reports, the current role of p53 as a potential biomarker for disease progression in BE is unclear. A single molecular marker will surely not have the sufficient predictive power, and further limitations derive from a lack of standardization of methodologies, the choice of techniques, and paucity of prospective trials. Substantial efforts therefore need to be undertaken to create a risk score by combining several clinical and biomarker variables.

- Numerous cellular processes and molecules have been implicated in Barrett neoplastic progression. Those related to cell cycle regulation and genetic instability are among the best-studied. Models of neoplastic progression based on the comparison of frequencies of an event across various histological categories are somewhat limited because of challenges in reproducible histological assessment. Studies that assess multiple, biologically relevant genetic and epigenetic events in mapped mucosal biopsies are preferable.

---

1. The value of claudin 4 expression in GERD acid-exposed squamous epithelium

Wang Jun, Zhao Jing-jing, Zhang Ya-fei, Yang Shi-ming, and Fang Dian-chun
fangdianchun@hotmail.com

GERD is the most common gastrointestinal diagnosis recorded during visits to outpatient clinics. The spectrum of injury includes erosive esophagitis (EE), stricture, the development of columnar metaplasia in place of the normal squamous epithelium (BE), and adenocarcinoma (ACC). Cell adhesion plays an important role in cancer development and progression. Claudins (CLDNs) are thought to be the major constituents of tight junctions (TJ) responsible for cell–cell adhesion, cell polarity, and control of paracellular ion transport.[1] It has been shown that the expression of claudin 4 in BE and ACC was significantly higher than that in esophageal squamous epithelium.[2,3] Reflux of gastric content into the esophagus has been suggested to be responsible for the development of Barrett's epithelium. Much less is known about the role of the esophageal acid exposure on expression of claudin 4 in esophageal squamous epithelium of GERD. The aim of this study was to evaluate the correlation between esophageal acid exposure and expression of claudin 4 in esophageal squamous epithelium of GERD.

Materials and methods

A total of 48 patients with endoscopically proved endoscopy negative gastroesophageal reflux disease (NERD) and EE were enrolled in the study. All patients underwent upper endoscopy to determine the presence of NERD or EE, and then biopsy specimens were obtained from 3 cm above the gastroesophageal junction. All patients underwent ambulatory 24-h esophageal pH monitoring after endoscopic examination. This study was approved by the human subjects committee of the Southwest Hospital.

Reverse transcription-polymerase chain reaction (RT-PCR) analysis

Total RNA was extracted from biopsy specimens using Trizol reagent (Gibco BRL) and cDNA was synthesized from 2 μg of total RNA using Superscript reverse transcriptase (Life Technologies, Inc.) as per the manufacturer's instructions. The cDNA was subjected to PCR using Primers for claudin 4: sense 5′-ATGGGTGCCCCTCGCTCTAC-3′ and antisense 5′- TCAGTCCAGGGAAGAACAAG-3′ (204 bp), and primers for the housekeeping gene GAPDH: sense 5′-ACCACAGTCCATGCCATCAC-3′ and antisense 5′-TCCACCACCCTGTTGCTGTA- 3′ (804 bp).

Ambulatory 24-hour esophageal pH monitoring

After an overnight fast, a pH probe with lower esophageal sphincter identifier (Synectics Medical, Digitrapper MK III, Stockholm, Sweden) was inserted via the nose. The pH probe was placed 5 cm above the upper margin of the lower esophageal sphincter and was connected to a digital portable recorder. A reference electrode was attached to the upper chest. Patients were instructed to keep a diary recording meal times, position changes, and time and type of symptoms. The following parameters were measured: total percentage of the time of the pH less than 4, the pH less than 4 when the subject was upright and supine, total number of GER episodes longer than 5 min, the time of the longest GER episode, and a composite score based on these parameters (DeMeester score).

Statistical analysis

Statistical analysis was performed using SPSS 13.0 software (SPSS Inc., Chicago, IL, USA). *P*-values less than 0.05 were considered statistically significant.

Results

There was no significant difference between the ages and sex of the two groups. There was a significant difference in DeMeester score between patients with NERD (23.26 ± 11.3) and those with EE (44.6 ± 10.9) ($P = 0.008$). There was also a significant difference in claudin 4 mRNA expression levels between NERD (0.22 ± 0.095) and RE (0.41 ± 0.210) patients ($P = 0.001$) (Fig. 1). Acid exposure parameters of patients with NERD and EE are summarized in Table 1. The percentage of the time pH < 4, the time pH < 4 when the subject was supine, number of GER

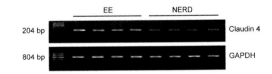

Figure 1.

Table 1. The acid exposure parameters in patients with NERD or EE

Group	n	Time pH < 4 (%)	Time of upright GER (%)	Time of supine GER (%)	Longest GER episode (min)	No. of GER episodes	No. of lasting ≥ 5 (min)	DeMeester score
NERD	24	3.45 ± 2.85	5.28 ± 4.31	2.25 ± 2.08	20.5 ± 9.83	94.57 ± 63.35	7.42 ± 6.21	23.26 ± 11.3
EE	24	14.24 ± 8.53	9.87 ± 8.22	6.88 ± 5.49	36.72 ± 67.81	119.57 ± 110.37	12.8 ± 7.21	44.6 ± 10.9
P	–	0.028	0.083	0.012	0.125	0.014	0.352	0.008

episodes, and the DeMeester scores in patients with RE were greater than these in patients with NERD ($P < 0.05$). There was a significant correlation between DeMeester score and the level of the claudin 4 mRNA expression r = 0.53, $P = 0.04$ and between the percentage of the time pH < 4 in patients with supine GER, no. of GER episodes and the claudin 4 expression ($r = 0.41$, $P = 0.04$ and $r = 0.58$, $P = 0.03$, respectively).

The esophageal TJ is responsible for the paracellular sealing of the esophageal epithelium. This TJ is considered to be one of the protective factors. The role of TJ proteins in the progression of GERD is still poorly understood. Tobey *et al.*[4] and Calabrese *et al.*[5] have shown that the intercellular space diameter was significantly greater in specimens from patients with heartburn than in specimens from controls. In a preliminary study, we found the expression of claudin 4 in patients with RE was increased compared with the patients with NERD. It is postulated that the alteration in TJ protein most likely increase the permeability of the esophageal epithelium, thereby impairing its defense mechanism. Our preliminary, unpublished findings may provide new insights for the understanding of the development of reflux esophagitis and possibly the generation of reflux symptoms.

The development of EAC is a multistep process that starts with the mucosal injury of the squamous epithelium of the distal esophagus and progresses through intestinal metaplasia, dysplasia, and finally to cancer. Although several molecular events associated with the progression from metaplastic to cancer tissue have been identified in recent years, little is known about the molecular changes that occur in the beginning of disease. This first step, conversion of squamous mucosa to columnar mucosa, is perhaps the most critical one because adenocarcinoma cannot develop within squamous mucosa. Our preliminary, unpublished data indicate that claudin 4

expression was significantly correlated with exposure of the distal esophagus to acid reflux, suggesting alteration of claudin 4 expression to be one of the earliest specific changes in the earliest stage of GERD.

2. The phenotypic and molecular changes observed during *in vitro* transformation of benign Barrett's epithelium by acid and bile

Kiron M. Das and Manisha Bajpai
daskm@umdnj.edu

Barrett's epithelium is a sequel of inflammation of the distal esophagus/gatresophageal junction due to chronic gastroesophageal reflux disease (GERD) that results in metaplasia of normal squamous epithelium of the esophagus to columnar epithelium. Epidemiological studies indicate a strong relationship between GERD, BE, and EAC. Clinical challenges include finding cost-effective ways to identify patients with BE and stratifying them according to their cancer risk, and improving the diagnostic potential of endoscopic sampling. Patients with BE have a 30- to 125-fold higher risk of developing EAC than those without BE. The conversion rate from BE to EAC is 0.5–1% per year.[6] The incidence of EAC has the highest rate of rise amongst all cancers in the U.S. and in Western Europe during the last two to three decades. The timely diagnosis and intervention is critically dependent upon proper understanding of the pathogenesis of and molecular mechanism of conversion of BE to EAC.

The molecular mechanism for the transition from BE to cancer is unclear. Acid and bile directly affect cell proliferation and differentiation in BE. We have recently shown that telomerase (hTERT)-immortalized benign Barrett cells (BAR-T), transformed to neoplastic phenotype following exposure to acid, HCL (pH4) (A) plus bile salt (glycochenodeoxycholic acid, 200 μM) and (B) 5 min/day for 65 weeks.[7] The BAR-T cell line is a hTERT-immortalized, benign, human Barrett's metaplastic cells that appears to recapitulate the various stages of neoplastic progression when exposed to a controlled acid and bile environment (A+B) close to the clinical physiological situation. Based on the physical characteristics, we have identified at least three stages in the progression of benign BAR-T cells to neoplasia in this novel model: *stage 1*, phenotype changes to colonic phenotype at 2 weeks (evidenced by monoclonal antibody, mAb Das-1 reactivity)[8]; *stage 2*, distinct morphological changes

around 40 weeks; and *stage 3*, neoplastic changes (transformation: contact inhibition as evident by colony formation in soft agarose in around 65 weeks of A+B exposure, foci formation, and growing tumor in A+B nude mice).[7]

Repeated exposure to acid and bile selectively induces a colonic phenotype expression in BAR-T cells

The BAR-T cells are a heterogeneous population of cells with about 30% reacting with mAb DAS-1, which is specific for colonic phenotype.[8] Chronic A + B, pH 4 treatment for 5 min/day, 5 days a week for two weeks significantly increased the number of mAb Das-1 reactive cells, suggesting an increase

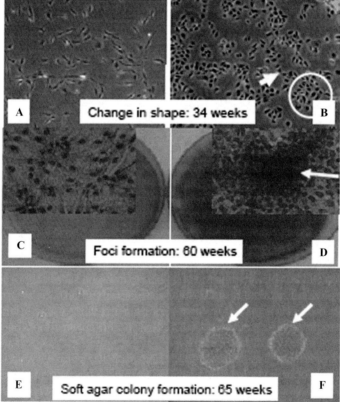

Progressive tumorigenic changes in BAR-T cells upon chronic exposure to A+B

CONTROL   **A+B TREATED**

A   Change in shape: 34 weeks   B

C   Foci formation: 60 weeks   D

E   Soft agar colony formation: 65 weeks   F

Figure 2. Chronic (>65) week treatment (5 min/day) of BAR-T cells with A + B, pH 4 transformed the benign BAR-T cells to neoplastic cells.[7] The control cells grown in parallel without any such treatment did not develop neoplastic phenotype. (A) Untreated cells, in contrast, are spindle shaped, sparse, and are evenly spread on the plate. (B) At 34 weeks of treatment, BAR-T cells developed distinct phenotypic changes, growing round or oval cells as clumps and acinar-like formations. Foci assay showed that the transformed cells, from 60 weeks onward, formed foci (D) in monolayer cultures, whereas untreated cells did not (C).

in the expression of colonic phenotype cells.[9] The proportion of the colonic phenotype cells increased to about 2.5-fold at 6 weeks and remained high at 65 weeks.

Repeated acid and bile exposure over 65 weeks causes transformation of benign Barrett's epithelial cells to neoplastic phenotype

Chronic (>65) week treatment (5 min/day) of BAR-T cells with A + B, pH 4 transformed the benign BAR-T cells to neoplastic cells.[7] The control cells grown in parallel without any such treatment did not develop neoplastic phenotype (Fig. 2).

Morphologic changes

At 34 weeks of treatment, BAR-T cells developed distinct phenotypic changes, growing round or oval cells as clumps and acinar-like formations (Fig. 2B). Untreated cells, in contrast, are spindle-shaped, sparse, and are evenly spread on the plate (Fig. 2A). Foci assay showed that the transformed cells, from 60 weeks onward, formed foci (Fig. 2D) in monolayer cultures, whereas untreated cells did not (Fig. 2C). At 58 weeks onwards, colony formation was observed in soft agar, which became more prominent at 65 weeks (Fig. 2F). Colony formation progressively increased in number and size with longer exposure. BAR-T cells, cultured in parallel without A + B treatment did not show any colony formation (Fig. 2E).

Molecular changes.

We observed changes in expression of COX-2, TC22, and p53 (Fig. 3). TC22 is a novel

tropomyosin isoform that is expressed in neoplastic, but not in normal colon epithelium.[10] Molecular changes were measured by real-time RT (RT)-PCR assay. TC22 gene and protein increased by threefold at 22 weeks, and sustained at 42 and 62 weeks, when compared to untreated controls cultured in parallel.[7] However, normal colon epithelial tropomyosin isoform 5 (hTM5) remained unchanged (data not shown). COX-2 gene expression increased and varied at 10- to 20-fold higher than control untreated cells during weeks 22–62.

Expression of apoptosis pathway genes and products

p53 protein expression doubled initially, but at around 40 weeks onwards, it declined, and by 54 weeks, it fell to the same level of p53 expression seen in untreated cells. Parallel changes in mRNA of p53 and related p21 and mdm2 genes (activated by p53 to regulate duration/extent of p53 activation), and perp (activated only in p53-mediated apoptosis, not cell cycle arrest) were seen. Untreated cells did not show any changes.[7] The molecular modulations paralleled the morphologic changes and colony growth in soft agar. It is not yet known if p53 has been mutated at this stage, if these cells have acquired LOH17p, or to what degree p53 protein levels are altered in BAR-T cells treated with A + B.

The transformed cells have increased Cdx2 mRNA expression, increased proliferation, and reduced apoptosis.[7] We also examined the ATM/ATR checkpoint molecular events at a series of time points that correlate with the evolutionary process of tumorigenesis. Acute induction of the ATM/ATR checkpoint components: RB, E2F, Cyclin E, Cdc25A, and BRCA1, as well as the tumor suppressor p53 in BAR-T cells, was observed at 20 weeks of A + B, pH 4-treated cells when compared to untreated cells (Table 2). Activation of the ATM-checkpoint is sustained in later stages at 40, 60, and 80 weeks, although at lower levels. P53, however, declined below baseline of untreated cells. Overexpressed cyclin E, Cdc25A, and E2F1 can promote unscheduled S-phase entry. Therefore, it is possible that the activated DNA damage response machinery might play an important role in tumorigenesis in BE.

Further studies on this model will not only help to understand the role of genomic and molecular changes during neoplastic progression but also help to identify novel biomarker(s) for cancer risk

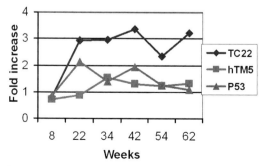

Expression of mRNA in BAR-T cells treated with Bile at PH 4 *

Figure 3. Observed changes in expression of COX-2, TC22, and p53.[7]

Table 2. Expression of selected apoptosis and cell cycle regulatory genes compared to untreated BAR-T cells of same duration in culture.

	20 weeks	40 weeks	60 weeks	80 weeks
RB1	2.18	Not done	1.45	1.45
E2F1	5.55	2.62	Not done	2.11
CCNE1	6.56	3.85	2.37	2.93
CDC25A	8.24	2.34	No change	No change
BRCA1	3.82	2.09	1.61	No change
TP53	2.2	2.14	−1.40	−1.3
CHEK2	2.13	3.65	1.77	1.68

stratification in BE as well as identify new targets for chemoprevention of neoplastic progression.

3. The role of NADPH oxidase NOX5-S in acid induced progression from Barrett's esophagus to esophageal adenocarcinoma

Weibiao Cao
wcao@hotmail.com

Gastroesophageal reflux disease complicated by BE is a major risk factor for EAC. Acid reflux may play an important role in the progression from metaplasia to dysplasia and to adenocarcinoma in patients with BE. However, the mechanisms whereby acid reflux may accelerate the progression from BE to EAC are not known.

ROS may be an important factor mediating acid reflux-induced damage. ROS may damage DNA, RNA, lipids, and proteins, leading to increased mutation and altered functions of enzymes and proteins. High levels of ROS are present in BE and in EAC. Low levels of ROS, seen in nonphagocytic cells, were thought to be byproducts of aerobic metabolism. More recently, however, superoxide-generating homologues of phagocytic NADPH oxidase catalytic subunit gp91[phox] (NOX1, NOX3-NOX5, DUOX1, DUOX2) have been found in several cell types, suggesting that ROS generated in these cells may have distinctive cellular functions related to immunity, signal transduction and modification of the extracellular matrix. NOX5 has α, β, δ, and γ and NOX5-S isoforms.[11] We have shown that NOX5-S is the major isoform of NADPH oxidase present in EAC cells[12] and that the expression of NOX5-S mRNA was significantly higher in EAC cells

than in esophageal squamous epithelial cells. NOX5 mRNA is also significantly higher in EAC tissues and in Barrett's tissues with high-grade dysplasia (LGD), when compared with Barrett's tissues without dysplasia.[13]

We have also shown that pulsed acid treatment significantly increases H_2O_2 production in FLO EAC cells, which is blocked by knockdown of NOX5 by NOX5 siRNA.[12] Acid treatment increases mRNA expression of NOX5-S, intracellular calcium, and phosphorylation of cAMP response element-binding protein (CREB). Acid-induced NOX5-S expression and H_2O_2 production are significantly inhibited by removal of extracellular calcium and by knockdown of CREB using CREB siRNA. These data indicate that acid-induced NOX5-S expression depends on an increase in intracellular calcium and activation of CREB.[13] We have reported that NOX5-S may contribute to increased proliferation and decreased apoptosis of EAC cells. The mechanisms of NOX5-S–mediated increase in cell proliferation are not fully understood. We have identified two mechanisms involved in NOX5-S–mediated increase in cell proliferation.

One mechanism may be through activation of cyclooxygenase-2 (COX2) because: (1) acid-induced increase in prostaglandin E2 (PGE2) production and COX2 expression was inhibited by the COX2 inhibitor NS-398, but not by the COX-1 inhibitor valeryl salicylate; (2) blockade of intracellular Ca^{2+} increase inhibited acid-induced increase in COX2 expression and PGE2 production; (3) knockdown of NOX5-S or NF-κB1 p50 by their siRNAs significantly inhibit acid-induced COX2 expression and PGE$_2$ production; (4) overexpression of NOX5-S in Barrett's cells significantly increases hydrogen peroxide production, COX2 expression, PGE$_2$ production, and thymidine incorporation; and (5) the increase in thymidine incorporation occurring in NOX5-S–overexpressing Barrett's cells or induced by acid treatment was significantly decreased by COX2 inhibitors or siRNA.[14]

A second mechanism may be via *p16* hypermethylation, which inactivates *p16*. Hypermethylation of the *p16* gene promoter is present at a much higher frequency in BE with dysplasia and EAC than in Barrett's intestinal metaplasia. Detection of *p16* hypermethylation has been reported to be used to predict the neoplastic progression.[15] Therefore, hypermethylation of *p16* gene promoter

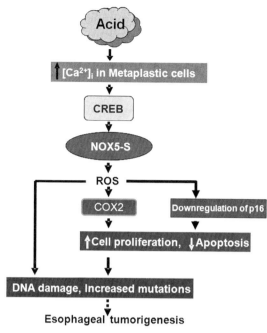

Figure 4. NOX5-S mediates acid-induced increase in cell proliferation and decrease in apoptosis.

is an important mechanism inactivating *p16*. Our data support this second mechanism because (1) exogenous H_2O_2 significantly increases *p16* promoter methylation and cell proliferation; (2) acid treatment significantly increases *p16* promoter methylation and decreases *p16* mRNA level; (3) knockdown of NOX5-S significantly increases *p16* mRNA, inhibits acid-induced downregulation of *p16* mRNA, and blocks acid-induced increase in *p16* methylation and cell proliferation; and (4) overexpression of NOX5-S significantly decreases *p16* mRNA and increases *p16* methylation and cell proliferation.[12]

The data indicate that NOX5-S is present in BE cells and EAC cells and mediates acid-induced H_2O_2 production and cell proliferation. Acid exposure upregulates NOX5-S in Barrett's metaplastic cells by an increase in intracellular calcium and activation of CREB. NOX5-S–derived ROS enhance PGE2 production via over-expression of COX2 and downregulation *p16* via hypermethylation of the *p16* gene promoter (Fig. 4). Upregulation of COX2 and downregulation of *p16* increase cell proliferation and decrease apoptosis in these cells. Persistent acid reflux present in BE patients may cause changes including high levels of ROS, increased cell proliferation, and decreased apoptosis, which may lead to DNA damage and increased mutations and

thereby contribute to the progression from metaplasia to dysplasia and to EAC. [these studies are supported by NIDDK R01 DK080703].

4. How does abnormal methylation contribute to neoplastic progression in Barrett's esophagus?

Usha Malhotra, Ajlan Atasoy, Ali Zaidi, Katie Nason, Blair Jobe, and Michael Gibson.
malhotrau@upmc.edu

BE is the most significant known risk factor for development of EAC. The sequence of progression from LGD, HGD, and EAC is accompanied by various changes at the genetic and epigenetic levels. The role of abnormal methylation in cancer has been well studied and reported in the literature. Hypomethylation or hypermethylation of CPG islands in the promoter regions leads to a number of downstream events like defects in DNA repair, angiognesis, entry in to the cell cycle, etc., which eventually contribute to the process of tumorigenesis. Hypermethylation of several genes has been observed in BE and EAC including p16 hypermethylation and APC inactivation.

Hypermethylation of p16 is highly prevalent in BE

p16 inhibits the function of cyclins and cyclin-dependent kinases (cdks), interferes with the cell cycle, thereby preventing cellular proliferation. Hypermethylation leads to silencing of this tumor suppressor gene. This event appears to be an early event in BE,[16] and its frequency increases on progression from LGD, HGD, to EAC.[17] The exact mechanism of this epigenetic event in context of BE and EAC is unclear though NADPH oxidase NOX5-S has been proposed to be involved.[12]

Methylation panels have been evaluated in various retrospective studies

In one study,[18] hypermethylation of p16, RUNX3, and HPP1 was found to be an early event in the sequence of progression, and was also postulated to be an independent risk factor for progression to HGD or EAC. Further studies evaluating more extensive panels have also reported a high predictive power and have proposed a potential role of these panels in clinical settings.[19]

A number of genes that have been shown to have altered expression due epigenetic changes in EAC/BE are currently being studied. These include TIMP3, TERT, CDKN2A, SFRP1, ID4, MGMT, RBP1, etc. Based on available data, there has been a lot of interest in this field, and the utility of combining these panels with clinical variables is also being explored.

In answer to the question, "how does abnormal methylation contribute to neoplastic progression in Barrett's esophagus?" (1) abnormal methylation is a frequent event in Barrett's progression, (2) various candidate genes have been evaluated, and (3) there is preliminary evidence supporting predictive value based on small and retrospective studies highlighting the need for systematic prospective analysis.

5. What are the genetic alterations that occur early in the stromal cells in the metaplasia–dysplasia cancer sequence?

George Triadafilopoulos
vagt@stanford.edu

The role of genetics and molecular biology in BE and EAC is multifaceted: in-depth knowledge in these domains will ultimately help to abort the development of BE in patients with GERD, prevent development of dysplasia and cancer from BE, regress LGD and HGD, and possibly arrest the spread of adenocarcinoma once it is detected. The stromal compartment is increasingly recognized to play a role in cancer. However, its role in the transition from preinvasive (BE) to invasive disease (adenocarcinoma) is unknown and has been the subject of recent investigations.

DNA microarrays that enable a genome-wide assessment of gene expression enhance the identification of specific genes as well as gene expression patterns that are expressed by BE and adenocarcinoma compared with normal tissues. BE length has also been identified as a risk factor for progression to adenocarcinoma, but whether there are intrinsic biological differences between short- and long-segment BE can also be explored with microarrays.

In a pioneering study by Hao *et al.*,[20] gene expression profiles for endoscopically obtained biopsy specimens of BE or EAC and associated normal esophagus and duodenum were identified for 17 patients using DNA microarrays. Unsupervised and

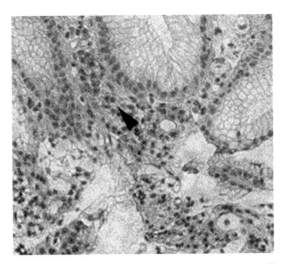

Figure 5. *In situ* hybridization for the collagen 5A2 (stromal) gene shows positive staining in Barrett's esophagus. Originally published in Ref. 20.

supervised approaches for data analysis defined similarities and differences between the tissues as well as correlations with clinical phenotypes. Each tissue displayed a unique expression profile that distinguished it from others. BE and EAC expressed a unique set of stromal genes that is distinct from normal tissues but similar to other cancers (Fig. 5).

Adenocarcinoma also showed lower and higher expression for many genes compared with BE. No difference in gene expression was found between short- and long-segment BE.

Taking tissues from BE at all levels of histological transformation, applying laser microdissection, then performing RNA extraction, amplification, and hybridization allows investigators to obtain specific and unique gene signatures. They can then proceed to perform protein analysis (expression level as well as localization) followed by functional analysis that explores the exact functional correlate to these genetic events.

A group of U.K. investigators[21] conducted supervised clustering of gene expression profiles from microdissected stroma and identified a gene signature that could distinguish between Barrett's metaplasia, dysplasia, and EAC. Cancer patients overexpressing any of the five genes (TMEPAI, JMY, TSP1, FAP-α, and BCL6) identified from this stromal signature had a significantly poorer outcome. Gene ontology analysis identified a strong inflammatory component in BE progression, and key pathways included cytokine–cytokine receptor interactions and

TGF-β. Increased protein levels of inflammatory-related genes significantly upregulated in cancer compared with preinvasive stages were confirmed in the stroma of independent samples, and *in vitro* assays confirmed functional relevance of these genes. Gene set enrichment analysis of external datasets demonstrated that the stromal signature was also relevant in the preinvasive to invasive transition of the stomach, colon, and pancreas cancers. These data implicate inflammatory pathways in the genesis of gastrointestinal tract cancers, which can affect prognosis.

In conclusion, the genome-wide assessment provided by current DNA microarrays reveals many candidate genes and patterns not previously identified. Stromal gene expression in BE and adenocarcinoma is similar, indicating that these changes precede malignant transformation. There is a distinct stage-specific stromal signature in Barrett's carcinogenesis, with predominance of inflammation- and TGF-β–related genes. Increased expression of one or more of five stromal genes is associated with a poor prognosis and has functional relevance.

6. Biomarker evaluation and neoplastic progression in Barrett's esophagus: can order be brought to a disordered process?

Robert M. Najarian
rnajaria@bidmc.harvard.edu

The identification of molecular biomarkers associated with the progression of BE from metaplasia to dysplasia to adenocarcinoma is inherently appealing for multiple reasons. Among these is the potential reduction in the number of invasive surveillance biopsy procedures, the identification of high risk patients with increased chromosomal instability whom may progress swiftly to carcinoma, and, potentially, the development of targeted therapies directed against molecules that may impact such neoplastic progression. Numerous challenges exist, however, in the application of these biomarkers including their nonspecificity, the genotypic and phenotypic heterogeneity of BE and its spectrum of neoplastic lesions, and the clinical applicability of the molecular methods used to detect such biomarkers. Although many potential biomarkers have been studied in early phase research trials, p16, p53, and chromosomal aneuploidy are the most well-studied biomarkers of interest and are discussed briefly.

The inactivation of the tumor suppressor gene p16 (also known as CDKN2A) on chromosome 9p has proven to be a biomarker in that it is expressed early in BE, with expression demonstrated in both metaplastic epithelium, as well as in dysplastic lesions and adenocarcinoma.[22] The mechanism of inactivation has proven to be multifactorial with hypermethylation of its promoter, loss of heterozygosity (LOH), and mutation being the most commonly demonstrated alterations. Although several studies have demonstrated changes in p16 to be exceedingly common in dysplasia and carcinoma in the setting of BE, this marker occurs at such a high frequency in nonneoplastic tissue that it is ineffective as a biomarker of progression to carcinoma.

Our attention next shifts to p53, a tumor suppressor gene whose alterations are nearly ubiquitous in the development of solid tumors of both epithelial and mesenchymal origin. Numerous studies have shown that LOH at the p53 gene locus on chromosome 17p occurs within dysplastic foci in the setting of BE with high frequency, whereas select investigations have additionally shown p53 abnormalities within nondysplastic Barrett's epithelium. The utility of p53 as a biomarker of progression to dysplasia and adenocarcinoma in the setting of Barrett's has been shown in phase 4 studies to be a strong predictor of carcinoma progression with a relative risk of 16.[23] A follow-up case-control study has proven its utility to be most robust when used in a panel of biomarkers, including proliferation marker Ki67 and chromosomal aneuploidy, as well as when it is used as a supplement to a tissue biopsy diagnosis of low-grade glandular dysplasia.[24] p53 is also attractive as a potential biomarker given the availability of immuno-peroxidase antibody identification methods for use on formalin-fixed, paraffin-embedded mucosal biopsy specimens that can serve as a surrogate for molecular changes conventionally assessed by methods that require fresh tissue specimens.

Chromosomal aneuploidy and tetraploidy have also been extensively studied for use as biomarkers of progression and have shown great promise. By definition, aneuploidy is the presence of an abnormal number of chromosomes rather than the expected diploid number of 46, with tetraploidy defined as 96 total chromosomes per cell nucleus.

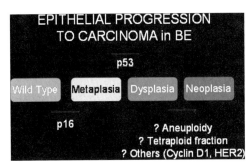

Figure 6. More study is needed to elucidate the potential predictive and therapeutic roles for molecular biomarkers in the process of carcinogenesis in BE.

Early studies have documented an increased risk of adenocarcinoma ranging from 4- to 11-fold, with a relative risk of 20 if both aneuploidy and tetraploidy were present in Barrett's epithelial cells by flow cytometric analysis.[25] Later studies using similar techniques demonstrated that expanded neoplastic clones gave rise to adenocarcinoma with increased amounts of clonal diversity that was correlated with adenocarcinoma risk.

Despite strong evidence for the predictive value of biomarkers used in panels and in concert with evaluation of a mucosal biopsy, there are several limitations to the use of individual biomarkers alone to evaluate a given patient's risk for BE-associated neoplasia. In addition to the obvious technical challenges of performing high volume molecular diagnostic testing, as well as the technical expertise required to apply such technology on a large scale, there are several basic molecular limitations. Just as a given segment of esophageal tissue can be histologically heterogeneous, so too can the molecular changes associated with such tissue. This was demonstrated elegantly in a study by Leedham *et al.*,[26] who showed that individual crypts of Barrett's epithelium with multiple degrees of dysplasia exhibited variable biomarker abnormalities that could potentially be masked if whole biopsy specimens were utilized in the analysis. In addition, the role played by environmentally induced damage from acid reflux and ingested irritants in the development of carcinoma is poorly understood, although may explain why the above molecular abnormalities are neither specific for nor sufficient for the development of adenocarcinoma. In short, more study is needed to elucidate the potential predictive and therapeutic roles for molecular biomarkers in the process of carcinogenesis in BE (Fig. 6).

7. What is the role of IGF in progression to adenocarcinoma?

Laura J. Hardie
l.j.hardie@leeds.ac.uk

Factors that are involved in the host response to reflux-induced injury and epithelial healing may play a pivotal role in the development of EAC. This includes components of the IGF system that comprises two ligands, IGF-I and IGF-II; three receptors, IGF-IR, the insulin receptor (IR), and IGF-IIR; and six high-affinity binding proteins, IGFBP-1–IGFBP-6. Circulating IGF-I and IGF-II are produced primarily by hepatocytes in response to growth hormone released from the pituitary gland. IGF-I and IGF-II may also be synthesized locally and act in an autocrine or paracrine fashion. In this regard, it should be noted that salivary glands synthesize IGF-1 resulting in the esophageal epithelium being continuously bathed in salivary IGF-1.

Binding of IGF-1 to IGF-1R is tightly regulated by IGFBPs—more than 95% of IGF-1 is complexed to IGFBP-3 in the circulation. Binding of IGF-I to IGF-1R results in autophosphorylation of the receptor via its intrinsic protein tyrosine kinase activity. This triggers a cascade of complex phosphorylation events, which result in enhanced protein synthesis through mTOR activation, increased cellular proliferation through enhanced Raf-1/MEK/ERK signaling, and inhibition of apoptosis via inactivation of Bad. Differentiation is also modulated through altered integrin signaling and changes to cytoskeleton-related proteins, including p130Cas and paxillin. In epithelial tissue, both epithelial and stromal cells can express the IGF-1R. Human esophageal epithelial cells express IGF-1R, and treatment with IGF-1 stimulates proliferation and outgrowth of new mucosa in cultured esophageal explants. IGFBP-3 has recognized activities that are independent of regulating IGF-1 bioavailability. IGFBP-3 has been shown to enhance apoptosis following UV-induced DNA damage in esophageal cells. This response may be important, given the DNA damaging and proapoptotic effects of reflux constituents such as deoxycholate.

During EAC development, a number of changes occur in the IGF axis at the tissue level. A study by Iravani *et al.* showed that levels of IGF-1R increase in a stepwise fashion during progression from Barrett's to dysplasia and adenocarcinoma.[27] Di Martino *et al.* demonstrated that mRNA for several IGFBPs was elevated in Barrett's tissue of EAC cases compared with uncomplicated Barrett's cases, providing additional evidence to link this pathway to disease progression at a tissue level.[28]

To date, only one study has examined circulating levels of IGF-I and IGFBP-3 and risk of EAC development.[29] Siahpush *et al.* tested whether circulating levels of IGF-1 and IGFBP-3 were associated with markers of progression in a cohort of BE patients. Although sample sizes were limited, risk of aneuploidy was approximately threefold higher among Barrett's patients with IGFBP-3 levels above the median. Cancer as an outcome was not significantly affected, but this could reflect the power of the study.

Genetic variation in the IGF axis has also been shown to modify risk of EAC development. A recent systematic genetic analysis of the IGF axis showed that a 17 CA microsatellite repeat in IGF-I was associated with an odds ratio of 7.3 for esophagitis, homozygosity for the A allele at rs6214 SNP in the IGF-I gene halved the risk of Barrett's, and presence of a C allele in the growth hormone receptor gene at SNP rs6898743 reduced the odds ratio for adenocarcinoma to <0.3.[30] IGF-II is also a ligand for the IGF-1R and has potent proproliferative and antiapoptotic effects. The IGF-II gene usually exhibits genomic imprinting with only the paternal allele expressed—the maternal allele is silenced via CpG methylation. Loss of imprinting is associated with re-expression of the maternal allele and associated gain of allelic gene expression (GOAGE). GOAGE of the IGF-II gene is observed in a number of cancers and recent studies have shown that GOAGE of IGF-II is common in Barrett's and EAC development.[31]

In conclusion, there is increasing evidence to support a link between the IGF axis and development of EAC. Given this pathway is regulated by energy balance, disruption to the IGF axis may provide a mechanistic link between obesity and EAC development and awaits detailed investigation.

8. Is confocal laser endomicroscopy, allowing subsurface analysis of the mucosa, a reliable tool for detection of BE associated neoplasia?

Charles J. Lightdale
cjl18@columbia.edu

CLE has emerged as an endoscopic method that offers extremely high magnification and resolution (<1 μm) approximating white light microscopy and providing *in vivo* histology or "optical biopsy" during ongoing endoscopy. Both dedicated endoscope (eCLE, Pentax) and probe-based (pCLE, Mauna Kea Technologies, Paris, France) devices have been used in BE surveillance, and both have been highly successful in initial studies in detecting HGD and early cancer (EC) in BE.

eCLE in Barrett's esophagus

Initial studies with eCLE in BE surveillance were by Kiesslich *et al.* Against the standard of mucosal biopsy and light microscopy, eCLE (with a resolution of 0.7 μm) had a sensitivity of 92.9% and specificity of 98.4% based on postprocedure analysis.[32] A recent single-center BE surveillance trial compared standard endoscopy with four-quadrant random biopsies to eCLE with optical biopsy analyzed in real time. The diagnostic yield of mucosal biopsies was increased from 17.2% to 33.7% in patients with suspected nonlocalized HGD. In the routine surveillance group, using eCLE, almost two thirds were able to forgo all mucosal biopsies as no areas suspicious for neoplasia were found.[33]

pCLE in Barrett's esophagus

BE surveillance with pCLE offers the flexibility of using any standard endoscope with the 2.7-mm-diameter mini-probe.[34] In a study using an early version of the probe, sensitivity for HGD or EC was 80% and 94%. The negative predictive value in the low-risk population studied was 98.8%, allowing nearly risk-free elimination of random mucosal biopsies when pCLE was negative.[35] The recently completed DON'T BIOPCE study utilized a newer probe with a resolution of 1.0 μm in a multicenter international randomized trial of white light or narrow band imaging or pCLE compared to pathology results of targeted mucosal abnormalities and four-quadrant random biopsies. For high-definition white light endoscopy (WLE) the diagnostic sensitivity was 32.8% and specificity 92.8% compared to 67.2%/88.0% with the addition of pCLE ($P < 0.001$). WLE + NBI had sensitivity/specificity of 44.0%/88.2% compared to 75%/84.3% with the addition of pCLE ($P < 0.001$).[36]

In conclusion, CLE, allowing subsurface analysis of the mucosa, is a reliable tool for detection of BE associated neoplasia. CLE has the potential to decrease the number of biopsies taken for BE surveillance, making surveillance more cost-effective, and has the potential for immediate guidance of endoscopic therapy.

9. What can be expected from statins, inducing apoptosis in BE adenocarcinoma cells, as adjuvant chemotherapeutic agents?

Ian L. P. Beales

i.beales@uea.ac.uk

Esophageal carcinoma remains a devastating disease and great attention continues to be paid to ways of preventing the development of cancer from the precursor lesion, BE. However, it must be appreciated that most patients with BE do not develop esophageal cancer and only a small proportion actually die from the malignancy. For instance in the follow up of a cohort of Barrett's patients by Van der Burgh *et al.*, although overall mortality was 50% higher than expected, only 2.5% died from esophageal cancer, whereas over 25% of deaths were due to circulatory diseases.[37] Therefore, it behooves us to take a holistic approach and consider the wider implications of any chemo-preventative strategies. For example, the COX-2 inhibitors seem attractive agents based on experimental and clinical data, but the likely increased cardiovascular risk militates against their use for widespread chemoprevention.

Statins (HMG-CoA reductase inhibitors) have an established place in the prevention of circulatory disease linked mainly to the reduction in cholesterol. However, by inhibiting this early step in the mevalonate–cholesterol synthetic pathway, statins also have the ability to modify other cellular processes. Several important biosynthetic intermediates are produced via this process including farnesylpyrophosphate and geranyl pyrophosphate, these are important in the posttranslational modification of small signaling G proteins (Ras, Rac, Rho, and cdc42), the addition of the hydrophobic prenylation motif localizes these proteins to the cell membrane where they control signaling via many growth and cell survival factors.

We have shown that in three different EAC cell lines that statins inhibit cell proliferation and induce apoptosis in a concentration dependent manner.

Similar effects were seen with simvastatin, pravastatin, and lovastatin, and the anticancer effects were additive to inhibition of COX-2 with either NS-398 or celecoxib. The effects of statins were mimicked by a farnesyl transferase inhibitor, reversed by the addition of farnesyl pyrophosphate and statins, reduced growth factor-stimulated Ras activation. This inhibition of Ras activation was linked with a downstream reduction in the activities of the ERK and Akt protein kinases that are known to promote cell division and survival and in keeping with this statins upregulated the proapoptotic proteins Bad and Bax.[38]

One criticism of most laboratory studies with statins is that the concentrations used were suprapharmacological. However our most recent studies have shown that significant pro-apoptotic effects can be induced in cancer and nonmalignant Barrett's cells with rosuvastatin at concentrations achievable *in vivo*. Importantly, these effects were synergistically enhanced by inhibition of PGE2 production using either pharmacological inhibition or RNA interference against mPGES-1, the enzyme responsible for PGE2 production distal COX-2 in the biosynthetic pathway (Fig. 7). The latter seems a viable chemo-preventative target because mPGES-1 inhibition does not reduce endothelial prostacyclin (PGI2) production and, theoretically, should have fewer cardiovascular side effects.[39]

Against this promising laboratory background, clinical studies are emerging, which also support a beneficial chemo-preventative role of statins. A cohort study using the review of the UK QResearch database,[40] (over two million patients), predominantly looking for adverse effects of statins, actually reported a significant reduction in esophageal cancer incidence in both men (odds ratio 0.65, 95% CI = 0.56–0.75) and women (odds ratio 0.74, 95% = 0.59–0.94). Although interesting, the lack of data on the accuracy of the diagnoses and comorbidity and other drug therapies means these data cannot be considered definitive.

Nguyen *et al.*[41] examined a cohort of overwhelmingly male patients with BE and showed that filling prescriptions for statins was also associated with a significant reduction in the development of esophageal cancer (odds ratio 0.55, 95% CI = 0.36–0.86). Interestingly, this effect was apparent even within the first year of statin therapy. Our own case–control study, comparing EAC cases with cancer-free controls attending for diagnostic

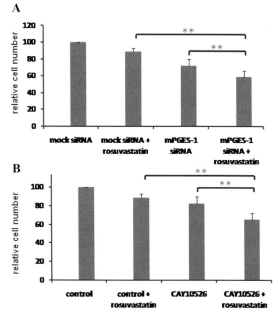

Figure 7. Combined effect of rosuvastatin and mPGES-1 inhibition on viable Barrett's esophageal cell numbers. FLO cells were treated with siRNA directed against mPGES-1 or control siRNA and then exposed to rosuvastatin (0.1 μM). After 48 h, relative cell numbers were assessed. $**P < 0.05$ for the comparison. The combination of mPGES-1 silencing and rosuvastatin was significantly more effective than either alone. QhERT Barrett's cells were treated with rosuvastatin (0.1 μM) and the mPGES-1 inhibitor CAY 10526 (10 μM) and relative cell numbers assessed after 48 h. $**P < 0.05$ for the comparison. A combination of mPGES-1 silencing and rosuvastatin was significantly more effective than either alone.

gastroscopy, has also found a significant reduction in cancer incidence in statin users. Statin use was associated with a significant 68% reduction in cancer incidence (odds ratio 0.42, 95% CI = 0.19–0.89), and this significance was maintained after correction for aspirin and NSAID use and was equally apparent in those with and without reflux symptoms. The beneficial chemo-preventative effect of statins and aspirin were additive (odds ratio 0.11, 95% CI = 0.01–0.82).

Therefore, statins seem to offer exciting potential as chemo-preventative agents in BE. Statins alter intracellular signaling pathways to induce apoptosis and inhibit proliferation. Statins would be expected to have a beneficial effect on the excess circulatory mortality associated with Barrett's esophagus, and preliminary clinical studies have consistently shown a significant reduction in EAC in statin users. Combination therapy with aspirin or mPGES-1 in-

hibitors offers great potential for chemoprevention, and deserves much wider study.

10. What is the value of macroscopic markers in defining a subset of Barrett's patients at high risk of HGD and adenocarcinoma?

Valter Nilton Felix

v.felix@terra.com.br

Biopsy specimens of the mucosa or brush cytology should be indicated especially if there is irregular or deep ulceration, presence of a mass lesion or nodularity, or an irregular or malignant-appearing stricture representing high risk of HGD and adenocarcinoma. Here, the new developments in endoscopic detection of early neoplastic lesions can be useful.

Today, it has been valued that one common aspect among the major risk factors for BE and EAC is the existence of chronic inflammation, both in the esophageal epithelium as well as systemically. It has been hypothesized that telomere length in leukocytes of people with BE might serve as an integrative measure of a person's long-term history of inflammation and oxidative damage, as factors such as insulin resistance, obesity, and smoking have been shown to reduce telomere length.[42,43]

Longitudinal analysis of baseline blood samples in a Barrett's esophagus cohort revealed that shorter telomere length was associated with increased risk of progression to EAC (adjusted hazard ratio comparing extreme quartiles: 3.45; 95% CI = 1.35–8.78).[42] These observations were replicated in a case–control study that found overall telomere length, as well as 17p and 12q telomere lengths, but not 11q and 2p telomere lengths, were associated with increased EAC risk.[43] These results suggest the importance of chronic systemic inflammation in the development of BE and EAC and raise the possibility that telomere length may be a useful component to a biomarker panel designed to stratify risk in people with Barrett's esophagus.

However, the endoscopic and/or histopathologic changes of esophageal mucosal injury and inflammation remain the main focus of Barrett's diagnosis and surveillance. The detection of HGD or EC has been shown to have the potential to improve survival in patients with BE. In long-term management of Barrett's patients, endoscopy is recommended with fair evidence that it improves important outcomes (Grade B evidence), and biopsies should target any areas of suspected dysplasia.

When BE is defined, biopsy specimens of the mucosa should be specially obtained under the following circumstances that predict the development of EAC: the presence of irregular or deep ulceration, proximal distribution of esophagitis, presence of a mass lesion or nodularity, or an irregular or malignant-appearing stricture. Glandular dysplasia arising in a background of BE typically shows scattered atypical cells with some, but not all, features of adenocarcinoma. Adenocarcinomas typically show groups and clusters of neoplastic epithelial cells.

Nodularity is defined as a subtle mucosal elevation of ≤1 cm. In one study, 63% of the patients with HGD and nodularity had cancers as compared with 13% without nodularity. Nodularity was associated with a 2.5-fold risk of cancer compared with those without it after adjusting for extent of dysplasia. Moreover, 36% of the patients with diffuse HGD and 7% of those with focal HGD had cancer at esophagectomy.[44]

Any mucosal abnormality, as ulcers or nodular area, must be carefully investigated and removed, if possible, by endoscopic mucosal resection. In patients with stenosis, esophageal dilatation may be required to allow for a standard endoscope (outer diameter of 9.8 mm) traversing the obstructed lumen. Alternatively, an ultrathin endoscope (outer diameter 5.3–6 mm) may pass through the stenosis and allow completion of the examination. Biopsy specimens are required for histological confirmation and the diagnostic yield reaches high rates when six or more samples are obtained using standard endoscopic biopsy forceps. EUS miniprobes may have a role in more accurate T staging than low-frequency probes in these patients, and stenotic lesions may be traversed without dilation. As an adjunct, brush cytology can be helpful in sampling tight malignant strictures, which may not be easily accessible to conventional biopsy techniques. However, the morphologic analysis of brush cytology specimens is difficult and, in fact, inferior to standard histology.

There have been several new developments in the endoscopic detection of early neoplastic lesions in BE patients. Thus, chromoendoscopy using methylene blue or indigo carmine dye, for example, involves topical application of dyes during endoscopy in an effort to enhance the detection of mucosal pattern or lesions on the basis of staining characteristics. Today, magnification endoscopy, which enhances mucosal detailing, is generally used in combination with chromoscopy.[45] The mucosal details, as seen with magnification endoscopy, can be further increased by using narrow band imaging without out the use of dyes. Fluorescence endoscopy has been clinically evaluated with promising results in distinguishing nondysplastic areas from areas with HGD or cancer.[46]

11. What should be the current interpretation of p53 mutations for identification of Barrett's patients at high risk for cancer?

Patryk Kambakamba, Georg Lurje, and Paul M. Schneider
paul.schneider@usz.ch

BE is the most significant risk factor for the development of EAC. EAC is thought to develop through progression of metaplasia to dysplasia and finally invasive carcinoma. Routine endoscopic surveillance of patients with BE is an expensive practice due to the low rate of progression to EAC in patients without dysplasia.[47]

Identification of factors predicting progression to EAC would help in focusing surveillance programs, thereby improve cost-effectiveness and detect patients when the disease can be cured. p53 is an evolutionary ancient transcription factor and in vertebrates it acts as an important tumor-suppressor, and either its or its attendant upstream or downstream pathways are functionally inactivated in virtually all cancers.[48] Schneider *et al.* and the group of A.G. Casson reported p53 mutations in approximately 50% of EAC or HGD lesions and much less frequently in BE without or LGD.[49–51] Mutations in EAC were independently associated with poor survival following potentially curative resections.[50,51] Mutation analysis of p53 was performed by DNA sequencing. Mutations were located in exons 4–10 and the predominant type (54–78%) were transition-type missense mutations with the majority being G:C > A:T base substitutions at CpG dinucleotides.

Despite the enthusiasm triggered by these reports, the current role of p53 as a potential biomarker for disease progression in BE is unclear. In a recent comprehensive review, Prasad *et al.*[47] summarized

Table 3. Synopsis of phases III and IV studies evaluating p53 in Barrett's esophagus (adapted from Ref. 47)

Authors	Biomarkers	Phase	Sample size	Technique	Endpoint	Predictive value
Reid *et al.*[23]	p53 LOH	IV	325	Locus specific PCR	EAC	RR 16 (6.2–39)
Younes *et al.*[52]	p53 staining	III	25 LGD	IHC	HGD/EAC	Sens. 100%, Spec. 93%, PPV 56%
Weston *et al.*[53]	p53 staining	IV	48 LGD	IHC	HGD/EAC	RR 5.7%
Murray *et al.*[54]	p53 staining	III	197	IHC	EAC	OR 11.7 (1.93–2.2), Sens. 32%

IHC, immunohistochemistry; PCR, polymerase chain reaction; EAC, esophageal adenoacarcinoma; LGD, low-grade dysplasia; HGD, high-grade dysplasia; RR, relative risk; Sens., sensitivity; Spec., specificity; PPV, positive predictive value; OR, odds ratio.

the current evidence on risk factors for progression in subjects with known BE. Literature was classified according to the Early Detection Research Network (EDRN) guidelines for the validation of markers (phases I–V) with phase V consisting of population based-studies that show an impact of biomarker detection on disease burden and cancer control.

Only two phase III and IV studies regarding p53 LOH ($n = 1$) and immunohistochemistry (IHC) ($n = 3$) were reported within this context, and results are summarized in Table 3. The phase IV study by Weston *et al.* analyzed p53 IHC expression in BE with LGD and found a significant correlation ($P < 0.002$) between progression of LGD and p53 expression.[53] However, only 5 of 48 (10.4%) patients showed a progression to HGD or cancer. Two further phase III trials using IHC for p53 analysis showed huge variations in sensitivities (32–100%) to identify patients at risk for disease progression. LOH describes the loss of normal function of the second allele of a gene, which in combination with mutations in the other allele leads to severe or complete dysfunction of the gene. Reid *et al.* demonstrated in a phase IV study including 325 patients with baseline endoscopic biopsies that p53 LOH was the strongest predictor of risk for progression to EAC (relative risk: 16; $P < 0.0001$).[23]

Several unresolved issues regarding molecular marker studies including p53 analysis are evident. Among them are the number of biopsies and the size and number of clones needed to be analyzed. With respect to p53 analysis, it is likely that direct DNA sequencing of the complete open reading frame is necessary to unequivocally prove the presence of mutations as 20–30% of mutations are not identified by IHC.

In summary, identification of biomarkers with predictive value for BE progression would be helpful to improve screening and surveillance programs. Until now, only few factors (aneuploidy, p53, LOH) have shown a predictive potential with significantly increased odds ratios for BE progression in phase III and IV biomarker studies. A single molecular marker such as p53, however, will surely not have the sufficient predictive power. Besides, further limitations derive from a lack of standardization of methodologies, the choice of techniques (e.g., DNA sequencing, LOH, or IHC for p53 analysis), and paucity or absence of prospective phase III/IV trials. Substantial efforts therefore need to be undertaken to create a risk score by combining several clinical and biomarker variables. Creation of such a score, which might include p53 mutations, will have the potential to improve outcomes and make the management of patients with BE cost-effective.

12. Can the sequence of molecular events interacting in malignant progression in Barrett's mucosa be more precisely defined?

Andrew M. Bellizzi
abellizzi@partners.org

Molecular events in Barrett's esophagus

A variety of cellular processes and molecules have been implicated in the neoplastic progression of BE. Table 4 lists those processes and molecules discussed in the plenary sessions at the OESO 10th World Congress. Research in these areas is in various states of maturity. This brief review will discuss the epistemology of sequence and a model of neoplastic progression encompassing those best-studied events.

How do we infer sequence?

A spectrum of histologic changes is seen in progression to Barrett's-associated adenocarcinoma, from columnar metaplasia without or with goblet cells, to dysplasia, which can be separated into low and high grades, to adenocarcinoma. It has been historically assumed that these histologic changes represent steps in a linear progression to cancer. Given this assumption, one way to infer the sequence of neoplastic progression is to compare the frequencies of an event across the various histologic categories—normal (nl), BE, negative for dysplasia (neg), LGD, HGD, and adenocarcinoma (AdCa). For example, Younes *et al.* determined the frequency of p53 overexpression as follows: neg 0%, LGD 9%, HGD 55%, and AdCa 87%.[52] Based on these data, p53 overexpression would appear important in the transition from LGD to HGD and from HGD to AdCa. Giménez *et al.*, performing a similar study, found p53 overexpression in 0% neg, 61.5% LGD, 100% HGD, and 78.5% AdCa.[55] Based on this study, p53 overexpression would appear important in the development of LGD.

These disparate results highlight several limitations of this investigatory model. Although dysplasia assessment remains the "gold standard" method for cancer risk assessment in patients with BE, interobserver reproducibility is modest at best. Studies are difficult to compare because of variation in technique and thresholds for a "positive" result. For example, Younes *et al.* considered any nuclear staining of any intensity and Giménez *et al.* "intense" nuclear staining in at least 1% of lesional nuclei as "positive." One should ask whether a study is interrogating a biologically relevant analyte. In the above studies "overexpression" of p53 as assessed by IHC was a surrogate for inactivating *TP53* mutations, but p53 expression is an imperfect surrogate, and p53 is also inactivated by LOH. Finally, this model assumes linear progression. Interestingly, while the rate of progression to AdenoCa at five years follow-up for HGD is on the order of 50%, the rate for LGD is only 5–10%. Could it be that LGD, rather than representing an obligate precursor to HGD, is instead the histologic manifestation of a separate, indolent neoplastic pathway? An alternative means of inferring sequence, taking advantage of the topography of the Barrett's segment, is the simultaneous assessment of multiple genetic and epigenetic events in mapped mucosal biopsies. In this model,

Table 4. Cellular processes and molecules in Barrett progression

Processes	Molecules
Oxidative stress	CDX-2
DNA damage	p16
Apoptosis	p53
Inflammation	Cyclin D1
Genetic instability	Telomerase
DNA methylation	microRNA
Cell cycle	IGF
	COX
	Adipocytokines
	AMACR
	Rab11a

a specific change (e.g., a distinct *TP53* point mutation), detected in multiple contiguous biopsy levels, is assumed to occur before a different change occupying a smaller area of mucosa. Because Barrett's segments, especially those without HGD, are generally left *in situ*, the logical extension of this approach is its application in individual patients over time.

Model of neoplastic progression

Of the processes and molecules listed in Table 4, the data regarding cell cycle dysregulation through inactivation of p16 and p53 and genetic instability are most compelling. A model encompassing these is shown in Figure 8. p16 (cyclin-dependent kinase inhibitor 2A) may be inactivated by promoter methylation, mutation, or 9p LOH. Inactivation of p16 is an early event in BE. Wong *et al.* analyzed negative, indefinite/LGD, and HGD biopsies and found LOH, mutation, and promoter methylation in 49%, 7%, and 66% of biopsies without dysplasia and found similar rates of any type of inactivation across the three histologic categories (88%, 87%, and 86%, respectively).[56] Because clonal p16 abnormalities may be found in Barrett segments even without dysplasia, many investigators consider BE, negative for dysplasia to represent a neoplasm (albeit one with a very low overall risk for progression to malignancy). As mentioned earlier, p53 is inactivated by mutation and LOH. Analyzing 782 mapped mucosal biopsies from 211 patients, Maley *et al.* found that, in all but one case, p53 lesions occurred within or were coextensive with p16 lesions.[57] Intact p53

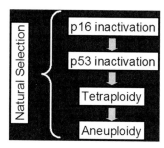

Figure 8. Model of neoplastic progression in Barrett's esophagus. p16 inactivation is an early event, occurring in Barrett epithelium before the development of dysplasia. Inactivation of p53 follows. It is permissive to the expansion of tetraploid clones, which lead to aneuploidy by subsequent chromosomal losses. Natural selection operates throughout.

function inhibits the expansion of genetically unstable clones, which trigger a DNA damage checkpoint. Aneuploidy is defined as an abnormal chromosome number. Aneuploid clones with the highest rate of progression to cancer have DNA contents between triploid (3N) and tetraploid (4N). As such, a "tetraploid intermediate" may be the precursor to most such aneuploid clones (rather than a diploid precursor). Loss of p53 function is permissive to the development of tetraploidy. Galipeau *et al.* found the mean 4N fraction increased from 2.7% to 9.5% with 17p allelic loss. They further showed that patients with increased 4N fractions (>6%) went on to develop aneuploidy 73% of the time (versus 11%).[58] In this model, natural selection is at work throughout, with aneuploidy serving as a rich source of genetic diversity.

Conclusion

Numerous cellular processes and molecules have been implicated in Barrett neoplastic progression. Those related to cell cycle regulation and genetic instability are among the best studied. Models of neoplastic progression based on the comparison of frequencies of an event across various histologic categories are somewhat limited because of challenges in reproducible histologic assessment and especially because they assume a linear progression. Studies that assess multiple, biologically relevant genetic and epigenetic events in mapped mucosal biopsies are preferable. Inactivation of p16 is an early event in neoplastic progression, detectable in nearly 90% of BE, negative for dysplasia. Inactivation of p53 follows, which permits the development of tetraploidy and subsequent aneuploidy.

Acknowledgments

These studies are supported by National Institute of Diabetes and Digestive and Kidney Diseases (NIDDK) Grant R01 DK080703.

Conflicts of interest

The authors declare no conflicts of interest.

References

1. Matsuda, M., A. Kubo, M. Furuse & S. Tsukita. 2004. A peculiar internalization of claudins, tight junction- specific adhesion molecules, during the intercellular movement of epithelial cells. *J. Cell. Sci.* **117**(Pt 7): 1247–1257.
2. Györffy, H., A. Holczbauer, P. Nagy, *et al.* 2005. Claudin expression in Barrett's esophagus and adenocarcinoma. *Virchows. Arch.* **447**: 961–968.
3. Montgomery, E., A.J. Mamelak, M. Gibson, *et al.* 2006. Overexpression of claudin proteins in esophageal adenocarcinoma and its precursor lesions. *Appl. Immunohistochem. Mol. Morphol.* **14**: 24–30.
4. Tobey, N.A., S.S. Hosseini, C.M. Argote, *et al.* 2004. Dilated intercellular spaces and shunt permeability in nonerosive acid-damaged esophageal epithelium. *Am. J. Gastroenterol.* **99**: 13–22.
5. Calabrese, C., A. Fabbri, M. Bortolotti, *et al.* 2003. Dilated intercellular spaces as a marker of esophageal damage: comparative results in gastro-esophageal reflux disease with or without bile reflux. *Aliment. Pharmacol. Ther.* **18**: 525–532.
6. Wang, K.K. & R.E. Sampliner. 2008. Updated guidelines 2008 for the diagnosis, surveillance and therapy of Barrett's esophagus. *Am. J. Gastroenterol.* **103**: 788–797.
7. Das, K.M., Y. Kong, M. Bajpai, *et al.* 2011. Transformation of benign Barrett's epithelium by repeated acid and bile exposure over 65 weeks: a novel in vitro model. *Intl. J. Cancer* **128**: 274–282.
8. Das, K.M., S. Sakamaki, M. Vecchi & B. Diamond. 1987. The production and characterization of monoclonal antibodies to a human colonic antigen associated with ulcerative colitis: cellular localization of the antigen by using the monoclonal antibody. *J. Immunol.* **139**: 77–84.
9. Bajpai, M., J. Liu, X. Geng, *et al.* 2008. Repeated exposure to acid and bile selectively induces colonic phenotype expression in a heterogenous Barrett's epithelial cell line. *Lab. Invest.* **88**: 643–651.
10. Lin, J.L.-C., X. Geng, S. Das-Bhattacharya, *et al.* 2002. Isolation and sequencing of a novel tropomyosin isoform preferentially associated with colon cancer. *Gastroenterology* **123**: 152–162.
11. Lambeth, J.D. 2004. NOX enzymes and the biology of reactive oxygen. *Nat. Rev. Immunol.* **4**: 181–189.
12. Hong, J., M. Resnick, J. Behar, *et al.* Acid-induced p16 hypermethylation contributes to development of esophageal adenocarcinoma via activation of NADPH oxidase NOX5-S. *Am. J. Physiol. Gastrointest. Liver Physiol.* **299**: G697–G706.
13. Fu, X., D.G. Beer, J. Behar, *et al.* 2006. cAMP-response element-binding protein mediates acid-induced NADPH

oxidase NOX5-S expression in Barrett esophageal adeno-carcinoma cells. *J. Biol. Chem.* **281:** 20368–20382.

14. Si, J., X. Fu, J. Behar, *et al.* 2007. NADPH oxidase NOX5-S mediates acid-induced cyclooxygenase-2 expression via activation of NF-kappaB in Barrett's esophageal adenocarcinoma cells. *J. Biol. Chem.* **282:** 16244–16255.

15. Kawamata, Y., R. Fujii, M. Hosoya, *et al.* 2003. A G protein-coupled receptor responsive to bile acids. *J. Biol. Chem.* **278:** 9435–9440.

16. Bian, Y.S., M.C. Osterheld, C. Fontolliet, *et al.* 2002. p16 inactivation by methylation of the CDKN2A promoter occurs early during neoplastic progression in Barrett's esophagus. *Gastroenterology* **122:** 1113–1121.

17. Klump, B., C.J. Hsieh, K. Holzmann, *et al.* 1998. Hypermethylation of the CDKN2/p16 promoter during neoplastic progression in Barrett's esophagus. *Gastroenterology* **115:** 1381–1386.

18. Schulmann, K., A. Sterian, A. Berki, *et al.* 2005. Inactivation of p16, RUNX3, and HPP1 occurs early in Barrett's-associated neoplastic progression and predicts progression risk. *Oncogene* **24:** 4138–4148.

19. Jin, Z., Y. Cheng, W. Gu, *et al.* 2009. A multicenter, double-blinded validation study of methylation biomarkers for progression prediction in Barrett's esophagus. *Cancer Res.* **69:** 4112–4115. Epub 2009 May 12.

20. Hao, Y., G. Triadafilopoulos, P. Sahbaie, *et al.* 2006. Gene expression profiling reveals stromal genes expressed in common between Barrett's esophagus and adenocarcinoma. *Gastroenterology* **131:** 925–933.

21. Saadi, A., N.B. Shannon, P. Lao-Sirieix, *et al.* 2010. Stromal genes discriminate preinvasive from invasive disease, predict outcome, and highlight inflammatory pathways in digestive cancers. *Proc. Natl. Acad. Sci. U S A* **107:** 2177–2182.

22. Barrett, M.T., C.A. Sanchez, L.J. Prevo, *et al.* 1999. Evolution of neoplastic cell lineages in Barrett's esophagus. *Nat. Genet.* **22:** 106–109.

23. Reid, B.J., L.J. Prevo, P.C. Galipeau, *et al.* 2001. Predictors of progression in Barrett's esophagus II: baseline 17 p (p53) loss of heterozygosity identifies a patient subset at increased risk for neoplastic progression. *Am. J. Gastroenterol.* **96:** 2839–2848.

24. Sikkema, M., M. Kerkof, E.W. Steyerburg, *et al.* 2009. Aneuploidy and overexpression of Ki67 and p53 as markers for neoplastic progression in Barrett's esophagus: a case-control study. *Am. J. Gastroenterol.* **104:** 2673–2680.

25. Rabinovitch, P.S., G. Longton, P.L. Blount, *et al.* 2001. Predictors of progression in Barrett's esophagus III: baseline flow cytometric variables. *Am. J. Gastroenterol.* **96:** 3071–3083.

26. Leedham, S.J., S.L. Preston, S.A. McDonald, *et al.* 2008. Individual crypt heterogeneity and the origin of metaplastic epithelium in human Barrett's esophagus. *Gut* **57:** 1041–1048.

27. Iravani, S., H.Q. Zhang, Z.Q. Yuan, *et al.* 2003. Modification of insulin-like growth factor 1 receptor, c-Src, and Bcl-X-L protein expression during the progression of Barrett's neoplasia. *Human Pathol.* **34:** 975–982.

28. Di Martino, E., C.P. Wild, O. Rotimi, *et al.* 2006. IGFBP-3 and IGFBP-10 (CYR61) up-regulation during the development of Barrett's oesophagus and esophageal adenocarci-

noma: potential biomarkers of disease risk. *Biomarkers* **11:** 547–561.

29. Siahpush, S.H., T.L. Vaughan, J.N. Lampe, *et al.* 2007. Longitudinal study of insulin-like growth factor, insulin-like growth factor binding protein-3, and their polymorphisms: risk of neoplastic progression in Barrett's esophagus. *Cancer Epidemiol. Biomarkers Prevent.* **16:** 2387–2395.

30. McElholm, A.R., A.J. McKnight, C.C. Patterson, *et al.* 2010. A population-based study of IGF axis polymorphisms and the esophageal inflammation, metaplasia, adenocarcinoma sequence. *Gastroenterology* **139:** 204–212.

31. Feagins, L.A., N. Susnow, H.Y. Zhang, *et al.* 2006. Gain of allelic gene expression for IGF-II occurs frequently in Barrett's esophagus. *Am. J. Physiol. Gastrointest. Liver Physiol.* **290:** G871–G875.

32. Kiesslich, R., L. Gossner, M. Goetz, *et al.* 2006. In vivo histology of Barrett's esophagus and associated neoplasia by confocal laser endomicroscopy. *Clin. Gastroenterol. Hepatol.* **4:** 979–987.

33. Wallace, M.B. & P. Fockens. 2009. Probe-based confocal laser endomicroscopy. *Gastroenterology* **136:** 1509–1513.

34. Dunbar, K.B., P. Okolo, III, E. Montgomery & M.I. Canto. 2009. Confocal laser endomicroscopy in Barrett's esophagus and endoscopically apparent Barrett's neoplasia: a prospective, randomized, double-blind, controlled, crossover trial. *Gastrointest. Endosc.* **70:** 645–654.

35. Pohl, H., T. Rosch, M. Vieth, *et al.* 2008. Miniprobe confocal laser microscopy for the detection of invisible neoplasia in patients with Barrett's oesophagus. *Gut* **57:** 1648–1653.

36. Sharma, P., A. Meining, E. Coron, *et al.* 2010. Detection of neoplastic tissue in Barrett's esophagus with in vivo probe-based confocal endomicroscopy (DONT BIOPCE). Final results of a prospective international randomized controlled trial: image-guided versus 4-quadrant random biopsies (Abstract) Digestive Disease Week 2010 #1071.

37. Van Der Burgh, A., J. Dees, W. Hop & M. Van Blankenstein. 1996. Esophageal cancer is an uncommon cause of death in patients with Barrett's oesophagus. *Gut* **39:** 5–8.

38. Ogunwobi, O.O. & I.L. Beales. 2008. Statins inhibit proliferation and induce apoptosis in Barrett's esophageal adenocarcinoma cells. *Am. J. Gastroenterol.* **103:** 825–837.

39. Beales, I.L. & O.O. Ogunwobi. 2010. Microsomal prostaglandin E synthase-1 inhibition blocks proliferation and enhances apoptosis in esophageal adenocarcinoma cells without affecting endothelial prostacyclin production. *Int. J. Cancer* **126:** 2247–2255.

40. Hippisley-Cox, J. & C. Coupland. 2010. Unintended effects of statins in men and women in England and Wales: population based cohort study using the QResearch database. *BMJ* **340:** c2197.

41. Nguyen, D.M., P. Richardson & H.B. El-Serag. 2010. Medications (NSAIDs, statins, proton pump inhibitors) and the risk of esophageal adenocarcinoma in patients with Barrett's esophagus. *Gastroenterology* **138:** 2260–2266.

42. Risques, R.A., T.L. Vaughan, X. Li, *et al.* 2007. Leukocyte telomere length predicts cancer risk in Barrett's esophagus. *Cancer Epidemiol., Biomarkers. Prev.* **16:** 2649–2655.

43. Xing, J., J.A. Ajani, M. Chen, *et al.* 2009. Constitutive short telomere length of chromosome 17p and 12q but not 11q

and 2p is associated with an increased risk for esophageal cancer. *Cancer Prev. Res.* **2:** 459–465.

44. Buttar, N.S., K.K. Wang, T.J. Sebo, *et al.* 2001. Extent of high-grade dysplasia in Barrett's esophagus correlates with risk of adenocarcinoma. *Gastroenterology* **120:** 1630–1639.

45. Wang, K.K., M. Wongkeesong & N.S. Buttar. 2005. American Gastroenterological Association Technical Review on the role of the gastroenterologist in the management of esophageal carcinoma. *Gastroenterology* **128:** 1471–1505.

46. Georgakoudi, I., B.C. Jacobson, J. Van Dam, *et al.* 2001. Fluorescence, reflectance, and light-scattering spectroscopy for evaluating dysplasia in patients with Barrett's esophagus. *Gastroenterology* **120:** 16.

47. Prasad, G.A., A. Bansal, P. Sharma & K.K. Wang. 2010. Predictors of progression in Barrett's esophagus: current knowledge and future directions. *Am. J. Gastroenterology* **105:** 1490–1502.

48. Junttila, M.R. & G.I. Evan. 2009. p53—a Jack of all trades but master of none. *Nat. Rev. Cancer* **9:** 821–829.

49. Schneider, P.M., A.G. Casson, B. Levin, *et al.* 1996. Mutations of p53 in Barrett's esophagus and Barrett's cancer: a prospective study of ninety-eight cases. *J. Thorac. Cardiovasc. Surg.* **111:** 323–331; discussion 331–3.

50. Madani, K., R. Zhao, H.J. Lim & A.G. Casson. 2010. Prognostic value of p53 mutations in esophageal adenocarcinoma: final results of a 15-year prospective study. *Eur. J. Cardiothorac. Surg.* **37:** 1427–1432.

51. Schneider, P.M., O. Stoeltzing, J.A. Roth, *et al.* 2000. P53 mutational status improves estimation of prognosis in pa-

tients with curatively resected adenocarcinoma in Barrett's esophagus. *Clin. Cancer Res.* **6:** 3153–3158.

52. Younes, M., R.M. Lebovitz, L.V. Lechago & J. Lechago. 1993. p53 protein accumulation in Barrett's metaplasia, dysplasia, and carcinoma: a follow-up study. *Gastroenterology* **105:** 1637–1642.

53. Weston, A.P., S.K. Banerjee, P. Sharma, *et al.* 2001. p53 protein overexpression in low grade dysplasia (LGD) in Barrett's esophagus: immunohistochemical marker predictive of progression. *Am J Gastroenterol* **96:** 1355–1362.

54. Murray, L., A. Sedo, M. Scott, *et al.* 2006. TP53 and progression from Barrett's metaplasia to oesophageal adenocarcinoma in a UK population cohort. *Gut* **55:** 1390–1397.

55. Giménez, A., A. Minguela, P. Parrilla, *et al.* 1998. Flow cytometric DNA analysis and p53 protein expression show a good correlation with histologic findings in patients with Barrett's esophagus. *Cancer* **83:** 641–651.

56. Wong, D.J., T.G. Paulson, L.J. Prevo, *et al.* 2001. p16(INK4a) lesions are common, early abnormalities that undergo clonal expansion in Barrett's metaplastic epithelium. *Cancer Res.* **61:** 8284–8289.

57. Maley, C.C., P.C. Galipeau, X. Li, *et al.* 2004. Selectively advantageous mutations and hitchhikers in neoplasms: p16 lesions are selected in Barrett's esophagus. *Cancer Res.* **64:** 3414–3427.

58. Galipeau, P.C., D.S. Cowan, C.A. Sanchez, *et al.* 1996. 17p (p53) allelic losses, 4N (G2/tetraploid) populations, and progression to aneuploidy in Barrett's esophagus. *Proc. Natl. Acad. Sci. U S A* **93:** 7081–7084.

Ann. N.Y. Acad. Sci. ISSN 0077-8923

ANNALS OF THE NEW YORK ACADEMY OF SCIENCES

Issue: *Barrett's Esophagus: The 10th OESO World Congress Proceedings*

Barrett's esophagus: prevalence and incidence of adenocarcinomas

Helen M. Shields,[1] Gerardo Nardone,[2] Jingjing Zhao,[3] Wen Wang,[4] Zheng Xing,[5] Dianchun Fang,[3] Brian C. Jacobson,[6] Yvonne Romero,[7] Katerina Dvorak,[8,9] Aaron Goldman,[9] Carlos A. Pellegrini,[10] Elizabeth L. Wiley,[11] David A. Peura,[12] Roger P. Tatum,[13] and Thomas G. Schnell[14]

[1]Gastroenterology Division, Harvard Medical School and Beth Israel Deaconess Medical Center, Boston, Massachusetts. [2]Department of Clinical and Experimental Medicine, Gastroenterology Unit, University "Federico II," Naples, Italy. [3]Department of Gastroenterology, Southwest Hospital, Third Military Medical University, Chongqing, China. [4]Department of Gastroenterology, 536 Hospital of PLA, Xining, China. [5]Department of Gastroenterology, Fuzhou PLA General Hospital, Fuzhou, China. [6]Section of Gastroenterology, Boston University Medical Center, Boston, Massachusetts. [7]Division of Gastroenterology and Hepatology, Department of Otolaryngology, and GI Outcomes Unit, Mayo Clinic, Rochester, Minnesota. [8]Department of Cell Biology and Anatomy, College of Medicine, The University of Arizona, Tucson, Arizona. [9]Arizona Cancer Center, The University of Arizona, Tucson, Arizona. [10]Department of Sugery, University of Washington School of Medicine, Seattle, Washington. [11]Department of Pathology, University of Illinois Chicago, Chicago, Illinois. [12]Division of Gastroenterology, University of Virginia Medical Center, Charlottesville, Virginia. [13]Department of Veterans Affairs Medical Center, University of Washington, Seattle, Washington. [14]Department of Medicine, Hines Veterans Affairs Hospital, Hines, Illinois.

The following on prevalence and incidence of adenocarcinomas in Barrett's esphophagus (BE) includes commentaries on the mechanisms of a potential protective effect of proton pump inhibitors (PPIs) on progression of BE to high-grade dysplasia; evaluation of the role of PPIs in decreasing the risk of degeneration; the geographical variations of incidence of BE; the role of the nonmorphologic biomarkers; the relationship between length of BE and development of cancer; the confounding factors in incidence rates of BE; the role of the increase of cell differentiation and apoptosis induced by PPIs in the diminution of cancer risk; the frequency of occult neoplastic foci and unsuspected invasive cancer in surgical specimens; the influence on the indications of endoscopic therapy; the overestimation of regression in surgical series; attempts to evaluate the reasons for variations of cancer incidence in the literature; and progress in screening and surveillance for BE.

Keywords: Barrett's epithelium; proton pump inhibitor therapy; low-grade dysplasia; adenocarcinoma; oxidative stress; cytokines; Barrett's esophagus; *Helicobacter pylori*; adipocytokines; esophageal cancer; cyclooxygenase; occult neoplasia; submucosal invasion; endoscopic treatment; esophagectomy; intramucosal carcinoma; high-grade dysplasia; short-segment and long-segment Barrett's esophagus; metaplasia; antireflux surgery

Concise summaries

- Compared with Western data, the endoscopic incidence of Barrett's esophagus (BE) is lower in the Chinese, but the average age of diagnosis is younger. The incidence of Barrett's adenocarcinoma among Chinese is similar to reports from Western countries.

- When interpreting incidence data, practice variation over time, quality control, and biology, like the trend for prolonged life expectancy and diminished competing causes of death, must be taken into account.

- The majority of the data compiled indicates that there is a trend for the highest risk of cancer to be associated with the longest lengths of Barrett's epithelium, but no large, prospective study demonstrates a definitively significant risk for cancer with longer lengths of Barrett's compared to shorter segments.

- The two most likely risk factors that might account for this rise in incidence of esophageal adenocarcinoma are the declining number of people infected with *Helicobacter pylori* and the growing number of overweight and obese

doi: 10.1111/j.1749-6632.2011.06054.x

individuals worldwide, and the most important public health steps to be taken to decrease the numbers of esophageal carcinoma cases in the future appear to be interventions aimed at reducing obesity.

- The results of studies investigating the effects of proton pump inhibitors (PPIs) on apoptosis are controversial and quite contradicting. PPIs inhibit H^+/K^+ ATPase, but potential other mechanisms of PPIs at cellular and molecular levels need to be further explored, especially in the context of long-term treatment.

- PPI treatment in BE provides not only the short-term benefit of symptom reduction and healing of esophagitis, but also the long-term chemoprevention benefits of reduced progression of dysplasia and cancer. The mechanisms through which PPIs affect the inflammatory immune response and related molecular alteration underlying the Barrett's metaplasia–dysplasia sequence are various and go beyond gastric acid inhibition.

- Randomized controlled trials are needed to provide definitive effects of acid suppressing medications in BE as chemopreventative agents against dysplasia and adenocarcinoma. The eagerly awaited randomized trial of PPIs in Barrett's called the Aspirin Esomeprazole Chemoprevention Trial (AspECT) is in progress, with the results due out in 2014.

- In patients with BE containing high-grade dysplasia (HGD), the risk of submucosal invasive adenocarcinoma is not as often as historically thought, which makes a trial of endoscopic therapy and follow-up surveillance more acceptable than esophagectomy. However, the presence of occult neoplasia with submucosal invasion in surgical specimens is probably not overestimated, but it remains important to understand what the diagnosis of HGD means in each individual case.

- The information comparing surgery and endoscopic treatment of HGD and early esophageal adenocarcinoma is scant and uncontrolled. Yet what is available suggests that expert endoscopists and expert surgeons can achieve similar short- and likely long-term, cancer-free survival rates, and one needs to balance the higher morbidity of surgery with the higher carcinoma recurrence of endoscopic therapy.

- For now, PPIs should be used to control symptoms or in conjunction with endoscopic treatment of patients with BE. More information is necessary to determine to what degree, if any, PPI use can obviate esophageal adenocarcinoma.

- The regression of low-grade dysplasia (LGD) to uncomplicated Barrett's metaplasia after antireflux surgery (ARS) is relatively common; even if the sample sizes are small in every report, the relatively high rates of LGD regression appear to be credible, confirming that ARS is a good option for the patient with Barrett's and LGD, with an expected chance of conversion to uncomplicated metaplasia somewhere in the vicinity of 67%.

- The interplay of several factors for the evaluation of cancer incidence can become quite complex as one factor may increase while another factor may decrease the incidence rate. Thus, it becomes easy to conclude that the reasons for the drastic variations of cancer incidence per patient year of follow-up in the literature are as varied as the incidence figures themselves. Most screening or surveillance studies have felt that the potential problems of lead time, length bias, and cost effectiveness have led to a rather pessimistic outlook on our ability to reduce mortality from esophageal cancer.

1. What is the effect of PPI therapy on the risk of neoplastic progression in patients with BE?

Helen M. Shields
hshields@bidmc.harvard.edu

Despite the fact that PPI therapy use has risen significantly over the past 15 years, the risk of adenocarcinoma of the esophagus has also risen significantly over the same time period. If PPIs were effective in decreasing the risk of neoplastic progression, why have we not seen a reduction rather than an increase in cancers of the esophagus in patients with Barrett's epithelium?

In 2004, El-Serag reported a retrospectively analyzed cohort of Barrett's patients from a single endoscopist's practice between 1981 and 2000 at the Southern Arizona Healthcare System.[1] These patients' pharmacy records regarding acid suppressive medication were retrieved.[1] A pathologist used standard criteria to identify dysplasia in biopsies.[1] The authors found that 56 patients were documented as having dysplasia, with 42 having LGD and 14 having HGD. Dysplasia developed in 9 of 19 patients on no PPI medication or H2RA, 25 of 64 patients on H2RA, and 22 of 155 patients on PPI therapy after the initial diagnosis of BE diagnosis.[1] These results indicated a highly significant diminution ($P < 0.001$) in the risk of developing dysplasia if the patient was on PPI therapy.[1] The same year, a study published from Australia, with Dr. Lybus Hillman as first author, examined in a prospective database, 350 patients with BE.[2] Patients who delayed beginning a PPI for two years after the diagnosis had 5.6 times the risk for developing LGD compared to those who used a PPI in the first year of the study.[2] Unfortunately, this study and El-Serag's were not randomized controlled trials.[1,2]

The diagnosis of LGD has been called into question by Curvers *et al.* recently as an "overdiagnosed and yet underestimated entity."[3] In their review of the diagnosis of LGD in BE, 85% of the patients with LGD were downgraded to nondysplastic or indefinite for dysplasia.[3] Only 15% of the patients kept the diagnosis of LGD.[3] Of these patients with a consistent diagnosis of LGD, the cumulative risk of progressing to HGD or carcinoma was 85% in 109 months compared with 4.6% in 107 months for patients who were down-staged to nondysplastic BE.[3]

In 2009, Nguyen *et al.* examined 344 patients with 236 patients coming from their original paper by El-Serag in 2004, along with 118 new patients added to the study and more follow-up time.[1,4] The authors concluded that PPI therapy significantly reduces the risk of cancer or HGD in patients with BE. Douglas Corley, in the editorial accompanying this paper, noted that randomized controlled trials are needed to accurately answer this question, and that the duration for the PPI therapy was only five years and one month, which may be too short an interval for the antineoplastic effects to be noted.[5] Corley felt that there was insufficient evidence to support the routine use of PPI therapy beyond that needed for symptom relief and mucosal healing.[5]

In summary, randomized controlled trials are needed to provide definitive effects of acid suppressing medications in BE as chemopreventative agents against dysplasia and adenocarcinoma. Why? Because the available studies have largely been retrospective with small numbers of patients who develop dysplasia, unclear starting points, not long enough intervals of PPI therapy, and not yet certain benefit.[5] The eagerly awaited randomized trial of PPIs in Barrett's called the AspECT is in progress with the results due out in 2014. At present, physicians should discuss with an individual patient what is known about PPIs and their possible effects on the risk of dysplasia, factor in the cost, and estimate specific risks of side effects over time for each patient, making an informed decision with the patient's help until better data are available.[5]

2. What are the mechanisms by which PPIs may exert a protective effect on the progression of BE, HGD, and carcinoma?

Gerardo Nardone
nardone@unina.it

The transformation of BE into EA occurs through a low and a high rate of cell dysplasia. This cellular transformation is triggered and sustained by gastric acid reflux that, through a complex inflammatory and immune response, induces a series of molecular alterations involving proliferation, apoptosis, cell differentiation, and angiogenesis. A large body of epidemiological data suggests that the reduction of esophageal acid exposure through chronic gastric acid inhibition, e.g., with long-term therapy with PPIs, decreases mucosal inflammation and might reverse metaplasia and the incidence of dysplasia and cancer. However, apart from gastric acid inhibition, the mechanisms through which PPIs may affect this cascade of molecular and cellular events are still poorly understood.

An important role in the progression of gastroesophageal reflux disease (GERD) has been attributed to the esophageal immunoregulatory environment and the response to oxidative stress.[6] Activation of the immune response leads to the release of cytokines and the related inflammatory mediators that trigger molecular and cellular alterations. Four and eight weeks of rabeprazole treatment in patients with esophagitis induced a significant decrease in the number of CD3$^+$ and CD8$^+$ T lymphocytes, in addition to mast cells and CD68 that are implicated in oxidative stress. Moreover, the mRNA level of interleukin 8 (IL-8), the main mediator of mucosal damage, which is upregulated in patients with GERD and is closely related to the severity of esophagitis, decreased dramatically after eight weeks of lansoprazole.[7] It is likely that PPIs suppress nuclear factor κ-B (NF-κB) signal transduction that upregulates the transcription and upregulation of IL-8.

Upregulation of IL-8 induces strong recruitment and activation of neutrophils. The activated neutrophils adhere to postcapillary venules and subsequently migrate to the interstitium. Among the adhesion molecules expressed on leucocytes, the CD11/CD18 integrin family plays a major role in the adhesion and transendothelial migration of neutrophils in *in vitro* and *in vivo* systems. In an *in vitro* system, lansoprazole and omeprazole, but not ranitidine or famotidine, suppressed the adhesion of polymorphonuclear leukocytes to the endothelium and their extravascular migration by inhibiting the expression of CD11b and CD18 on neutrophils and neutrophil adherence to endothelial cells. Although, the exact mechanism is still unclear, it is possible that PPIs exert a direct effect on NF-κB signal transduction pathways or on translocation and conformational changes of the CD11b/CD18 complex. In addition, recent studies have demonstrated that these effects are prevalently related to the blocking of vascular-type ATPase that, in turn, suppresses the intracellular calcium metabolism.

This finding suggests that PPIs exert antiinflammatory activity. As a consequence of chronic esophageal inflammation, reactive oxygen species (ROS) are generated, which in turn promote oxidative stress. Oxidative stress may result in the formation of DNA adducts that can initiate and promote carcinogenesis. Increased levels of DNA adducts have been observed along the metaplasia–dysplasia–adenocarcinoma sequence in Barrett's epithelium. However, four and eight weeks of rabeprazole did not affect levels of DNA adducts, quantified by measurement of 8-hydroxy-2-deoxyguanosinea in esophageal bioptic samples. Therefore, short-term PPI therapy in patients with esophagitis reduces the esophageal cellular immune response, but does not change oxidative DNA damage. This observation may partly explain why EA is found even after successful medical and surgical treatment for GERD.

As Barrett's epithelium progresses to dysplasia and adenocarcinoma, there is increased and uncoordinated cell proliferation and decreased cell differentiation. In BE, after six months of PPI therapy, a significant decrease of esophageal epithelia cell proliferation, measured by immunohistochemistry of the expression of proliferating nuclear cell antigen, was observed only when exposure to esophageal acid was well controlled.[8] Moreover, compared with H$_2$ receptor antagonists and antacids, PPI-induced acid suppression was associated with significantly lower expression levels of the key cell cycle proteins cyclin D1 and cyclin E, and higher levels of the cell death markers p16 and p21. Thus, in patients with BE, acid suppression decreased cell proliferation and induced apoptosis. Furthermore, effective intraesophageal acid suppression induced cell differentiation. The inverse relationship between cell proliferation and cell differentiation induced by effective intraesophageal acid suppression could, theoretically, lead to restoration of the cells that are altered in BE, that is, the areas of metaplasia and dysplasia. Indeed, a small, but statistically significant regression of BE in terms of both length and surface area was observed in patients treated with omeprazole (40 mg twice daily) with respect to patients treated with ranitidine (150 mg twice daily). Furthermore, PPI therapy is associated with a significant reduction in the risk of developing dysplasia in patients with BE. However, more studies are required to confirm this finding.

Therefore, the mechanisms through which PPIs affect the inflammatory immune response and related molecular alterations underlying the Barrett's metaplasia–dysplasia sequence are various and go beyond gastric acid inhibition. However, it is well known that a common side effect of long-term PPI therapy is hypergastrinemia that in turn may induce cell proliferation in BE metaplasia via prevention of apoptosis, activation of CCKR-2, and upregulation of cyclooxygenase-2 (COX-2).[9] An increased level of COX-2 has been reported in patients with BE treated with PPI.

Moreover, in an *in vitro* model, acid exposure exerted p53-mediated antiproliferative effects in a nonneoplastic Barrett's epithelial cell line. These findings contrast with the results of earlier studies and suggest that PPIs could be detrimental in patients with GERD in dosages beyond those required to heal mucosal damage. However, a recent study conducted with sophisticated *ex vivo, in vivo,* and *in vitro* approaches has shown that, while short-term treatment with gastrin enhances epithelial restitution in BE, there is no clinical evidence that BE length expands over time in patients treated with PPI.[10]

In conclusion, PPI treatment in BE not only provides the short-term benefit of symptom reduction and healing of esophagitis, but also the long-term chemoprevention benefits of reduced progression of dysplasia and cancer.

3. The endoscopic and clinico-pathological characteristics of BE in the Chinese population

Jingjing Zhao, Wen Wang, Zheng Xing, and Dianchun Fang
fangdianchun@hotmail.com

BE is characterized by the development of columnar line esophageal mucosa and is thought to be a premalignant condition that increases the esophageal adenocarcinoma (EAC) 30–40-fold.[11] EAC among white men has been increasing in incidence since the mid-1970s, and has replaced squamous cell carcinoma as the most common type of esophageal cancer in the United States and western Europe. Meta-analyses suggest that the risk for conversion from BE to EAC is 0.5% per year, and this conversion is thought to occur up to 15 years after diagnosis.[12] The rapid rise in the incidence of EAC has evoked greatly increased interest in BE, and it is being seen as a growing public health problem in Western countries. BE is considered to be one of the complications of GERD. In recent years, the prevalence of this disease is increasing in China, partly because of increasing usage of endoscopy and also due to a concomitant rise in GERD. However, in contrast with numerous studies about BE in industrialized countries, the endoscopic and clinico-pathological data on BE in China are very limited.

The aim of our preliminary study was to investigate the endoscopic and clinico-pathological characteristics of BE in Chinese patients undergoing an endoscopy for upper gastrointestinal symptoms in our three medical centers. A total of 253,542 consecutive patients undergoing an endoscopy for upper gastrointestinal symptoms in our three medical

centers from May 1, 2006 to December 30, 2008 were enrolled in the study. The frequencies of reflux symptoms, including heartburn and acid regurgitation were recorded. Other characteristic clinical data, including gender and, age were also recorded. All patients who agreed to participate in the study signed their informed consent. This study was approved by the Human Subjects Committee of the Third Military Medical University.

Endoscopy and biopsy samples
The upper endoscopy was performed by experienced endoscopists, who were blinded to the medical history and symptoms of patients and had reached a consensus about endoscopic assessment for BE. When a suspected CLE was found based on salmon-pink mucosa either in the circumferential upward shift of the SCJ or in the adjacent mucosal tongue or island samples were taken from the tubular esophagus including the mucosal tongue or island. In case of a circumferential segment, biopsy samples were taken from each of the four quadrants; at least one every 2 cm, and at least two samples from each tongue or island, respectively. The samples were fixed in 4% buffered formalin. The slides were stained with a combination of hematoxylineosin and Alcian Blue at pH 2.5, and then examined by an experienced pathologist. The diagnosis of BE was made according to the Montreal definition, any columnar epithelium (intestinal or nonintestinal) above the gastroesophageal junction was to be considered as BE.[13] The statistical analysis was performed using SPSS 13.0 software (SPSS Inc., Chicago, IL, USA). P-values less than 0.05 were considered statistically significant.

Results
Of 253,542 consecutive patients who received an endoscopy during the study period 4868 were diagnosed as BE. The prevalence of BE was 1.92%. Of these 4,868 BE patients 3,298 were males 1,570 were females with a ratio of 2.1:1. The age of BE patients was from 18~84 years with the average 51.2 years. The analysis of symptoms showed that only 74.5% of the subjects with BE had reflux symptoms, and there were no reflux symptoms in 25.5%.

Endoscopic characteristics
At endoscopy, BE was classified into circumferential type, island type, and tongue type. The percentage of circumferential-type was 25.7%, island-type BE was 54.5%, and tongue-type was 19.8%. Based

Table 1. The endoscopic-pathological characteristics of 4,868 BE cases.

Characteristics	Number of cases (%)
Endoscopic characteristics	
LSBE	1,051 (21.6)*
SSBE	3,797 (78.4)
Circumferential-type	1,251 (25.7)
Island-type	2,653 (54.5)**
Tongue-type	964 (19.8)
Pathological characteristics	
gastric fundic-type	1,724 (35.4)
cardiac-type	1,601 (32.9)
specialized intestinal metaplasia type	1,543 (31.7)

*Compared with SSBE, $P < 0.05$.

**Compared with tongue-type and circumferential-type BE, $P < 0.05$.

on the length of metaplasia columnar epithelium, the BE was divided into long segment BE (LSBE $\geq$ 3 cm in length) and short segment BE (SSBE less than 3 cm in length). The percentage of LSBE was 21.6% and SSBE was 78.4% (Table 1).

Histological characteristics

Three types of columnar epithelia could be detected in the columnar-lined esophagus: gastric-fundic type epithelium, cardiac type epithelium and distinctive specialized intestinal metaplasia (SIM)-type epithelium. The percentage of gastric fundic-type was 35.4%, cardiac-type was 32.9%, and SIM was 31.7% (Table 1). We also found that there were more males with SIM than females, with a ratio of 2.2 : 1. Furthermore, SIM was most common in tongue-type BE, in contrast with the island-type and the circumferential-type, and it was more observed in LSBE than in SSBE. The incidence of low-grade dysplasia in BE patients was 6.8%.

Complications and concomitant diseases

Of 4,868 patients hiatus hernia was found in 925 (19.0%) cases esophageal ulcer in 775 (15.9%) cases and esophageal stenosis in 1,457 (31.1%) cases. Endoscopic follow up ranged from 12.1 months to 4 years, and incidence of EAC was 0.43% (21/4,868).

We have performed a preliminary study and found that the prevalence of BE in 253,542 Chinese patients undergoing an endoscopy for upper gastrointestinal symptoms was 1.92%, lower than that in developed countries. The probable causes of

the difference are racial differences, variation in diet and lower prevalence of GERD, but other reasons may not be excluded, such as the higher prevalence of *H. pylori* infection in China, which may confer protection against development of BE. BE is a metaplasia that occurs in response to exposure to damaging agents, namely refluxate. About 10–15% of patients with GERD develop BE. In this study, although 74.5% of patients were found presenting GERD symptoms, there were 25.5% subjects without GERD symptoms (unpublished data). Therefore, it is crucial to avoid missed diagnosis for patients with BE without GERD symptoms. BE was more common in males than females, with a ratio of 2.1:1, similar to the European ratio of 2:1.[14] The median age of endoscopically diagnosed BE was 51.2 years in Chinese subjects, younger than in Europeans[14] (about 60 years), which should be considered with attention. In this study, island-type BE and SSBE were predominant, which is similar to the reports from other countries (unpublished data).

In recent years, a controversy has emerged about the clinical significance of SSBE. Although the LSBE with intestinal-type metaplasia is the most important identified risk factor for EAC, SSBE can also evolve to dysplasia and cancer, but the incidence of the development of cancer in SSBE is not fully defined. It is still argued for neglecting surveillance in SSBE, considering that SSBE represents a high proportion of BE. BE consists of a mixing of different epithelial cell types including gastric fundic, cardiac, and SIM types. There is a debate about the requirement for the presence of intestinal type cells to diagnose BE. The close relationship between SIM-type BE and EAC has been well investigated. In this study, the incidence of SIM was 31.7%. We also found that SIM was more common in males than in females, and most are tongue-type BE (unpublished data). Moreover, it was more often observed in LSBE than in SSBE. These results were consistent with others. BE represents an accepted risk factor for EAC, and the goal of the endoscopic follow up of patients with BE is to detect curable neoplasia; a follow-up was carried out in this study for one to four year and the incidence of EAC was 0.43% similar to 0.54% reported by Conio.[15] The data from our preliminary study suggest that more endoscopic surveillance on Barrett's patients, especially with dysplasia, is needed in the aim of decreasing the incidence of EAC in China.

In conclusion, compared with Western data, the endoscopic incidence of BE is lower in the Chinese, but the average age of diagnosis is younger (unpublished data). The incidence of BE developing EAC among the Chinese is similar to reports from Western countries. BE is more frequent in males than in females, and about a quarter of patients have no symptoms of GERD. Intestinal metaplasia is especially frequent in tongue-type BE and LSBE.

4. The rising incidence of adenocarcinoma of the esophagus

Brian C. Jacobson
brian.jacobson@bmc.org

Is there indeed a rising incidence of esophageal adenocarcinoma (EAC), and, if so, can we explain this rise? Is it possible that the observed increase in EAC incidence is simply due to greater use of surveillance endoscopy or a change in classifications of gastric cardia cancers to EAC?

If the former were true, we would expect to observe a shift to diagnoses made at earlier stages, or in younger patients. However, data show that there is indeed a rising incidence in EAC for all stages and for all age groups.[16] Furthermore, we have seen a rise in both cardia cancers and EAC simultaneously, making it unlikely that EAC has simply replaced what was called cardia cancer in the past.[17]

What factors might account for this rise in incidence of EAC? BE is the precursor lesion accounting for the overwhelming majority of EAC. We also know that the incidence of BE is rising, even after accounting for possible detection biases due to increased use of upper endoscopy. Therefore, what might account for increasing numbers of patients with BE?

The two most likely risk factors are the declining number of people infected with *H. pylori* and the growing number of overweight and obese individuals worldwide.

Chronic *H. pylori* infection results in atrophic gastritis, decreased acid production, and thus a lower likelihood for severe GERD. In fact, meta-analyses have shown that *H. pylori* infection is associated with lower rates of BE and EAC, particularly when considering the more virulent CagA-positive strain of the bacteria.[18] Therefore, as global rates of

H. pylori infection fall further, we may expect to see even greater numbers of patients with EAC.

Excess body fat, especially centrally located or visceral fat, is associated with greater risk for both BE and EAC.[19,20] This may relate to mechanical factors associated with greater intraabdominal fat, such as greater gastroesophageal pressure gradients, more frequent transient lower esophageal sphincter relaxations, or a greater likelihood for developing a hiatal hernia. However, there may also be hormonal reasons for this association. Adipocytokines produced predominantly by visceral fat have a host of properties potentially associated with neoplasia. Some examples include the angiogenic and antiapoptotic properties of leptin and the proliferative properties of adiponectin. Given the fact that men have much more visceral fat than women, these potential associations are an attractive explanation for why men are six to seven times more likely to develop EAC than women. Therefore, the rising incidence of EAC may also be explained by the global trend toward higher body mass index and increasing rates of obesity.

In summary, there is a very real rise in the incidence of EAC, and the most likely explanations include the obesity epidemic and declining rates of chronic *H. pylori* infection. Given the fact that the decrease in *H. pylori* probably accounts for the tremendous drop in gastric cancer observed over the last century, it is unlikely we will see proponents suggesting a return to greater rates of infection. Therefore, the most important public health steps to be taken to decrease the numbers of EAC cases in the future appear to be interventions aimed at reducing obesity.

5. What are the possible confounding factors that may influence cancer incidence rates?

Yvonne Romero
romero.yvonne@mayo.edu

As stated on the National Institutes of Health National Cancer Institute web site, "a cancer incidence rate is the number of new cancers of a specific site or type occurring in a specified population during a year, usually expressed as the number of cancers per 100,000 population at risk."[21] In developed countries, the incidence of adenocarcinoma

Table 2. Average human life expectancy over time

Period	Years
Neolithic	20
Roman	28
Medieval Britain	30
Early 20th century	30–45
Current world average	67.2

Adapted from Ref. 23.

of the esophagus and gastroesophageal junction have been exponentially increasing over the past 40 years.[22] It is not clear, however, if the incidence of BE, the neoplastic precursor of EAC, has changed. Although it is tempting to think of incidence as a simple and rigid mathematical construct, there are many potential confounding factors that influence the frequency with which a specific type of tumor is diagnosed. Two such factors are extended life expectancy and competing causes of death.

As demonstrated in Table 2, human life spans have been increasing in duration over time, particularly over the past 100 years, especially in developed countries.[23] Advances in clinical care, such as the advent of coronary artery bypass surgery and stenting, and societal changes in behavior, such as diminished use of tobacco products, have altered the natural history of the people most at risk for these neoplasms. In the United States in the 1950s, white non-Hispanic males commonly died in their fifth and sixth decade of life of acute coronary ischemic events. Given that these people now survive their atherosclerotic disease, they remain in the denominator (also termed the "population at risk") and are available to experience an esophagus cancer event with advancing age.

Additional confounding factors that have introduced bias into calculations of the incidence of specific upper gastrointestinal cancers over the past four decades have included changes in the clinical practice of gastroenterologists, surgeons, pathologists, and their staff;[24] physician awareness; and advances in technology.

In the 1970s, squamous cell carcinoma was the predominant histologic type of esophageal neoplasm. Investigators of the time chose to pool adenocarcinoma cases with squamous cell carcinoma cases, perhaps based on the assumption that adenocarcinoma would always be a rare neoplasm, perhaps because there were no tissue-specific treatment options, perhaps due to a sense of futility given the poor survival rates of both neoplasms, or perhaps because of the faulty assumption that pooling the different tumor types would increase their statistical power. Likewise, over the past 20 years, as the adenocarcinoma phenotype has become more common, there has been a trend for investigators to pool tubular esophageal neoplasms, with and without obvious background intestinal metaplasia with goblet cells (BE), with those of the gastric cardia and gastroesophageal junction, with the assumption that the neoplasms share identical underlying mechanisms and risk factors. It is potentially erroneous to assume that no insights will be gleaned by differentiating the location and histologic type of each neoplasm. With individualized medicine in the forefront, only time will show which assumptions were correct.

Physician and patient awareness of the association between GERD symptoms and esophagus cancer risk has altered the threshold for recommendation of endoscopy, and may contribute to diagnosis of esophagus cancer at an early asymptomatic and perhaps incidental stage, if the patient is destined to die from a competing cause (lead time bias).

Patient health care seeking behavior, and access to healthcare and endoscopy alter diagnosis and, hence, incidence rates. As endoscopes have improved their resolution over time, beginning with fiberoptic scopes, progressing to video endoscopes, high resolution endoscopy, and now narrow band imaging, autofluorescence imaging, and confocal microscopy, the endoscopist's ability to detect neoplasm has changed. These advances have not only altered the frequency with which neoplasm can be diagnosed, they have added to the complexity of assessing the incidence of BE. Beyond the scope of this presentation, epidemiologic factors, such as the prevalence of obesity and *H. pylori*, have altered the biology of disease.

Therefore, in conclusion, when interpreting incidence data, we must take practice variation over time, quality control, and biology, like the trend for prolonged life expectancy and diminished competing causes of death, into account. With these sources of bias in mind, there remains convincing evidence that the incidence of adenocarcinoma of the tubular esophagus and gastroesophageal junction both continue to increase in developed countries at this point in human history.

6. Is there a clear relationship between length of BE and cancer development?

Helen M. Shields
hshields@bidmc.harvard.edu

Although the early studies on length and BE indicated a clear relationship between length and cancer risk, these studies now appear flawed because they used an endoscopic diagnosis rather than histological diagnosis of Barrett's epithelium. More recent studies do not support an obvious linear relationship between length and cancer risk. Instead, they indicate variability of collected data from around the world and trends rather than definitive results.

A major study that looked at length, dysplasia and cancer risk was performed by Hirota in 1999.[25] His group found that 889 patients had twice the prevalence of dysplasia and/ or cancer in long segments of BE (greater than 3 cm) compared to short segment Barrett's ($P = 0.043$). A year later, Rudolph,[26] after studying 309 patients, noted that segment length was not related to risk for cancer. The risk for adenocarcinoma in short segment BE was not significantly lower than in patients with long segment Barrett's. However, a 5 cm difference in segment length was associated with a small increase in the risk for aneuploidy ($P = 0.06$, for trend). Rudolph suggested that, until more data were available, the frequency of endoscopic surveillance should be selected without regard to segment length.

In 2003, Gopal reviewed 309 patients records from a multicenter consortium where 90% of the patients were men.[27] Gopal found that the length of BE was significantly longer in patients with dysplasia. Those patients with ≥ 3 cm of Barrett's epithelium had a significantly greater prevalence of dysplasia compared to length <3 cm ($P = 0.0001$). Rising age was also a risk factor for increased chance of dysplasia. In 2004, Hage[28] from Rotterdam, the Netherlands, looked at all patients with >3 cm of length diagnosed between 1973 and 1984 who had had intestinal metaplasia diagnosed by histology. A longer length of Barrett's was associated with an increased risk of progression to cancer or adenocarcinoma ($P = 0.02$). When the risk of progression to cancer alone was evaluated, the results did not quite reach significance ($P = 0.06$).

In 2010, Wong and colleagues[29] reported that after evaluating 248 patients, between 1999 and 2005, a length of >3 cm was associated with the development of dysplasia ($P = 0.004$).

The risk of developing adenocarcinoma was also increased in patients with a length >3 cm ($P = 0.001$). In a abstract presented at the OESO meeting, Gatenby's group,[30] using the UK National BE Registry (UKBOR) from the United Kingdom, showed a trend in 828 patients for an increased incidence of adenocarcinoma with an increase in segment length ($P = 0.054$). The development of HGD plus adenocarcinoma did reach significance ($P = 0.031$).

In summary, the majority of the data compiled indicates that there is a trend for the highest risk of cancer to be associated with the longest lengths of Barrett's epithelium. Some variability of data is evident from the different countries reporting on this topic. No large, prospective study demonstrates a definitively significant risk for cancer with longer lengths of Barrett's compared to shorter segments. Shorter lengths and medium lengths can harbor a cancer or HGD. Thus, length has an effect on cancer risk in BE, but at present it is still not entirely clear how much of an effect length this is.

7. Might the effects of PPIs, by increasing cell apoptosis as well as reduction of COX-2 expression, be an indication of their role in the diminution of cancer risk?

Katerina Dvorak and Aaron Goldman
kdvorak@email.arizona.edu

BE is a premalignant condition that is linked to GERD and is associated with 30–125-fold increased risk of developing EA.[31] PPIs are very effective drugs that are mostly used for treatment of acid related disorders, including GERD, peptic and duodenal ulcers, and also BE. PPIs reduce acid secretion through inhibition of H^+/K^+ ATPase in parietal cells.

The majority of clinical studies show that PPI use is associated with a decreased risk of EAC or HGD development and suggest the beneficial effects of PPIs in Barrett's patients, including mucosal healing and possibly partial regression of BE.[32] However, several studies indicate that PPIs may increase risk of gastric and esophageal cancer. Therefore, it is important to evaluate in detail the acute and long-term effects of PPIs on signaling, proliferation, and cell death pathways in esophageal cells.

Apoptosis is a tightly controlled process of programmed cell death, and its dysregulation is linked to cancer development. Avoidance of apoptosis is one of the major characteristics of cancer. It is hypothesized that the normal squamous epithelium is exposed to gastric acid and/or hydrophobic bile acids during esophageal reflux. Although a short-term effect of bile acid exposure is induction of apoptosis, a longer-term effect of repeated high exposure to apoptosis-inducing agents appears to be selection for apoptosis resistant cells. These cells resistant to apoptosis have a growth advantage in the presence of agents that ordinarily induce apoptosis and will tend to proliferate to form a field of apoptosis resistant cells.

The results of studies investigating the effects of PPIs on apoptosis are controversial and quite contradictory. Several studies suggest that PPIs are potent antioxidants and protect gastric mucosa against inflammation and apoptosis by scavenging hydroxyl radicals.[32] On the other hand, Yeo *et al.* reported that lansoprazole at a concentration of 500 μM induces apoptosis in gastric cancer cells.[33]

Other studies show that PPIs induce apoptosis in Jurkat cells, B cell tumor cells, or hepatocytes. However, all these studies use relatively high concentrations of PPIs that are not physiological (~200 μM). After 40 mg oral dose of omeprazole, plasma peak concentrations are only ~1–2 μM. One study directly related to EAC reported that in neoplastic BE cells, 35 μM esomeprazole induces apoptosis through production of ROS.[34]

It is possible that PPIs' effects are specific to cancer cells. PPIs may produce an apoptotic response by dysregulation of intracellular pH. In cancer cells proton extrusion, activity is upregulated, and tumor cells are characterized by acidic extracellular pH and alkaline intracellular pH. Proteins that regulate intracellular pH are often upregulated in cancer cells such as H^+ ATPases and Na^+/H^+ exchanger. PPIs, by inhibiting proton pumps, decrease cytosolic pH, and this event can lead to caspase activation and, consequently, to apoptosis. It was shown that acidification precedes mitochondrial dysfunction and damaged mitochodria then may produce ROS. Furthermore, since PPIs are weak bases, the active protonated form of the drug will target the most acidic sites in the body, therefore, it is possible that PPIs may accumulate in acidic extracellular tumor environment where they induce apoptosis.

Now, the question is what are the long-term effects of PPIs on apoptosis in BE? The majority of cells adapt to stress conditions, such as oxidative stress, by upregulation of proteins and pathways that can inhibit apoptosis resulting from these stresses. PPIs therefore may be useful drugs for short-term treatment but not for long-term treatment, because apoptosis-resistant phenotype may develop in malignant and premalignant cells. In addition, if the mechanism of PPI-induced apoptosis indeed involves ROS in long-term scenarios, PPI-derived ROS may damage DNA and contribute to cancer progression.

As far as the effects of PPIs on COX-2 expression, from the literature, it appears that PPIs do not have any direct effect on the COX-2 expression in esophageal tissue. However, one study suggests that lansoprazole-induced mucosal protection through gastrin receptor-dependent upregulation of COX-2 in rats.[35]

In summary, PPIs are widely regarded as safe and effective drugs for the treatment of BE, however their effects on apoptosis induction are not exactly clear. PPIs inhibit H^+/K^+ ATPase, but potential other mechanisms of PPIs at the cellular and molecular level need to be further explored, especially in the context of long-term treatment.

8. Is the presence of foci of occult neoplasia with submucosal invasion in surgical specimens of esophagectomy for HGD overestimated?

Eelco B. Wassenaar and Carlos A. Pellegrini
pellegri@u.washington.edu

The easiest answer to the question posed above is that it is unknown. There are, however, a number of practical issues that should help the gastroenterologist and surgeon treating a patient with HGD. First, HGD may be a "marker" for the presence of EA. Chances of harboring an EAC in the presence of HGD are increased if the mucosa has nodules, if the HGD is multifocal, and whether it is the first examination in that patient.

Second, HGD also has the potential to develop into EAC. The debate currently is how to treat this entity. Intramucosal cancer is considered an endoscopically treatable disease, although the risk of lymph node involvement is not zero (3–4%).

Deeper invasion gives a higher risk of lymph node involvement.

In a case series from the Cleveland Clinic, 111 patients had esophagectomy for HGD, and 50 (45%) were found to have EAC.[36] Most of these were intramucosal cancers, but 20% had deeper invasion. There was no operative mortality. Occult neoplasia, including intramucosal lesions, in HGD specimens are found in approximately 40% of patients; and invasion of the submucosa is found in 7–17% of patients. In a recent review, submucosal or deeper invasion was reported in 12.7% of specimens.[37] It was shown that visible lesions increase the risk of submucosal invasion.

It is generally accepted that endoscopic treatment is less morbid than esophagectomy. Esophagectomy for HGD, on the other hand, has been shown to result in excellent quality of life with very low mortality and morbidity rates.[38,39] These rates seem to be lower compared to esophagectomy for EAC. Survival of these patients is excellent.

Many issues influence the decision process whether esophagectomy or endoscopic treatment gives a patient the best chance for a cure. The natural history of HGD is to progress to EAC, but regression has also been shown to occur. The pathologic diagnosis of HGD is not always clear or easy to establish.[40] Diagnosis is generally made through biopsies and is therefore a sample of the actual lesion with risk of underestimation. As mentioned before, a visible (nodular) lesion increases the risk of deeper invasion. The role of endoscopic ultrasound in diagnosing local disease and lymphadenopathy is not yet clearly defined. Once the diagnosis of HGD has been made, a weighing of the risks and benefits of the intervention has to be made taking into consideration the characteristics of the lesion and the individual patient.

The presence of occult neoplasia with submucosal invasion for HGD is probably not overestimated, but it remains important to understand what the diagnosis of HGD means in each individual case.

9. What is the true prevalence of unsuspected invasive cancer (submucosal invasion) in the esophageal specimens resected for HGD?

Yi Zhou and Elizabeth L. Wiley
ewiley@uic.edu

In patients with BE with a biopsy diagnosis of HGD, and then treatment with esophagectomy, the risk of having an unsuspected invasive EAC is thought to be around 40%. It is so high that performing a prophylactic esophagectomy has been one of the main management options. However, the role of surveillance versus esophagectomy on this topic has been debated in the literature for years, mainly because of the concern of the mortality rate from esophagectomy.

The good news now is that endoscopic ablative therapy and endoscopic mucosal resection are beginning to show success with eradication of the lesion in patients with BE with HGD, or intramucosal carcinoma (IMC). Although these treatment options may provide a nice compromise between esophagectomy and surveillance, a high risk of occult invasive adenocarcinoma would make these options less effective.

Recently, several studies have shown that by using strict and standardized definition, the risk of occult invasive EA in specimens resected for HGD is much lower than we thought. One review[41] of 23 studies on this topic in 2008 from the University of Chicago has shown that although the overall pooled average rate for invasive adenocarcinoma in the 23 studies was 39.9%, among 441 patients who underwent esophagectomy due to HGD, only 14 studies had differentiated submucosal invasion versus IMC. Of those 14 studies, 12.7% of the 213 patients actually had submucosal invasion at esophagectomy.

In 2009, another study[42] from Brigham and Women's Hospital and the UCLA medical center reported that, over a 20 year period, in 60 patients with BE containing HGD or IMC treated with esophagectomy, the overall rate of submucosal invasive cancer was 6.7%. Interestingly, of those 60 patients, 19 patients had preoperative biopsy diagnosis of IMC, only two (11%) of them were found to have submucosal invasive cancer. It is still far less than "40%" prevalence.

Both studies applied strict definitions of invasive EA. It is important to highlight the difference between intramucosal and submucosal disease, because submucosal invasion confers a risk of node metastasis around 25%, which makes local therapy inappropriate. Although IMC invoving the esophagus is unique, there is small risk of nodal metastasis of 3–4%; however, it is considered minimal. Furthermore, thanks to the better imaging surveillance, we know that visible lesions in BE with HGD are associated with high risk of submucosal invasion, which will enable physicians to individualize risk of cancer. Better imaging screening surveillance has decreased the rate of unsuspected invasive EAC in specimens resected for BE with HGD.

In summary, in patients with BE containing HGD, the risk of submucosal invasive adenocarcinoma is around 12%, not as often as historically thought, which makes a trial of endoscopic therapy and follow-up surveillance more acceptable than esophagectomy.

10. In spite of the current dramatic increase in the incidence of adenocarcinoma, has a lower prevalence of concomitant adenocarcinoma in HGD led to a shift in treatment favoring endoscopic therapy? Is the compared rate of long-term cancer development with PPI therapy alone or associated to endoscopic treatments currently available?

David A. Peura
dap8v@virginia.edu

The incidence of EAC has been on the rise in Western countries, but recent data suggest that the rate increase may have peaked. The reason for this is unclear, but it is possible that the impact of things such as GERD and obesity has reached its limit. Other possible explanations include a changing natural history of transition to EAC, more frequent exposure to possible protective factors (PPIs), or better detection of early stage disease prompting more timely intervention.

GERD is a recognized risk factor for EAC, with BE serving as an intermediary stage in carcinogenesis. Metaplastic Barrett's epithelium appears to progress through stages of dysplasia (which may be reversible) and mucosal cancer before transformation to later stage invasive malignancy. The time course and events involved in this sequence are not completely understood but periodic endoscopic surveillance and reduction of esophageal acid exposure are key components to BE management. The hope is that acid reduction might slow progression to dysplasia and endoscopy might detect dysplasia and EAC at an early stage when potential cure is still possible.

Traditionally, HGD and EAC have been managed surgically (esophagectomy), an approach that is associated with significant morbidity, mortality, and reduced quality of life even when operations are performed in centers of excellence. Emerging endoscopic technologies permit more accurate diagnosis of BE (narrow band, high resolution, and magnified imaging), enable better tissue sampling and staging (endoscopic mucosal resection and ultrasonography), and allow for ablation of metaplasia, dysplasia, and even mucosal EAC (photodynamic therapy, cryotherapy, and radiofrequency ablation). These techniques are all better tolerated than surgery, but they are relatively new, and their clinical utility and long term effectiveness in the management of BE are being defined.

Confusion surrounding BE confounds any comparative evaluation of management strategies. For example, more endoscopic screening/surveillance, better tools, and different definitions can influence prevalence and clinical outcomes. Is BE defined by columnar or specialized intestinal epithelium? Is the risk for HGD/EAC similar with long and short segment BE? Are the implications of flat, nodular, focal, and diffuse dysplasia the same? Poor agreement with the histologic diagnosis of dysplasia (even BE itself) make clinical progression difficult to assess. Is the reported variability in the natural history of HGD ($<15\%$ to $>50\%$ progression to EAC) due to progression, regression, or incomplete sampling?

The information comparing surgery and endoscopic treatment of HGD and early EAC is scant and uncontrolled. Yet, what is available suggests that expert endoscopists and expert surgeons can achieve similar short- and likely long-term cancer free survival rates. One needs to balance the higher morbidity of surgery with the higher EAC recurrence of endoscopic therapy. The results in the hands for "nonexpert" surgeons and endoscopists are not known.

Ablative therapy (most often followed by maintenance PPI treatment) can achieve complete sustained remission of Barrett's dysplasia (both HGD and LGD) in approximately 80% of cases during one to two years of follow-up. Complete remission of metaplastic Barrett's epithelium is also possible about 70% of the time using endoscopic ablation. Persistent IM, dysplasia, and possible subsquamous IM, carry a residual cancer risk albeit reduced. Therefore, lacking long-term controlled data to determine how effectively endoscopic treatments will prevent EAC, continued surveillance will still be needed for most individuals whose BE is managed endoscopically.

Similarly, there are insufficient long-term data with PPIs used alone to determine if they significantly affect development of EAC. PPIs may prevent (but not totally) or slow progression of BE to dysplasia and EAC. Used alone, they can possibly promote regression of HGD but not entirely prevent its progression to EAC. For now, PPIs should be used to control symptoms or in conjunction with endoscopic treatment of patients with BE. More information is necessary to determine to what degree if any PPI use can obviate EAC (Selected reading: see Refs. 43–45).

11. May the inappropriate consideration of inflammation as LGD be a reason for overestimation of regression rates in surgical series?

Roger P. Tatum
rtatum@u.washington.edu

Over the last 20 or more years, numerous reports have examined the issue of whether or not ARS results in the regression or eradication of Barrett's metaplasia over time. While symptomatic relief persists in 75% or more of patients with Barrett's after ARF in long-term follow-up,[47–52] improvement or disappearance of metaplasia is observed in a relative minority of subjects. In fact, most series claim a rate of regression for Barrett's metaplasia to normal epithelium in 14–33% of patients after one or more years of follow-up after surgery.[49–51,53,54] In general, those patients with short-segment (i.e., ≤3 cm) Barrett's appear to be far more likely to experience complete regression than those with long-segment disease,[47,51] and regression correlates with effective acid reflux control as demonstrated on follow-up pH testing.[50]

In Barrett's patients who are found to have LGD, the question of regression more typically involves a change from findings of dysplasia prior to surgery to findings of intestinal metaplasia alone. While the implications of such an improvement are significant in the potential to reduce the progression of metaplasia to EAC, this likely represents a less dramatic transformation than the eradication of metaplasia

altogether. In those series in which such a transformation is reported, therefore, the percentage of patients who go from having a histologic diagnosis of Barrett's with LGD to uncomplicated Barrett's metaplasia alone after ARF is typically much higher, anywhere from 44% to 93%.[48,49,51,53–55] Such variability in the regression rates of LGD may be attributable to a number of factors, not the least of which is that all of these studies tend to include only a small subset of patients who have LGD. This is not surprising, as only approximately 10% of patients with Barrett's have histologic findings consistent with LGD in the first place.[55]

Further complicating this issue is the fact that there is frequent disagreement amongst pathologists as to what LGD represents. The histologic classification of Barrett's can be divided into negative for dysplasia; indefinite for dysplasia, in which there are nuclear alterations but typically there is associated inflammation; LGD, in which there are also nuclear changes but little to no inflammation; and HGD, with striking nuclear alterations as well as many other abnormal cell characteristics. Interobserver agreement between different pathologists tends to be relatively high for the ends of the spectrum, but for indefinite and LGD, agreement is substantially lower, with κ scores of 0.15 and 0.32, respectively.[56]

Thus, the presence of inflammatory changes within a biopsy specimen can indeed make a determination of LGD difficult, particularly if a specimen is only reviewed by a single pathologist.

Therefore, when reviewing studies reporting the regression of LGD to Barrett's negative for dysplasia, perhaps some caution in the interpretation of the results is warranted. This is ameliorated to a large degree, however, in those studies in which the method of histologic diagnosis is well described, particularly in those in which either the same pathologist reviewed all specimens or when some measure was taken to control for interobserver variability. For example, in the report of Rossi *et al.* demonstrating a 93.8% regression rate, the same pathologist reviewed each specimen twice, with one of the examinations being performed in blinded fashion;[55] in a series from O'Riordan *et al.*, in which six of eight patients with LGD exhibited regression, two independent pathologists evaluated each biopsy.[50] Another notable feature of some studies is that progression to LGD from nondysplastic metaplasia is also reported in a small percentage of patients, typically 6% or less,[47,48,50] thus giving the impression that the diagnosis of LGD is somewhat balanced, and not simply overdiagnosed in the preoperative setting.

In conclusion, the regression of LGD to uncomplicated Barrett's metaplasia after ARS is relatively common, seen in over half of patients with LGD reported in surgical series of the last decade. Notably, the sample sizes are small in every report, with a maximum of less than 20 LGD patients, reflecting the relatively small subset of Barrett's patients with this histologic finding. Inflammatory changes in the mucosa can make the histologic diagnosis difficult, often leading to an indefinite diagnosis of dysplasia, and interobserver agreement for the finding of LGD is historically low in comparison to HGD.

However, in those studies in which the histologic method of diagnosis is well described, and, in particular, where steps have been taken to account for interobserver variability, which includes those with higher numbers of LGD patients, the relatively high rates of LGD regression appear to be credible and likely representative of the true state of affairs, confirming that ARS is a good option for the patient with Barrett's and LGD, with an expected chance of conversion to uncomplicated metaplasia somewhere in the vicinity of 67%.

12. What are the reasons for the drastic variations of cancer incidence per patient year of follow-up in the literature?

Thomas G. Schnell

thomas.schnell@va.gov

This question implies that there truly is a wide variation in the reported incidence of adenocarcinoma of the esophagus (if there is not then this will be a very brief report.) Fortunately for the author, the reported incidence of adenocarcinoma of the esophagus does vary from a high of 4.0%/year to a low of 0 cases/year.[57]

For some of the reasons to be discussed, an incidence of 0%, while limiting worry about getting cancer to only the most neurotic patients, is unlikely to be true: while a 4% incidence of cancer/year would alarm even the most stoic of patients and is also not likely true. The most frequently quoted estimate of cancer incidence is in the range of 0.5–0.6%/year, with many studies clustering around this estimate.[57,58]

Some of this variation may represent real differences in incidence rates from one population to another, and some of the variation may be due to differences in the methodology of the study. It is important to realize that depending on population related factors (i.e., the population studied), there may be no single correct answer or rate.

To understand the reasons for the variation it is necessary to look beyond the bottom line of the reported rate and look at the details of the study. While it would take an exhaustive tome to cover all of the factors that could play a role, the most important factors can be found on an "Epidemiology 101" level. Although most of these are obvious, the obvious can get overlooked if only the bottom line of the cancer incidence rate is looked at.

For this brief discussion, it is convenient to lump the various factors into the groups of population-based differences and study or paper-related differences. For example, it is known that sex, race, and age make large differences in cancer risk in this disease.[59]

Adenocarcinoma in BE is known to be a cancer of white middle-aged and older males, so for studies to be comparable the proportion of these groups in the population studied should be comparable. There is also a wide geographic variation with a reported incidence of 0.6% in Scotland and 0% in Thailand in southeast Asia.[60] On the population level, it is important to note whether the study is a true population based study or a single center study. A study from a referral center might be expected to have a larger proportion of patients referred because they were felt to be at risk for cancer (referral bias), and thus a higher incidence rate, whereas a study done from a more primary care type of center might be expected to more closely reflect the rate of the population in that area.

While population based differences are easier to notice, the study or paper-related factors may be a bit more subtle. As the saying goes, the "devil is in the details," and many potential devils must be looked at. Is the study prospective or retrospective? Obviously, prospective studies are subject to fewer biases, but true prospective studies take time, while retrospective studies can be done on already existing data.

A very basic question is what the definition of Barrett's is? Is it a visual Barrett's or a histological Barrett's, including any type of columnar mucosa or only intestinal metaplasia? Although there is some controversy, the presence of intestinal metaplasia is felt to carry the highest risk, so, in ascending order of expected incidence rates, studies with visual Barretts, studies using any type of columnar mucosa, and those using only intestinal metaplasia would be expected to show differing incidence rates.

Since the length of the Barretts segment may be a risk factor, does the study include any length of Barrett's or only so-called long (>3 cm with presumably higher risk) segments? What are the starting and ending points? A study that includes only Barrett's with no dysplasia would be expected to have a lower cancer incidence than one including patients with preexisting dysplasia. A study with an end point of invasive cancer would be expected to have a lower incidence than one with an end point that included HGD, and a study that used only clinically symptomatic cancers would have an even lower cancer incidence. Also playing into this factor is how hard the authors looked for the cancers? As the maxim goes, "seek and ye shall find."

Studies with regular surveillance would be expected to yield a higher cancer incidence than a study that included only clinically evident cancers.[61] How incidence is defined also plays a role. If a study includes all cancers noted within a brief time after the diagnosis, then some of these cancers were likely prevalence cancers that were present, but missed, on the initial EGD. Including the prevalent cancers would inflate the cancer incidence. Most would consider one year a reasonable period to separate prevalent from incident cancers. How large is the study? While bigger is not always better, based on the number alone, studies with smaller numbers show a wider range of incidence rates than larger studies.[58] Publication bias, or the tendency to publish studies with extreme or newsworthy results, may also play a role, but this question has no definite answer at present.[57,58] While not as well documented, there are some hints that treatment with PPIs may decrease the cancer risk and, thus, the expected cancer incidence.

The interplay of these factors can become quite complex as one factor may increase while another factor may decrease the incidence rate. Thus it becomes easy to conclude that the reasons for the drastic variations of cancer incidence per patient year of follow-up in the literature are as varied as the incidence figures themselves.

13. Given the best screening/surveillance possible, how much could we expect to decrease esophageal cancer mortality?

Thomas G Schnell

thomas.schnell@va.gov

Given the high mortality rate of EAC, which, in most cases, is felt to arise from BE, screening to find patients with Barrett's, and then surveillance at regular intervals to find early curable cancer or its dysplastic precursors, seems a logical pursuit. As with all screening and surveillance programs, there are the potential problems of lead time and length bias and no fewer than 59 other types of potential biases that must be overcome.

However, the main problems arise due to the low prevalence of esophageal cancer as compared to breast, prostate, or colorectal cancer, which makes screening and surveillance less likely to be cost effective for large populations. In addition, the split between squamous and adenocarcinomas of the esophagus is usually felt to be approximately 50/50, which eliminates half of the cancers from consideration, since at least in the Western world, there are no currently available guidelines for screening for or surveillance of squamous cancer of the esophagus.

The next problem faced is that it is widely held that up to 40% of patients with adenocarcinoma have no symptoms of GERD that would lead them to be screened in the first place. The next hurdle is that, even with screening and surveillance, not all cancers will be detected at a curable stage. Even cancers that can be resected for cure carry the high mortality of esophagectomy (2% in centers, 10–15% in low volume hospitals). It is no surprise then that most screening or surveillance studies have felt that such efforts would not be cost effective and would have little impact on mortality from esophageal cancer.[62] These difficulties have lead to a rather pessimistic outlook on our ability to reduce mortality from esophageal cancer. Is there a way to look at currently available data and come up with a more optimistic view?

Using cancer data from the United States, there are predicted to be 16,640 cases of esophageal cancer and 14,400 deaths from esophageal cancer in 2010.[63] Using the pessimistic numbers, half of these would be squamous cancers for which no screening/surveillance has even been contemplated in the

United States, thus, leaving us with 7,200 deaths to be prevented. If 40% of these cases are asymptomatic, we have no way of finding them for screening and surveillance, leaving us with 4,320 deaths to be prevented.

This small number can be made even smaller by factoring in the less than perfect success rates reported from existing surveillance programs, the mortality rates for esophagectomy, and other factors that are beyond this brief review. However, these numbers, although extremely important to the patients with the cancers, are too small to be deemed cost effective in any large scale screening/surveillance programs.

It is known that in Western countries the proportion of esophageal cancers that are adenocarcinomas has been rising, and in one recent report adenocarcinoma comprised 83% of esophageal cancers resected.[64] The widely quoted figure that 40% of patients with adenocarcinoma of the esophagus have no symptoms of reflux comes from two important studies. In the landmark study by Lagergren *et al.*,[65] patients were only asked about GERD symptoms in the last five years. Since it is known that in some patients the presence of Barretts decreases the acid sensitivity of the esophagus, it is possible that some of the "asymptomatic" patients had GERD symptoms in the more distant past. In the study by Ronkainen *et al.*,[66] patients were considered symptomatic if they had symptoms that were "at least troublesome during the past three months," thus excluding symptoms from an earlier time. While it is difficult to be certain of the exact percentage of these strictly defined "asymptomatic" patients who had some GERD symptoms, it is certainly lower than the widely quoted 40%.

Using the 85% adenocarcinoma figure, and a more optimistic estimate that only 20% of patients who have adenocarcinoma of the esophagus have no preceding GERD symptoms, leaves us with 9,792 deaths (or 68% of the total esophageal cancer deaths) that may be preventable. Although still small compared to the deaths expected from the more common cancers, such a number would make cost effectiveness estimates closer to acceptable even in groups larger than the known risk group (white males aged 50 or greater with chronic GERD symptoms).[67]

While not yet proven, there is some evidence that patients diagnosed while on a surveillance program do have reduced mortality from EAC. Progress is being made in attempting to identify high risk groups within the larger population of patients with Barrett's (methylation markers and improvements in flow cytometry), which will make surveillance more effective and efficient.

Widespread screening based on GERD symptoms has much more progress to be made. Given the plethora of newer imaging and potential screening techniques being evaluated, screening should become more effective in the future. Combining more optimistic estimates with progress in screening and surveillance and the newer endoscopic techniques for treating early stage cancers and dysplasia (which should reduce the need for high risk esophagectomies), there is room for some optimism in this thus far dark field.

Conflicts of interest

The authors declare no conflicts of interest.

References

1. El-Serag, H. B., T. V. Aguirre, S. Davis, *et al.* 2004. Proton pump inhibitors are associated with reduced incidence of dysplasia in Barrett's esophagus. *Am. J. Gastroenterol.* **99:** 1877–1883.

2. Hillman, L.C., L. Chiragakis, B. Shadbolt, *et al.* 2004. Proton pump inhibitor therapy and the development of dysplasia in patients Effect of proton pump inhibitors on markers of risk with Barrett's oesophagus. *MJA* **180:** 3871–3391.

3. Curvers, W. L., F.J. ten Kate, K. K. Krishnadath, *et al.* 2010. Low-grade dysplasia in Barrett's esophagus: overdiagnosed and underestimated *Am. J. Gastroenterol.* **109:** 1523–1530.

4. Nguyen, D.M., H.B. El-Serag, L. Henderson, *et al.* 2009. Medication usage and the risk of neoplasia in patients with Barrett's esophagus. *Clin. Gastroenterol. Hepatol.* **7:** 1299–1303.

5. Corley, D. 2009. Chemoprevention in Barrett's esophagus: are we there yet, are we there yet...? *Clin. Gastroenterol. Hepatol.* **7:** 1266–1268.

6. Yoshida, N. 2007. Inflammation and oxidative stress in gastroesophageal reflux disease. *J. Clin. Biochem.* **40:** 13–23.

7. De Jonge, P.J.F., P.D. Siersema, S.G.J. Van Breda, *et al.* 2008. Proton pump inhibitor therapy in gastro-oesophageal reflux disease decreases the oesophageal immune response but does not reduce the formation of DNA adducts *Aliment. Pharmacol. Ther.* **28:** 127–136.

8. Quatu-Lascar, R., R.C. Fitzgerald & G. Triadafilopoulos. 1999. Differentiation and proliferation in Barrett's esophagus and the effcts of acid suppression. *Gastroenterology* **117:** 327–335.

9. Umansky, M., W. Yasui, A. Hallak, *et al.* 2001. Proton pump inhibitors reduce cell cycle abnormalities in Barrett's esophagus. *Oncogene* **29:** 7987–7991.

10. Obszynska, JA., P.A. Atherfold, M. Nanji, *et al.* 2010. Long-term proton pump induced hypergastrinaemiadoes induce lineage-specific restitution but not clonal expansion in benign Barrett's oesophagus in vivo. *Gut* **59:** 156–163.

11. Shaheen, N.J. & J.E. Richter. 2009. Barrett's oesophagus. *Lancet* **373:** 850–861.

12. Brown, L.M., S.S. Devesa & W.H. Chow. 2008.Incidence of adenocarcinoma of the esophagus among white Americans by sex, stage, and age. *J. Natl. Cancer Inst.* **100:** 1184–1187.

13. Vakil, N., S.V. van Zanten, P. Kahrilas, *et al.* 2006. Global Consensus Group. The Montreal definition and classification of gastroesophageal reflux disease: a global evidence-based consensus. *Am. J. Gastroenterol.* **101:** 1900–1920.

14. Caygill, C.P., A. Watson, P.I. Reed, *et al.* 2003. Characteristics and regional variations of patients with Barrett's oesophagus in the UK. *Eur. J. Gastroenterol. Hepatol.* **15:** 1217–1222.

15. Conio, M., S. Blanchi, G. Lapertosa, *et al.* 2003. Long-term endoscopic surveillance of patients with Barrett's esophagus. Incidence of dysplasia and adenocarcinoma: a prospective study. *Am. J. Gastroenterol.* **98:** 1931–1939.

16. Brown, L.M., S.S. Devesa & W.H. Chow. 2008. Incidence of adenocarcinoma of the esophagus among white Americans by sex, stage, and age. *J. Natl. Cancer Inst.* **100:** 1184–1187.

17. Pohl, H. & H.G. Welch. 2005. The role of overdiagnosis and reclassification in the marked increase of esophageal adenocarcinoma incidence. *J. Natl. Cancer Inst.* **97:** 142–146.

18. Islami, F. & F. Kamangar. 2008. *Helicobacter pylori* and esophageal cancer risk: a meta- analysis. *Cancer Prev. Res.* **1:** 329–338.

19. Edelstein, Z. *et al.* 2007. Central adiposity and risk of Barrett's esophagus. *Gastroenterology*. **133:** 403–411.

20. Whiteman, D. *et al.* 2008. Combined effects of obesity, acid reflux and smoking on the risk of adenocarcinomas of the oesophagus. *Gut*. **57:** 173–180.

21. http://www.cancer.gov/statistics/glossary/incidence.

22. Pohl, H. *et al.* 2005. *J. Natl. Cancer Inst.* **97:** 142–146; doi:10.1093/jnci/dji024.

23. Dean koontz, life expectancy, Wikipedia 2010. http://en.wikipedia.org/wiki/life_expectancy.

24. Crane, S.J., G.R. III Locke, W.S. Harmsen, *et al.* 2007. Subsite-specific risk factors for esophageal and gastric adenocarcinoma. *Am. J. Gastroenterol.* **102:** 1596–1602. UI: 17459024.

25. Hirota, W.K., T.M. Loughney, D.J. Lazas, *et al.* 1999. Specialized intestinal metaplasia, dysplasia, and cancer of the esophagus and esophagogastric junction: prevalence and clinical data. *Gastroenterology* **116:** 277–285.

26. Rudolph, R.E., T.L. Vaughan, B.E. Storer, *et al.* 2000. Effect of segment length on Risk for neoplastic progression in patients with Barrett esophagus. *Ann. Intern. Med.* **132:** 612-620.

27. Gopal, D.V., D.A. Lieberman, N. Magaret, *et al.* 2003. Risk factors for dysplasia in patients with Barrett's esophagus.(BE). Results from a multicenter consortium. *Dig. Dis. Sci.* **48:** 1537–1541.

28. Hage, M., P.D. Siersema, H. van Dekken, *et al.* 2004. Oesophageal cancer incidence and mortality in patients with long-segment Barrett' s oesophagus after a mean follow-up of 12.7 years. *Scand. J. Gastroenterol.* **39:** 1175–1179.

29. Wong, T., J. Tian & A.B. Nagar. 2010. Barrett's surveillance identifies patients with early esophageal adenocarcinoma. *Am. J. Med.* **123:** 462–467.

30. Gatenby, P., J. Ramus, C. Caygill, *et al.* 2010. Columnar-lined esophagus segment length and high-grade dysplasia and adenocarcinoma risk. OESO Abstract, Boston.

31. Falk, G.W. 2002. Barrett's esophagus. *Gastroenterology* **122:** 1569–91.

32. Kedika, R.R., R.F. Souza, S.J. Spechler. 2009. Potential anti-inflammatory effects of proton pump inhibitors: a review and discussion of the clinical implications. *Dig. Dis. Sci.* **54:** 2312–2317.

33. Yeo, M., D.K. Kim, Y.B. Kim, *et al.* 2004. Selective induction of apoptosis with proton pump inhibitor in gastric cancer cells. *Clin. Cancer Res.* **10:** 8687–8696.

34. Hormi-Carver, K.K., X. Zhang, X. Huo, *et al.* 2010. W1881 in neoplastic Barrett's epithelial cells, esomeprazole induces apoptosis through the production of reactive oxygen species: a potential role for PPIs in the chemotherapy of Barrett's Cancer. *Gastroenterology* **138:** S-758.

35. Tsuji, S., W.H. Sun, M. Tsujii, *et al.* 2002. Lansoprazole induces mucosal protection through gastrin receptor-dependent up-regulation of cyclooxygenase-2 in rats. *J. Pharmacol. Exp. Ther.* **303:** 1301–1308.

36. Rice, T.W. 2006 Pro: esophagectomy is the treatment of choice for high-grade dysplasia in Barrett's esophagus. *Am. J. Gastroenterol.* **101:** 2177–2179.

37. Konda, V.J., A.S. Ross, M.K. Ferguson, *et al.* 2008. Is the risk of concomitant invasive esophageal cancer in high-grade dysplasia in Barrett's esophagus overestimated? *Clin. Gastroenterol. Hepatol.* **6:** 159–164.

38. Williams, V.A., T.J. Watson, F.A. Herbella, *et al.* 2007. Esophagectomy for high grade dysplasia is safe, curative, and results in good alimentary outcome. *J. Gastrointest. Surg.* **11:** 1589–1597.

39. Chang, L.C., B.K. Oelschlager, E. Quiroga, *et al.* 2006. Long-term outcome of esophagectomy for high-grade dysplasia or cancer found during surveillance for Barrett's esophagus. *J. Gastrointest. Surg.* **10:** 341–346

40. Overholt, B.F., C.J. Lightdale, K.K. Wang, *et al.* 2005. Photodynamic therapy with porfimer sodium for ablation of high-grade dysplasia in Barrett's esophagus: international, partially blinded, randomized phase III trial. *Gastrointest. Endosc.* **62:** 488–498.

41. Kinda, V.J., A.S. Ross, M.K. Ferguson, *et al.* 2008. Is the risk of concomitant invasive esophageal cancer in high-grade dysplasia in Barrett's esophagus overestimated? *Clin. Gastroenterol. Hepatol.* **6:** 128–129.

42. Wang, V.S., J.L. Hornick, J.A. Sepulveda, *et al.* 2010. Low prevalence of submucosal invasive carcinoma at esophagectomy for high-grade dysplasia or intramucosal adenocarcinoma in Barrett's esophagus: a 20-year experience. *Gastrointest. Endosc.* **71:** 429.

43. Pohl, H., B. Sirovich & H.G. Welch. 2010. Esophageal adenocarcinoma incidence: are we reaching the peak? *Cancer Epidemiol. Biomarkers Prev.* **19:** 1468–1470.

44. Yousef, F., C. Cardwell M.M. Cantwell, *et al.* 2008. The incidence of esophageal cancer and high-grade dysplasia in

Barrett's esophagus: a systematic review and meta-analysis. *Am. J. Epidemiol.***168:** 237–249.

45. Shaheen, N.J. & D.J. Frantz. 2010. When to consider endoscopic ablation therapy for Barrett's esophagus. *Curr. Opin. Gastroenterol.* **26:** 361–366.

46. El-Serag, H.B., T.V. Aguirre, S. Davis, *et al.* 2004. Proton pump inhibitors are associated with reduced incidence of dysplasia in Barrett's esophagus. *Am. J. Gastroenterol.* **99:** 1877–1883.

47. Bowers, S.P., S.G. Mattar, C.D. Smith, *et al.* 2002. Clinical and histologic follow-up after antireflux surgery for Barrett's esophagus. *J. Gastrointest. Surg.* **6:** 532–538; discussion 539.

48. Hofstetter, W.L., J.H. Peters, T.R. DeMeester, *et al.* 2001. Long-term outcome of antireflux surgery in patients with Barrett's esophagus. *Ann. Surg.* **234:** 532–538; discussion 538–539.

49. Desai, K.M., N.J. Soper, M.M. Frisella, *et al.* 2003. Efficacy of laparoscopic antireflux surgery in patients with Barrett's esophagus. *Am. J. Surg.* **186:** 652–659.

50. O'Riordan, J.M., P.J. Byrne, N. Ravi, *et al.* 2004. Long-term clinical and pathologic response of Barrett's esophagus after antireflux surgery. *Am. J. Surg.* **188:** 27–33.

51. Oelschlager, B.K., M. Barreca, L. Chang, *et al.* 2003. Clinical and pathologic response of Barrett's esophagus to laparoscopic antireflux surgery. *Ann. Surg.* **238:** 458–464; discussion 464–6.

52. Zaninotto, G., G. Portale, M. Costantini, *et al.* 2007. Long-term results (6–10 years) of laparoscopic fundoplication. *J. Gastrointest. Surg.* **11:** 1138–1145.

53. Zaninotto, G., M. Cassaro, G. Pennelli, *et al.* 2005. Barrett's epithelium after antireflux surgery. *J. Gastrointest. Surg.* **9:** 1253–1260; discussion 1260–1261.

54. Biertho, L., B. Dallemagne, J.M. Dewandre, *et al.* 2007. Laparoscopic treatment of Barrett's esophagus: long-term results. *Surg. Endosc.* **21:** 11–15.

55. Rossi, M., M. Barreca, N. de Bortoli, *et al.* 2006. Efficacy of Nissen fundoplication versus medical therapy in the regression of low-grade dysplasia in patients with Barrett esophagus: a prospective study. *Ann. Surg.* **243:** 58–63.

56. Montgomery, E. 2005. Is there a way for pathologists to decrease interobserver variability in the diagnosis of dysplasia? *Arch. Pathol. Lab. Med.* **129:** 174–176.

57. Yousef, F., C. Cardwell, M.M. Cantwell, *et al.* 2008. The incidence of esophageal cancer and high-grade dysplasia in Barrett's esophagus: a systematic review and meta-analysis. *Am. J. Epidemiol.* **168:** 237–249 [Epub 2008 Jun 12].

58. Shaheen, N.J., M.A. Crosby, E.M. Bozymski & R.S. Sandler 2000. Is there publication bias in the reporting of cancer risk in Barrett's esophagus? *Gastroenterology* **119:** 333–338. Review. PMID: 1093 0368.

59. Corley, D.A., A. Kubo, T.R. Levin, *et al.* 2009. Race, ethnicity, sex and temporal differences in Barrett's oesophagus diagnosis: a large community-based study, 1994–2006. *Gut.* **58:** 182–188 [Epub 2008 Oct 31.PMID: 18978173].

60. Corley, D. & P. Buffler 2001. Oesophageal and gastric cardia adenocarcinomas: analysis of regional variation using the Cancer Incidence in Five Continents database. *Int. J. Epidemiol.* **30:** 1415–1425.

61. Fitzgerald, R.C., I.T. Saeed, D. Khoo, *et al.* 2001. Havering, Rigorous surveillance protocol increases detection of curable cancers associated with Barrett's esophagus. *Dig. Dis. Sci.* **46:** 1892–1898.

62. Inadomi, J.M. 2009. Surveillance in Barrett's esophagus: a Failed Premise: *Keio. J. Med.* **58:** 12–18 1.

63. http://www.cancer.gov/cancertopics/types/esophageal, Accessed 08/15/10.

64. Hofstetter, W., S.G. Swisher, A.M. Correa, *et al.* 2002. Treatment outcomes of resected esophageal cancer. *Ann. Surg.* **236:** 376–384; discussion 384–385. PMID: 12192324.

65. Lagergren, J., R. Bergstrom, A. Lindgren, *et al.* 1999. Symptomatic gastroesophageal reflux as a risk factor for esophageal adenocarcinoma. *N. Engl. J. Med.* **340:** 825–831.

66. Ronkainen, J., P. Aro, T. Storskrubb, *et al.* 2005. Prevalence of Barrett's esophagus in the general population: an endoscopic study. *Gastroenterology* **129:** 1825–1831.

67. Inadomi, J.M., R.E. Sampliner, J. Lagergren, *et al.* 2003. Screening and surveillance for barrett esophagus in high-risk groups: a cost-utility analysis. *Ann. Intern. Med.* **138:** 176–186.

Ann. N.Y. Acad. Sci. ISSN 0077-8923

ANNALS OF THE NEW YORK ACADEMY OF SCIENCES
Issue: *Barrett's Esophagus: The 10th OESO World Congress Proceedings*

Barrett's esophagus: treatments of adenocarcinomas I

Srinadh Komanduri,[1] Pierre H. Deprez,[2] Ajlan Atasoy,[3] Günther Hofmann,[4] Peter Pokieser,[5,6] Ahmed Ba-Ssalamah,[6] Jean-Marie Collard,[7] Bas P. Wijnhoven,[8] Roy J.J. Verhage,[9] Björn Brücher,[10] Christoph Schuhmacher,[11] Marcus Feith,[12] and Hubert Stein[13]

[1]Feinberg School of Medicine, Division of Gastroenterology/Hepatology, Northwestern University, Chicago, Illinois. [2]Cliniques Universitaires Saint-Luc, Université Catholique de Louvain, Brussels, Belgium. [3]Division of Hematology Oncology, UPMC Cancer Pavillion, University of Pittsburgh, Pittsburgh, Pennsylvania. [4]Photo Dynamic Therapy LLC, Vienna, Austria. [5]Department of Medical Education, University of Vienna, Vienna, Austria. [6]Department of Radiology, Medical University of Vienna, Vienna, Austria. [7]Department Chirurgie de l'Appareil Digestif, Louvain Medical School, Brussels, Belgium. [8]Department of Surgery, Erasmus University Medical Center, Rotterdam, the Netherlands. [9]University Medical Center Utrecht, Department of Surgery, Utrecht, the Netherlands. [10]Department of Surgery, University of Tübingen, Tübingen, Germany. [11]Chirurgischen Klinik and Poliklinik, Technical University of Munich, Munich, Germany. [12]Chirurgische Klinik und Poliklinik, Technische Universität München, Munich, Germany. [13]Klinik für Allgemein, Viszeral, und Thoraxchirurgie, Klinikum Nürnberg Nord, Nürnberg, Germany

The following on the treatments of adenocarcinomas in Barrett's esophagus contains commentaries on endo mucosal resection; choice between other ablative therapies; the remaining genetic abnormalities following stepwise endoscopic mucosal resection and possible recurrences; the Fotelo–Fotesi PDT; the CT TNM classification of early stages of Barrett's carcinoma; the indications of lymphadenectomy in intramucosal cancer; the differences in lymph node yield in transthoracic versus transhiatal dissection; video-assisted lymphadenectomy; and the importance of the length of proximal esophageal resectipon; and indications of sentinel node dissection.

Keywords: endoscopic mucosal resection; Barrett's esophagus; intramucosal cancer; high-grade dysplasia; EMR; ESD; submucosal dissection; stepwise radical endoscopic resection (SRER); esophageal adenocarcinoma; photonic therapy; surveillance; computer tomography; endosonography; PET multislice detector scanner; spiral CT; esophageal cancer; lymph nodes; transhiatal; transthoracic; minimally invasive esophagectomy; robot-assisted thoracolaparoscopic esophagectomy; lymphadenectomy; histological differentiation; squamous cell carcinoma; Will Rogers phenomenon; sentinel node concept; resection margin; sentinel lymph nodes

Concise summaries

- The improvement of and high efficacy of ablative strategies and improved imaging modalities has led to the concept of a staging endoscopic mucosal resection (EMR) as a diagnostic strategy to ensure no evidence of invasive cancer that should be referred for esophagectomy. The overall recurrence rate of EMR for Barrett's esophagus (BE)–associated mucosal advanced neoplasia appears to be extremely low. The addition of radiofrequency ablation appears to be even superior to EMR alone in recurrence risk.

- Band ligation-EMR is the easiest method to use, but may induce bridging and may be complicated due to poor viewing and bleeding. The most popular method therefore remains the cap-EMR, quite easy to learn and perform and allowing large specimens to be resected. Both techniques can be used to remove a superficial cancer occurring in Barrett's mucosa or also to resect the full Barrett's mucosa in a stepwise radical resection. For lesions larger than 15 mm, endoscopic submucosal dissection seems to be preferable, and may provide *en bloc* removal.

- Stepwise radical endoscopic resection (ER) seems to be an effective approach to eradicate BE and early neoplasia with lower short-term recurrence rates compared to focal resection.

- Ablation may have in some way eradicated the underlying genetic properties inherent to that

doi: 10.1111/j.1749-6632.2011.06055.x

Ann. N.Y. Acad. Sci. 1232 (2011) 248–264 © 2011 New York Academy of Sciences.

mucosa and prevent recurrence of neoplasia. However, even if it appears that the neosquamous epithelium is free of genetic abnormalities, this is limited by the fact that we are unclear which markers are meaningful in prediction of neoplasia.

- The photonic tumor therapy system provides with its novel model a cost-effective modality, minimally invasive, repeatable if required without dose limitation, with no interaction with other treatment modalities.
- Multislice detector scanner, the current standard CT technique, serves as a basic staging tool for all stages of Barrett's carcinoma, especially to detect distant metastasis and concomitant abnormalities.
- Its combination with FDG PET is still under investigation, but can be estimated as a future standard in the diagnostic work up of esophageal carcinoma.
- The clear diagnosis of a submucosal lesion is a formal indication of a three-field esophagectomy with radical lymph node dissection from the neck down to the abdomen.

- Lymphadenectomy is warranted for achievement of complete oncological clearance, and such extensive surgery can be facilitated by minimally invasive or video-assisted techniques in the hands of experienced endoscopic surgeons, taking into account the Will Rogers Phenomenon.
- The incidence of tumor recurrence at the anastomotic site after esophagectomy varies with respect to the length of the resection margin, and a margin above three cm should be aimed for.
- The increased morbidity of a transthoracic (TT) approach should be weighted against a less morbid transhiatal (TH) approach. Hopefully, more accurate staging techniques will be developed to better tailor the surgical treatment and lymph node dissection to the individual patient, enabling to perform the most radical operation with the lowest morbidity and mortality.
- If the sentinel lymph node concept holds true, lymphadenectomy with its associated morbidity could be safely omitted in most patients with early adenocarcinoma without compromising the cure rates.

---

1. What are the current results of EMR in lesions confined to the mucosa?

Srinadh Komanduri
koman1973@gmail.com

EMR in the setting of BE-associated high-grade dysplasia (HGD) and intramucosal (IMC) cancer has been very effective.[1,2] The treatment paradigm has been evolving with the improvement and high efficacy of ablative strategies such as RFA and improved imaging modalities. Integral to this strategy is identifying depth of penetration. This can be done with EUS before resection but, at times, can only be determined by surgical pathology with the resected specimen. This has led to the concept of a staging EMR as a diagnostic strategy to ensure no evidence of invasive cancer, which should be referred for esophagectomy.

In superficial lesions, strategies of utilization of EMR include circumferential resection of all Barrett's in the setting of HGD/IMC to resection visible areas of nodularity, ulceration, or superficial mass lesions, then followed by ablation of the remainder of flat IM. More recently, data suggest EMR of all identifiable lesions under HD white light or NBI, followed by RFA, may be the optimal strategy, avoiding the higher stricture rates (>30%) associated with circumferential mucosal resection. In 2009, Chennat *et al.*[3] published a series of 49 patients with HGD/IMC who underwent circumferential or complete EMR with 96.9% complete response to nearly two years. However they did have 37% symptomatic stricture rate. Recent data with the EURO-1 trial demonstrated EMR with RFA in the setting of HGD/IMC yielded 100% eradication of dysplasia and 96% CR-IM with no significant complications in 24 patients. Our center has experienced similar results without complications. Prasad *et al.* also compared patients treated with surgery or EMR (178 patients) and determined overall survival to be comparable and unrelated with very low recurrence rates.[5]

What is the rate of recurrence in the mucosa remaining after ER?

In the study by Chennat *et al.*,[3] only 1 of 32 patients had any recurrence of disease to two years. In the EURO-1 trial with EMR followed by RFA no patients recurred after treatment. Finally, in the largest study by Prasad *et al.*,[5] 16 of 132 patients had endoscopic recurrence by two years. Fifteen out of sixteen patients had nodules resected with CR by EMR. The overall recurrence rate of EMR for BE-associated mucosal advanced neoplasia appears to be extremely low. The addition of RFA following EMR appears to be superior to EMR alone in lowering the risk of recurrence.

2. What are the criteria for a logical choice between EMR and other ablative techniques?

Pierre H. Deprez
pdeprez@uclouvain.be

Endoscopic treatment of superficial digestive tumors may be divided into resection and ablation techniques. Resection remains the gold standard management since it provides a pathological specimen that will allow adequate and optimal correct staging. EMR was developed in the 1990s for the resection of esophageal and gastric neoplasms and now includes a large variety of techniques either aimed at lifting or sucking a lesion before snaring it. The most popular EMR methods nowadays are the band-ligation EMR and the cap-assisted EMR.[6] More recently, endoscopic submucosal dissection (ESD) has been developed by Japanese authors. The rationale for ESD is that there is no size limit for *en bloc* resection, while it is difficult to achieve *en bloc* resection of specimens larger than 15–20 mm with EMR, and that piecemeal resection by EMR leads to local recurrence rates of about 15%. Experience in the Western world, however, is still limited, and ESD is only performed in a few select centers, with low volumes of cases, no description of training programs, and few published reports.[7] The criteria to choose between the different EMR techniques and ESD are the following: ease of use, efficacy in terms of R0 resection, safety, cost, indications, and previous endoscopic or surgical treatments.

Ease of use

EMR or mucosectomy is, in fact, an inappropriate word, since all techniques involve resection of the muscularis mucosae and part of the submucosa. It is an easy method to apply in the esophagus, although Barrett's mucosa may be "tricky" to remove due to thickening of mucosa consecutive to chronic inflammation, ulceration, and scarring. Band ligation-EMR is the easiest method to use, very similar to the technique applied for variceal banding. It provides effective piecemeal resection of the lesion and Barrett's mucosa, but may induce bridging and may be complicated due to poor viewing and bleeding. The most popular method, therefore, remains the cap-EMR, quite easy to learn and perform and allowing for large specimens of more than 2 cm to be resected. Both techniques can be used to remove a superficial cancer occurring in Barrett's mucosa or also to resect the full Barrett's mucosa in a stepwise radical resection.[8]

Efficacy

ER should match the surgical standards and aim at complete resection of the tumor (R0) with free deep and lateral margins. Piecemeal resection doesn't provide adequate pathological analysis when considering not only the lateral margins, but also possibly deep margins, due to bridging and coagulation effects. The risk of recurrence after piecemeal ER has been shown in many other sites (esophageal squamous cell carcinoma, gastric adenocarcinoma, and colorectal lateral spreading tumors) to be mainly related to the size of the tumor and piecemeal rather than *en bloc* resection. *En bloc* and R0 resection should, therefore, be performed, and for lesions larger than 15 mm, this can only be accomplished by ESD removal. Table 1 summarizes the results of a prospective randomized trail comparing EMR and ESD in esophageal superficial cancer resection, showing higher R0 rates with ESD but with a procedure of longer duration and higher cost.[9]

Safety

Safety should always remain a major concern for endoscopists. Several studies have shown that band ligation is safer than cap-assisted EMR and ESD. The main complications observed after EMR and ESD are early or delayed bleeding, perforation, and esophageal stricture. Risk of perforation is lower than 5% in most reports on esophageal EMR, but may reach 10% with ESD, especially in the Western world where training and expertise is still lacking. The immediate and delayed bleeding risk is below 10% and might even be lower with ESD than EMR

Table 1. Prospective comparison of EMR-cap and ESD in the removal of superficial esophageal cancer

	EMR-Cap	ESD	*P*
En bloc resection	None (1–11 pieces)	96%	<0.0001
Surface resected (mm^2)	1,488 (185–3194)	2,453 (600–5400)	<0.01
Procedure duration (min)	61 (20–130)	150 (64–334)	<0.001
Devices costs (€)	264 (60–515)	486 (247–1019)	<0.001
R0 (free lat & deep margins)	24%	64%	<0.05
Follow-up (months)	21.5 (7–42)	21 (6–41)	NS
CR neoplasia	84%	92%	NS
CR intestinal metaplasia	52%	68%	NS

CR, complete remission.

due to a more precise control of hemostasis during dissection of the submucosa. In our prospective trial comparing EMR and ESD, bleeding and perforation rates were not significantly different, but strictures were observed in more than 50% of patients treated by ESD, due to a significantly broader surface resected compared with cap-EMR.[9]

Cost

Cost may also be an issue and a criterion to consider when choosing the technique to resect a Barrett's mucosa or a superficial lesion. Lift and cut EMR will only cost 25€, while ligation cost will rise to 100–150€ for a variceal single use band ligator, or even 250€ with the Duette™ system (Wilson-Cook). Cap-assisted EMR costs will depend on the number of snares and the hemostatic device employed, but should not exceed 520€. ESD cost is related to the type of knife used, the most popular being TT-knife™, Flex-knife™, Insulated tip-knife™, Hook-knife™ (all from Olympus Corporation), Flush-knife™ (Fujinon Corporation), Safe-knife™ (Pentax Corporation), and Hybrid-knife™ (ERBE Corporation), with a cost varying between 250 and 500€. During ESD, the cost of endoscopic hemostasis achieved with a hemostatic forceps such as the Coag-grasper™ (Olympus Corporation) or/and hemoclips could add 20–400€.

Specific indications

The choice between EMR and ESD may also depend on the size of the lesion: small tumors less than 15 mm may be easily removed with band or cap-assisted EMR, and lesions larger than 15 mm by ESD may require *en bloc* removal (Table 2). In case of a short-segment Barrett's with no visible

Table 2. Criteria to choose EMR and ESD in removal of Barrett's superficial cancer

	Band-EMR	Cap-EMR	ESD
Ease of use	+++	++	−
R0	Only for lesions <15mm	Only for lesions <15 mm	+++
Bleeding risk	−	++	+
Perforation risk	−	+	+++
Strictures	+	+	++
Cost	+	+	++
Specific indications	−	−	Lesions that might involve the submucosa tumors > 15 mm
Previous treatment	−	−	Previous EMR Scars Ulcers Previous surgery

EMR, endoscopic mucosal resection; ESD, endoscopic submucosal dissection.

lesions, band- and cap-assisted EMR may provide quick and easy removal of the entire Barrett's mucosa in a single session, but long Barrett's may need one to three sessions to be fully resected. ESD may sometimes be of help if lifting cannot be obtained, due to scarring consecutive to previous EMR. Tumors that might involve the submucosa (suspected on endoscopic mucosal pattern or EUS staging) should be resected by ESD to provide *en bloc* resection and adequate staging. Finally, ESD will be necessary in some cases in whom scarring, ulceration, previous surgery (antireflux surgery, partial esophagectomy), or previous radiotherapy ablation may prevent mucosal lifting, which is necessary to apply the various lift and suck EMR techniques.[10]

In conclusion, band-EMR is the easiest and safest technique for removal of small tumors and short Barrett's mucosa. Cap-EMR remains, however, the gold standard since it allows for better viewing during resection and lower bridging rates during piecemeal resection of large segments of Barrett's mucosa. ESD needs more expertise and should be used in specific indications: tumors larger than 15 mm, risk for submucosal involvement, and poor lifting lesions due to scarring, ulceration, previous EMR, ablation, or surgery.

3. Can it be assumed that, following stepwise radical ER of BE, the neosquamous epithelium is free of genetic abnormalities?

Srinadh Komanduri
koman1973@gmail.com

J. Bergman's group demonstrated this by assessing p53 overexpression in nine patients undergoing stepwise radical endoscopic resection (SRER). DNA-FISH was used to evaluate numeric abnormalities on chromosomes 1 and 0 and losses of p16 and p53. All genetic abnormalities were eradicated postresection. Further studies have validated SRER in efficacy in dysplastic BE. Furthermore, it does appear that ablation leads to complete eradication of disease and associated genetic abnormalities. Jacques Bergman *et al.* assessed Ki-67, p53, and various genetic abnormalities by DNA-FISH of chromosomes 1,9, p16, and p53, before and after ablative therapy.[12] All 22 patients with clear genetic

abnormalities in the setting of HGD/IMC showed no abnormalities after ablative therapy.[11]

This finding suggests that ablation may have in some way eradicated the underlying genetic properties inherent to that mucosa and prevent recurrence of neoplasia. At this point, it appears that after SRER of BE, the neosquamous epithelium is free of genetic abnormalities; however this is limited by a lack of multiple studies, and the simple fact that we are unclear which markers are meaningful in predicting neoplasia.

4. Can long-term recurrence rate after stepwise radical ER be evaluated?

Ajlan Atasoy
atasoya@upmc.edu

ER of early esophageal adenocarcinoma is promising. It provides tissue specimens for accurate histopathologic diagnosis, and it is therapeutic at the same time. Morbidity and mortality rates are significantly less than with surgical resection. Long-term results were investigated in a prospective study of 100 consecutive patients with early esophageal adenocarcinomas;[13] the five-year survival rate was 98%. During a mean follow-up of 36.7 months, 11% of patients had recurrent or metachronous carcinomas, and they were all treated successfully with ER. Other studies on ER of focal lesions reported recurrence rates of up to 30%. Treating the remaining Barrett's mucosa may reduce the rate of recurrent or metachronous carcinomas. Ablation methods such as photodynamic therapy (PDT) have been successfully used to treat early neoplasia in BE. However, there is a concern for remaining areas of intestinal metaplasia buried under neosquamous epithelium.

Stepwise radical ER of the complete BE seems to be a promising alternative. It has the advantage of complete removal of all BE and allows histological correlation. SRER may give rise to less remaining buried Barrett's and may eliminate the oncogenic alterations of the epithelium, and may lead to a lower recurrence rate. There are, however, a limited number of studies on SRER. In a prospective study from the Netherlands published in 2006, SRER sessions were performed in 37 patients.[14] Complete eradication was achieved with a median of three sessions. Follow-up was scheduled every three months during the first year and annually thereafter. There was no recurrence in a median follow up of 11 months. In a retrospective study including 34 patients with a median follow up of 23 months, high grade intraepithelial neoplasia (HGIN)/early cancer recurred in 9% of patients.[15] In another cohort of 169 patients, complete eradication was achieved in 97%.[8] After a median follow up of 32 months, complete eradication of neoplasia was sustained in 95% of patients.

In summary, SRER seems to be an effective approach to eradicate BE and early neoplasia, with lower short-term recurrence rates compared to focal resection. Further prospective studies are needed to evaluate long-term outcomes.

5. What are the cost-benefit advantages of the photonic tumor therapy system in the endoscopic treatment of adenocarcinoma?

Günther Hofmann
gh@pdt.at

Basically, photonic tumor therapy is an effective, safe, and patient-friendly treatment modality for the minimally invasive procedure in precursors to, early stage, developed, and late stage of certain tumors, that is, in the gastrointestinal tract and especially in the esophagus. The modality summarized as interventional oncology (IO) causes tumor cell death by light in the optical red of the spectra. With the aid of an intravenously administered photon transformer, which accumulates in abnormal altered cells, reactive oxygen in these cells is activated by intelligently, modulated, and locally applied laser light, and subsequent tumor cell death by apoptosis and necrosis is induced.

Photonic tumor therapy is available throughout the EU for the healthcare institutions as CE-certified clinical service with hands-on support of field specialists for providing the best possible treatment support, and technique-related backup for the clinicians performing the procedure.

The photonic tumor therapy system provides the following advantages:

1. the CE-certified clinical service with well-trained field specialists;
2. the Standard Operating Procedures (SOP) for the individual procedure referring to the in- and out-criteria for patients' selection, staging, and patients' consent; the therapy light application with recommendations for treatment parameters, sedation, and monitoring; and finally, guidelines for follow-up and recommended surveillance;
3. the involved technical equipment contains the therapy laser, the photon transformer, and the light applicator, with a variety of sizes available for the optimized fit to the treatment area, allowing for homogenous irradiation, and adapted to the shortest possible treatment time;
4. the pay-per-use approach avoids time-consuming negotiations and delays due to equipment investments, and allows for highly effective allocation of administration resources (Table 3);
5. the hospital administration support in terms of billing and reimbursement.

Conclusion

The proprietary photonic tumor therapy system, with its novel CE-certified model, provides a cost-effective modality that is minimally invasive, repeatable if required without dose limitation, and

Table 3. The pay-per-use approach avoids time-consuming negotiations and delays due to equipment investments, and allows for highly effective allocation of administration resources

Cost advantages	RF-Ablation*	Mucosectomy*	Photonic tumor therapy
Number of procedures required	3–4	2–3	1
Cost/procedure (€)	9,000	750	3,860
Cost/hospitalization (€)	7,500	6,250	1,000
Over all cost (€)	16,500	7,000	4,860
Cost disadvantage (%)	340	168	0

*Figures are courtesy of Prof. A. Puespoek, MD, Head of Endoscopy, Medical University Hospital Vienna, Internal Medicine III, August 2010.

with no interaction with other treatment modalities, low complication rate, and a favorable side effect profile.

6. What is the role of CT in the evaluation of TNM classification of early stages in Barrett's carcinoma?

Peter Pokieser and Ahmed Ba-Ssalamah
peter.pokieser@meduniwien.ac.at

Technique

Scanning parameters: for computer tomography, multislice detector scanners (MDCT) with 16, 64 (or higher) channel technology are required, with an image reconstruction of about 2 mm. The contrast injection targets to the arterial phase for the upper abdomen and chest and for the portal venous phase for the entire abdomen (after ingestion of 1–1.5 L of water for distention of the gut (Hydro-MDCT)). By this protocol, a double phase investigation of the liver are lymph nodes are included.

Evaluation procedure

The review of axial, sagittal, and coronal sections *in cine* display must be performed by specialized radiologists, who are members of an interdisciplinary clinical working group on esophageal carcinoma. The report refers to the highest stage in any imaging plane. The presentation of every staging procedure during the rounds of the interdisciplinary working group allows for the continuous correlation of the study with endosonography, PET, endoscopy, and clinical course of patients. Preexisting outpatient CTs are repeated or completed to the needs of the standard protocol.

- most T1 and T2 tumors show a smooth outer border, whereas T3 and T4 tumors present with irregular outer borders and infiltration of the peri-esophageal fat,[16,17,50,51] (Fig. 1 and Table 4).
- CT Criteria for involvement of lymph nodes are the diameter and the longitundinal/transverse ratio: N1= ≥ 6/≥ 10 mm for regional/distant lymph nodes, L/T-ratio <1.5 (more or less round); an enhancement more than that of muscle tissue is classified as suspicious.
- CT Criteria for distant metastasis: M1– suspicious lesions of the liver, lungs, adrenal glands, kidneys, bones, brain, or peritoneum other sites (rare ∼1%).

Hydro-MDCT, ideally combined with PET, is a basic test for surgical staging of esophageal carcinoma. MDCT has an accuracy from 60% to 90% for M1/M0. Furthermore, MDCT gives information about concomitant diseases, like liver cirrhosis, lung diseases, or anatomic variants. The multiplanar reconstruction allows additional topographic considerations for operation planning. MDCT is used in a complementary manner, with interdisciplinary correlation, and with other imaging modalities.

EUS is superior to CT in locoregional differentiation between T1a and T1b. Mallery *et al.* reported an EUS Accuracy for T1 = 86% and for T2 = 73%.[18] MDCT and spiral-CT cannot differentiate wall layers and so have a very low accuracy for T1 and T2 tumors. The study of Yuan *et al.*[19] demonstrated promising results for PET/CT for N staging, with a sensitivity of 94% ($P = 0.032$), specificity of 92%, and accuracy of 92% ($P = 0.006$), superior to FDG-PET alone (82%, 87%, and 92%).

Conclusion

MDCT, the current standard CT technique, serves as a basic staging tool for all stages of Barrett's carcinoma, especially to detect distant metastasis and concomitant abnormalities. MDCT serves as

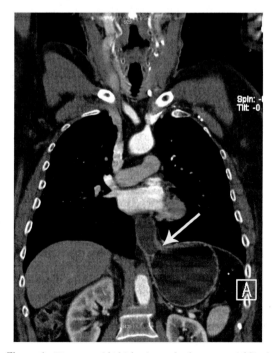

Figure 1. T1 tumor with thickening and enhancement of distal esophageal wall of ≤ 10 mm and length of ≤ 20 mm and a smooth outer border.

Table 4. T staging criteria for CT analysis

	Width	Enhancement	Outer border	Stenosis
T1	>3–≤10 mm	+	smooth	−
T2	>10–≤15 mm	+	Smooth/stranding for <1/3 of the tumour extension.	+/−
T3	>15 mm	+	Irregular/stranding for >1/3 of the tumour extension.	+
T4	>15 mm	+	Infiltrarion of adjecnt organs[*]	+

[*]Defining the site of infiltration

a complementary investigation to other tests for T & N classification. MDCT is not accurate for differentiating T1a and T1b tumors; the combination of MDCT with FDG PET is a promising tool in particular for evaluating responses to neoadjuvant chemotherapy.

7. Is lymphadenectomy justified for intra-mucosal disease?

Jean-Marie Collard
jean-marie.collard@uclouvain.be

Long-term outcome of esophageal cancer depends on the presence of metastatic regional lymph nodes in the resected specimen with five-year survival rates after Japanese-like esophagectomy approaching 50% when fewer than five lymph nodes are involved, and of about 20% in the presence of more

than five metastatic lymph nodes.[20–22] To reduce the price to pay for getting cured, minimally invasive techniques such as EMR or vagus-sparing esophagectomy (VSE) have been introduced—all techniques to be used in patients who are unlikely to have metastatic regional lymph nodes.

Likelihood of metastatic lymph nodes
Thorough review of the literature (1,865 patients) indicates that the prevalence of metastatic lymph nodes nears zero in HGD, is about 4% in mucosal cancers, and reaches 40% in submucosal cancers. Further subclassification of so-called superficial esophageal cancers shows that this prevalence increases from 0% in m1 tumors, to 1.5% in m2 lesions, and to 8.8% in m3 cancers. As for submucosal lesions, this prevalence is 21.5%, 31.5%, and 54.2% in sm1, sm2, and sm3, respectively. In addition, it is higher in squamous-cell carcinomas (SCC)

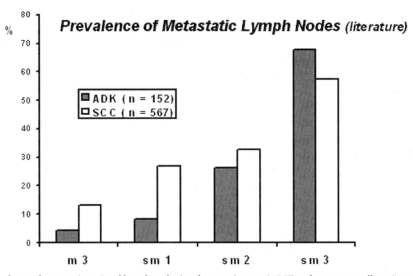

Figure 2. Prevalence of metastatic regional lymph nodes in adenocarcinomas (ADK) and squamous cell carcinomas (SCC) of the esophagus (meta-analysis of the literature).

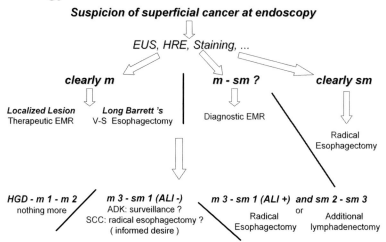

Figure 3. Therapeutic strategy before an esophageal cancer suspected to be superficial at upper gastro-intestinal endoscopic examination based on objective data from literature.

($n = 567$) than in adenocarcinomas (ADK) ($n = 152$) (Fig. 2). As reported by Ancona *et al.*,[23] the likelihood of metastatic lymph nodes is substantially higher in the presence of angio-lymphatic invasion (ALI) in the resected specimen, namely in sm1 tumors (ALI positive: 21.4% vs. ALI negative: 0%). Interestingly, as pointed out by Bolschweiler *et al.*,[24] metastatic lymph nodes accompanying superficial esophageal cancers may be far distant from the primary, i.e., in the neck or the abdomen (SCC: 9% vs. ADK: 23%).

Multifocality of superficial esophageal cancers

As demonstrated by Altorki *et al.*,[25] multiple neoplastic lesions are concomitantly present in the esophagus of 13% (short-segment Barrett's ADK), 50% (long-segment Barrett's ADK), and 33% (SCC) of the patients in whom a superficial cancer has been detected.

Therapeutic strategy

The clear presence without any shadow of doubt of a single lesion strictly confined to the mucosa at endoscopic ultrasonography combined to high-resolution endoscopy and mucosal staining techniques is a good indication for therapeutic EMR, except in long Barrett's ADK, where VSE should be considered due to the high prevalence of concomitant microscopic neoplastic lesions. If the endoscopist hesitates between a mucosal and a submucosal lesion, diagnostic EMR has to be performed

to get more tissue material to be at the disposal of the Pathologist. On the other hand, the clear diagnosis of a submucosal lesion is a formal indication of a Japanese-like esophagectomy with radical lymph node dissection from the neck down to the abdomen. Once the clinician has got further histological information from therapeutic or diagnostic EMR, or from VSE, the therapeutic strategy needs a careful reassessment. HGD, m1, and m2 lesions do not need any additional therapy. Radical esophagectomy (after EMR) or additional lymphadenectomy (after VSE) have to be performed for lesions classified m3 (ALI +), sm1 (ALI +), sm2, and sm3. As for lesions classified m3 (ALI −) or sm1 (ALI −), endoscopic surveillance versus radical esophagectomy are to be discussed with the patient, preferably recommending endoscopic surveillance in ADK and a radical esophagectomy in SCC. Another critical factor to influence the decision-making process is the general status of the patient, as to whether he is likely to tolerate or not a radical esophagectomy (Fig. 3).

Conclusion

In the 21st century, proper management of any esophageal cancer requires a multidisciplinary approach and the decision-making process must be based on both objective arguments and clinical good sense, keeping in mind that the early detection of an esophageal cancer is a unique opportunity to get cured.

8. What is the lymph node yield with TT versus TH dissection?

Bas P.L. Wijnhoven, Hugo W. Tilanus, and Jan J.B. van Lanschot
b.wijnhoven@erasmusmc.nl

In the previous editions of the UICC–AJCC–TNM staging manual for esophageal cancer, the location of lymph nodes was used for staging and prognostication. In the recent 7th edition, the N classification relies on the number of involved lymph nodes. Also, the number of involved nodes divided by the number of lymph nodes resected (i.e., the lymph node ratio) has been found to more accurately predict prognosis. Hence, the debate of which surgical approach for esophageal cancer yields the highest number of resected lymph nodes is still timely.

When reviewing published papers on the outcome of esophageal cancer after TH and TT esophagectomy, the number and location of the resected and examined lymph nodes is often poorly defined. Most studies are retrospective cohort studies, and the inclusion and exclusion criteria of the patients under study are poorly defined. Details of the surgery (especially which nodal stations were dissected) are absent in many studies as well as the methods of pathological examination of the specimens. Therefore, a comparison of the lymph node yield between TH and TT esophagectomy is fraught with bias. The best available evidence comes from a randomized controlled trial performed in the Netherlands.[26] There are more data coming from large comparative cohort studies, but limitations in interpretation, as mentioned previously, should be kept in mind.

Approximately twice as many lymph nodes are resected when a TT esophagectomy is peformed (Table 5). The right paratracheal nodes, the nodes in the aortic-pulmonary window as well as the subcarinal nodes can be dissected when performing a right-sided thoracotomy. The left thoracophrenotomy achieves similar results although the paratracheal nodes are more difficult to dissect. On the contrary, when performing a TH esophagectomy, only the distal posterior mediastinal nodes can be dissected easily and the subcarinal nodes are mostly out of reach, even for the experienced surgeon. The lymph node yield after minimally invasive TT and TH esophagectomy is comparable to the open procedures.[29] However, differences in patient de-

Table 5. Mean number of lymph nodes resected with transthoracic (TT) versus transhiatal (TH) esophagectomy

	TT	TH	Remarks
Dutch trial[26]	31	16	RCT
Comparative cohort studies[27,28]			
	28	16	Mediastinum 16 vs. 3
	52	22	
	30	19	After neoadj. treatment
	13	13	After neoadj. treatment
Minimally invasive techniques[29]	17	11	Review paper
Robotic esophagectomy[30]	29	14	Noncomparative studies

RCT, randomized controlled trial.

mographics and tumor stage exist between comparative studies on open esophagectomy versus minimally invasive techniques and this may bias the results on the number of lymph node dissected. European, American, and Japanese studies on three-field esophagectomy (with the third-field being the bilateral nodal dissection in the neck) show that a mean number 50–70 lymph nodes can be resected. Three-field lymph node dissection improves staging accuracy, but if survival is superior as compared to two-field nodal dissection is still debatable.

An important question to address is whether a patient's survival improves when more nodes are taken out by the surgeon. First of all, achieving a tumor-free resection margin (R0) is likely to be one of the most important predictors of survival. Patients that underwent an R1 resection have generally a poor prognosis and frequently suffer from recurrence of tumor. The number of lymph nodes involved with tumor cells and the lymph node ratio are also very strong independent predictors of survival. In the Dutch RCT, no significant difference in survival was observed between TT and TH esophagectomy after five years of follow-up.[26] However, a subgroup analysis showed that TT esophagectomy was beneficial in patients who had between one and eight positive lymph nodes. More evidence in favor of an extended lymphadenectomy comes from a recent study that examined the relationship between the number of resected nodes and survival.[31] It was found that the optimal number of lymph nodes that needs to be removed is around 23. If more nodes are resected, this likely does not lead to an increased chance of surviving. However, if less that 23 nodes are being removed, patients' predicted survival was at risk. Is this true for all patients with esophageal cancer? Probably not because in patients with >8 lymph nodes involved, systemic disease is almost invariably present and survival is very poor. In these patients, an extensive lymph node sampling is not of benefit and only leads to increased morbidity.

Therefore, extended TT esophagectomy with mediastinal lymph node clearance is the treatment of choice for Siewert type I esophageal cancers and in patients without evidence of massive nodal involvement. However, the increased morbidity of a TT approach should be weighted against a less morbid TH approach, as reported by the Dutch RCT.[26] Unfortunately, with the current diagnostic modalities, we cannot accurately predict the number and location of positive lymph nodes preoperatively. Hopefully more accurate staging techniques will be developed to better tailor the surgical treatment and lymph node dissection to the individual patient. This will enable us to perform the most radical operation but with the lowest morbidity and mortality.

The treatment of esophageal cancer has changed in recent years. Meta-analyses of randomized controlled trials on neoadjuvant chemoradiotherapy/chemotherapy versus surgery alone show a survival benefit in favor of neoadjuvant therapy followed by esophagectomy. It is hypothesized that neoadjuvant therapy, and especially radiotherapy, reduces the number of examined nodes after surgery. This has been shown in studies on rectal cancer. Moreover, the theoretical benefit of performing a lymph node dissection in the chest could be questioned because of the pretreatment of the tumor and locoregional lymph nodes stations by chemoradiotherapy.

One study from the United Kingdom did not find a difference in the number of lymph nodes removed by TT versus TH esophagectomy (both a median number of 13), nor in the overall survival after neoadjuvant chemoradiotherapy.[32] However, a TT *en bloc* esophagectomy proved to be superior compared to THE in an another study, even after neoadjuvant treatment.[28] We will have to await more studies to further guide the surgeon as to what surgical approach and extent of lymph node

dissection is optimal in patients after neoadjuvant treament.

9. What are the indications and limits of video-assisted lymphadenectomy in the surgical treatment of esophageal cancer?

Roy J.J. Verhage and Richard van Hillegersberg
R.J.J.Verhage@umcutrecht.nl

Rapidly increasing incidence of esophageal adenocarcinoma has boosted research in this rapidly evolving field of cancer medicine. However, survival remains relatively poor. A probable explanation for this low survival is that lymph node involvement in esophageal cancer is common, and already occurs in early stage disease. Lymph node metastases are found in less than 2% of T1a tumors, but for T1b disease this number goes up to 20%. For T3 tumors, the number of patients with positive lymph nodes is even 80%. These figures support ER for T1a stage disease, but warrant surgical treatment with extensive lymphadenectomy for higher stage disease to accomplish oncological clearance.

Current diagnostic strategies are lacking enough predictive value for identifying patients with and without lymph node involvement. Endoscopic ultrasound for the detection of N stage has a sensitivity of 80% and specificity of 70% for regional lymph nodes.[33] Computed tomography is an unreliable tool to detect small lymph node metastases, which are frequently observed during pathological assessment of tumor specimens. Surgical treatment should, therefore, be directed towards a radical tumor resection as well as proper lymphadenectomy. In our own series, the robot-assisted thoracolaparoscopic approach yielded a median of 29 lymph nodes per patient (Fig. 4A).[34] From 47 patients, 35 had a distal tumor in the lower third of the esophagus or at the gastro-esophageal junction. One third of the positive lymph nodes in these patients were found proximally in the mediastinum (Fig. 4B). These lymph nodes would not have been resected when a TH procedure was performed. This further illustrates the need for extensive lymphadenectomy, even when distal tumors are concerned.

The limits in diagnostics and the high rate and location of lymph node involvement warrant lymph node dissection for esophageal cancer. Several surgical strategies exist, which can be grouped in the open

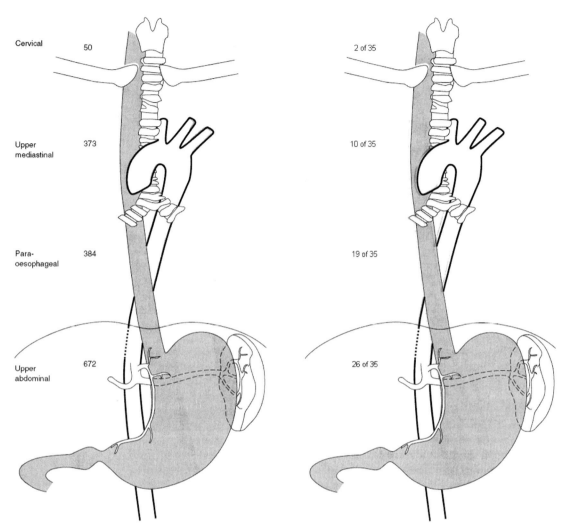

Figure 4. (A) Distribution of 1,479 lymph nodes dissected in 47 patients who underwent robot-assisted thoracolaparoscopic esophagectomy. (B) Location of lymph node metastases in 35 patients with a distal or gastro-esophageal junction tumor. With permission from Boone *et al.*[34]

TH approach and the TT approach and their minimally invasive counterparts, laparoscopic, and thoracolaparoscopic esophagectomy. The largest trial to date showed improved survival in patients who underwent TT esophagectomy when compared to TH surgery. Long-term results showed significantly improved five-year survival for patients with one to eight positive lymph nodes when operated on through the TT approach.[27] These results support that more extensive surgical lymphadenectomy improves oncological outcome.

However, TT surgery is associated with higher morbidity than TH surgery. To limit surgical trauma and morbidity, while at the same time achieving oncological clearance, thoracoscopic techniques offer an alternative. Data from randomized trials are not available yet, but review of current literature supports that minimally invasive esophagectomy reduces trauma and morbidity (Table 6).[35] Furthermore, minimally invasive techniques improve the surgeon's vision of the operative field. Several other studies have also shown that lymph node harvest in video-assisted lymphadenectomy is at least comparable to open surgery.[34,36] For the surgeon, the advantage of minimally invasive esophagectomy with extended lymphadenectomy lies in the improved magnified vision through angles that cannot be reached at open surgery. For the patient, the

Table 6. Average short-term postoperative outcomes for open transthoracic esophagectomy versus thoracolaparoscopic esophagectomy

		TTE	TLSE
	n	203	78
Operating time total	min	331	384
EBL	mL	630	317
ICU stay	days	4.1	4.4
Hospital stay	days	18.2	14.9
Lymph nodes	*n*	16.1	17.4
Pulmonary complications	%	26.5	15.3
Complications	%	67.3	57.1
Perioperative mortality	%	3.8	

Values represent weighted means (adapted from Verhage *et al.*,[35] with extra data added from Smithers *et al.* 2007). EBL, estimated blood loss; ICU, intensive care unit; TTE, transthoracic esophagectomy; TLSE, thoracolaparoscopic esophagectomy; *n*, number; mL, milliliters; min, minutes.

advantages include reduced blood loss, reduced postoperative pain, shorter recovery, less postoperative morbidity, and improved cosmetics.

Some important limits to minimally invasive techniques for esophagectomy must be mentioned. This type of surgery requires a surgeon with advanced endoscopic skills. The learning curve for developing these skills is far from steep. Much training is necessary before a surgeon is able to perform at such an advanced level. However, with the advent of robot-assisted surgery, esophagectomy has become less demanding for the surgeon. Ergonomics are significantly improved, and the surgeon is provided with a three dimensional vision, further improving the view of the operative field. In addition, the surgeon is able to control articulating instruments with great precision devoid of tremor. Robot-assisted surgery overcomes many limits of conventional endoscopic surgery and is a suitable technique for performing complex procedures such as *en bloc* esophagectomy with extensive lymphadenectomy.[34]

In conclusion, lymphadenectomy in patients with esophageal cancer is warranted for achievement of complete oncological clearance. Such extensive surgery can be facilitated by minimally invasive or video-assisted techniques in the hands of an experienced endoscopic surgeon. Further improvements

in this field might be achieved with robot-assisted surgery.

10. Is it justified to enlarge the extent of the mediastinal lymphadenectomy?

Björn Brücher
bjoern.bruecher@med.uni-tuebingen.de

The extent of lymphadenectomy in esophageal cancer has been a subject for discussion for many years.[37] Mediastinal lymphadenectomy in EC by itself is not an independent therapeutic principle, but it represents the most independent therapy-related prognostic factor[38,39] and can lead to a R0 resection within the so-called fourth dimension.

The histological differentiation is of great importance: esophageal squamous cell carcinoma (ESCC) versus Barrett-Carcinoma (AEG Type I), cause T1a tumors that rarely metastasize into the lymph nodes in AEG Type I, in which ESCC is already associated with a positive lymph node status of 7–10%.[40] This shows that the vast majority of patients with early tumor categories must undergo lymphadenectomy, but not an extended one. Within a large series of AEG tumors, about 45% of the Type I tumors showed a pN1-stage, increasing in Type II (~66%) and in Type III tumors (~79%). In addition, it had been shown that a microinvolvement of pN0-staged AEG Type I tumors can be proven in about 6–7% of cases. Moreover, the prior tumor stage before the existence of positive lymph nodes is extremely important, leading to the inclusion of lymphatic vessel invasion within the TNM classification.[41] There is a bias in judging the literature where the "Will Rogers Phenomenon" has to be taken into account: the more lymph nodes that are removed and examined, the more positive lymph nodes will be determined, and patients will be classified into higher tumor categories (stage migration). The initial tumor category is cleared, and therefore prognosis is improved (pseudo-prognostic benefit). Due to tumor heterogeneity, we can assume that this also can be found within lymph nodes. Although the sentinel concept might be helpful in experienced hands, so far we do not know which lymph node should be taken or not.

Another point of interest in judging literature is the surgical approach: compared to the TT approach, the TH approach reveals a smaller number of lymph nodes with less morbidity but comparable mortality; an actual literature reveals a higher failure rate and lower disease-free survival. An actual PubMed search for the terms "quality, histopathological examination" retrieves no results.

In conclusion, enlargement of the extent of mediastinal lymphadenectomy does not seem to be necessary in early AEG–Type-I, but mandatory in early tumor categories of ESCC, with a greater benefit than in AEG–Type-I. The TT approach seems to be favorable for judging the extent of mediastinal lymphadenectomy, but the Will Rogers Phenomenon has to be taken into account. Basic histopathological studies are warranted.

11. Following R0 resection for Siewert types I, II, and III, what is the influence of proximal esophageal resection margin on survival of patients?

Christoph Schuhmacher, Marcus Feith, Andre Mihaljevic, and Helmut Friess
schuhmacher@chir.med.tu-muenchen.de

The prognosis after surgical treatment of gastrointestinal carcinomas is mainly related to a curative, so-called R0 resection.[42] By definition, an R0 resection is achieved even if there is only one layer of non-malignant cells between the carcinoma and resection margin. Without doubt, the diameter of this safety zone is a matter of discussion. Here, we try to evaluate the existing data, which might help us define the optimal safety margin for tumors of the esophagogastric junction (AEG I–III).

From a biological viewpoint, one might postulate that the wider the safety margin, the better it is in terms of prognosis. From a practical and technical viewpoint, the size of the luminal resection margin is limited. The reconstruction of the passage after a TH extended gastrectomy depends on the length and mobility of the jejunal mesenteric root, resulting in the pull up of a well-perfused small bowel segment. Only in AEG type I (Barrett carcinoma), where the reconstruction is usually performed with a gastric tube, the upper resection margin is almost never a matter of concern. Resection margins in AEG type II and III, on the other hand, which are reconstructed with an end-to-side jejunoesophagostomy, are naturally restricted by technical means of the interposed bowel and by the TH access.

Table 7. Incidence of anastomotic recurrence (AR[*]) with respect to length of resection margin after esophagectomy for esophageal cancer

Resection margin (cm)	AR
0–2	7/54 (13%)
2–<4	15/203 (7.4%)
4–<6	5/132 (3.8%)
6–<8	1/55 (1.8%)
≥8	0/80 (0%)

According to results from an Asian center of upper GI surgery, the incidence of tumor recurrence at the anastomotic site after esophagectomy varies with respect to the length of the resection margin. Margins below 2 cm exhibited anastomotic recurrences in 13% of cases. The recurrence rate decreased when the length of the resection margin was extended. It was 7.4% for margins between 2 and 4 cm, 3.8% for margins between 4 and 6 cm, and 1.8% for margins between 6 and 8 cm. No anastomotic recurrence was notified in cases with resection margins larger than 8 cm (Table 7).[43]

For tumors of the gastroesophageal junction (AEG), a more recent publication revealed a cut-off value of 3.8 cm to be significantly correlated with improved survival after resection ($P = 0.0004$).[44] Interestingly, in this group of patients, the prognostic benefit of an extended resection margin disappeared ($P = 0.48$) if more than six lymph nodes were metastatic.

As a consequence, if technically feasible, resection with a margin above 3 cm should be aimed for. Since the metastatic lymph node involvement cannot be assessed with sufficient accuracy preoperatively, the recommendation would be to rather go for changing the resection strategy from a TH gastrectomy to an abdomino-thoracic esophagectomy or even an esophagogastrectomy in cases were the lower tumor clearance is not possible by performing a gastric tube for reconstruction, to achieve adequate resection margins. Only a proven advanced nodal involvement may leave room for making compromises towards limited proximal resection. In addition the "third dimension," that is, the analysis of the resection margin in the area of the tumor bed (retroperitoneal space), is of interest for future studies.

12. What are the indications of the sentinel node dissection?

Hubert Stein and Marcus Feith
feith@chir.med.tu-muenchen.de

In early cancer of the esophagus, complete residual tumor-free resection and lymph node infiltration are the leading prognostic factors. More than 85% of all positive lymph nodes in early adenocarcinoma of the esophagus (Barrett's cancer) were located in close anatomic proximity to the primary tumor site.[45] The focus in these patients should be guided toward accurate pretherapeutic identification of patients with or without lymph node metastases. The results of endoscopic ultrasound with fine needle aspiration of lymph nodes are disappointing, and positron emission tomography has, so far, not met the promise of accurate lymph node staging in esophageal cancer.

The most attractive current practice is the application of the sentinel lymph node concept for early adenocarcinoma of the esophagus. A number of reports have shown that the identification of the sentinel lymph node and reliable prediction of the lymph node status based on histopathological and immunhistochemical evaluation of the sentinel lymph nodes may be possible.[45,46] The currently used techniques, however, report nearly the same predictive results for endoscopic blue dye markers, ^{99m}Tc-labeled colloids with radioguided detection, and near-infrared fluourescent lymph node tracers, and have become highly feasible for and accurate in staging esophageal cancer.[46,48]

To answer the question, what the indications of sentinel lymph node dissection in 2010 are, the possible consequences of the treatment of the patients with early Barrett's cancers are important to consider. The major disadvantages of radical esophagectomy and lymphadenectomy are its invasiveness,

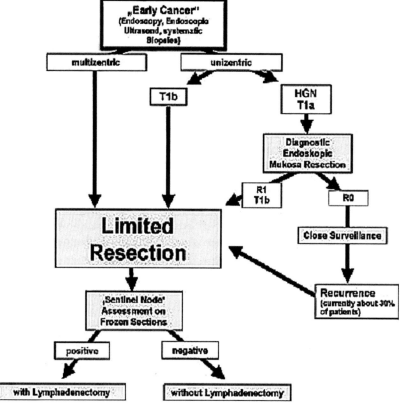

Figure 5. Flowchart outlining the concept for early carcinoma of the esophagus, including the sentinel lymph node concept to the tailored therapeutic approach.

morbidity, mortality, and poor postoperative quality of life. We believe that the EMR as a staging modality to identify true mucosal Barrett cancers, which will not need lymphadenectomy, is a promising concept. However, the endoscopic mucosa resection is compromised by the frequent persistence of premalignant lesions with BE, the high rate of recurrence and/or metachronous lesions, and the continued need of for medical acid suppression and surveillance. With a limited surgical resection of the distal esophagus and regional lymphadenectomy, an oncologically adequate alternative approach is established. In addition, limited surgical resection with jejunal interposition abolishes underlying gastroesophageal reflux and provides a good quality of life.[49] If the sentinel lymph node concept holds true, lymphadenectomy with its associated morbidity could be safely omitted in most patients with early adenocarcinoma without compromising the cure rates. Figure 5 illustrates the current concept for patients with early cancer limited to mucosa or submucosa in our department of surgery.

Conflicts of interest

The authors declare no conflicts of interest.

References

1. Van vilsteren, F.G., R.E. Pouw, S. Seewald, *et al.* 2011. Stepwise radical endoscopic resection versus radiofraquency ablation for Barrett's oesophagus with high-grade dysplasia or early cancer: a multicentre randomised trial. *Gut.*

2. Moss, A., M.J. Bourke, L.F. Hourigan, *et al.* 2010. Endoscopic resection for Barrett's high-grade dysplasia and early esophageal adenocarcinoma: an essential staging procedure with long-term therapeutic benefit. *Am. J. Gastroenterol.* **105:** 1276–1283 [Epub 2010 Feb 23].

3. Chennat, J., V.J. Konda, A.S. Ross, *et al.* 2009. Complete Barrett's eradication endoscopic mucosal resection: an effective treatment modality for high-grade dysplasia and intramucosal carcinoma—an American single-center experience. *Am. J. Gastroenterol.* **104:** 2684–2692 [Epub 2009 Aug 18].

4. Pouw, R.E., K. Wirths, P. Eisendrath, *et al.* 2010. Efficacy of radiofrequency ablation combined with endoscopic resection for Barrett's esophagus with early neoplasia. *Clin. Gastroenterol. Hepatol.* **8:** 23–29 [Epub 2009 Aug 11].

5. Prasad, G.A., T.T. Wu, D.A. Wigle, *et al.* 2009. Endoscopic and surgical treatment of mucosal (T1a) esophageal adenocarcinoma in Barrett's esophagus. *Gastroenterology* **137:** 815-823 [Epub 2009 Jun 12].

6. Inoue, H., M. Endo, K. Takeshita, *et al.* 1991. Endoscopic resection of early-stage esophageal cancer. *Surg. Endosc.* **5:** 59–62.

7. Deprez, P.H., J.J. Bergman , S. Meisner, *et al.* 2010. Current practice with endoscopic submucosal dissection in Europe: position statement from a panel of experts. *Endoscopy* **41:** 853–858.

8. Pouw, R.E., S. Seewald, J.J. Gondrie, *et al.* 2010. Stepwise radical endoscopic resection for eradication of Barrett's oesophagus with early neoplasia in a cohort of 169 patients. *Gut* [Epubahead of print].

9. Deprez, P.H., H. Piessevaux, T. Aouttah, *et al.* 2010. ESD in Barrett's esophagus high grade dysplasia and mucosal cancer: Prospective comparison with CAP mucosectomy. *Gastrointest. Endosc.* **71:** AB126–AB126.

10. Van Den Eynde, M., A. Jouret-Mourin, Ch. Sempoux, *et al.* 2010. Endoscopic mucosal or submucosal resection of early neoplasia in Barrett's esophagus after antireflux surgery. *Gastrointest. Endoscopy* **72:** 855–861.

11. Schneider, P.M., O. Stoeltzing, J.A. Roth, *et al.* 2000. P53 mutational status improves estimation of prognosis in patients with curatively resected adenocarcinoma in Barrett's esophagus. *Clin. Cancer Res.* **6:** 3153–3158.

12. Peters, F.P., K.K. Krishnadath, A.M. Rygiel, *et al.* 2007 Stepwise radical endoscopic resection of the complete Barrett's esophagus with early neoplasia successfully eradicates preexisting genetic abnormalities. *Am. J. Gastroenterol.* **102:** 1853–1861 [Epub 2007 May 17].

13. Ell, C., A. May, O. Pech, *et al.* 2007. Curative endoscopic resection of early esophageal adenocarcinomas (Barrett's cancer). *Gastrointest. Endosc.* **65:** 3–10.

14. Peters, F.P., M.A. Kara, W.D. Rosmolen, *et al.* 2006.Stepwise radical endoscopic resection is effective for complete removal of Barrett's esophagus with early neoplasia: a prospective study. *Am. J. Gastroenterol.* **101:** 1449–1457.

15. Pouw, R.E., F.P. Peters, C. Sempoux, *et al.* 2008. Stepwise radical endoscopic resection for Barrett's esophagus with early neoplasia: report on a Brussels' cohort. *Endoscopy* **40:** 892–898.

16. Ba-Ssalamah, A., J. Zacherl, M. Iris, *et al.* 2009. Dedicated multi-detector CT of the esophagus: spectrum of diseases. *Abdom Imaging*: 343–418.

17. Wu, L.F., B.Z. Wang, J.L. Feng, *et al.* 2003. Preoperative TN staging of esophageal cancer: Comparison of miniprobe ultrasonography, spiral CT and MRI.World. *J. Gastroenterol.* **9:** 219–224.

18. Mallery, S., J. Van Dam. 2000. Gastrointest Endosc. EUS in the evaluation of esophageal carcinoma **52:** S6–11.

19. Yuan, S., Y. Yu, K.S. Chao, *et al.* 2006.Additional value of PET/CT over PET in assessment of locoregional lymph nodes in thoracic esophageal squamous cell cancer. *J. Nucl. Med.* **47:** 1255–1259.

20. Collard, J.M. 2002. Surgery for high-grade dysplasia in Barrett's esophagus : the case for esophagectomy. *Chest. Surg. Clin. N. Am.* **12:** 77–92.

21. Collard, J.M., J.B. Otte, R. Fiasse, *et al.* 2001. Skeletonizing en-bloc esophagectomy for cancer. *Ann. Surg.* **234:** 25–32.

22. Collard, J.M. 2001. Exclusive radical surgery for esophageal adenocarcinoma. *Cancer* **91:** 1098–1104.

23. Ancona, E., S. Rampado, M. Cassaro, *et al.* 2008. Prediction of lymph node status in superficial esophageal carcinoma. *Ann. Surg. Oncol.* **15:** 3278–3288.

24. Bollschweiler, E., S.E. Baldus, W. Schröder, *et al.* 2006. High rate of lymph node metastasis in submucosal esophageal squamous cell carcinomas and adenocarcinomas. *Endoscopy* **38:** 149–156.

25. Altorki, N.K., P.C. Lee, Y. Liss, *et al.* 2008. Multifocal neoplasia and nodal metastases in T1 esophageal carcinoma: implications for endoscopic treatment. *Ann. Surg.* **247:** 434–439.

26. Omloo, J.M., S.M. Lagarde, J.B. Hulscher, *et al.* 2007. Extended transthoracic resection compared with limited transhiatal resection for adenocarcinoma of the mid/distal esophagus: five-year survival of a randomized clinical trial. *Ann. Surg.* **246:** 992–1000.

27. Junginger, T., I. Gockel, S. Heckhoff. 2006. A comparison of transhiatal and transthoracic resections on the prognosis in patients with squamous cell carcinoma of the esophagus. *Eur. J. Surg. Oncol.* **32:** 749–755.

28. Rizzetto, C., S.R. Demeester, J.A. Hagen, *et al.* 2008. En bloc esophagectomy reduces local recurrence and improves survival compared with transhiatal resection after neoadjuvant therapy for esophageal adenocarcinoma. *J. Thorac. Cardiovasc. Surg.* **135:** 1228–1236.

29. Decker, G., W. Coosemans, P. De Leyn, *et al.* 2009. Minimally invasive esophagectomy for cancer. *Eur. J. Cardiothorac. Surg.* **35:** 13–20.

30. Boone, J., M.E. Schipper, W.A. Moojen, *et al.* 2009. Robot-assisted thoracoscopic oesophagotomy for cancer. *Br. J. Surg.* **96:** 878–886.

31. Peyre, C.G., J.A. Hagen, S.R. Demeester, *et al.* 2008. The number of lymph nodes removed predicts survival in esophageal cancer: an international study on the impact of extent of surgical resection. *Ann. Surg.* **248:** 549–556.

32. Morgan, M.A., W.G. Lewis, A.N. Hopper, *et al.* 2007. Prospective comparison of transthoracic versus transhiatal esophagectomy following neoadjuvant therapy for esophageal cancer. *Dis. Esophagus.* **20:** 225–231.

33. Van Vliet, E.P., M.H. Heijenbrok-Kal, M.G. Hunink, *et al.* 2008. Staging investigations for oesophageal cancer: a meta-analysis. *Br. J. Cancer.* **98:** 547–557.

34. Boone, J., M.E. Schipper, W.A. Moojen, *et al.* 2009. Robot-assisted thoracoscopic oesophagotomy for cancer. *Br. J. Surg.* **96:** 878–886.

35. Verhage, R.J., E.J. Hazebroek, J. Boone, *et al.* 2009. Minimally invasive surgery compared to open procedures in esophagectomy for cancer: a systematic review of the literature. *Minerva. Chir.* **64:** 135–146.

36. Puntambekar, S.P., G.A. Agarwal, S.N. Joshi, *et al.* 2010. Thoracolaparoscopy in the lateral position for esophageal cancer: the experience of a single institution with 112 consecutive patients. *Surg. Endosc.* **24:** 2407–2414.

37. Herrera, L.J. 2010. Extend of lymphadenectomy in esophageal cancer: how many lymph nodes is enough? *Ann. Surg. Oncol.* **17:** 676–678.

38. Siewert, J.R., F. Lordick, K. Ott, *et al.* 2006. Curative versus palliative strategies in locoregional recurrence of gastrointestinal malignancies. *Chirurg.* **77:** 227–235.

39. Brücher, B.L.D.M. 2009. Esophageal squamous cell carcinoma: Pre-operative combined radiochemotherapy from a surgical oncological viewpoint. *Chirurg.* **80:** 1011–1018.

40. Stein, H.J., M. Feith, B.L.D.M. Brücher, *et al.* 2005. Early esophageal squamous cell and adenocarcinoma: Pattern of lymphatic spread and prognostic factors for long term survival after surgical resection. *Ann. Surg.* **242:** 566–573.

41. Brücher, B.L.D.M., H.J. Stein, M. Werner, *et al.* 2001. Lymphatic vessel infiltration as an independent prognostic factor in primary resected esophageal squamous cell carcinoma. *Cancer* **92:** 2228–2233.

42. Hoelscher, A.H., E. Bollschweiler, R. Bumm, *et al.* 1995. Prognostic factors of resected adenocarcinoma of the esophagus. *Surg.* **118:** 845–855.

43. Law, S., C. Arcilla, K. Chu, *et al.* The significance of histologically infiltrated resection margin after esophagectomy for esophageal cancer. *Am. J. Surg.* **176:** 286–290.

44. Barbour, A., N. Rizk, M. Gonen, *et al.* 2007. Adenocarcinoma of the gastroesophageal junction. Influence of esophageal resection margin and operative approach on outcome. *Ann. Surg.* **246:** 1–8.

45. Stein, H.J., M. Feith, B.L.D.M. Bruecher, *et al.* 2005. Early Esophageal Cancer: Pattern of Lymphatic Spread and Prognostic Factors for Long-Term Survival After Surgical Resection. *Ann. Surg.* **242:** 566–575.

46. Burian, M., H.J. Stein, A. Sendler, *et al.* 2004. Sentinel node detection in Barrett's and cardia cancer. *Ann. Surg. Oncol.* **11:** 255–258.

47. Lamb, P.J., S.M. Griffin, A.D. Burt, *et al.* 2005. Sentinel node biopsy to evaluate the metastatic dissemination of oesophageal adenocarcinoma. *Br. J. Surg.* **92:** 60–67.

48. Grotenhuis, B.A., B.P. Wijnhoven, R. Van Marion, *et al.* 2009. The sentinel node concept in adenocarcinomas of the distal esophagus and gastroesophageal junction. *J. Thorac. Cardiovasc. Surg.* **138:** 608–612.

49. Stein, H.J., M. Feith. Surgical strategies for early esophageal adenocarcinoma. *Best Pract. Res. Clin. Gastroenterol.* **19:** 927–930.

50. Ba-Ssalamah, A., W. Matzek, S. Baroud, *et al.* 2011. Accuracy of hydro-multidetector row CT in the local T staging of oesophageal cancer compared to postoperative histopathological results. *Eur Radiol.* Jun 28. DOI: 10.1007/s00330-011-2187-2.

51. Hsu, P.K., Y.C. Wu, T.Y. Chou, C.S. Huang, W.H. Hsu. 2010. Comparison of the 6th and 7th editions of the American Joint Committee on Cancer tumor-node-metastasis staging system in patients with resected esophageal carcinoma. *Ann Thorac Surg.* **89:** 1024–1031.

Ann. N.Y. Acad. Sci. ISSN 0077-8923

ANNALS OF THE NEW YORK ACADEMY OF SCIENCES

Issue: *Barrett's Esophagus: The 10th OESO World Congress Proceedings*

Barrett's esophagus: treatments of adenocarcinomas II

William S. Twaddell,[1] Peter C. Wu,[2] Roy J.J. Verhage,[3] Marcus Feith,[4] David H. Ilson,[5] Christoph P. Schuhmacher,[6] James D. Luketich,[7] Björn Brücher,[8] Daniel Vallböhmer,[9] Wayne L. Hofstetter,[10] Mark Jonathan Krasna,[11] Daniela Kandioler,[12] Paul M. Schneider,[13] Bas P.L. Wijnhoven,[14] and Stephen J. Sontag[15]

[1]Anatomic Pathology, University of Maryland Medical Center, Baltimore, Maryland. [2]VA Puget Sound Health Care System, Surgical and Perioperative Care, Seattle, Washington. [3]University Medical Center Utrecht, Department of Surgery, Utrecht, the Netherlands. [4]Department of Surgery, Technische Universität München, Klinikum Rechts der Isar, Munich, Germany. [5]Department of Medicine, Gastrointestinal Oncology, Memorial Sloan-Kettering Cancer Center, New York, New York. [6]Chirurgischen Klinik and Poliklinik, Klinikum rechts der Isar, Technical University of Munich, Munich, Germany. [7]Department of Cardiothoracic Surgery, University of Pittsburgh Medical Center, Pittsburgh, Pennsylvania. [8]Comprehensive Cancer Center Tübingen Department of Surgery, University of Tübingen, Tübingen, Germany. [9]Department of General, Visceral, and Cancer Surgery, University of Cologne, Cologne, Germany. [10]The University of Texas, M.D. Anderson Cancer Center, Houston, Texas. [11]Division of Thoracic Surgery, St. Joseph Medical Center, Towson, Maryland. [12]Department of Surgery, Medical University of Vienna, Vienna, Austria. [13]Division of Visceral and Transplantation Surgery, University Hospital Zurich, Zurich, Switzerland. [14]Department of Surgery Erasmus Medical Center MC, Rotterdam, the Netherlands. [15]Veterans Administration Hospital, Hines, Illinois

The following topics are explored in this collection of commentaries on treatments of adenocarcinomas related to Barrett's esophagus: the importance of intraoperative frozen sections of the margins for the detection of high dysplasia; the preferable way for sentinel node dissection; the current role of robotic surgery and of video-endoscopic approach; the value of the Siewert's classification of adenocarcinomas; the indications of two-step esophagectomy; the evaluation of pathological complete response; the role of PET scan in staging and response assessment; the role of p53 in the selection of adenocarcinomas patients; chemotherapy regimens for adenocarcinomas; the use of monoclonal antibodies in the control of cell proliferation; he attempt to define a stage-specific strategy, and the possible indications of selective therapy; and changes in mortality rates from esophageal cancer.

Keywords: sentinel node; gamma probe; PET tracer; esophageal cancer; minimally invasive esophagectomy; lymphadenectomy; robot assisted thoracolaparoscopic esophagectomy; robotic surgery; sentinel lymph nodes; Barrett's esophagus; neoadjuvant chemotherapy; radiotherapy; chemoradiotherapy; adenovirus vector; adenocarcinoma; prognosis; Siewert 's classification; AEG; two-stade esophagectomy; high risk patients; FDG PET scan; integrated PET/CT scan; chemoradiation; residual disease; molecular markers; gefitinib; R0 resection; p53; cisplatin; 5-FU; FOLFOX; EGFR; HER2; submucosal invasion; multimodality therapy

Concise summaries

- Drawbacks of frozen section are relatively minor in most cases. The procedure is somewhat time-consuming and may add slightly to the time of the operation. Although permanent histology is slightly altered by the process of freezing, in most cases this does not impair final interpretation. The high accuracy of frozen section for esophageal adenocarcinoma (EAC) must be considered against the relatively low frequency of positive margins. However, given the importance for patient outcome of complete resection, intraoperative frozen section for margins may be justified in a great number of cases.

- Further studies are needed to define the prognostic significance of esophageal micrometastases and optimize the intraoperative evaluation of harvested sentinel nodes to identify the

doi: 10.1111/j.1749-6632.2011.06056.x

presence of micrometastases that can influence surgical decision-making during esophagectomy.

- The best candidates for sentinel lymph node (SLN) dissection in Barrett's cancer are the non-pretreated early adenocarcinomas, in an experienced center with blue dye or ^{99m}Tc techniques. The pathologist needs experience with fresh frozen section of SLNs, and a limited surgical approach for complete resection of the lesion and prelesion should be available. The role of SLN biopsy for early-stage tumors remains however unproven with a need for prospective validation studies.

- Robotic systems have been developed to overcome the limitations of standard minimally invasive procedures. Robot-assisted thoracoscopic esophagectomy in conjunction with conventional laparoscopy has shown to be technically feasible providing oncological clearance whilst minimizing blood loss. Minimally invasive and robot assisted esophagectomy offer promising results with outcomes that are at least comparable to conventional open surgery. Esophagectomy can be safely performed using a minimally invasive approach in experienced centers and is associated with acceptable morbidity, low mortality, and potentially equivalent oncologic results.

- Two-stage esophagectomy is a surgical approach reducing mortality and should be taken into account for high-risk patients. Comparing the different types of adenocarcinomas of the esophagogastric junction of all stages, Siewert type I tumors seem to have the best prognosis and type III the worst. The reason for this prognostic difference might be ascribed to the fact that proximal lesions, due to the limited passage diameter, might be symptomatic in earlier stages.

- The goal of neoadjuvant therapy in EAC is to identify responders, improve tolerance of toxicity associated with therapy, downstage the tumor, enhance resectability, improve local control, and potentially improve survival. Targeted therapy based on molecular markers for sensitivity/resistance and prognosis may help with the decision to use combined modality therapy in the future.

- Most thoracic surgical and medical oncologists accept the premise that neoadjuvant therapy should be employed in esophageal carcinoma staged either T3 or node positive by endoscopic ultrasound. An argument can also be made to treat T2 staged tumors given the poor survival achieved with surgery alone.

- A recent phase I/II trial attempted direct delivery of therapy into the primary tumor of patients receiving chemoradiotherapy for esophageal cancer. Weekly intratumoral injections with an adenovirus vector carrying the TNF gene linked to a radiation inducible promoter was performed in patients receiving cisplatin, 5-FU, and radiation therapy. Viral markers were detectable in resected tumor tissue and regional lymphatics, indicating the therapy could permeate regional lymphatics.

- Non-5-FU–based regimens have been explored in combined chemoradiotherapy phase II trials, including paclitaxel or docetaxel with cisplatin or carboplatin, irinotecan/cisplatin, and docetaxel/irinotecan.

- Clinical variables seem not to be effective for response prediction in the multimodality therapy of esophageal cancer. Data of molecular variables is promising, but to date not a single marker is available in clinical practice.

- FDG–PET currently cannot accurately predict pathologic complete response. Correlation with prognosis is likely, but is of questionable importance as that information is not currently used to alter treatment. PET can detect interval metastatic disease but a cost-benefit model is lacking. p53 may predict response to neoadjuvant chemotherapy in esophageal cancer patients, and therefore could be relevant for the choice of therapy.

- Targeted therapies with mAbs directed against growth factor receptors in combination with chemotherapy or chemoradiation already demonstrated a promising potential in phase I–II trials. Data regarding associated toxicities are currently difficult to interpret and deserve careful monitoring. The development of novel mAbs against various targets, application of mAb combinations and molecular and proteomics analysis appear to have a promising potential to improve treatment results.

- There are many potential targets for treatment in esophageal cancer and the number increases with our understanding of the pathophysiology of cancer, but the possible benefit of targeted treatments must be weighed against toxicity. A possible stage specific paradigm, with a role for adjuvant therapy, can be proposed for adenocarcinoma of the esophagus, especially

when found to be locally advanced after surgical resection.

- The future of treatment for this disease will probably depend on molecular targets with therapy being given on a personalized approach.

---

1. What is the accuracy of intraoperative frozen sections?

William S. Twaddell
wtwaddell@umm.edu

EAC is increasing in incidence in the developed world. Surgical resection is central to the treatment of established esophageal carcinoma, with completeness of resection correlating significantly with survival.[1] The use of frozen section may be helpful in assessing apparently uninvolved margins for the presence of cryptic tumor.

Despite the development of numerous nonsurgical and neoadjuvant modalities for the therapy of EAC, surgery remains the mainstay for curative treatment. Therefore, intraoperative consultation with frozen section may be pursued to ensure complete resection. Our experience (unpublished data) demonstrates a frequency of 1.6% (1 of 61 cases) of detection of high-grade or invasive carcinoma at the frozen section margin. This is also associated with 2 of 61 cases (3.3%) that were not identified as positive margins intraoperatively (one of which was interpreted as negative at the time of surgery, the other was diagnosed as indefinite and deferred to permanent section), but for which final pathology ultimately showed adenocarcinoma at the margins, for an overall accuracy of 96.7% and a negative predictive value of 96.6% (counting the indefinite case as a false negative).

When frozen sections were not evaluated, high-grade dysplasia or adenocarcinoma was identified at the permanent margin in 4 of 70 cases (5.7%), for an accuracy of gross evaluation for tumor of 94.3%. In addition, a single case had pools of mucin without associated malignant cells identified at the proximal margin. This is a somewhat lower percentage than has been reported previously in the absence of frozen sections,[2] although that study did not include any patients who had received neoadjuvant chemo- or radiation therapy.

There is a paucity of previously published data on the subject of intraoperative accuracy for margins in the resection of EACs. To some degree, an analogy may be made with frozen sections performed on other sites. Frozen sections in margins taken for resection of squamous cell carcinoma of the vocal cord were confirmed by permanent sections in approximately 95% of cases (97 patients).[3] Similarly, Shen *et al.*[4] had 97% accuracy in 66 cases treated for gastric adenocarcinoma. Drawbacks of frozen section are relatively minor in most cases. The procedure is somewhat time-consuming and may add slightly to the time of the operation. Although permanent histology is slightly altered by the process of freezing, in most cases this does not impair final interpretation. There is an increased cost to the payer associated with the performance of frozen section.

Based on our unpublished findings, and in line with similar reports for other operative procedures, frozen section for EAC has a high accuracy. However, this must be considered against the relatively low frequency of positive margins, even in cases in which no frozen section was performed. However, given the importance for patient outcome of complete resection, intraoperative frozen section for margins may be justified in many cases.

---

2. What are the indications and techniques of sentinel node biopsy for esophageal cancer?

Peter C. Wu
pcwu@u.washington.edu

The term *sentinel node* was first introduced by Cabanas in 1977 to describe metastatic lymph nodes associated with penile cancer and is defined as the first draining lymph node from a primary tumor and represents the first site of metastasis. Morton and colleagues at the John Wayne Cancer Institute are credited with first introducing in 1992 the concept of lymphatic mapping using intradermal injections of blue dye in patients with early stage melanoma. Shortly afterwards, Alex and Krag described the use of technetium-99 sulfur colloid with an intraoperative handheld gamma-detecting probe to localize sentinel nodes in melanoma patients. SLN biopsy has since become widely accepted as a minimally invasive and highly accurate and reliable technique for detecting occult nodal metastases in breast cancer and cutaneous melanoma, and has been validated as an independent prognostic factor.

There are several reasons that have been proposed to support the use of SLN staging in patients diagnosed with early stage esophageal cancer. Lymph node status has been shown to be a strong predictor of survival, and patients with immuno-histochemistry detected micrometastases in histologically negative nodes have a higher risk of locoregional and systemic relapse and decreased survival.[5] Current staging modalities are limited by their ability to detect nodal disease with one study comparing FDG PET versus combined CT and endoscopic ultrasound, which showed an accuracy of only 48% versus 69% and sensitivity of 22% versus 83%, respectively.[6] Considering the prognostic significance of detecting nodal micrometastases and existing limitations of current staging studies, SLN biopsy may offer a more precise methodology to identify lymph node metastases and has been shown to upstage 13–36% of colon cancer cases.[7] Considering the morbidity associated with radical esophagectomy, it seems reasonable that SLN staging could be used to spare patients with early stage disease from unnecessary radical multifield lymphadenectomy, individualize treatment by selective lymph node dissection (LND) or modified radiation fields, or select patients for esophagus-preserving therapy (e.g., endoscopic mucosal resection) or limited esophageal resection (e.g., the Merendino procedure).

On the other hand, there are several drawbacks that have limited widespread adoption of SLN procedures for esophageal cancer. Due to the diffuse multidirectional and longitudinal lymphatic drainage of the esophagus, several studies have reported unpredictable sites of lymph node metastases for thoracic esophageal squamous cell cancer that can occur widely throughout the cervical, mediastinal, and/or abdominal lymph node basins. Interestingly, Feith *et al.* showed a more predictable

pattern of lymphatic spread in patients with distal EAC (Barrett's cancer) with > 95% of cases of solitary lymph node metastases occurring in the lower mediastinum and upper abdomen.[8] Compared to other cancers, early experience with esophageal cancer has shown a higher number of SLNs (median > 4), multiple nodal sites in 20% of cases, and "skip" metastases to distant nodal sites in 50–60% of cases. Furthermore, identification of mediastinal lymph nodes often requires extensive mobilization of the esophagus, which disrupts the lymphatic channels limiting the efficacy of intra-operative localization with blue dye. Finally, blue dye injection is less effective due to frequently dark-pigmented anthracotic mediastinal lymph nodes.

To date, there have been nine published studies totaling 312 patients that have undergone successful SLN biopsy for potentially curable esophageal cancer. The greatest experience has been reported from Japanese centers, with individual case series reported from the United Kingdom, Germany, Netherlands, Australia, and India (Table 1). Seven studies used the technique of endoscopic submucosal peritumoral injection of radiocolloid ranging from 0 to 18 hours prior to surgical resection, while two studies used blue dye alone. SLN detection rates ranged from 81% to 100% with a sensitivity of 77–100%, accuracy of 75–100%, and false-negative rate of 0–15%, which is comparable to early reports of SLN biopsy in melanoma and breast cancer.

Gamma probes are currently available in a variety of configurations that can be adapted for both laparoscopic and thoracoscopic procedures to harvest abdominal and mediastinal nodes, respectively. New technologies that may improve localization of esophageal SLN include the use of PET tracers. When a PET tracer (e.g., [18F]FDG) decays, a positron is emitted that interacts with a nearby electron. Both are annihilated, creating gamma photons that are detected by PET scan systems. Several gamma-PET probes are currently being marketed to detect the gamma photons emitted from targeted tissue. This has been successfully reported in pilot studies for the intraoperative localization of both recurrent and metastatic solid tumors. Experimental animal studies using [18F]FLT probes designed to target tissue based upon cellular proliferation rather than cellular metabolism show promising results with improved discrimination between malignant and inflammatory tissue. Preclinical studies

Table 1. Summary of SLN studies for esophageal cancer

Study	Year	Method	Patients	Detection Rate	Sensitivity	Accuracy	False-negative rate
Kitagawa[9] (Japan)	2000	^{99m}Tc tin colloid	27	93%	88%	92%	
Kato[10] (Japan)	2003	^{99m}Tc rhenium colloid	25	92%	87%	91%	9%
Burian[11] (Germany)	2004	^{99m}Tc colloid, + blue dye (N = 10)	20	85%			
Lamb[12] (UK)	2005	^{99m}Tc nanocolloid	57	100%	95%	96%	5%
Arima[13] (Japan)	2006	^{99m}Tc tin colloid	19	95%	78%	78%	
Takeuchi[14] (Japan)	2009	^{99m}Tc tin colloid	75	95%		94%	
Grotenhuis[15] (Netherlands)	2009	Patent blue V	40	98%	77%	85%	15%
Bhat[16] (India)	2010	Methylene blue	32	81%	86%	75%	
Thompson[17] (Australia)	2010	^{99m}Tc antimony colloid	17	88%	100%	100%	0%

have also been reported using near-infrared fluorescent tracers that have the ability to fluoresce brightly against a low background that have the advantage of minimizing shine-through effect from the primary tumor site, do not stain the operative field, and eliminates the need for a specialized probe.

The treatment of esophageal cancer continues to evolve with improvements in technology and surgical technique, better understanding of genomics and tumor biology, and refinements in combined modality therapy. However, the role of SLN biopsy for early stage tumors remains unproven with a need for prospective validation studies. There is currently no standardized operative approach, and SLN identification can be accomplished through the use of both laparoscopic transhiatal and thoracoscopic mediastinal techniques. Further studies are needed to define the prognostic significance of esophageal micrometastases and optimize the intraoperative evaluation of harvested SLNs to identify the presence of micrometastases that can influence surgical decision-making during esophagectomy. The specific role of surgery will likely change with the introduction of novel therapies, but traditional esophagectomy currently remains the mainstay treatment for potentially curable esophageal cancer.

3. What is the role of robotic surgery in the treatment of esophageal cancer?

Roy J.J. Verhage and Richard van Hillegersberg
r.j.j.verhage@umcutrecht.nl

Radical surgical resection of the esophagus and surrounding lymph nodes offers the best chance for cure in patients with locoregional disease.[18] Optimal treatment for esophageal cancer, therefore, consists of transthoracic en bloc esophagectomy with an extensive mediastinal LND. This approach through thoracotomy is accompanied by significant morbidity, mainly consisting of cardiopulmonary complications. To reduce surgical trauma and morbidity of open transthoracic esophagectomy, minimally invasive esophagectomy (MIE) techniques have been introduced. An international survey showed that thoracic esophagectomy with a two-field LND is the most commonly applied extent of LND.[19] The survey also revealed that 40% of the surgeon responders routinely use minimally invasive techniques for esophagectomy. With regard to MIE, a review of the literature shows a substantial decrease in blood loss, complication rate, and hospital stay.[20] However, conventional scopic techniques have important limitations, such as a two-dimensional view, a disturbed eye–hand coordination, and a

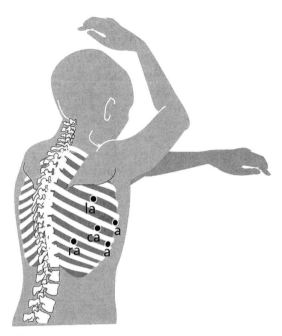

Figure 1. Trocar arrangement during robot-assisted thoraco-scopic phase. la, left robotic arm; a, assistant port; ca, robotic camera arm; ra, right robotic arm (Boone *et al.*[22]).

decrease in degrees of freedom due to large, rigid instruments.

Robotic systems have been developed to over-come the limitations of standard minimally invasive procedures.[21] The Da Vinci™ robotic system pro-vides a three-dimensional, 10-fold-magnified view of the operating field. It filters the tremor of the surgeon, restores the natural eye–hand coordina-tion axis as a result of the ergonomically designed surgeon's console, and offers more degrees of free-dom through its articulating scopic surgical instru-ments. During esophagectomy, the robotic platform enables the surgeon to perform an accurate me-diastinal dissection of the esophagus with sur-rounding lymph nodes in a confined surgical field.

In our tertiary referral center, the robot-assisted thoracolaparoscopic approach is routinely used for patients with resectable cancer of the esophagus. The patient is positioned in the left lateral decubitus position and tilted 45° toward the prone position (Fig. 1). The robotic system is placed at the dor-socranial side of the patient. Three robotic and two assistant's instrument ports are placed. After the pulmonary ligament has been divided, the pari-

etal pleura is dissected at the anterior side of the esophagus from the diaphragm up to the azygos arch. The azygos arch is ligated, and dissection of the parietal pleura continues above the arch for a right paratracheal LND. Subsequently, the pari-etal pleura is dissected at the posterior side of the esophagus cranially to caudally along the azygos vein, including the thoracic duct to avoid postop-erative chyle leakage. At the level of the diaphragm, the thoracic duct is clipped with a 10-mm endo-scopic clipping device (Endoclip™ II). A Penrose drain is then placed around the esophagus to fa-cilitate esophageal mobilization. In this way, the esophagus can be resected *en bloc* with the sur-rounding mediastinal lymph nodes and the thoracic duct from the diaphragm up to the thoracic inlet. For LND, the robotic system provides an excellent view at angles that cannot be reached during open surgery. LND includes the right-sided paratracheal (lymph node station 2R), tracheobronchial (lymph node station 4), aortopulmonary window (station 5), carinal (station 7), and periesophageal (station 8)

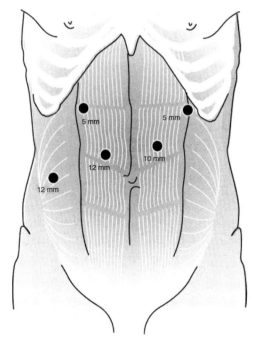

Figure 2. Trocar arrangement during conventional laparo-scopic phase. The camera is inserted through the 10-mm trocar port, and two 5-mm trocars are used as working ports. The liver retractor is inserted through the 12-mm right pararectal trocar port and the harmonic scalpel introduced through the 12-mm paraumbilical port (Boone *et al*[22]).

lymph nodes. The abdominal phase of the operation is performed with conventional laparoscopy (Fig. 2), dissecting the greater and lesser curvature of the stomach, crux, and celiac trunk. LND includes lymph nodes surrounding the left gastric artery and the lesser omental lymph nodes. The resected specimen is removed through a 7 cm transverse transabdominal incision. Linear staplers (GIA 80, 3.8 mm) are used to create a gastric conduit 3–4 cm wide with oversewing of the staple line. Through a left-sided vertical incision along the sternocleidoid muscle, a handsewn end-to-side anastomosis is created between the gastric tube and the cervical esophagus using 3/0 polydioxanone single-layer running sutures. No formal cervical LND is carried out unless lymph node metastases are suspected macroscopically.

Our first series reported 47 patients who underwent robot-assisted thoracolaparoscopic esophagectomy (RTE).[22] Conversion to thoracotomy was necessary in seven patients. Median operating time was 450 min (360–550). Median blood loss during thoracoscopy was 250 mL (0–800) and 625 mL (150–5300) for the entire procedure. A learning curve was observed, illustrated by a significant decrease in total blood loss between the first 23 and second 24 patients (median 900 mL vs. 450 mL, respectively; $P < 0.001$) and a reduction of operating time (median 7.5 hours vs. 7.0 hours; $P = 0.024$). Patients were ventilated for a median of one day (0–126). Median intensive care unit (ICU) stay was three days (0–136) and hospital stay 18 days (10–182). Though not significant, the first 23 patients had a higher pulmonary complication rate than the last 24 (13 of 23 vs. 8 of 24; $P = 0.147$). A median of 29 (range 8–68) lymph nodes was dissected, and R0 resection was achieved in 36 patients. Twenty-three patients had stage IVa disease. After a median follow-up of 35 months, median disease-free survival was 15 months (95% CI 12–18).

Robot-assisted thoracoscopic esophagectomy in conjunction with conventional laparoscopy has shown to be technically feasible providing oncological clearance while minimizing blood loss. Despite their short history in the field of esophagectomy, MIE and robot-assisted esophagectomy offer promising results with outcomes that are at least comparable to conventional open surgery. Future research will focus on long-term outcomes and the comparison of MIE with open surgery.

4. Can the sentinel node concept be still considered following chemoradiotherapy? What are the characteristics of the best candidate for sentinel node dissection?

Marcus Feith and Daniel Reim
feith@chir.med.tu-muenchen.de

Locally advanced Barrett's carcinoma is a highly malignant tumor, with a poor prognosis despite the advances in surgery or the introduction of neoadjuvant treatment. Current meta-analysis showed the benefit of neoadjuvant treatment in esophageal carcinoma.[23] In advanced adenocarcinoma of the esophagus, even after neoadjuvant treatment, the complete residual tumor-free resection and the lymph node infiltration are the leading prognostic factors.[24]

Results for the SLN detection after neoadjuvant treatment in esophageal cancer are small. Mostly investigated is the experience in breast cancer and SLN detection after preoperative chemoradiotherapy. However, the results are divergent with a safe and accurate SLN detection as diagnostic tool on one side,[25] and a higher rate of false-negatives with the increasing tumor stage on the other side.[26] The limitations for SLN detection after neoadjuvant chemoradiotherapy in esophageal carcinoma are that mostly advanced tumor stages receive the neoadjuvant therapy, with high rates of lymph node metastases up to 80%. The detection rate of lymph nodes is reduced after radiochemotherapy and currently no limitations of the surgical approach are oncologically adquate in advanced carcinomas. Only a small group of patients will benefit from reduced radical lymphadenectomy, with higher rates of tumor recurrence.[27]

The best candidates for SLN dissection in Barrett's cancer are the non-pretreated early adenocarcinomas in an experienced center with Blue dye or ^{99m}Tc techniques. The pathologist needs experience with fresh frozen section of SLNs, and a limited surgical approach for complete resection of the lesion and prelesion should be available.

5. The role of neoadjuvant therapy in esophageal cancer and the potential for "lymphatic-directed" therapy

David H. Ilson
ilsond@mskcc.org

In 2010, most thoracic surgical and medical oncologists accept the premise that neoadjuvant therapy should be employed in esophageal carcinoma staged either T3 or node positive by endoscopic ultrasound. An argument can also be made to treat T2-staged tumors given the poor survival achieved with surgery alone. Neoadjuvant therapy with preoperative chemotherapy has achieved mixed results, with British and French trials (MAGIC, FFCD) of preoperative ECF or CF improving survival by a 13–14% increment at five years; older British and U.S. studies (MRC OEO-2, INT-113) either failed to improve or achieved marginal survival improvements.[28,29] Smaller trials of preoperative chemoradiotherapy followed by surgery have also achieved mixed results, with only two of the five published trials reporting a survival improvement.

A recent meta-analysis of trials of preoperative chemotherapy and chemoradiotherapy indicated a superior mortality reduction (10% vs. 19%) and a superior two-year survival improvement (7% vs. 13%) favoring preoperative chemoradiotherapy over chemotherapy alone.[30] A head-to-head comparison of preoperative chemotherapy versus chemoradiotherapy was conducted in a recent German trial (POET); this phase III trial treated EUS and laparoscopically staged Siewert I-III adenocarcinomas.[31] Poor accrual led to closure of the trial at 119 of 360 planned patients. Chemoradiotherapy trended superior to chemotherapy in three-year overall survival (47% vs. 28%, $P = 0.07$) and local tumor control (77% vs. 59%, $P = 0.06$). Additional evidence supporting the benefit of preoperative chemoradiotherapy versus surgery alone comes from the recently presented CROSS trial from the Netherlands.[32] Surgery alone was compared to preoperative chemoradiotherapy with weekly paclitaxel, carboplatin, and 41.4 Gy of radiotherapy in 363 patients with EUS-staged esophageal cancer. The majority had adenocarcinoma (74%), mid or distal tumors (85%), or stage T3N0–1 (75–80%). Preoperative therapy was well tolerated and resulted in improved rates of R0 resection (92% compared

to 67%, $P < 0.002$) and a pathologic complete response rate of 27%. Median survival was improved by nearly two years ($P = 0.011$) and three-year overall survival by 11% with chemoradiotherapy. These results may establish this therapy as a new preoperative standard of care.

Taxane/platinum chemoradiotherapy is now under study in the United States in two RTOG trials, one nonoperative trial comparing chemoradiotherapy with or without the EGFr-targeted agent cetuximab, and the other an operative trial comparing HER2 + EAC treated with chemoradiotherapy with or without trastuzumab followed by surgery. A recent phase I/II trial attempted direct delivery of therapy into the primary tumor of patients receiving chemoradiotherapy for esophageal cancer. Weekly intratumoral injections with the agent TNFerade, an adenovirus vector carrying the TNF gene linked to a radiation inducible promoter, were performed in patients receiving cisplatin, 5-FU, and radiation therapy.[33] Viral markers were detectable in resected tumor tissue and regional lymphatics, indicating that the therapy could permeate regional lymphatics. Pathologic complete responses in 6 of 15 patients were observed. Further study of this agent is under consideration.

6. Does Siewert's classification allow for distinction of patients with different life expectancy?

Christoph Schuhmacher, Marcus Feith, Andre Mihaljevic, and Helmut Friess
schuhmacher@chir.med.tu-muenchen.de

The classification of adenocarcinoma of the esophagogastric junction (AEG) by J.R. Siewert[34] was primarily intended to be used as a technical guideline in terms of the extent of resection for surgeons. According to this classification, tumors having contact to the center of the cardia in the area of the esophagogastric (EG) junction but growing toward the esophagus should be treated as esophageal carcinomas. The histopathology of these tumors show, in most cases (97%), an intestinal metaplasia (BE). Tumors with their center at the cardia (AEG II) and tumors that grow toward the stomach (AEG III) classify as gastric carcinomas. AEG II and III rarely show intestinal metaplasia (9.8% and 2.0%) and more often Laurens diffuse type growth

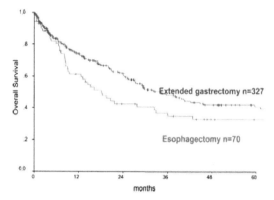

Figure 3. Survival of patients (Kaplan–Meier) undergoing either a transhiatal extended gastrectomy or esophagectomy. Due to the nonrandomized comparison of a series of prospectively collected data (Department of Surgery, Technische Universität Münich), the results are preliminary and need further evaluation on the basis of a randomized trial.

pattern.[34] The surgical treatment of AEG type II and III tumors should be carried out according to the standards of gastric cancer. A transhiatal extended gastrectomy is the procedure of choice for these cases (Fig. 3).

Siewert's classification, however, is usually not employed as a predictive score. For this purpose, the depth of infiltration of the primary tumor, the nodal status, and the absence of metastasis are the main factors used. These tumor categories, expressed in the TNM system and in the UICC stage of the disease, are used to predict the prognosis of the disease (Fig. 4).

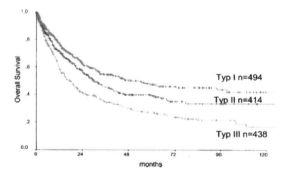

Figure 4. There seems to be a survival difference in patients depending on the localization of the adenocarcinoma of esophagogastric junction after R0-resection (AEG I, II and III; all UICC stages).

(i) It is without doubt that, in AEG type I, esophagectomy is the procedure of choice to achieve curative resection. The results of a randomized trial[35] are in favor of the transthoracic approach in AEG type I, compared to a transhiatal esophagectomy from an abdominal incision. Reconstruction is usually carried out using a gastric tube.

(ii) AEG type II, despite being gastric tumors, are presently in the focus of a debate, especially in obese patients with a short mesenterium where reconstruction using the proximal jejunum might be difficult. Here, the abdomino-thoracic approach, as applied in AEG type I, is the safer technique. As a standard recommendation, for AEG type II the transhiatal gastrectomy is the resection of choice.

In both cases, transhiatal extended gastrectomy and the abdomino-thoracic approach, a radical dissection of the lymph nodes (D2), especially at the celiac trunk, is mandatory. In cases of AEG II tumors, where the exact upper tumor margin is not sufficiently diagnosed by preoperative endoscopy, there is the recommendation to start the procedure at the esophageal hiatus with an early transsection proximal to the tumor. Thus, after frozen section of the resection margin, both options of resection are still feasible. This is not the case after dissecting the duodenum and the vasa gastroepiploica. A nonrandomized comparison of both techniques in a selected series of patients at the surgical department of the TUM did show some prognostic advantage for the extended gastrectomy in these cases.[36]

(i) Transhiatal gastrectomy is the treatment of choice for AEG type III tumors.

Comparing the different types of AEG I-AEG III of all stages, there is a prognostic difference. AEG type I seem to have the best prognosis and AEG type III the worst.[34] The reason for this prognostic difference might be ascribed to the fact that proximal lesions due to the limited passage diameter might be symptomatic in earlier stages. AEG type III are more often of diffuse type growth pattern, a fact that might contribute to an earlier dissemination of tumor cells, especially around the cardia and its close anatomical structures.

7. The advantages of MIE

Arjun Pennathur and James D. Luketich

luketichjd@upmc.edu

The incidence of esophageal cancer has increased dramatically in the Western population in the last two decades due to the increasing incidence of adenocarcinoma of the esophagus. The reasons for this dramatic increase in the incidence of adenocarcinoma are not entirely clear, but gastroesophageal reflux disease, obesity, and Barrett's esophagus have been identified as risk factors. Surgery is an important component of treatment for esophageal cancer. However, there has been concern about the morbidity of esophagectomy for esophageal neoplasm. Esophagectomy performed in a minimally invasive fashion has the potential to decrease the perioperative morbidity of the procedure. Over the last two decades, the techniques of MIE have been refined, and in this article we will discuss MIE and some recent developments.

MIE

In 2003, we published our analysis of 222 consecutive patients who had undergone MIE at the University of Pittsburgh.[37] Esophagectomy was performed with thoracoscopy, laparoscopy, and cervical anastomosis. Although early in the series we selectively performed MIE on patients with smaller tumors and no previous therapy, 35% of the patients in this series had been treated with chemotherapy and 16% treated with radiation. In addition, 25% of patients had undergone prior open abdominal surgery.

We were able to complete the MIE as planned in 206 (93%) patients. No emergent conversions to an open procedure were necessary for bleeding. There were three deaths in the series (1.4% mortality). This very low mortality rate compares favorably with the largest series of open esophagectomy. MIE is also safe for treatment of early stage tumors. We recently published our experience of 100 consecutive patients with T1 tumors who were treated with esophagectomy.[38] A minimally invasive approach was used in 80% of the patients. There was no operative mortality. In addition, we evaluated quality of life postoperatively with the GERD-HRQL instrument, which indicated that the quality of life was preserved.

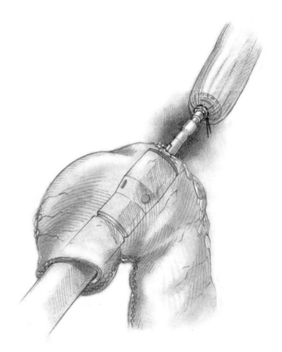

Figure 5. Creating the anastomosis during an Ivor Lewis MIE. © Heart, Lung, and Esophageal Surgery Institute, University of Pittsburgh Medical Center.

New developments in MIE; minimally invasive Ivor Lewis esophagectomy

The standard MIE performed at the University of Pittsburgh has traditionally been a three-field operation, with a cervical anastomosis. More recently, however, we reported our initial experience with a minimally invasive Ivor Lewis esophagectomy.[39] Early in our adoption of the Ivor Lewis MIE, we performed the operation as a hybrid procedure, combining laparoscopic mobilization of the stomach with a mini-thoracotomy for creation of the anastomosis. With increasing experience, we have turned to a completely minimally invasive approach for performing the Ivor Lewis esophagectomy. The Ivor Lewis MIE is a particularly useful option, especially for patients with extensive involvement of the cardia in whom the conduit may not reach to the neck (Figs. 5 and 6).

ECOG 2202 multicenter trial: MIE

In 2009, at the American Society for Clinical Oncology (ASCO) Annual Meeting, the preliminary results of the Eastern Cooperative Oncology Group (ECOG) multicenter Phase II trial on MIE (ECOG

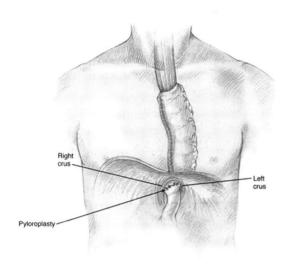

Figure 6. Schematic representation of the completed MIE. © Heart, Lung, and Esophageal Surgery Institute, University of Pittsburgh Medical Center.

2202) were presented.[40] This trial is sponsored by ECOG, with participation of multiple centers across the United States and the University of Pittsburgh serving as the lead center. A total of 106 patients from 16 institutions in the United States (84% men; 22% women; median age 64, range 36–83) entered into the study. MIE was performed in 99 patients. The operative mortality was less than 2%. The median ICU stay was two days. At a mean follow-up of 19 months, the estimated three-year overall survival for the entire cohort was 50% (95% confidence interval 35–65%). Stage-specific survival was similar to open series. This initial analysis of the ECOG 2202 trial demonstrated that MIE is safe and feasible in multiple centers, with low perioperative mortality and morbidity.[40] Oncologic outcomes were similar to open esophagectomy.

Conclusion

Esophagectomy can be safely performed using a minimally invasive approach in experienced centers and is associated with good results. The preliminary results of a Phase II trial of MIE (ECOG 2202), with participation of multiple centers across the United States, are encouraging and showed a low morbidity and mortality with a minimally invasive approach. In summary, MIE can be performed with acceptable morbidity, low mortality, and potentially equivalent oncologic results.

8. What are the indications of two-step esophagectomy?

Björn Brücher
bjoern.bruecher@med.uni-tuebingen.de

The two-stage procedure is not a new approach, as it was successfully performed for the first time in 1913 by the German Franz Torek.[41] By definition, a two-stage esophagectomy is a right thoracic esophagectomy with a left cervical esophageal fistula. The reconstructive surgery of the gastroinstinal tract is done afterwards as a two-stage procedure. This rationale minimizes patients' risk of death in high-risk patients by anastomozing the esophagus safely. Therefore, the two-stage esophagectomy is a prophylaxis of mediastinitis. Therefore the two-stage esophagectomy is one principle in reducing mortality in esophageal cancer, in association with preoperative preparation (e.g., coronary bypass/stenting, chemotherapy, pulmoary training, alcohol and nicotin-withdrawal, etc.), possibly leading to avoid surgery in high-risk patients (e.g. liver cirrhosis, poor compliance, etc.). Esophageal patients of high risk are esophageal emergencies (trauma by perforation or ingestion), elderly patients with co-morbidities, esophageal squamous cell carcinoma[42] (compared to other histologies), and those patients who underwent multimodal treatment.[43] In addition, surgery is, by itself, a risk factor. In particular, ESCC patients nonresponding after neoadjuvant radiochemotherapy have a significantly worse survival compared to those responding.[44]

In conclusion, two-stage esophagectomy is a surgical approach reducing mortality and should be taken into account for high-risk patients.

9. Is it conceivable to identify clinical variables or biomarkers predictive of pathological complete response?

Daniel Vallböhmer, Arnulf H. Hölscher, and J. Brabender
daniel.vallboehmer@uk-koeln.de

Despite advances in preoperative staging, surgical techniques, and postoperative care, the overall survival of patients with esophageal cancer remains low.[45] In particular, the poor prognosis of patients with locally advanced esophageal cancer prompted the assessment of neoadjuvant treatment options to improve patients' survival.[46] However, it has been well established that only patients with a complete pathological response to neoadjuvant therapy will have a significant survival benefit.[46] Therefore, predictive markers to allow a tailored multimodality treatment are needed.

To date, there is still a great lack in clinical variables or biomarkers for response assessment in patients with esophageal cancer undergoing multimodality treatment. The most potential but invasive method for response assessment is the histomorphologic regression grading system, suggested by several groups, including ours.[46] By using histopathologic criteria, this system classifies tumor regression in the surgical specimen based on the estimated percentage of vital residual tumor cells that was demonstrated to be of significant prognostic importance.[46] As opposed to this, noninvasive imaging modalities, such as endoscopy, endoscopic biopsies, computed tomography (CT), and endoscopic ultrasound (EUS), have been shown to be highly inaccurate to evaluate response to neoadjuvant therapy in patients with esophageal cancer.[47]

Interestingly, recent studies suggest that ^{18}F-fluoro-deoxyglucose-positron emission tomography (FDG PET) seems to be the best available noninvasive tool for response assessment in esophageal cancer. For example, Lordick *et al.* assessed in a prospective single-center study, including 119 patients with locally advanced EAC, the feasibility of a PET response-guided treatment algorithm.[48] Indeed, the authors were able to demonstrate that FDG PET is useful for early response prediction in the course of multimodality treatment, suggesting this diagnostic tool to have great impact in response assessment of esophageal cancer patients. However, quite the opposite results were reported just recently by our own working group.[49] We failed to show significant differences between responders and nonresponders in patients with esophageal cancer using FDG PET for response assessment, so that the role of FDG PET in the multimodality treatment of esophageal cancer remains to be determined in further studies.

Finally, potential predictive/prognostic factors have been characterized for response assessment in esophageal cancer patients by innovative molecular-based technologies.[50] These factors include growth-factor receptors, enzymes of angiogenesis, tumor suppressor genes, cell cycle regulators, enzymes involved in the DNA-repair system, in apoptosis, and in the degradation of extracellular matrix.[50] The results of these mostly retrospective studies are promising, but this research topic still fails to provide a reliable and inexpensive molecular tool for response assessment.

In conclusion, clinical variables seem not to be effective for response prediction in the multimodality therapy of esophageal cancer. Data on molecular variables are promising, but to date not a single marker is in clinical practice so that prospective/multiinstitutional studies are needed.

10. What role does PET scan play in response assessment and restaging in esophageal cancer?

Wayne L. Hofstetter
Whofstetter@mdanderson.org

Patients with locally advanced esophageal cancer are commonly offered combined concurrent chemoradiation. However, not all patients respond equally to therapy and, as a result, patients derive a differential outcome benefit from neoadjuvant therapy. Patients who have achieved a complete pathologic response enjoy greater overall survival compared to patients who are incomplete responders. Therefore, there is a potential benefit to accurately predicting response. Theoretically, patients found to have a complete response could consider observation rather than surgery and incomplete responders would be offered surgery without delay. Unfortunately, up to this point, detection of complete pathologic response (pCR) has been a surgical phenomenon. The role of FDG PET, and more recently, integrated PET/CT scan as a reliable predictor of treatment response, has been evaluated and is the topic of this discussion. What role does PET scan currently play in response assessment and restaging in esophageal cancer?

Reasons for obtaining a PET/CT during or after treatment include the following:

1. Predict pCR;
2. Predict prognosis; and
3. Alteration in management.

In fact, there are many published studies on the accuracy of PET in treatment response. A PubMed search reveals over 150 papers evaluating potentially optimal metrics for response: mean/max SUV, completely negative PET, ΔSUV, tumor/liver ratios, volumetric PET, and number of abnormalities seen on PET scan. One senses that the modality has promise but that its potential is still being actively sought. What exactly is the appropriate PET metric that best evaluates response? This is not completely understood, and prospective studies are not yet completed.

Studies investigating the potential to predict pathologic complete response

Many retrospective studies and reviews are searchable within PUBMED on this topic. A few will be used as example. A 2004 study from MD Anderson reviewed 83 patients who received posttreatment PET scans. These were retrospectively analyzed surgical patients, and the authors report that PET could identify with 95% specificity the patients who had pathologically confirmed residual tumor.[51] These patients had SUVmax of four or higher. However, other patients with residual disease manifested low SUV. Therefore, for residual disease the specificity of PET with SUV cut-off of four was high but the sensitivity was low (26%), indicating that PET could be a reliable predictor of residual disease, but not necessarily pCR. In contrast, two years later the same group of authors contradicted their previous publication because in a different sample set, 6 of 19 patients who had high SUVmax actually had a confounding finding of an ulcerated esophagus leading to a false-positive result.[52] Surgical pathology revealed no evidence of tumor. This publication questions the reliability of PET alone in the assessment of residual disease. Another angle is to explore whether a completely negative PET scan is predictive of pCR. A group from Moffitt looked at 81 patients, and among 20 patients with a completely negative PET, 13 patients had residual disease at resection; 7 had no disease.[53] Therefore, and summarizing other available literature, neither positive (range 24–93%) nor negative predictive value (range 33–95%; overall accuracy range 29–79%) of PET for pCR has proven to be valuable thus far.

Predicting prognosis

Our group recently reviewed data on ΔSUVmax and found that there is a cut-off point at about 52% decrease between pretreatment and posttreatment SUV in terms of overall prognosis.[54] However, this is retrospective, nonvalidated data in a single in-

stitution, and although it shows we may identify differences in prognosis, these data do not lead to changes in therapy.

Alteration in management

 (i) Detect interval metastatic disease before taking the patient for surgical resection
 (ii) Surgical planning—i.e., plan timing of surgery; if severe pneumonitis on PET/CT would one take patients immediately to surgery or delay?
(iii) Treatment planning—used as an interval treatment scan; patients that are nonresponsive referred directly to surgery, responders continue with neoadjuvant therapy to completion

FDG PET can detect interval metastatic disease that manifests over the neoadjuvant treatment duration. In one study of 88 patients, new metastatic lesions were detected in seven patients (8%), but in review of CT scans, only two were occult retrospectively.[55] Therefore, the PET focused the radiologist on where to look at the CT FDG uptake in the pulmonary parenchyma after neoadjuvant chemoradiotherapy has been shown to correlate with radiation pneumonitis symptoms,[56] but no correlation of FDG avid radiation pneumonitis to complications is known. In our practice, we use this finding as an indicator to delay surgery and treat the pneumonitis.

In regards to treatment planning and interval response, review studies show that the positive and negative predictive values are variable. A very good evidence-based medicine review from March 2010 in *Radiology* shows that sensitivity and specificity in existing publications ranges from 33% to 100% and 30% to 100%, respectively for treatment response,[57] but there are very few studies that show high sensitivity and high specificity on both; this indicates that accuracy is very limited (Fig. 7).

In conclusion, FDG PET currently cannot accurately predict pathologic complete response. Correlation with prognosis is likely but is of questionable importance as that information is not currently used to alter treatment. PET can detect interval metastatic disease but a cost-benefit model given its usefulness is lacking. Utilizing PET for surgical planning around radiation pneumonitis is possible, but there may be no benefit of PET above CT and patient symptoms.

Study/Reference No./Year	Sensitivity (%)	Specificity (%)
Schmidt et al/6/2009	48 (30, 67)	100 (90, 100)
Smith et al/7/2009	78 (40, 97)	42 (15, 72)
Cerfolio et al/8/2009	65 (47, 80)	82 (68, 91)
Roedl et al/9/2008	86 (64, 97)	67 (47, 83)
McLoughlin et al/10/2008	40 (26, 56)	68 (49, 83)
Smithers et al/11/2008	71 (29, 96)	76 (58, 89)
Lordick et al/12/2007	100 (88, 100)	72 (60, 82)
Mamede et al/13/2007	75 (35, 97)	59 (33, 82)
Port et al/14/2007	90 (55, 100)	45 (31, 60)
Bruzzi et al/15/2007	83 (66, 93)	30 (12, 54)
Gillham et al/16/2006	44 (25, 65)	40 (5, 85)
Ott et al/17/2006	80 (44, 97)	78 (64, 89)
Levine et al/18/2006	92 (62, 100)	37 (16, 62)
Westerterp et al/19/2006	75 (35, 97)	75 (35, 97)
Song et al/20/2005	37 (19, 58)	100 (48, 100)
Brink et al/21/2004	86 (42, 100)	77 (46, 95)
Wieder et al/22/2004	93 (68, 100)	88 (47, 100)
Kroep/23/2003	100 (40, 100)	86 (42, 100)
Arslan et al/24/2002	33 (4, 78)	61 (36, 83)
Brücher et al/25/2001	85 (55, 98)	82 (48, 98)

Note.—Data in parentheses are 95% CIs. Pooled estimates of sensitivity and specificity were 67% (95% CI: 62%, 72%) and 68% (95% CI: 64%, 73%), respectively.

Figure 7. Accuracy of [^{18}F]FDG–PET in the prediction of tumor response to neoadjuvant therapy. [56]

11. What are advantages of neoadjuvant therapy in locoregional EAC?

Mark J. Krasna
markkrasna@catholichealth.net

Introduction

The goal of neoadjuvant therapy in EAC is to identify responders, improve tolerance of toxicity associated with therapy, downstage the tumor, enhance resectability, improve local control, and potentially improve survival. Targeted therapy based on molecular markers for sensitivity/resistance and prognosis may help with the decision to use combined modality therapy in the future.

Review of data and guidelines

Management of esophageal cancer with chemoradiation was described by Hershkovics in the landmark RTOG study where radiation therapy (XRT) versus chemoradiation (CXRT) was used.[58] The findings included a 32% versus 12% five-year survival (YS). An update showed 20% versus 0% 10 YS, and a later report demonstrated similar results among randomized and nonrandomized patients in the trial. Local recurrence rates, however, were significant ranging from 20% to 40%.

The use of neoadjuvant chemotherapy for esophageal cancer has been studied: Kelsen described the results of 413 PTS in a RCT (INT 0113) using chemo/surgery/chemo versus surgery. The regimen included 5FU 1,000 mg/CIS 100 mg. Resectability was (65%); 1/2 YS = (62/40%). Mortality was 6.4% versus 4%. [59] Walsh *et al.* reported the first positive trial of trimodality versus surgery alone in 113 patients with adenocarcinoma. Increased survival/downstaging was noted, although there was a high mortality and low survival in surgery alone patients.[60] CALGB 9781 also studied trimodality versus surgery in 56 carefully staged patients. Grade 3 toxicities included heme (54%) and GI (40%). Fourteen (SURG) and 17 (TRI) patients had surgical complications; two postsurgical deaths occurred in the surgery arm. The postoperative length of stay (los) was 11.5 (SURG) and 10 (TRI) days. There was an 80% partial response rate and 40% pathological complete response (pCR). Survival was 4.5 years (TRI) versus 1.8 years (SURG), $P = 0.02$. five-year survival was 39% versus 16% for trimodality therapy. Stratifications by N stage, staging, and histology demonstrated a *P* value of 0.005.[61]

A RCT of 556 patients with resected adenocarcinoma of the stomach or GEJ using an adjuvant regimen of 425 mg 5FU/20 mg leucovorin followed by 4500 cGy of XRT was reported. The median OS for the surgery group was 27 months versus 36 months in the CRT group (HR 1.35, $P = 0.005$). The hazard ratio (HR) for relapse was 1.52 ($P < 0.001$). One percent died from CRT toxicity. Based on these results, it was recommended that postoperative CRT should be considered for all patients at high risk for recurrence of adenocarcinoma of the stomach or GEJ who have undergone curative resection. Trimodality therapy was recently reported by Koshy, Krasna, and Suntharalingam *et al.* in 164 patients over 14 years. Squamous cell cancers occurred in 52 and adenocarcinomas in 112. The pCR was 41%. OS was 46% (58% for those with pCR). Locoregional control (LRC) was 79%. Squamous cancers did better with improved LRC (100%) and higher pCR (54%). M1a (celiac nodal) or residual disease portended a poor prognosis.[62] A recent meta-analysis showed significant benefit with trimodality. Eleven RCTs including 1,308 patients were reviewed. Neoadjuvant CRT significantly improved the overall survival compared with surgery alone. Odds ratio (OR) was 1.28 ($P = 0.05$) for one-year survival, 1.78 ($P = 0.004$) for three years; and 1.46 ($P = 0.02$) for five-year survival. Postoperative mortality increased in patients treated by neodjuvant CRT ($P = 0.04$), and postoperative complications were similar. Neoadjuvant (NA) CRT lowered local-regional cancer recurrence ($P = 0.04$), and the incidence of distant cancer recurrence was similar. Squamous cell carcinoma did not benefit from neoadjuvant CRT in this meta-analysis with an OR of 1.16 ($P = 0.34$) for one-year survival, 1.34 ($P = 0.07$) for three-year survival, and 1.41 ($P = 0.06$) for five-year survival.[63]

NACRT with "targeted therapy" was described in a series from the Cleveland Clinic. To reduce distant metastases, gefitinib was added to the standard regimen. Patients included T3, N1, or M1a patients staged by EUS and PET/CT. 80 patients were enrolled and received four-day continuous i.v. cis (20 mg/m/day) and 5FU (1,000 mg/m/day) with preoperative XRT (30 Gy and 1.5 Gy bid). Surgery followed in four to six weeks and then an identical course of CRT was given six to ten weeks postoperatively. Gefitinib, 250 mg/day, was given with preoperative CRT for four weeks and then restarted postoperatively for two years. Gefitinib did not increase toxicity except for development of rash in 42 (53%) and di-

arrhea in 44 (55%) patients. OS improved (42% vs. 28%, $P = 0.06$) and intolerance for Gefit maintenance occurred in 48%. Of note, diarrhea patients appeared to have improved outcomes.[64] The standard approach should be combined modality treatment, including XRT, if a neoadjuvant approach is pursued. If XRT is not given preoperatively, additional chemotherapy should be given. The role of surgery postchemoradiation includes definitive restaging, prevention of local recurrences, identifying responders, selecting patients for molecular targeted therapies, and allowing better oral nutrition. Also, at this juncture there is no way to accurately predict preresection the degree of response.

In conclusion, the role of surgery post chemoradiation depends on whether one ascribes to one of the following two hypotheses. Hypothesis 1: surgery is only for residual disease—this assumes that chemoradiation is curative and assumes the role of surgery as salvage will increase survival. Hypothesis 2: surgery is best used when there is an apparent pCR to chemoradiation, then surgery can deal only with microscopic disease—still have some (micro) disease in at least 50%.

12. Can p53 mutations be of help to select patients for certain therapies?

Daniela Kandioler
daniela.kandioler@meduniwien.ac.at

It is generally accepted that a normal p53 gene is required to induce apoptosis in response to DNA damage. A number of chemotherapeutic drugs interact with DNA (e.g., cisplatinum, 5 FU), and DNA damage is the strongest trigger for p53 activation. Based on this hypothesis, p53 has been suggested as a potential marker predicting response to treatment.[65] The robustness of the p53 hypothesis has been approved in a number of experimental and clinical settings. However, inconsistent results arose from the widespread use of inadequate testing methods, which may have resulted in an underreporting of the p53 mutations frequencies in the international databases.[66]

In esophageal cancer, the five-year survival rates range between 15% and 25% and postoperative radio- and/or chemotherapy did not prove to increase survival. In an attempt to prevent systemic spread and to improve the chance for complete

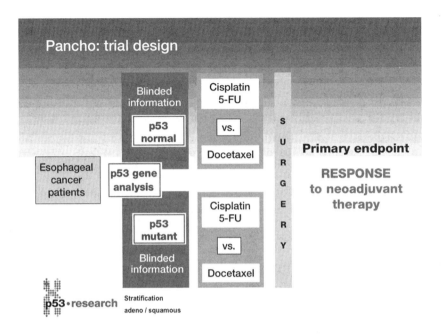

Figure 8. The pANCHO trial is an academic-driven trial with thirteen affiliated centers in Austria, recruiting around 50 patients per year. Primary operable esophageal cancer patients who are staged >T1 are eligible. Patients are stratified for adeno- and squamous cell carcinoma. Based on the study design, patients are separated into two groups by the marker test.[68] Within each group, patients receive randomly one of two different chemotherapy drugs preoperatively. After three cycles, tumors are surgically removed and response is assessed pathohistologically.

resection, neoadjuvant treatment strategies were investigated in clinical trials during the last decade. Meta-analysis produced conflicting results concerning the overall survival benefit. Only in those few patients (15–20%) who manage to experience complete pathological remission, a dramatic survival benefit and an enhanced chance for cure could be consistently observed.[67] Thus, a prospective randomized clinical trial has been initiated to test whether p53 is a useful marker for guidance in choosing optimal preoperative treatment in oesophageal cancer.

The pANCHO trial is an academic-driven trial with 13 affiliated centers in Austria, recruiting around 50 patients per year. Primary operable esophageal cancer patients who are staged >T1 are eligible. Patients are stratified for adeno- and squamous cell carcinoma. Based on the study design, patients are separated into two groups by the marker test.[68] Within each group, patients receive randomly one of two different chemotherapy drugs preoperatively. After three cycles, tumors are surgically removed and response is assessed pathohistologically (Fig. 8). The pANCHO trial tests for the first time the hypothesis that p53 may predict response to neoad-

juvant chemotherapy in esophageal cancer patients, and therefore could be relevant for the choice of therapy.

13. What are the indications of chemotherapy without 5-FU and without cisplatin?

David H. Ilson
ilsond@mskcc.org

The mainstay of chemotherapy in esophageal cancer in the past combined a four- or five-day infusion of 5-FU with high-dose cisplatin, used both in metastatic disease and with concurrent radiotherapy in locally advanced disease. The toxicity of this regimen at this dose and schedule, however, is substantial, with significant mucositis, diarrhea, nausea/vomiting, and myelosuppression. The diminishing use of this regimen is analogous to the 5-FU/leucovorin Mayo Clinic regimen, no longer used in colorectal cancer because of its toxicity. Adding a third drug to high-dose cisplatin/infusional 5-FU, docetaxel, results in even greater toxicity and slight increases in response rate and survival in metastatic disease. In the United Kingdom, a modified schedule of 5-FU/cisplatin employs lower-dose cisplatin, a protracted low-dose infusion of 5-FU, and epirubicin, the ECF regimen. ECF, is tolerable and active, has proven to improve survival as preoperative chemotherapy in gastric and gastroesophageal junction (GEJ) cancers.

Non-cisplatin–containing regimens, including modifications of the FOLFIRI regimen used in colorectal cancer, and combining irinotecan with taxanes, have shown acceptable activity in phase II and III trials in metastatic disease. Colorectal cancer dosing and scheduling of chemotherapy, using regimens such as FOLFOX, and 5-FU/cisplatin scheduled like FOLFOX, appear to have improved therapy tolerance and acceptable activity. A recent CALGB phase II trial combining the EGFr-targeted agent cetuximab, with either FOLFOX, ECF, or irinotecan/cisplatin, indicated the best activity, progression free and overall survival for the FOLFOX and ECF regimens.[70] Toxicity favored FOLFOX as the regimen to take forward as the backbone to add targeted agents in future studies. Recent trials also indicate activity and tolerance for 5-FU/oxaliplatin–based chemoradiotherapy. Non-cisplatin-based regimens, using paclitaxel and 5-FU with radiotherapy, have been tested and shown to be active.

Non-5-FU–based regimens have been explored in combined chemoradiotherapy phase II trials, including paclitaxel or docetaxel with cisplatin or carboplatin, irinotecan/cisplatin, and docetaxel/irinotecan. The recent CROSS trial conducted in the Netherlands combining weekly carboplatin, paclitaxel, radiotherapy and surgery indicated superior survival compared to surgery alone.[69] This trial establishes this easy to administer and well tolerated regimen as a potential new therapy standard for definitive and preoperative chemoradiotherapy. Taxane/platinum-based chemoradiotherapy regimens are now employed in ongoing national cooperative group trials in the United States. RTOG trial 0436 administers to nonsurgical patients primary chemoradiotherapy with paclitaxel, cisplatin with or without cetuximab. RTOG trial 1010 will test the addition of trastuzumab to preoperative chemoradiotherapy in HER2$^+$ esophageal and GE junction cancers, using weekly carboplatin and paclitaxel as the chemotherapy backbone.

14. Are there new advances for the use of *specific* monoclonal antibodies in patients with esophageal carcinoma?

Sophia F. Kaiser and Paul M. Schneider
paul.schneider@usz.ch

Cancer of the esophagus (EC) and GEJ are among the 10 most common malignancies worldwide, and EAC is one of the fastest increasing malignancies in Western countries in the last four decades. Once diagnosed, the five-year survival rate is about 10%. Surgery is the treatment of choice for most localized esophageal cancers. Despite complete tumor resection (R0) and extensive lymphadenectomy, systemic and local recurrences are common, and five-year survival rates range from 15% to 39%.[71] Current treatment concepts for locally advanced, resectable tumors contain preoperative chemotherapy or chemoradiation. In randomized trials, it has been demonstrated that multimodality therapy increases resectability and decreases local relapse compared with surgical resection alone, but the effect on overall survival is still not certain. Recent meta-analyses of randomized trials showed modest but significant survival advantages for patients that received neoadjuvant chemotherapy or particularly chemoradiation. Increasing evidence exists that major histopathologic tumor regression (<10% residual tumor cells or pathologic complete response) following neoadjuvant treatment and complete resection (R0) identifies patients that clearly benefit from these potentially harmful and expensive treatment strategies.[71]

In an effort to increase the frequency of major histopathologic responders, novel treatment strategies need to be exploited. In the past few years, an emerging understanding of molecular pathways that are important in cancer biology led to the identification of several new molecular targets. This, coupled with innovations in the field of drug development, has led to the introduction of several new classes of agents that target specific molecular sites or pathways. Among those, the growth factor receptors ERBB1 (EGFR) and ERBB2 (HER2) appear to be very attractive since they are overexpressed in many malignancies including esophageal cancer. The EGFR and HER2 signal transduction has an essential role in different tumorigenic processes, including cell cycle control, angiogenesis, metastasis, and protection from apoptosis.[72]

Table 2. Summary of mAb trials against EGFR or HER2 in esophageal cancer

Study	Phase	Patients	EGFR	Chemotherapy	Radiation	Response Rate	Toxicities
Pinto et al.[91]	II	25	Cetuximab	FOLFIRI	No	Radiological PR 42%	Grades 3–4: 63%
Suntharalingam et al.[92]	II	37	Cetuximab	Paclitaxel, carboplatin	No	Complete responders 67%	Grade 3: 20% grade 4: 0%
Ruhstaller et al.[74]	Ib-II	28	Cetuximab	Cisplatin, docetaxel	45 Gy	68% Pathological major response	No dose-limiting toxicities
Safran et al.[93]	I-II	10*	HER2/neu Trastuzumab	Paclitaxel, cisplatin	50.4 Gy	50% Endoscopic complete responders	Cardiotoxicity /esophagitis: no increase
Bang et al.[76]	III	478[a],**	±Trastuzumab	Cisplatin/5-FU or cisplatin/ capecitabine	No	Overall (p < 0.001) 47%[b] vs. 35%[c], complete response 5%[b] vs. 2%[c]	Grades 3–4: 68% no difference

5-FU, 5-fluorouracil; PR, partial response. *HER2 positive tumors by immunohistochemistry or ** ± fluorescence *in situ* hybridization.
[a]106 Patients with gastroesophageal junction carcinomas.
[b]Trastuzumab + Chemotherapy.
[c]Chemotherapy alone.

Targeting those transmembrane receptors at the extracellular binding site of their natural ligands with specific monoclonal antibodies (mAb) is therefore one of the most promising novel treatment options.[73]

Cetuximab (Erbitux[TM], C255), a chimeric IgG1 antibody, is already very advanced in terms of clinical testing and selected phase I-II studies in esophageal cancer are summarized in Table 2. When used as a single agent, antitumor efficacy is very low however, in combination with chemotherapy or chemoradiation, a clear synergistic effect occurs.[73] Ruhstaller *et al.* (SAKK 75/06) investigated cetuximab added to preoperative chemoradiation for resectable, locally advanced EC in a phase Ib-II trial. 28 patients (15 AC, 13 SCC) were included and received two cycles of induction chemoimmunotherapy (cisplatin, docetaxel, and cetuximab) followed by chemoimmunoradiation (CIRT). R0-resection was performed in 25 of 28 (89%) patients. Trimodality treatment was completed by 24 of 28 (86%) patients. There were no perioperative deaths at 30 days and no treatment-related mortality after one year, and 19 patients (68%) showed complete/near complete histopathological tumor regression. The treatment appeared to be safe and did not compromise the feasibility of this trimodal approach.[74] These results, however, are in contrast to the findings of the ECOG 2205 trial, which evaluated the addition of cetuximab to preoperative chemoradiation and was prematurely closed because of excess toxicity.[90] As the sample size of the SAKK trial was small, efficacy results should also be interpreted with caution. The results of this study however, are promising and induced the initiation of a phase III randomized trial (SAKK 75/08).

Two newer anti-EGFR mAbs, matuzumab (EMD72000), a humanized IgG1 mAb, and panitumumab (ABX-EGF), a fully human IgG2 mAb, both with high affinities for EGFR, are currently under investigation.[75] Trastuzumab (Herceptin™) is a humanized IgG1 mAb that is approved for use in HER2 overexpressing breast cancer and recent trials in EC and GEJ are summarized in Table 2. Based on preclinical data suggesting synergy with the combination of trastuzumab with cisplatin, paclitaxel, and radiation, a phase I trial including 10 of 30 (33%) patients with EAC that overexpress HER2 by immunohistochemistry was conducted. Full doses of trastuzumab were delivered in combination with chemoradiation without any increase in esophagitis or cardiotoxicity. In posttreatment endoscopic biopsies, 5 of 10 patients in the trastuzumab arm in HER2 overexpressing tumors achieved an endoscopic complete response (eCR). Eight patients with eCR underwent surgical resection and three patients had a pathologic CR.[93]

The recent ToGA (trastuzumab for gastric cancer) trial,[76] an international multicenter randomized controlled study, was performed in patients with gastric ($n = 478$) or GEJ ($n = 106$) cancers if tumors showed overexpression of HER2 protein by immunohistochemistry or gene amplification by fluorescence *in situ* hybridization. Median overall survival was 13.8 months in patients assigned to trastuzumab plus chemotherapy compared with 11.1 months in those treated with chemotherapy alone ($P = 0.0046$).

Conclusion

In summary, targeted therapies with mAbs directed against EGFR or HER2 in combination with chemotherapy or chemoradiation already demonstrated a promising potential in phase I–II trials. Data regarding associated toxicities are currently difficult to interpret and deserve careful monitoring. The future outlook in EC multimodality treatment using mAb therapy against growth factor receptors depends on randomized phase III trials, which have already started. The development of novel mAbs against various targets, application of mAb combinations and molecular (e.g., mRNA expression, microarrays) and proteomics analysis, especially activity-based profiling and metabolomics for response prediction and monitoring, seems to have a promising potential to improve treatment results in future studies.

15. Can a valid stage-specific therapy for esophageal cadenocarcinoma be defined?

Mark J. Krasna

markkrasna@catholichealth.net

Introduction

The goal of staging esophageal cancer is to prognosticate, decrease morbidity, and avoid unnecessary surgery/chemoradiation therapy. In short, we must change the mindset in esophageal cancer to allow us to compare treatment results and develop a stage-specific approach for each patient. The new WECC Staging System modified the existing AJCC staging system with the following essential changes: inclusion of tumor grade and addition of N1 and N2 categories based on the number of LN involved (<5 or ≥ 5).[77–79]

Review of data and literature

Recent data have shown that using the new staging system greater extent of LND is associated with increased survival for all patients with esophageal cancer except at the extremes (TisN0M0 and > or = 7 regional lymph nodes positive for cancer) and well-differentiated pN0M0 cancer.[80] Recent data on SLN biopsy for esophagogastric cancer have been reported. Four hundred and thirty-three patients with early gastric cancer, T1 or T2N0M0 with tumors <4 cm, had radioactive colloid and blue dye injected with detection rates of SLN 387 of 397 (97.5%). The mean number of SLN was 5.6 per case. The sensitivity to detect metastases based on SLN status was 93%.[81] Further development of the SLN concept is ongoing; the goal is to reduce the extent of resection in treatment of very early stage esophageal and gastric cancers. Laparoscopy pretreatment in 198 patients showed peritoneal or visceral metastases designated as M1; the remaining 93 patients had M0cyt+ disease, (cytology indicative of metastatic tumor but with no visible visceral or peritoneal metastases). M0cyt+ tumors had a longer disease-specific survival (DSS) than those with m1cyt+ disease ($P < 0.0001$). M0cyt+ patients who received subsequent chemotherapy resulting in a conversion of their cytology to negative at subsequent laparoscopy had better survival.[82]

Esophageal cancer treatment options include surgery alone and multimodality therapy (chemoradiation therapy or chemotherapy f/b surgery,

surgery f/b radiation therapy, surgery followed by chemoradiation, or chemoradiation f/b surgery). The following is a stage-specific approach to treatment based on recent data.

Medically inoperable: any stage

Chemoradiation if tolerable as per the results of the RTOG trial showing a 32% versus 12% 5YS, and 20% versus 0% 10 years with a local recurrence rate of 20–40%.

Early stage esophageal cancer (stage 1/2)

In these patients, the impact of tumor length on pT1 adenocarcinoma was reported in 133 resections. pT1 tumors greater than 3 cm decreased long-term survival and higher risk of LN involvement ($P < 0.001$), even when controlled for submucosal involvement, LN involvement, and lymphatic/vascular invasion status.[83] In these patients, MIE has been advocated for esophagogastric cancer resection. Mortality and morbidity were identical for each cohort (transthoracic open-TTO vs. MIE) with a mortality of 3% versus 2% and morbidity of 50% versus 48%. Pulmonary related complications were higher in the open group (23% vs. 8%; $P = 0.05$). The incidence of gastric-conduit related complications was similar between the two cohorts (13% vs. 18%; $P = 0.52$). Survival at one and two years was 86% and 58% in the TTO group and 94% and 74% in the MIE group. For patients with more locally advanced disease, the use of neoadjuvant-combined modality therapy has been the most popular option. A recent report showed that post CRT, the percent (%) decrease in standard uptake value (SUV) on PET/CT from baseline correlated with OS and pathologic response.[84]

Stage T3–4N0M0 or T1–4N1M0 EAC

These are best treated definitively with neoadjuvant therapy followed by esophagectomy. In patients in whom esophagectomy was performed for an alleged early stage tumor that returns as T2 or N1 or higher on final pathology, there may be a value with postoperative radiation. In 1,046 patients including 683 (65.3%) with surgery alone and 363 (34.7%) with postoperative radiation, significant improvement was found in median and three-year OS ($P < 0.001$) and DSS ($P < 0.001$), for AC in stage III.

For trimodality therapy-T3/N1, if recognized pretreatment, patients with locally advanced resectable esophageal cancer should be offered neoadjuvant therapy followed by surgery. No increase in morbidity or mortality or LOS was found in several recent studies and meta-analyses. An 80% PR, 40% pCR with a survival of 4.5 years versus 1.8 years, and $P = 0.02$ was noted. Stratifications by N stage, staging, and histology demonstrated a P-value of 0.005 for five-year survival (39% vs. 16%) for trimodality therapy.[85]

Possible stage-specific paradigms for adenocarcinoma of the esophagus can be proposed:

(i) Stage 0/ 1a: esophagectomy (MIE/ THE)
(ii) Stage 1b/2a: surgery alone/ NACRT
(iii) Stage 2b/3a: NACRT
(iv) Stage 3b 3c: chemoradiation alone/NACRT

Whether there is a role for adjuvant chemotherapy is unclear, although recent gastric cancer data would suggest that there is a role, especially in those patients who are HER2 Neu-positive (treated with herceptin). As noted above, there may be a role for adjuvant XRT, especially when found to be locally advanced after surgical resection. The future of treatment for this disease will probably depend on molecular targets with therapy being given on a personalized approach.

16. Are there promising targets for selective therapy?

B.P.L. Wijnhoven, H.W. Tilanus, and J.J.B. van Lanschot
b.wijnhoven@eramsusmc.nl

Despite neoadjuvant chemo(radio)therapy combined with radical surgery, about 30–50% of patients are diagnosed with locoregional and/or systemic recurrence within the first two years after treatment. Therefore, new therapeutic strategies to improve the outcome are needed. Targeted therapy is a new adjunctive mode of treatment that has been shown to be able to change the outlook of patients suffering from cancer. Targeted therapy is a type of medication that blocks the growth of cancer cells by interfering with specific molecules needed for tumor initiation and progression, whereas traditional chemotherapy interferes with all rapidly dividing cells. Therefore, targeted therapy may be more effective than current treatments, less harmful to normal cells, and less toxic. Many potential targets have already been identified in human cancers and drugs designed that are capable to interact. Mostly, these targets are tumor suppressor genes or proto-oncogens that likely play an important role in carcinogenesis. Relatively few studies have looked at the efficacy and safety of targeted agents for the treatment of esophageal cancer. Here, we briefly discuss some issues around the introduction of targeted therapy for the treatment of esophageal cancer.

An understanding of the pivotal genetic pathway(s) and targets that are dysregulated during esophageal carcinogenesis is important to search for suitable genes than can be targeted. When levels of expression of certain oncogenes and tumor suppressor genes correlate with tumor aggressiveness (e.g., tumor grade, stage, and survival or recurrence), targeting these genes will likely be effective. Most of the key regulators identified in esophageal cancer development and progression are involved in cell cycle control, proliferation, and invasion/dissemination.[86–89] Several drugs are already available that are capable of blocking these pathways or essential components of it.

Targeted agents can be divided into small molecules and monoclonal antibodies. Examples of small molecules are the tyrosine kinase inhibitors (e.g., erlotinib, imatinib). The monocolonal antibodies such as trastuzumab or panitumumab (human epithelial growth factor receptor blockers) block the receptor on the cell surface and thereby inhibit transduction of cell signaling. Trastuzumab improves overall and progression-free survival in breast and gastric cancer, but only for HER2 overexpressing tumors. So far, one phase I–II trial has studied trastuzumab in the setting of esophageal cancer.[88] Experimental studies can yield lots of important background information on the understanding and proof of principle of targeted therapy. *In vitro* studies with esophagogastric cancer cell lines describe the potential toxic and beneficial affects of targeted agents. In addition, a possible synergistic effect of some targeted agents added to radiotherapy has been acknowledged.

There is lot that can be learned from earlier trials in other tumor types using agents that one would like to study in the setting of esophageal cancer. What could be a starting dose? Is it safe to give these agents in combination with other chemotherapy agents and, maybe even more importantly, radiotherapy? We now know the side effects of bevacizumab (an angiogenesis inhibitor) in combination with radiotherapy, which leads to increased rates of gastro-intestinal perforations, bleeding, and thrombo-embolic complications. Since neoadjuvant chemoradiation is considered standard treatment for esophageal cancer, one should be well aware of these potential side effects. A thorough review of the literature to search for dose escalation studies, toxicity profiles, and efficacy is of utmost importance to anticipate this when designing trials.

Does the value of the new drug lie in inducing regression of the tumor prior to surgical treatment (i.e., to facilitate the radicality of resection) or to improve locoregional control by adding it to radiotherapy for its potential synergistic effect, to reduce metastases (systemic effect) or improve palliation? This is an important question to address because it will largely dictate the timing of administering the drug. If it will be combined with standard chemoradiotherapy, then one has to think about the potential interaction between the drugs and/or chemotherapy. For example, trastuzumab is a promising candidate drug for esophageal cancer. However, its cardiotoxic effects are well known from the breast cancer trials. Adding trastuzumab to the neoadjuvant radiotherapy regimen for esophageal cancer could induce an increase in cardiotoxicity. In addition, the surgeon needs to consider this toxic effect and its implications for the operability of the patients and timing for surgery. Finally, costs and quality of life are important outcome measures nowadays and should be incorporated in the design of new trials.

We now know that not every drug is as effective in every patient. Several factors may play a role such as the genomics of the patient and its metabolism/detoxification or tumor type. Identifying patients and tumor types that will benefit most from targeted agents by looking at genetic profiles will be crucial in the nearby future. For example, wild-type k-Ras colon cancer patients have no benefit from cetuximab (an EGFR-monoclonal antibody). Identification of subgroups of patients with certain molecular characteristics is crucial but also introduces a problem. Accrual of patients in trials will be difficult due to the stringent criteria with regard to the expression profile of cancer-related genes. Finally, when assessing the primary outcome, this should be a well-defined outcome and a clinically important outcome-measure. We have learned from GIST-tumors that plain CT scanning to measure response after initiation of imatinib is not appropriate and that the metabolic activity, as measured by FDG PET, is a better tool for measuring response to treatment. In the case of esophageal cancer, EUS, CT, and FDG PET have all been shown to have a poor accuracy for predicting outcome and response to neoadjuvant treatment.

In summary, there are many potential targets for treatment in esophageal cancer, and the number increases with our understanding of the pathophysiology of cancer. More new drugs will become available, and existing drugs should be tested for effectiveness in the setting of esophageal cancer. Among these are trastuzumab (HER2 receptor), bevacizumab (VEGF receptor), and RAD001 (mTOR receptor), and several phase I and II trials are underway.[89] However, important issues to address are the dose and timing of drug administration. This is also dictated by the goal of targeted treatment: to achieve the best palliation, to induce tumor shrinkage to facilitate a radical resection, or to reduce risk of disease-recurrence or progression. For sure, not all patients and tumor types are genetically similar; hence, pharmacogenomics and unraveling genetic pathways to predict response to treatment will become very important for the nearby future. Finally, the possible benefit of targeted treatments must be weighed against toxicity. We need well-designed trials and the help of funding bodies and the industry to move the promising field of targeted therapy forward in esophageal cancer.

17. Has the mortality rate from esophageal cancer really changed?

Stephen J.Sontag
sontagsjs@aol.com

"The only thing we have to fear. . .is fear itself."
Franklin Delano Roosevelt

There is little doubt that esophageal cancer is an entity worthy of fear. We are all familiar with the following statements:

- "The incidence of Barrett's is skyrocketing out of control."
- "The incidence of Barrett's without dysplasia is on the rise."

- "The incidence of Barrett's LGD is increasing by the hour."
- "The incidence of Barrett's HGD is the highest ever reported in the history of mankind."
- "The incidence of Barrett's adenocarcinoma is increasing by the minute."
- "The incidence of Barrett's without dysplasia threatens world stability."

For an opening sentence in a presentation, any one of the above will suffice. As an introduction to a manuscript, any two of the above will suffice. To justify a research project, any three of the above will suffice. However, when dealing with reality, we should be asking whether the stated and published increases in Barrett's adenocarcinoma (AdCa) are real.

Is esophageal squamous cell carcinoma (SCC) really decreasing while Barrett's AdCa is increasing? The literature is conflicting, and (at least for me) difficult to interpret. We reasoned that if changes in esophageal cancer rates are truly occurring as many reports indicate, they should be reflected in the annual mortality figures of esophageal cancer. So, where does one go to get these data?

The *Cancer Journal for Physicians*, published by the American Cancer Society, has been distributed to physicians every other month for the last 60 years, since January 1951. Each year, the January/February issue is dedicated to cancer statistics and contains the cancer data on prevalence, incidence, mortality, etc. Data on esophageal cancer was not published until 1970.

Therefore, to try to understand the changes that have taken place regarding esophageal cancer, we entered the statistical data from the journal tables into an Excel spread sheet. Because the data on esophageal cancer are not clearly delineated into SCC and AdCa, we had to make several assumptions—right or wrong:

Assumptions:

- Half the esophageal cancers are SCC.
- Half the esophageal cancers are AdCa,
  - Half the AdCa are Barrett's,
  - Half the AdCa are NOT Barrett's (GEJ without intestinal metaplasia, see Figs. 9 and 10).

Results

Since 1970, The mortality rate from esophageal cancer (SCC and AdCa) has increased from 6000 per year to 14,000 year. The annual mortality has

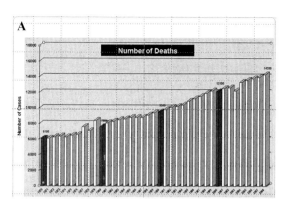

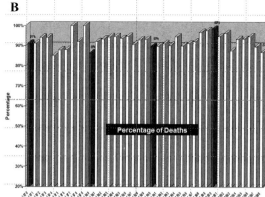

Figure 9. Esophageal cancer mortality (1970–2008). Numbers of deaths (A) and percentage of deaths (B).

remained stable at about 90% of new cases. The percentage increase in esophageal cancer deaths over the 40 year period is 134% (from 900 cases/year in 1970 to 2,200 cases/year in 2010). This figure translates into an absolute total number of 80,000 cases (or 80,000 patients over a 40-year period).

Using our assumptions, 40,000 patients had SCC and 40,000 had AdCa. Of the 40,000 AdCa, 20,000 were Barrett's cancers and 20,000 were non-Barrett's AdCa. Of the 20,000 non-Barrett's AdCa, it is generally thought that the cancers belong to the GE junction and that most are at a late, non-curable stage. Of the 20,000 Barrett's AdCa, is generally thought that half present with non-curable tumors and that

this half have absolutely no history of GER symptoms. In the end, we are left with 10,000 patients diagnosed over the last 40 years who had Barrett's AdCa that may have been curable or detectable at an early stage.

Based on these past data, what can we accomplish by looking forward? In the United States:

- 10,000 potentially curable patients over a 40 year period;
- 1,000 potentially curable patients over a 4 year period;
- 250 potentially curable patients over a 1 year period;
- Three patients every 2 days.

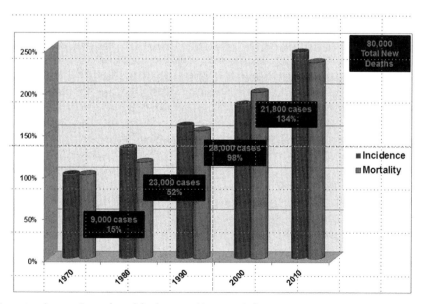

Figure 10. Percentage increase in esophageal deaths over a 40-year period.

Conflicts of interest

The authors declare no conflicts of interest.

References

1. Bonavina, L. *et al.* 2003. Results of surgical therapy in patients with Barrett's adenocarcinoma. *World J. Surg.* **27:** 1062–1066.

2. Casson, A.G. *et al.* 2000. What is the optimal distal resection margin for esophageal carcinoma? *Ann. Thorac. Surg.* **69:** 205–209.

3. Remacle, M. *et al.* 2010. Is frozen section reliable in transoral CO_2 laser-assisted cordectomies? *Eur. Arch. Otorhinolaryngol.* **267:** 397–400.

4. Shen, J.G. *et al.* 2006. Intraoperative frozen section margin evaluation in gastric cancer of the cardia surgery. *Hepatogastroenterology* **53:** 976–978.

5. Buskens, C.J., F.J. Ten Kate, H. Obertop, *et al.* 2008. Analysis of micrometastatic disease in histologically negative lymph nodes of patients with adenocarcinoma of the distal esophagus or gastric cardia. *Dis. Esophagus.* **21:** 488–495.

6. Lerut, T., P. Flamen, N. Ectors, *et al.* 2000. Histopathologic validation of lymph node staging with FDG-PET scan in cancer of the esophagus and gastroesophageal junction: a prospective study based on primary surgery with extensive lymphadenectomy. *Ann. Surg.* **232:** 743–752.

7. Aikou, T., Y. Kitagawa, M. Kitajima, *et al.* 2006. Sentinel lymph node mapping with GI cancer. *Cancer Metastasis. Rev.* **25:** 269–277.

8. Feith, M., H.J. Stein & J.R. Siewert. 2003. Pattern of lymphatic spread of Barrett's cancer. *World J. Surg.* **27:** 1052–1057.

9. Kitagawa, Y., H. Fujii, M. Mukai, *et al.* 2000. The role of the sentinel lymph node in gastrointestinal cancer. *Surg. Clin. North. Am.* **80:** 1799–1809.

10. Kato, H., T. Miyazaki, M. Nakajima, *et al.* 2003. Sentinel lymph nodes with technetium-99m colloidal rhenium sulfide in patients with esophageal carcinoma. *Cancer* **98:** 932–939.

11. Burian, M., H.J. Stein, A. Sendler, *et al.* 2004. Sentinel node detection in Barrett's and cardia cancer. *Ann. Surg. Oncol.* **11:** 255S-8S.

12. Lamb, P.J., S.M. Griffin, A.D. Burt, *et al.* 2005. Sentinel node biopsy to evaluate the metastatic dissemination of oesophageal adenocarcinoma. *Br. J. Surg.* **92:** 60–67.

13. Arima, H., S. Natsugoe, Y. Uenosono, *et al.* 2006. Area of nodal metastasis and radioisotope uptake in sentinel nodes of upper gastrointestinal cancer. *J. Surg. Res.* **135:** 250–254.

14. Takeuchi, H., H. Fujii, N. Ando, *et al.* 2009. Validation study of radio-guided sentinel lymph node navigation in esophageal cancer. *Ann. Surg.* **249:** 757–763.

15. Grotenhuis, B.A., B.P. Wijnhoven, R. van Marion, *et al.* The sentinel node concept in adenocarcinomas of the distal esophagus and gastroesophageal junction. *J. Thorac. Cardiovasc. Surg.* **138:** 608–612.

16. Bhat, M.A., Z.A. Naikoo, T.A. Dass, *et al.* 2010. Role of intraoperative sentinel lymph node mapping in the management of carcinoma of the esophagus. *Saudi. J. Gastroenterol.* **16:** 168–173.

17. Thompson, S.K., D. Bartholomeusz, P.G. Devitt, *et al.* 2010. Feasibility study of sentinel lymph node biopsy in esophageal cancer with conservative lymphadenectomy. *Surg. Endosc.*

18. Mariette, C., G. Piessen & J.P. Triboulet. 2007. Therapeutic strategies in oesophageal carcinoma: role of surgery and other modalities. *Lancet Oncol.* **8:** 545–553.

19. Boone, J., D.P. Livestro, S.G. Elias, *et al.* 2009. International survey on esophageal cancer: part I surgical techniques. *Dis. Esoph.* **22:** 195–202.

20. Verhage, R.J., E.J. Hazebroek, J. Boone & R. Van Hillegersberg. 2009. Minimally invasive surgery compared to open procedures in esophagectomy for cancer: a systematic review of the literature. *Minerva. Chir.* **64:** 135–146.

21. Ruurda, J.P., T.J. Van Vroonhoven & I.A. Broeders. 2002. Robot-assisted surgical systems: a new era in laparoscopic surgery. *Ann. R. Coll. Surg. Engl.* **84:** 223–226.

22. Boone, J., M.E. Schipper, W.A. Moojen, *et al.* 2009. Robot-assisted thoracoscopic oesophagectomy for cancer. *Br. J. Surg.* **96:** 878–886.

23. Courrech Staal, E.F., B.M. Aleman, H. Boot, *et al.* 2010. Systematic review of the benefits and risks of neoadjuvant chemoradiation for oesophageal cancer. *Br. J. Surg.* **97:** 1482–1496.

24. Feith, M., H.J. Stein & J.R. Siewert. 2006. Adenocarcinoma of the esophagogastric junction: surgical therapy based on 1602 consecutive resected patients. *Surg. Oncol. Clin. N. Am.* **15:** 751–764.

25. Newman, E.A., M.S. Sabel, A.V. Nees, *et al.* 2007. Sentinel lymph node biopsy performed after neoadjuvant chemotherapy is accurate in patients with documented node-positive breast cancer at presentation. *Ann. Surg. Oncol.* **14:** 2946–2952.

26. Gimbergues, P., C. Abrial, X. Durando, *et al.* 2008. Sentinel lymph node biopsy after neoadjuvant chemotherapy is accurate in breast cancer patients with a clinically negative axillary nodal status at presentation. *Ann. Surg. Oncol.* **15:** 1316–1321.

27. Stein, H.J., M. Feith & J.R. Siewert. 2009. Neoadjuvant therapy in the upper gastro-intestinal tract. Modern strategies for Barrett's cancer. *Chirurg* **80:** 1019–1022.

28. Boige, V., J. Pignon, B. Saint-Aubert, *et al.* 2007. Final results of a randomized trial comparing preoperative fluorouracil / cisplatin to surgery alone in adenocarcinoma of the stomach and lower esophagus: FNLCC ACCORD 07 –FFCD 9703 trial. *J. Clin. Oncol.* **25:** 4510.

29. Allum, W.H., S.P. Stenning, J. Bancewicz, *et al.* 2009. Long term results of surgery with or without preoperative chemotherapy in esophageal cancer. *J. Clin. Oncol.* **27:** 5062–5067.

30. Gebski, V., B. Burmeister, B.M. Smithers, *et al.* 2007. Survival benefits from neoadjuvant chemoradiotherapy or chemotherapy in esophageal carcinoma: a meta-analysis. *Lancet Oncol.* **8:** 226–234.

31. Stahl, M., M. Stuschke, N. Lehmann, *et al.* 2005. Chemoradiation with or without surgery in patients with locally advanced squamous cell carcinoma of the esophagus. *J. Clin. Oncol.* **23:** 2310–2317.

32. Gaast, A.V., P. Van Hagen, M. Hulsof, *et al.* 2010. Effect of preoperative concurrent chemoradiotherapy on survival

of patients with resectable esophageal or esophagogastric junction cancer: results of a multicenter randomized phase III trial. *J. Clin. Oncol.* **28**: (Abstract 4004).

33. Senzer, N., S. Swisher, T. Reid, *et al.* 2006. Long-term outcome in esophageal cancer after endoscopically delivered intratumoral injections of TNFerade with neoadjuvant chemoradiotherapy. *GI. Symposium. Abstract* **9**.

34. Feith, M., H.J. Stein & J.R. Siewert. 2006. Adenocarcinoma of the esophagogastric junction: surgical therapy based on 1602 consecutive resected patients. *Surg. Oncol. Clin. N. Am.* **15**: 751–764.

35. Hulscher, J.B.F., J.W. Van Sandick, A.G.E.M. De Boer, *et al.* 2002. Extended transthoracic resection compared with limited transhiatal resection for adenocarcinoma of the esophagus. *N. Engl. J. Med.* **347**: 1662–1669.

36. Siewert, J.R. & M. Feith. 2007. Adenocarcinoma of the esophagogastric junction: competition between Barrett and gastric cancer. *J. Am. Coll. Surg.* **205**: 49–53.

37. Luketich, J., M. Alvelo-Rivera, P. Buenaventura, *et al.* 2003. Minimally invasive esophagectomy: outcomes in 222 patients. *Ann. Surg.* **238**: 486–495.

38. Pennathur, A., A. Farkas, A.M. Krasinskas, *et al.* 2009. Esophagectomy for T1 esophageal cancer: outcomes in 100 patients and implications for endoscopic therapy. *Ann. Thorac. Surg.* **87**: 1048–1054; discussion 1054–5.

39. Bizekis, C., M. Kent, J.D. Luketich, *et al.* 2006. Initial experience with minimally invasive Ivor Lewis esophagectomy. *Ann. Thorac. Surgery.* **82**: 402–406; discussion 406–7.

40. Luketich, J., A. Pennathur, P.J. Catalano, *et al.* 2009. Results of a phase II multicenter study of minimally invasive esophagectomy (Eastern Cooperative Oncology Group Study E2202). *J. Clin. Oncol. (Meeting Abstracts)* **27**: 4516.

41. Torek, F. 1925. Carcinoma of the thoracic portion of the esophagus. *Arch. Surg.* **10**: 353–360.

42. Brücher, B.L.D.M. 2009. Esophageal squamous cell carcinoma: pre-operative combined radiochemotherapy from a surgical oncological viewpoint. *Chirurg*.

43. Brücher, B.L.D.M., S. Swisher, A. Königsrainer, *et al.* 2009. Response to Preoperative Therapy in Upper Gastrointestinal Cancers. *Ann. Surg. Oncol.* **16**: 878–886.

44. Brücher, B.L.D.M., K. Becker, F. Lordick, *et al.* 2006. The clinical impact of histopathological response assessment by residual tumor cell quantification in esophageal squamous cell carcinomas. *Cancer* **106**: 2119–2127.

45. Rice, T.W., V.W. Rusch, C. Apperson-Hansen, *et al.* 2009. Worldwide esophageal cancer collaboration. *Dis. Esophagus.* **22**: 1–8.

46. Schneider P.M., S.E. Baldus, R. Metzger, *et al.* 2005. Histomorphologic tumor regression and lymph node metastases determine prognosis following neoadjuvant radiochemotherapy for esophageal cancer: implications for response classification. *Ann. Surg.* **242**: 684–692.

47. Schneider, P.M., R. Metzger, H. Schaefer, *et al.* 2008. Response-evaluation by endoscopy, re- biopsy, and endoscopic ultrasound does not accurately predict histopathologic regression following neoadjuvant chemoradiation for esophageal cancer. *Ann. Surg.* **248**: 902–908.

48. Lordick, F., K. Ott, B.J. Krause, *et al.* 2007. PET to assess early

metabolic response and to guide treatment of adenocarcinoma of the oesophagogastric junction: the MUNICON phase II trial. *Lancet Oncol.* **8**: 797–805.

49. Vallböhmer, D., A.H. Hölscher, M. Dietlein, *et al.* 2009. 18F]-Fluorodeoxyglucose-positron emission tomography for the assessment of histopathologic response and prognosis after completion of neoadjuvant chemoradiation in esophageal cancer. *Ann. Surg.* **250**: 888–894.

50. Vallböhmer, D., J. Brabender, R. Metzger & AH Hölscher. 2010. Genetics in the pathogenesis of esophageal cancer: possible predictive and prognostic factors. *J. Gastrointest. Surg.* **14**(Suppl 1): S75–S80.

51. Swisher, S.G., J. Erasmus, M. Maish, *et al.* 2004. 2-Fluoro-2-deoxy-D-glucose positron emission tomography imaging is predictive of pathologic response and survival after preoperative chemoradiation in patients with esophageal carcinoma. *Cancer* **101**: 1776–1785.

52. Erasmus, J.J., R.F. Munden, M.T. Truong, *et al.* 2006. Preoperative chemo-radiation-induced ulceration in patients with esophageal cancer: a confounding factor in tumor response assessment in integrated computed tomographic-positron emission tomographic imaging. *J. Thorac. Oncol.* **1**: 478–486.

53. McLoughlin, J.M., M. Melis, E.M. Siegel, *et al.* 2008. Are patients with esophageal cancer who become PET negative after neoadjuvant chemoradiation free of cancer? *J. Am. Coll. Surg.* **206**: 879–886; discussion 86–87.

54. Javeri, H., L. Xiao, E. Rohren, *et al.* 2009. Influence of the baseline 18F-fl uoro-2-deoxy-D-glucose positron emission tomography results on survival and pathologic response in patients with gastroesophageal cancer undergoing chemoradiation. *Cancer* **115**: 624–630.

55. Bruzzi, J.F., S.G. Swisher, M.T. Truong, *et al.* 2007. Detection of interval distant metastases: clinical utility of integrated CT-PET imaging in patients with esophageal carcinoma after neoadjuvant therapy. *Cancer* **109**: 125–134.

56. Hart, J.P., M.R. McCurdy, M. Ezhil, *et al.* 2008. Radiation pneumonitis: correlation of toxicity with pulmonary metabolic radiation response. *Int. J. Radiat. Oncol. Biol. Phys.* **71**: 967–971.

57. Kwee, R.M. 2010. Prediction of tumor response to neoadjuvant therapy in patients with esophageal cancer with use of 18F FDG PET: a systematic review. *Radiology* **254**: 707–717.

58. Herskovic, A., K. Martz, M. al-Sarraf, *et al.* 1992. Combined chemotherapy and radiotherapy compared with radiotherapy alone in patients with cancer of the esophagus. *N. Engl. J. Med.* **326**: 1593–1598.

59. Kelsen, D.P., R. Ginsberg, T.F. Pajak, *et al.* 1998. Chemotherapy followed by surgery compared with surgery alone for localized esophageal cancer. *N. Engl. J. Med.* **339**: 1979–1984.

60. Walsh, T.N., N. Noonan, D. Hollywood, *et al.* 1996. A comparison of multimodal therapy and surgery for esophageal adenocarcinoma. *N. Engl. J. Med.* **335**: 462–467.

61. Tepper, J., M. Krasna , D. Niedzwiecki, *et al.* 2008. Phase III trial of trimodality therapy with Cisplatin, Fluoracil, radiotherapy, and surgery compared with surgery alone for esophageal cancer: CALGB 9781. *J. Clin. Oncol.* **26**: 1086–1092.

62. Koshy, M., B.D. Greenwald, P. Hausner, *et al.* 2010. Outcomes after trimodality therapy for esophageal cancer: the impact of histology on failure patterns. *Am. J. Clin. Oncol.* **3** [Epub ahead of print].

63. Jin, H.L., H. Zhu, T.S. Ling, *et al.* 2009.Neoadjuvant chemoradiotherapy for resectable esophageal carcinoma: a meta-analysis. *World J. Gastroenterol.* **15:** 5983–5991.

64. Rodriguez, C.P., D.J. Adelstein, T.W. Rice, *et al.* 2010. A phase II study of perioperative concurrent chemotherapy, gefitinib, and hyperfractionated radiation followed by maintenance gefitinib in locoregionally advanced esophagus and gastroesophageal junction cancer. *J. Thorac. Oncol.* **5:** 229–235.

65. Lowe, S.W., H.E. Ruley, T. Jacks, *et al.* 1993. p53-dependent apoptosis modulates the cytotoxicity of anticancer agents. *Cell* **74:** 957–967.

66. Kandioler-Eckersberger, D., S. Kappel, M. Mittlbock, *et al.* 1999. The TP53 genotype but not immunohistochemical result is predictive of response to cisplatin-based neoadjuvant therapy in stage III non-small cell lung cancer. *J. Thorac. Cardiovasc. Surg.* **117:** 744–750.

67. Urschel, J.D. & H. Vasan. 2003. A meta-analysis of randomized controlled trials that compared neoadjuvant chemoradiation and surgery to surgery alone for resectable esophageal cancer. *Am. J. Surg.* **185:** 538–543.

68. Sargent, D.J., B.A. Conley, C. Allegra, *et al.* 2005. Clinical trial designs for predictive marker validation in cancer treatment trials. *J. Clin. Oncol.* **23:** 2020–2027.

69. Enzinger, P., B. Burtness, D. Hollis, *et al.* 2010. CALGB 80403 / ECOG 1206: a randomized phase II trial of three standard chemotherapy regimens (ECF, IC, FOLFOX) plus cetuximab in metastatic esophageal and GE junction cancer. *J. Clin. Oncol.* **28:** 15s (Abstract 4004).

70. Gaast, A.V., P. Van Hagen, M. Hulsof, *et al.* 2010. Effect of preoperative concurrent chemoradiotherapy on survival of patients with resectable esophageal or esophagogastric junction cancer: results of a multicenter randomized phase III trial. *J. Clin. Oncol.* **28:** (Abstract 4004).

71. Schneider, P.M., S.E. Baldus, R. Metzger, *et al.* 2005. Histomorphologic tumor regression and lymph node metastases determine prognosis following neoadjuvant radiochemotherapy for esophageal cancer: implications for response classification. *Ann. Surg.* **242:** 684–692.

72. Hynes, N.E. & H.A. Lane. 2005. ERBB receptors and cancer: the complexity of targeted inhibitors. *Nat Rev Cancer.* **5:** 341–354.

73. Aklilu, M. & D.H. Ilson. 2007. Targeted agents and esophageal cancer—the next step? *Semin. Radiat. Oncol.* **17:** 62–69.

74. Ruhstaller, T., M. Pless, D. Dietrich, *et al.* Cetuximab in combination with chemoradiotherapy prior to surgery in patients with resectable, locally advanced esophageal carcinoma: a prospective, multicenter phase lb-ll trial (SAKK 75/06). *J. Clin. Oncol.* In press.

75. Pande, A.U., R.V. Iyer, A. Rani, *et al.* 2007. Epidermal growth factor receptor-directed therapy in esophageal cancer. *Oncology* **73:** 281–289.

76. Bang, Y.J., E. Van Cutsem, A. Feyereislova, et al.; ToGA Trial Investigators. 2010. TrastuzumAb in combination with chemotherapy versus chemotherapy alone for treatment of HER2-positive advanced gastric or gastro-oesophageal junction cancer (ToGA): a phase 3, open-label, randomised controlled trial. *Lancet* **376:** 687–697.

77. Rice, T.W., V.W. Rusch, C Apperson-Hansen, *et al.* 2009. Worldwide esophageal cancer collaboration. *Dis. Esophagus.* **22:** 1–8.

78. American Joint Committee on Cancer. 2010. In *Cancer Staging Manual.* 7th ed. S.B. Edge, D.R. Byrd, C.C. Compton, *et al.* Eds.: Springer. NY.

79. International Union Against Cancer. 2009. In *TNM Classification of Malignant Tumours*, 7th ed. L.H. Sobin, M.K. Gospodarowicz & C. Wittekind, Eds.: Wiley-Blackwell. Oxford, UK.

80. Rizk, N.P., H. Ishwaran, T.W. Rice, *et al.* 2010. Optimum lymphadenectomy for esophageal cancer. *Ann. Surg.* **251:** 46–50.

81. Javeri, H., L. Xiao, E. Rohren, *et al.* 2009. The higher the decrease in the standardized uptake value of positron emission tomography after chemoradiation, the better the survival of patients with gastroesophageal adenocarcinoma. *Cancer* **115:** 5184–5192.

82. Mezhir, J.J., M.A. Shah, L.M. Jacks, *et al.* 2010. Positive peritoneal cytology in patients with gastric cancer: natural history and outcome of 291 patients. *Ann. Surg. Oncol.* **17:** 3173–3180 [Epub 2010 Jun 29].

83. Grotenhuis, B.A., B.P. Wijnhoven, R. van Marion, *et al.* 2009. The sentinel node concept in adenocarcinomas of the distal esophagus and gastroesophageal junction. *J. Thorac. Cardiovasc. Surg.* **138:** 608–612.

84. Bolton, W.D., W.L. Hofstetter, A.M. Francis, *et al.* 2009. Impact of tumor length on long-term survival of pT1 esophageal adenocarcinoma. *J. Thorac. Cardiovasc. Surg.* **138:** 831–836.

85. Jin, H.L., H. Zhu, T.S. Ling, *et al.* 2009. Neoadjuvant chemoradiotherapy for resectable esophageal carcinoma: a meta-analysis. *World J. Gastroenterol.* **15:** 5983–5991.

86. Tew, W.P., D.P. Kelsen & D.H. Ilson. 2005. Targeted therapies for esophageal cancer. *Oncologist* **10:** 590–601.

87. Arkenau, H.T. 2009. Gastric cancer in the era of molecularly targeted agents: current drug development strategies. *J. Cancer Res. Clin. Oncol.* **135:** 855–866.

88. Dragovich, T. & C. Campen. 2009. Anti-EGFR-targeted therapy for esophageal and gastric cancers: an evolving concept. *J. Oncol.* **2009:** 804–808.

89. Ku, G.Y. & D.H. Ilson. 2010. Esophagogastric cancer: targeted agents. *Cancer Treat. Rev.* **36:** 235–248.

90. Gibson, M.K., P.J. Catalano, L. Kleinberg, *et al.* 2010. E2205: A phase II study to measure response rate and toxicity of neoadjuvant chemoradiotherapy (CRT) with oxaliplatin (OX) and infusional 5-fluorouracil (5-FU) plus cetuximab (C) followed by postoperative docetaxel (DT) and C in patients with operable adenocarcinoma of the esophagus. *J. Clin. Oncol.* **28:** 316s.

91. Pinto, C., F. Di Fabio, S. Siena, *et al.* 2006. Phase II study of cetuximab in combination with FOLFIRI as first-line treatment in patients with unresectable metastatic gastric or gastroesophageal junction (GEJ) adenocarcinoma (FOLCETUX study): Preliminary results. *J. Clin. Oncol.* **24:** 4031.

92. Suntharalingam, M., T. Dipetrillo, P. Akerman, *et al.* 2006. Cetuximab, paclitaxel, carboplatin and radiation for esophageal and gastric cancer. *J. Clin. Oncol.* **24:** 4029.

93. Safran, H., T. DiPetrillo, A. Nadeem, *et al.* 2004. Trastuzumab, paclitaxel, cisplatin, and radiation for adenocarcinoma of the esophagus: a phase I study. *Cancer Invest* **22:** 670–677.

Ann. N.Y. Acad. Sci. ISSN 0077-8923

ANNALS OF THE NEW YORK ACADEMY OF SCIENCES
Issue: *Barrett's Esophagus: The 10th OESO World Congress Proceedings*

Barrett's esophagus: natural history

Henry D. Appelman,[1] Asad Umar,[2] Roy C. Orlando,[3] Stephen J. Sontag,[4] Sanjay Nandurkar,[5] Hala El-Zimaity,[6] Angel Lanas,[7] Paolo Parise,[8] René Lambert,[9] and Helen M. Shields[10]

[1]Department of Pathology, University of Michigan, Ann Arbor, Michigan. [2]Division of Cancer Prevention, National Cancer Institute, Rockville, Maryland. [3]Department of Cell and Molecular Physiology, University of North Carolina School of Medicine, Chapel Hill, North Carolina. [4]Veterans Administration Hospital, Hines, Illinois. [5]Department of Gastroenterology, Box Hill Hospital, Box Hill, VIC, Australia. [6]University Health Network, Anatomic Pathology, Toronto General Hospital, Toronto, Canada. [7]Department of Digestive Diseases, University of Zaragoza, Aragón Health Research Institute, CIBERehd, Zaragoza, Spain. [8]Department of General Surgery IV, Regional Referal Center for Esophageal Pathology, Pisa, Italy. [9]International Agency for Research on Cancer, Lyon, France. [10]Gastroenterology Division, Harvard Medical School and Beth Israel Deaconess Medical Center, Boston, Massachusetts

The following on the natural history of Barrett's esophagus (BE) includes commentary on histological sequences of the development of Barrett mucosa; the transformation of esophageal cells from squamous to columnar phenotype; the stages of natural history of dysplasia; the difficulties of predicting progression of dysplasia to adenocarcinoma; the preferable biopsy protocols; the role of *Helicobacter pylori* infection and gastric atrophy in the risk of BE; the value of decrease of proton pump inhibitor efficacy following eradication of *H. pylori*; the place of antireflux surgery in the natural history of BE; the newest procedures for the endoscopic detection of early neoplasia; and the essential importance of a good understanding of the natural history for the best management of high-grade dysplasia.

Keywords: reflux; adenocarcinoma; CDX2; dilated intercellular spaces; bile salts; high-grade dysplasia; Barrett's esophagus; biopsy protocol; adenocarcinoma; gastric atrophy; *H. pylori*; GERD; endoscopic grading system; Cag A-postive strain; metaplasia; laparoscopic surgery; high resolution endoscopy; narrow band imaging; trimodal technology; bimodal protocol; esophageal metaplasia; radiofrequency ablation; endoscopic mucosal resection; interobserver reproducibility

Concise summaries

- The natural history of Barrett's esophagus (BE) with high-grade dysplasia (HGD) remains an enigma.
- Some patients have developed adenocarcinoma very rapidly after the diagnosis of the first HGD. Others have waxed and waned for years, with some regressing to lesser grades of dysplasia, some regressing to no dysplasia (ND), and still some others just living happily with continued HGD.
- It can be assumed that every esophageal mucosa in Barrett's patients started as out as normal squamous mucosa that was then severely damaged by reflux of acid, duodenal contents, or both. From a molecular and genetic standpoint, we know a great deal about the changes

that occur once Barrett's mucosa has developed during the dysplasia to carcinoma sequence, but we have hardly any information on comparable genetic and molecular changes in the squamous mucosa that turns it into columnar.

- Despite decades of research, current management of esophageal adenocarcinoma (EA) is still inadequate because at-risk patients are rarely identified. However, it now seems possible to develop a clinical risk classification tool that can probably be further refined and improved using molecular characterization including genetic and epigenetic alterations of early disease.
- Since it is present and to full length on the initial endoscopy, it can be inferred that BE phenotype is generated early in the course of disease. It is also a silent lesion even when exposed to high levels of pathologic acidity, which supports the

doi: 10.1111/j.1749-6632.2011.06057.x

view that BE is a form of "adaptive protection" for the defense of the host against ongoing acid damage to the esophageal wall.

- There is good evidence that has shown that mucosal irregularity, nodules, and ulcers with the Barrett's segment are highly associated with the presence of dysplasia and/or cancer. Thus, close scrutiny of the Barrett's segment to identify surface irregularity and getting targeted biopsies from those areas is extremely important before embarking on 4-quadrant biopsies lest those landmarks get obliterated by blood during sampling. Confocal laser endomicroscopy is a revolutionary technique that images subcellular tissue in real time (virtual biopsy). However, it samples only a highly limited surface area, is time consuming, and early reports to date have not shown it to be better than standard biopsy protocol.

- The trimodal endoscopic protocol requires a specialized material restricted to some reference centers, and random biopsies are still recommended in asymptomactic patients with BE for the detection of neoplasia in Western countries. In Japan, the detection of suspicious areas at the surface of the mucosa is completed by characterization through categories of the pit pattern and vascular pattern, and the best method of detection of flat areas of neoplasia relies on a *bimodal HRE-NBI protocol* coupled to magnification.

- Epidemiologic data suggest that a subset of *Helicobacter pylori*–infected patients may experience a lower risk of Barrett's carcinoma and, altogether, studies suggest that gastric atrophy associated with *H. pylori* infection may be responsible for the inverse association with esophageal disease. However, a negative association has been found in patients without atrophic gastritis, and *H. pylori* infection may increase gastric secretion in patients with antral gastritis.

- There are no studies to define whether *H. pylori* eradication worsens or improves BE after *H. pylori* eradication, but indirect evidence suggests that a potential decrease of proton pump inhibitor (PPI) efficacy should not preclude the indication for eradication.

- Even though antireflux surgery seems to better promote regression of BE or dysplasia than medical therapy, it has not demonstrably reduced the incidence rate of adenocarcinoma.

- The wise management of HGD is based on understanding that there is variability in the diagnosis of HGD by pathologists. At present, endoscopic mucosal resection therapy with or without radiofrequency ablation appears to be reasonable therapy for HGD or early esophageal carcinoma. Research data also favor the use of radiofrequency ablation compared to photodynamic therapy because of fewer complications and better efficacy.

---

1. What is proof that Barrett's mucosa develops in areas of damaged, previously normal squamous mucosa?

Henry D. Appelman
appelman@umich.edu

Someone must know the answer to this question, so I tried to find out who, and I felt that it was wise to start by asking the experts. To quote Kahrilas and Pandolfino, two acknowledged esophageal experts writing in a major gastroenterology textbook, "while the cause of Barrett's metaplasia is uncertain, it is clearly associated with gastroesophageal reflux disease (GERD) and believed to occur as a consequence of excessive esophageal acid exposure."[1] According to Spechler, Fitzgerald, Prasad,

and Wang, four more acknowledged esophageal experts, "long-segment BE is associated with GERD and the epithelial metaplasia characteristic of BE is widely regarded as a consequence of GERD."[2] According to the website of the Society of Thoracic Surgeons, "the exact reasons for the development of BE are unknown. Most physicians believe that the damage to the squamous mucosa, which leads to the development of BE is caused by chronic reflux of acid or other stomach contents."[3]

Therefore, we assume that every esophageal mucosa in Barrett's patients started out as normal squamous mucosa that was then severely damaged by reflux of acid, duodenal contents, both, or something else. The damaged squamous epithelium somehow was prevented from regenerating, and, instead, it was replaced by metaplastic columnar epithelium. One problem with this concept is that we pathologists commonly see significant damage to esophageal squamous mucosa in biopsies, including ulcers and erosions, and what we always see is regenerating squamous epithelium rather than replacement of the squamous epithelium by metaplastic columnar epithelium.

From a molecular and genetic standpoint, we know a great deal about the changes that occur once Barrett's mucosa has developed during the dysplasia to carcinoma sequence.[2] However, we have hardly any information on comparable genetic and molecular changes in the squamous mucosa that turns it into columnar.

There are some studies using *in vitro* esophageal squamous mucosal tissue or squamous cell cultures that indicate that acid and/or bile induce columnar type changes in these systems.[2] In one such study, CDX2, an intestinal differentiation factor, was upregulated in cultured squamous cells. In another study, the expression of CDX1, also an intestinal differentiation factor, was induced in cultured squamous cells. In a third study, there was increased BMP4 expression in stromal cells, which led to columnar cell keratin expression in the squamous cells. Then there was a study that indicated that there was upregulation of HB/EGF in lamina propria fibroblasts under damaged squamous epithelium, which promoted CDX2 in the squamous cells.

Thus, there are changes in squamous cells induced by reflux-type substances that might stimulate columnar metaplasia in the squamous mucosa in the laboratory, but we need to know if these factors actually cause this metaplasia in people. We can manipulate dog esophagi and gastro-esophageal junctions to produce columnar mucosa in the distal esophagus in response to acid, but these are animal models, and we don't have a comparable model in people. Therefore, we have some hints of the molecular and genetic determinants that might turn squamous cells into columnar cells in experimental models, but we do not know if these are the same determinants that work in people with Barrett's mucosa. We also have not identified the progenitor cells that lead to columnar metaplasia following damage to squamous epithelium. Presumably these are some type of stem cells, but we don't know that for a fact.

To summarize, Barrett's mucosa does occur. Epidemiologic evidence suggests that reflux of gastric acid and/or duodenal contents is important in its development. These reflux-type substances can produce molecular and genetic alterations in esophageal squamous cells in the laboratory, but we have no direct evidence that these substances cause columnar metaplasia of squamous mucosa in people.

2. In GERD patients, can the risks factors for development of Barrett's mucosa be determined? Is it possible to envisage a clinical risk classification tool?

Asad Umar
asad.umar@nih.gov

While the overall incidence and mortality rate of many cancers have declined in recent years, the incidence of esophageal adenocarcinoma (EA) has continued to rise. EA incidence has increased in the last three decades more than 600% in men aged 65 years and older and, notwithstanding progress in multimodality therapies, the overall five-year survival rate is still estimated at 15%.[4,5] It is estimated that more than 16,000 new cases of EA will be diagnosed in the United States alone in 2010. Furthermore, esophagectomy with or without neoadjuvant radiation therapy often incurs early postoperative complications and devastating long-term functional abnormalities. Likewise, medical therapies are still highly toxic, and remain unsatisfactory in response duration and overall survival benefit. The completion of any therapy for EA is most often followed by tumor recurrence or distant metastasis that leads to severe morbidities and eventual death. The natural course of the disease is insidious and debilitating, becoming clinically apparent only in advanced stages that are refractory to treatment and are resource intensive. Effective cancer preventive measures will benefit not only affected individuals but also the public at large.

Histologically, EA is thought to arise from the injury of the esophageal mucosa by frequent reflux of gastric contents that result in a sequence of metaplasia to low-grade dysplasia (LGD), HGD, and carcinoma. The metaplasia to dysplasia phase of this sequence is known as BE. BE is diagnosed in approximately 10% of patients who are referred to endoscopy for GERD symptoms.[6,7] BE, the only widely accepted precursor lesion to EA, is defined as the replacement of the normal squamous epithelium of the distal esophagus by columnar epithelium with intestinal metaplasia. Patients with BE are at least 30 times more likely to develop EA than patients without BE.

Currently, chronic GERD patients are screened for BE and, if diagnosed to have BE, they are subjected to endoscopic surveillance. Studies demonstrate that patients with malignancy detected at surveillance endoscopy have cancers at an earlier stage and better survival than those with no surveillance. The value of surveillance, however, is questioned by other studies demonstrating that only about 60% of patients diagnosed with EA have a prior diagnosis of GERD and less than 5% have BE. Furthermore, although the increased risk of EA in BE patients has been observed consistently, only 0.5% of endoscopically monitored BE patients progress to EA per year (with the HGD patients progressing at an annual rate of 5–20%). These findings suggest that despite decades of research, current management of EA neoplasia is still inadequate because at-risk patients are rarely identified. Moreover, criteria for screening and endoscopic surveillance still need to be established in a randomized trial. Given the threat of a highly lethal cancer, both patients and physicians typically opt for the most aggressive strategies for treatment and surveillance even with procedure-related risks.

Clinical risk classification tools need to be developed for better management of GERD of patients. Age, ethnicity, tobacco and/or alcohol use, obesity, and family history make for risk factors for GERD. It is estimated that over 60 million report heartburn or acid indigestion at least one time per month in the United States alone. Over 15 million individuals experience heartburn daily and frequent heartburns (two or more times per week) may be associated with GERD. This is significant, as approximately 10% of GERD patients develop BE, which eventually is a risk factor for esophageal cancer.[3,4] Gerson *et al.* used a multiple logistic regression analysis to predict BE using age, ethnicity, gender, dysphagea, heartburn, nausea, belching, nocturnal pain, odynophagi, and pain relief with food intake.[8] Therefore, using a scale of 0–550 total points, a score of 397.4 or higher was strongly associated with an increased risk of BE

while 351.3 for lower risk. This demonstrates that it is possible to develop a clinical risk classification tool, and it can probably be further refined and improved using molecular characterization including genetic and epigenetic alterations of early disease.

3. Can it be stated that BE follows a phenotypic presentation model in the natural history of GERD?

Roy C. Orlando
roy_orlando@med.unc.edu

The question posed in the title can be more succinctly stated as, "does BE evolve from GERD?" The answer succinctly stated is, "probably, yes!"

The case in support of this conclusion is based on the following observations:

- BE is more common in GERD (~10%) than in the general population, which has been estimated by a Swedish study to be in the range of 1.6%.[9]
- BE is located in the distal esophagus and associated with exposure of the region to pathologic levels of acid and bile reflux.
- BE exhibits a pattern of growth that appears to parallel those of reflux damage to the distal esophageal epithelium.
- BE has been reported to appear in areas of erosive esophagitis that biopsy did not previously show had evidence for its presence.
- BE has been observed to emerge in the proximal esophagus above an esophagogastric anastamosis following esophagectomy for BE.[10]
- BE has been observed to emerge in the esophagus of animal models of reflux-induced damage to native esophageal stratified squamous epithelium.[11] Further, and consistent with this *in vivo* data, are the observations *in vitro* that esophageal squamous cells exposed to acid and/or bile salts can express CDX2, a gene that favors transformation from squamous to the columnar phenotype.[12]
- The esophageal stratified squamous epithelium above BE has been reported to exhibit the lesion of dilated intercellular spaces.[13] This lesion is notable for being a feature of acid injury to both animal and human esophageal squamous

epithelium, and a histopathological correlate of the symptom of heartburn in GERD.

- When refluxate acidity is reduced by treatment with PPIs, islands of squamous epithelium reappear within regions of BE; and when reduced by PPI therapy, areas of distal esophagus from which BE has been ablated are repaired by a (neo)-squamous epithelium that phenotypically resembles the native esophageal squamous epithelium.

The three observations that prevent full acceptance of this concept include the fact the majority of patients with Barrett's have never been diagnosed with GERD before the diagnosis of BE; the fact that a significant number of those with BE are asymptomatic and have never had a history of GERD; and the fact that on endoscopy and irrespective of the presence or degree of active esophagitis, BE presents at its full length, a length that neither significantly increases nor decreases over time.

In summary, the weight of the evidence is that BE arises as a consequence of GERD. Since it is present and full length at the initial endoscopy, it can be inferred that BE phenotype is generated early in the course of disease, and, further, because there are large disparities in the frequency of BE among different ethnicities. The appearance of BE requires an inherent host susceptibility. BE is also a silent lesion even when exposed to high levels of pathologic acidity, which supports the view that BE is a form of "adaptive protection" for the defense of the host against ongoing acid damage to the esophageal wall.

4. Current knowledge on the natural history of Barrett's dysplasia regarding the best management of patients with HGD

Stephen J. Sontag
sontagsjs@aol.com

The natural history of BE with HGD remains an enigma. Some patients have developed adenocarcinoma very rapidly after the diagnosis of the first HGD. Others have waxed and waned for years, with some regressing to lesser grades of dysplasia, some regressing to ND, and still some others are living happily with continued HGD. We present unpublished data on two flat Barrett's HGD patients with

completely different courses during observation periods ranging from 9 to 18 years.

Patient number 1 was 63 years old when he was diagnosed with HGD at the first esophagogastroduodenoscopy (EGD). For the next 15 years, his course was as follows (Fig. 1, patient 1):

- 37 EGDs,
- 1,455 histologic specimens, and
- 43% of the 1,455 specimens had HGD.

After 15 years of continuous flat HGD, a small nodule developed and AdCa appeared for the first time. For the subsequent two years, Patient number 1 was treated with various ablative procedures. He is currently doing well at the age of 80.

Patient number 2 was a 66-year-old white male when he was diagnosed with HGD at two outside hospitals. In a three-month period, he was diagnosed with EGD by three different endoscopists at two different hospitals. HGD was diagnosed by three different pathologists. The patient self-referred himself to our hospital. After his initial diagnosis of HGD at the outside hospitals, his course for the next 11 years at our institution was as follows (Fig. 1, patient 2):

- 15 EGDs;
- 259 histologic specimens demonstrating either ND or no intestinal metaplasia; and
- absolutely no specimens demonstrating LGD, HGD, or AdenoCa.

This patient demonstrates the exact opposite of our first patient. After being diagnosed with HGD at three outside clinics (histologic samples confirmed by our pathologist as well as three outside pathologists), the patient never again showed any evidence of dysplasia on 15 EGDs and 259 specimens. As of this date, he is doing great.

Conclusion

The biologic influences controlling the fate of HGD are not understood. Our two examples (unpublished data) clearly demonstrate that not all patients with HGD have predictable responses, and the best management for one patient may not be the best management for another patient. Research is needed to discover the influencing factors, but, meanwhile, each patient with flat HGD needs to be assessed as an individual patient.

Patient 1

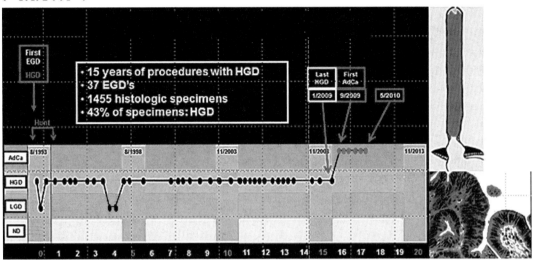

Patient 2

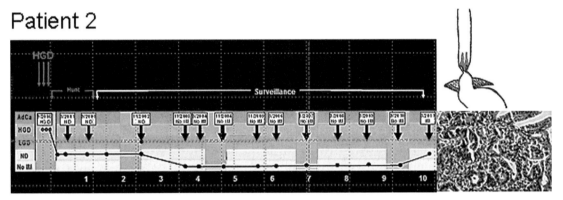

Figure 1.

5. Is it possible to predict which patients with HGD will progress to adenocarcinoma?

Stephen J. Sontag
sontagsjs@aol.com

BE remains a premalignant metaplasia of the esophageal mucosa with a spectrum of cellular behavior ranging from ND to LGD to HGD to cancer (AdCa). Current follow-up recommendations are usually ignored for (flat) HGD: follow-up every three months with EGD and biopsy until HGD disappears or develops into a lump and ablation therapy with any of five modalities.

Objectives

To offer safe, feasible, and evidence-based BE surveillance strategies comprising long-term follow-up guidelines with which physicians as well as patients can feel comfortable.

Methods

Our Veterans Association (VA) outpatient scope room was opened in 1979. Esophagogastroduodenoscopies (EGDs) were performed by one of three endoscopists using preestablished and agreed-upon clinical criteria for (1) EGD indications, (2) definitions, and (3) biopsy technique. Locations, configurations, and extent of BE and hiatal hernia were recorded and mapped by hand on to one of 22 diagram figures that adjusted for hiatal hernia (HH) size and shape. Attempts were made to biopsy the squamo-columnar junction (SCJ) regardless of its appearance. Biopsy specimens were taken as follows:

- Two for every 1 cm BE, or four for every 2 cm of BE (one from each quadrant).
- Targeted biopsies were taken of irregular or suspicious areas.
- Biopsy specimens (for all 26 years) were read in detail by one pathologist (GC).

Definitions

- BE: intestinal metaplasia (IM) from the tubular esophagus or from the GE junction area IF the biopsy contained, as one specimen, the squamo-IM junction.
- Prevalent HGD or AdenoCa: diagnosis at the first (or within 12 months of the first) EGD.
- Incident HGD or AdenoCa: diagnosis at least one year after the first EGD.
- Surveillance: time period beginning one year after the first EGD in patients with no current or past HGD or AdenoCa.

Protocol

Patients were categorized according to the most advanced lesion (e.g., HGD and AdCa occurring together were considered AdenoCa) and remained in the category until a more advanced lesion was found.

- For LGD: biopsy repeated once at one to two years and then every two to four years;
- For HGD: biopsy repeated at three-month intervals for one year ("the hunt");
- If no HGD was found on two consecutive biopsies, intervals became six months;
- After another year, intervals became 12 months, until and unless HGD was again noted.

Results (unpublished data)

During the 26 years, 1,664 patients were found with BE ranging from ND to AdenoCa:

- ND on first EGD ($n = 644$): not a single patient with ND progressed to AdenoCa;
- LGD on first EGD ($n = 968$);
- 946 LGD (97.7%) remained with LGD (or bounced: ND/HGD), but did not progress to AdenoCa;
- 13 LGD (1.3%) progressed through HGD to AdCa (incident AdenoCa from LGD through HGD);
- 10 LGD (1.0%) progressed directly to AdCa (incident AdenoCa from LGD without HGD);

- HGD on first EGD: ($n = 51$) (prevalent HGD);
- 43 HGD (84.3%) remained with HGD (or bounced: ND/HGD), but did not progress to AdenoCa; and
- 3 HGD (5.9%) progressed to AdenoCa (incident AdCa after The Hunt).

Discussion

Management strategies designed to detect Barrett's cancers must consider several factors:

1. AdenoCa rarely develops in patients with Barrett's and ND.
2. AdenoCa does develop in patients with a diagnosis of only LGD.
3. HGD found in flat Barrett's should be followed by the hunt.
4. With the one-year Hunt, it is guaranteed that your life will be meaningful.

   a. 10% of patients with flat HGD will be harboring a Barrett's cancer that will be detected and cured by your wise decision to employ the hunt.
   b. In the 15 years following the hunt, an additional 6% of patients with HGD found at first EGD will have a Barrett's cancer that will be detected and cured by your wise decision to perform "post-hunt" surveillance.
   c. Thus, if we find flat HGD during the first EGD, we can expect in the next 15 years that 16% will have a Barrett's cancer that will be cured as a result of our wisdom and intellectual prowess.

5. With the knowledge that ND is benign and that LGD can precede both HGD and AdCa, you can impress your patients with the following facts:

   a. Surveillance during the next 15 years is unlikely to detect anything meaningful if you have ND, but we'll do it anyway because I'm tired of talking about it.
   b. Surveillance during the next 15 years will detect curable AdCa in 2% of all patients with any Barrett's: dysplastic or nondysplastic.
   c. Surveillance during the next 15 years will detect curable AdCa in 2.5% of all patients with dysplastic Barrett's of LGD.

d. Surveillance during the next 15 years will detect curable AdCa in 3.0% of all patients with dysplastic Barrett's LGD and HGD. Surveillance during the next 15 years will detect curable AdCa in 19.0% of all patients who have HGD at any time.

6. Thirty of the 31 patients with AdCa detected on our program were curable, including those whose last EGD was three years earlier.

Conclusions

If the endoscopist has clearly visualized a flat Barrett's mucosa and has obtained appropriate biopsy specimens:

1. The hunt, followed by surveillance, is a safe and effective protocol for patients with flat HGD.
2. Patients with LGD (without HGD/AdCa) can safely be followed with EGD at two to three year intervals.
3. Patients with HGD should undergo the hunt, followed by surveillance EGD.
4. Yearly EGD (for LGD) and quarterly EGD (for HGD) is not necessary after the first intensive year if the endoscopist has clearly visualized a flat (no bumps) mucosa and has obtained appropriate biopsy specimens.
5. Surgical resection for Barrett's HGD is a thing of the past.

6. Which biopsy protocol is most likely to detect dysplasia in Barrett's mucosa?

Sanjay Nandurkar
sanjay.nandurkar@med.monash.edu.au

BE is a chronic condition characterized by a change in lining of esophageal mucosa from squamous epithelium to columnar metaplasia. The latter epithelium can develop dysplasia, which can lead to the development of adenocarcinoma. Thus, Barrett's is an important preneoplastic condition that confers a 30–50-fold increased risk of adenocarcinoma. The incidence of adenocarcinoma of the esophagus has increased significantly in the last two decades in the Western world.

Periodic endoscopic and histological surveillance has been recommended as a means to detect dysplasia or adenocarcinoma at an early stage, as instituting therapy at this point confers survival advantage. Barrett's segments can vary widely: some can be only a few centimeters long (short segment Barrett's) and others can extend more than 10 cm. Accurate sampling of mucosa to get a good representative pathological perspective of the entire Barrett's segment can pose a challenge. Most gastroenterology societies recommend taking a biopsy from four quadrants at 2 cm intervals. While this is logistically easy for short segment Barrett's, this can be quite time consuming for long segments.

A recent study from the Glasgow Royal Infirmary analyzed the biopsy practice between two groups of endoscopists; the surgeons adopted the systematic 4-quadrant approach in 1995, whereas the physicians continued to take fewer nonsystematic biopsies. The mean number of biopsies taken per patient was greater in the surgical group compared to the physicians (16 vs. 4, respectively). And this was evidenced by greater detection of LGD and HGD by the surgeons compared with the physicians (LGD: 18.9% vs. 1.6%; HGD: 2.8% vs. 0%). Advanced cancer was seen in three cases in the physicians group but none in the surgical group.[14] This study underscores the importance of a systematic approach to surveillance. Apart from not taking adequate biopsy samples, the other significant issue is the lack of follow up of many patients with BE. Data from a VA center in the United States analyzed a cohort of 472 patients with Barrett's between 1995 and 2005. They found that two-thirds of patients ($n = 305$) had only one endoscopy performed, and approximately 25% of patients with LGD missed their surveillance interval by more than six months.[15]

In spite of an adequate number of biopsies per protocol, endoscopic sampling only examines a very limited surface area. The standard biopsy forceps can obtain a 1.9 mm biopsy (with a depth of 1 mm). Biopsy forceps with a larger cup (jumbo forceps) can increase the surface area sampled (width = 3.3 mm, depth = 2 mm). Intuitively, it would appear more logical to use jumbo forceps to obtain greater tissue mass for analysis. One small study has shown improved dysplasia detection using jumbo forceps, but larger studies are needed.[16] There is good evidence that has shown that mucosal irregularity, nodules, and ulcers with the Barrett's segment are highly associated with the presence of dysplasia and/or cancer. Thus, close scrutiny of the Barrett's segment to identify surface irregularity and getting targeted biopsies from those areas is extremely important before embarking on 4-quadrant biopsies, lest those landmarks get obliterated by blood during sampling.

The presence of dysplasia, especially HGD, portends the presence of concomitant adenocarcinoma or the possibility of cancer developing in the immediate future. Thus, patients with HGD need closer observation at frequent intervals. Although some groups have campaigned for early resection in HGD to avoid missing a prevalent cancer, the Seattle group has shown quite convincingly that adequate biopsy sampling at close time intervals does not lead to missed cancers.[17] They advocated taking 4-quadrant biopsies at 1-cm intervals using jumbo forceps as well as taking multiple biopsies from any macroscopic abnormality. They showed that in patients with HGD who have a high probability of harboring cancer, their 1-cm-interval protocol detected all cancers, whereas a 2-cm protocol would have missed 50% of the cancers. The Cleveland group performed a retrospective analysis and found that in their hands the 1-cm protocol and the standard 2-cm protocol both performed badly and missed 30–40% of intramucosal cancers (although no submucosal cancers escaped detection). However, Cleveland study has been criticized by some as being retrospective for proactively identifying and targeting macroscopic irregularities that the Seattle group highlighted.

The use of acetic acid improves surface visualization and is quick and easy to apply. Preliminary data suggest that acetic acid target biopsies improve detection of dysplasia compared to the standard 2-cm protocol. Numerous investigators have evaluated the use of chromoendoscopy (usually methylene blue) to identify suspicious areas for targeted biopsies. However, it appears to be highly operator dependent, and the published reports are highly contradictory; hence, its use would difficult to advocate.

Newer imaging techniques such as narrow band imaging (NBI) and Fujinon intelligent color enhancement (FICE) can provide improved visualization of surface mucosa. There is a significant amount of published literature that has shown improvement in neoplasia detection using NBI technology. A recent meta-analysis of eight studies that included 446 patients and 2,194 lesions showed that the sensitivity and specificity for detection of HGD using NBI was 0.96 and 0.94, respectively.[18] Confocal laser endomicroscopy (CLE) is a revolutionary technique that images subcellular tissue in real time (virtual biopsy). However, it samples only a highly limited surface area, is time consuming, and early reports to date have not shown it to be better than standard biopsy protocol.

In summary, scheduled surveillance protocol with 2-cm protocol for Barrett's patients at average risk and 1-cm protocol (Seattle) for patients at high risk shows the best outcome. Adequate visualization of Barrett's surface mucosa is critical to identify mucosal irregularities which are associated with HGD and or cancer. Targeted biopsies using acetic acid and NBI and use of jumbo forceps to obtain larger samples appears to be beneficial. Use of chromoendoscopy cannot be routinely advocated, except in certain institutions.

7. Can gastric atrophy be an explanation of the inverse association of adenocarcinoma with *H. pylori* infection?

Hala El-Zimaity
hala.el-zimaity@uhn.on.ca

Until the mid 1970s, adenocarcinoma was a rare cancer type in the esophagus. Since then, the continuing decline in *H. pylori* infection in Western populations has been associated with a marked increase in GERD, BE, and EAC.[19] The question to answer here is, "can gastric atrophy be an explanation of the inverse association of adenocarcinoma with *H. pylori* infection?"

The explanation for the inverse association would come from clinical trials. Epidemiologic data suggest that a subset of *H. pylori*–infected patients may experience a lower risk of Barrett's carcinoma. Many studies use serology biomarkers to screen patients for gastric atrophy. Serum pepsinogen I is an indirect measure of corpus function. As PGI is secreted only by oxyntic glands, with advancing corpus atrophy, PG1 goes down. A low sPGI is a serologic marker of corpus atrophy. Most of Japanese Barrett's patients are *H. pylori* naïve with high serum pepsinogen levels.[20] *H. pylori* infection was present in four of 36 patients (11%) with Barrett's and in 80 of 108 controls (74%, *P* < 0.0001).[20] In

H. pylori–negative subjects, both serum pepsinogen I and pepsinogen II concentrations are significantly higher in Barrett's patients than in controls (mean pepsinogen I: Barrett's 51.0–14.0 ng/mL vs. control 38.9–13.5 ng/mL, $P = 0.0012$; mean pepsinogen II: Barrett's 10.8–4.0 ng/mL vs. control 7.9–2.0 ng/mL, $P = 0.0097$). Thus, in Japan, an inverse association exists between low pepsinogen I levels (a marker of advanced gastric atrophy) and Barrett's.[20]

Since 1969, Japanese physicians have used endoscopy to visualize changes in the gastric mucosa of gastritis patients.[21] Atrophic gastric mucosa is pale yellowish in color, with transparent blood vessels, and nonatrophic mucosa is homogeneously reddish and smooth. The atrophic border is the boundary between the antral and fundic glandular territories. At endoscopy, the atrophic border is recognized by discriminating between the differences in the color and height of the gastric mucosa. Japanese physicians incorporated the endoscopic atrophic border in an endoscopic grading system for atrophy.[21] Corpus atrophy begins at atrophic border (antrum–corpus border) in particular the incisura and extends proximally more rapidly up the lesser curve than the greater curvature. Atrophy in corpus biopsies high on the greater curvature are among the last to show atrophy. Following the Japanese endoscopic grading system, atrophy limited to the lesser curve is "closed." Atrophy extending high on the greater curvature is "open." Kim *et al.* showed the endoscopic grading of atrophic gastritis is inversely associated with gastroesophageal reflux and gastropharyngeal reflux.[22] GERD and gastropharyngeal reflux disease was significantly lower in the open type (advanced gastric atrophy) than in the closed type (less-advanced gastric atrophy) ($P < 0.001$, $P = 0.012$, respectively).[22]

The endoscopic grading system shows a good correlation with histological evaluation. Gastric background mucosa in patients with distal esophageal cancer has a higher prevalence of nonatrophic gastric mucosa when compared to gastric background mucosa in patients with distal gastric cancer. The latter are always associated with advanced gastric atrophy.[23] Altogether, studies suggest that gastric atrophy associated with *H. pylori* infection may be responsible for the inverse association between *H. pylori* infection and esophageal disease.

8. What are the arguments against the decrease of the risk of BE by *H. pylori* infection?

Angel Lanas
alanas@unizar.es

H. pylori infection has been associated with a decreased risk of GERD and related diseases. No clinical trials are available to answer this question. In general, epidemiological studies have found an inverse relationship between *H. pylori* infection and/or Cag-A–positive strains and BE and adenocarcinoma of the esophagus, but these findings have not been consistent in all studies, and two meta-analyses have come out with different conclusions. One, reported in 2007, concluded that in patients with BE there were inverse relationships with *H. pylori* infection overall and with Cag-A–positive strain (OR, 0.64; 95% CI, 0.43–0.94; OR, 0.39; 95% CI, 0.21–0.76, respectively).[24] However, a most recent one with a higher number of studies[25] concluded that there was no association between *H. pylori* infection and BE (Fig. 2). The overall prevalence of *H. pylori* infection between BE and controls was 42.9% versus 43.9% (OR = 0.74, 95% CI 0.40–1.37), but with significant heterogeneity. Further analyses were conducted based on the type of controls used as reference group. In nine studies, the prevalence of *H. pylori* infection was lower in BE than in endoscopically normal healthy controls (23.1% vs. 42.7%, OR = 0.50, 95% CI 0.27–0.93) with significant heterogeneity observed between studies. In contrast, *H. pylori* infection was significantly increased in BE patients in the three studies using healthy blood donors as "normal controls" (71.2% vs. 48.1%, OR = 2.21, 95% CI 1.07–4.55).

The question then may rely on who is the appropriate control for this type of studies. In principle, patients undergoing endoscopy for different indications should be excluded as controls since they may suffer of diseases linked to *H. pylori* infection. On the other hand, blood donors may represent a selected population. Controls should be as close as possible to the general healthy population and should be matched by age and sex, since *H. pylori* infection prevalence is age dependent, and BE is more frequent in males. Other factors that should be considered when interpreting these studies are geographical/race differences, definitions of

Outcome: Prevalence of *H. pylori* infection in BE and healthy controls

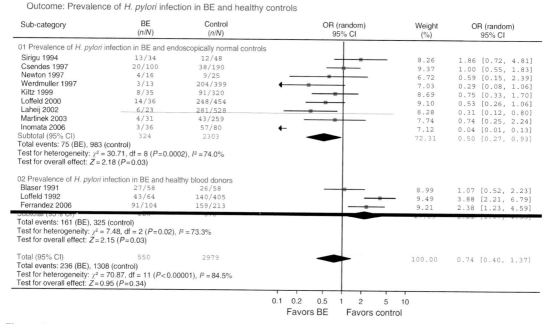

Figure 2. Meta-analysis of the prevalence of *Helicobacter pylori* in patients with BE versus controls.[25] With permission from Macmillan Publishers Ltd.

BE, using a retrospective versus a prospective approach, and the diagnostic tests used for *H. pylori* infection. Furthermore, confounding variables can explain negative results. No clear mechanistic explanation is available. The most frequent one has been linked to a reduced acid output due to the presence of corpus gastritis and different degrees of atrophy in *H. pylori*–infected individuals, but a negative association has been found in patients with negative atrophic gastritis. Also, *H. pylori* infection may increase gastric secretion in patients with antral gastritis.[26,27] Therefore, due to the low quality of most studies and the lack of an appropriate mechanistic explanation, we cannot conclude that there is a relationship between *H. pylori* and BE. Well-performed, larger studies with appropriate controls matched by age and sex should be conducted.

9. Should decrease of PPI efficacy following eradication of *H. pylori* be considered in the treatment of BE?

Angel Lanas
alanas@unizar.es

It has been shown that PPIs induce a higher degree of acid inhibition in *H. pylori*–infected in-

dividuals, which provides higher healing rates in erosive esophagitis patients treated with PPIs.[28] Patients with BE are recommended to be treated with high-dose PPI to reduce gastric acid and reduce esophageal acid exposure as much as possible. Patients with BE can undergo *H. pylori* eradication under different circumstances. This may reduce the capacity of PPIs to inhibit acid gastric acid secretion. However, no studies have addressed specifically this question in BE patients. There are no studies to define whether *H. pylori* eradication worsens or improves BE after *H. pylori* eradication. In one study, which included 24 cases of short-segment BE within a sample of 82 patients with peptic ulcer disease, it was shown that after *H. pylori* eradication, there were six new cases of short-segment BE after a mean follow-up of 24 months.[29] Another study showed that *H. pylori* infection did not influence esophageal acid reflux and symptoms in patients with BE, either at baseline or during low, as well as profound, acid suppressive therapy. The authors concluded that the dose of acid suppression does not have to be titrated upon *H. pylori* status in GERD patients (Fig. 3).[30] A systematic review of 27 studies concluded that *H. pylori* eradication in peptic ulcer patients does not induce esophagitis or worsen

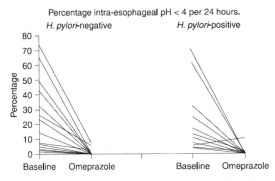

Figure 3. Individual values of percentage intraesophageal pH < 4 per 24 hours in *Helicobacter pylori* –negative and *H. pylori*–positive Barrett's esophagus patients at baseline and during therapy with omeprazole 40 mg b.d. at three months.[30] With permission from John Wiley & Sons.

GERD symptoms.[31] Also, it has been shown that patients with established GERD did not require increased doses of PPI after *H. pylori* eradication.[32]

Therefore, although no studies have specifically addressed this question in BE patients, indirect evidence suggests that a potential decrease of PPI efficacy should not preclude the indication for *H. pylori* eradication, and that this should not be of concern for patients with BE.

10. Is surgical treatment likely to modify the progression of natural history of BE?

Paolo Parise
p.parise@ao-pisa.toscana.it

The American College of Gastroenterology 2008 guidelines defines BE as a "change in distal esophageal epithelium of any length that can be recognized as columnar type mucosa at endoscopy and is confirmed to have intestinal metaplasia by biopsy of the tubular esophagus."[33] Patients with long-segment BE have a 30–125-fold increased risk of developing esophageal cancer,[34,35] but the real natural history of the sequence metaplasia–dysplasia–carcinoma is still unclear, because most of these patients undergo surgical or medical therapy. However, in this multistep sequence, dysplasia represents the best marker of the development of adenocarcinoma of the gastro-esophageal junction. In this cascade, some steps are thought to be very rarely reversible (BE normal epithelium) or never (adenocarcinoma–dysplasia), but others can and do regress. This represents the rationale for

the surveillance and medical or surgical treatment of BE.

In a prospective study in 1999, Weston and colleagues followed 108 patients affected by BE and who were treated with PPI for a mean period of 40 months. At baseline endoscopy, they found 80 patients with ND, 20 with LGD, and eight with HGD. Among the nondysplastic group, 2.5% progressed to cancer and 28.7% progressed to LGD with a subsequent regression rate of 78.2%. In the LGD group, 65% of patients regressed to ND, but 20% progressed to HGD, subsequently developing cancer or multifocal HGD in 50% cases and nondysplastic BE in the remaining 50% cases. Patients presenting with HGD developed cancer or multifocal HGD in 62.5% cases and regressed to LGD or ND in the other cases.[36]

In a retrospective study from the Netherlands, Hage and colleagues analyzed 105 patients affected by at least 3 cm BE without HGD or cancer at first endoscopy for a mean follow-up period of 12.7 years. LGD was present in 11 patients at entry endoscopy. At the end of follow-up, 6% patients had developed adenocarcinoma, which equals one cancer case per 221 patient-year or 0.45% per year. Tumors were interestingly diagnosed in a very wide range of time, from 4.6 to 15.9 years after index endoscopy. HGD was diagnosed in 5% of patients, which equals one cancer case per 266 patient-year or 0.38% per year. Similarly, diagnosis was made in wide period, ranging from 0.6 to 18.9 years. Regression from LGD to nondysplastic Barrett's epithelium was observed in 50% cases, but a progression to HGD was observed in 25% cases. A trend towards cancer development was observed for increasing lengths of BE.[37] But, with logistic regression analysis, other risk factors have been identified for development of multifocal HGD or adenocarcinoma: dysplasia at first endoscopy ($P < 0.001$), >3 cm hiatal hernia ($P < 0.02$), presence of dysplasia at any time during follow-up ($P < 0.03$), and Barrett's epithelium >2 cm ($P < 0.009$).[36]

The rationale of laparoscopic antireflux surgery in patients affected by BE is to prevent the progression to dysplasia–carcinoma and even to induce the regression to a nondysplastic Barrett's epithelium or a non metaplastic epithelium. It is commonly accepted that, once established, BE doesn't regress. This conclusion is supported by some endoscopic data that show no change in the length of the columnar-lined epithelium under therapy,[38] but in a study on 77 patients treated with antireflux surgery versus 14 patients treated with PPI, Gurski *et al.* observed a complete regression of the metaplastic epithelium in 36.4% of surgical patients versus 7.1% of medical patients ($P < 0.03$). Authors also evidenced that regression happened only in patients with short segment BE.[39] Even better results were reported in a recent study on 125 patients with short segment BE treated with laparoscopic Nissen fundoplication, duodenal switch, or duodenal diversion. Regression to nonmetaplastic mucosa was observed in 61% patients of the Nissen group, and 64% and 65%, respectively, in the other two groups.[40] Antireflux surgery also seems to be effective in inducing regression from LGD and preventing progression to HGD or cancer. Hofstetter and colleagues evaluated the long-term outcome (five years) of antireflux surgery in 97 patients affected by BE. LGD regressed to nondysplastic Barrett's in 44% cases and intestinal metaplasia was lost, regressing to cardiac mucosa, in 14%. No patient developed HGD or cancer in 410 patient-years of follow-up, but LGD developed in 6% patients.[41] In 2003, Parrilla published the results of a randomized study comparing medical and surgical treatment of BE patients. In the medical group, 2 of 3 patients regressed from LGD to ND, and in the surgical group, 5 of 5 regressed. In the medical arm, dysplasia *de novo* appeared in 8 of 40 patients (20%); two of these developed HGD. In the surgical arm, 3 of 53 patients (6%) developed dysplasia *de novo*, and two of these subsequently progressed to HGD, but these two showed a pH-metric recurrence of gastroesophageal reflux. No statistically significant differences were found between these two groups. If the patients with pH-metric failure are excluded, dysplasia *de novo* appeared only in 2% of patients and the surgical group showed a statistically significant difference respect the medical group ($P < 0.05$). The rate of malignancy was 0.8% per year in the medical group and 0.5% in the surgical group.[42] Similar good results were obtained in a little study from our institution, where medical (19 patients) versus surgical (16 patients) treatment were compared in LGD patients at 18 months follow-up. We observed a regression rate of 63.2% in the medical arm versus a 93.8% in the surgical arm ($P = 0.047$). The association between treatment and remission of LGD was examined using multiple logistic regression; laparoscopic Nissen fundoplication was the only variable associated with the probability of remission of LGD.[43]

These apparently better results of surgery respect medical therapy could be explained by the fact that the esophageal mucosa exposure to duodeno-gastric refluxate is higher in patients with BE and with dysplasia[44] and PPI are not able to block bile reflux; moreover, we know that even under PPI therapy about 60% patients have pathological esophageal exposure to bile, in a weakly acid environment that promotes the deconjugation of bile-salts.[45] Unfortunately, these results are not completely confirmed by large meta-analysis of the literature.[46,47] In fact, surgically treated patients demonstrated a higher incidence of regression from LGD to Barrett's epithelium (15.4%) when compared with medically treated patients (1.9%). Even when only controlled studies were analyzed, the probability of developing regression was greater in the surgically treated group (6.5% vs. 0.5%, $P = 0.024$).

The largest difference between surgical and medical therapy was demonstrated in the probability of regression from nondysplastic BE to normal squamous epithelium (17% vs. 0.4%). But, in regard of incidence of EA, when data from all included studies are pooled, the median incidence of cancer was 2.8 cases per 1,000 patient-years among the surgical group and 6.3 in the medical group ($P = 0.034$). When data from only controlled studies were pooled, the median incidence of adenocarcinoma in the surgical group did not significantly differ from that of the medical group: 4.8 cases per 1,000 patient-years versus 6.5, respectively ($P = 0.32$).

These conflicting results between the risk of cancer development and induction of regression could be explained with the fact that cellular and genetic alterations leading to adenocarcinoma may have already occurred before an antireflux procedure was performed; thus some cancers, particularly those that present during the first few postoperative years, probably do not represent progression of the disease.

Even though antireflux surgery seems to better promote regression of BE or dysplasia than medical therapy, it has not demonstrably reduced the incidence rate of adenocarcinoma, and therefore cannot be currently recommended as an antineoplastic procedure. Nevertheless, antireflux procedures should be proposed as a therapeutic alternative to all patients affected by BE with or without associated dysplasia, thus balancing the risks and benefits for each patient.

11. Is trimodal esophageal imaging (HRE-FI-NBI) the best tool for enhancement of detection of early neoplasia in Barrett's patients?

René Lambert
lambert@iarc.fr

Columnar metaplasia in the esophagus (Barrett's) occurs in relation to esophageal reflux and obesity in the young age. Three distinct types of gastric epithelium may develop in the distal esophagus: a cardiac type with mucous epithelial cells, a fundic type with chief and oxyntic cells, and an intestinal type with goblet cells and enterocytes with a brush border. The prevalence of Barrett's is higher in Caucasian males of Western countries; however, it has been overestimated, and based on a Swedish population of endoscopies performed in adults, it is now estimated at 1.6%. Multiple studies confirm an increased risk of adenocarcinoma in columnar metaplasia of the esophagus, but it has also overestimated, and recent evaluations account for one case per 200 patient-years. The risk has been correlated with the presence of intestinal cells in the metaplastic segment. However, recent studies conducted in the United States have shown that intestinal cells are found in only 48% of cases of Barrett's, and a study of small esophageal resected carcinomas has shown that the tumor develops more often (70%) in the vicinity of a cardiac type of epithelium. The risk of cancer is the same in the presence or absence of intestinal cells in the metaplastic segment; therefore, endoscopic exploration should aim to detect dysplasia rather than the intestinal type of epithelium.

In Western countries, attention given to the detection of early cancer in BE is justified by an increasing incidence of EA in recent decades;[48] as an example, the annual variation reaches +8.6% in men in the SEER registries of the United States during 1973–1995, but the worldwide incidence of adenocarcinoma is still very low as compared to that of squamous cell cancer in the esophagus. Overall, detection of early esophageal neoplasia in asymptomatic persons aims for curative treatment by endoscopic resection or by radiofrequency. As a rule, early neoplasia in the metaplastic mucosa of a BE is often missed during endoscopy, even with the help of chromoscopy, when a dye solution is projected at the surface of the mucosa (indigocarmine, methylene blue, or acetic acid). The poor efficacy of targeted biopsies explains the recommendation to adopt the time-consuming Reid protocol, with blind or random biopsies performed in quadrants at each length of 1 cm in the segment with columnar metaplasia.

In recent years, the dramatic progression in endoscopic imaging, and the cumulative impact of high resolution imaging (HRE), magnification, autofluorescence spectroscopy (AFI), and image processing modifies the diagnostic strategy of neoplasia in BE.

1. *High-resolution imaging* depends on the increased number of pixels in the charged coupled device (CCD) receiving the efferent photons and on the high (1,080 lines) definition of the image transmitted to the TV receptor.
2. *Magnification* with an optical zoom at a power of ×60 or ×80 describes with precision the microarchitecture of surface epithelium (pit pattern) and subepithelial capillaries (vascular pattern). An electronic zoom may also contribute to magnification.
3. *Autofluorescence imaging* requires a specific material: the AFI system proposed by Olympus Medical Systems consists of a light source (XCLV-260HP), a processor (XCV-260HP), a video monitor, and a dedicated videoendoscope (XCF-Q240FAI), which incorporates two CCDs, one for autofluorescence, the other for white light. In autofluorescence, the excitation light (390–470 nm) is provided by a rotation filter on the light source. The resulting image is artificially colored to green. A normal mucosa emits a bright autofluorescence and is colored in green. Fluorophores in the tumor absorb autofluorescence; the lesion appears in the complementary color of green–magenta. However, false-positive reactions in magenta are common.
4. *Image processing with the NBI technique* of Olympus is based on the restriction of the afferent light in two channels (blue and green); in the efferent image the micro-architecture of the epithelial crest is enhanced, and the subepithelial capillaries have greater contrast. Other methods in image processing have been developed by Fujinon (FICE) and Pentax (i-scan).

The increased efficacy of HRE endoscopy in white light combined to NBI has been stressed; both are proposed as red flag techniques for the detection of neoplasia in Barrett's.[49,50] Recently, a further progress in sensitivity and specificity is linked to the *trimodal technology*, combining HRE, AFI, and NBI, with or without magnification.[51,52] This protocol is proposed in a joint venture by endoscopy units based in the Netherlands (Amsterdam) and England (Manchester). The trimodal protocol significantly increases the sensitivity of HRE and more positive results are found. In addition, NBI reduces the false-positive rate of HRE + AFI from 71% to 48%; however, it is concluded that this protocol cannot substitute for the blind and random biopsies protocol in BE.[52]

In conclusion, the trimodal protocol requires specialized materials, is restricted to some reference centers, and, in Western countries, random biopsies are still recommended in asymptomatic patients with BE for the detection of neoplasia. However, in those countries, not enough room is attributed to magnification. Currently, in Japan, the detection of suspicious areas at the surface of the mucosa is completed by characterization through categories of the pit pattern and vascular pattern, and the best method of detection of flat areas of neoplasia relies on a bimodal HRE-NBI protocol coupled with magnification. Both protocols are currently available in this country with video-endoscopes and deserve to be spread around the world. Exploration of BE should rely on a protocol ensuring characterization after detection, while targeted biopsies could replace random biopsies.

12. The essential importance of natural history for the wise management of HGD

Helen M. Shields
hshields@caregroup.harvard.edu

HGD is not a fixed, well-defined entity. This is a major problem to address in the management of HGD in BE. Poor interobserver reproducibility is present in the diagnosis of HGD even when excellent pathologists, experienced in reading gastrointestinal biopsies, focus on diagnosing HGD on Barrett's slides from Barrett's patients.[53] Dr. Maru from the M.D. Anderson Cancer Center notes that 41% of outside cases called "HGD" are classified as adenocarcinoma

by their group of pathologists.[53] It is important to recognize this fact in making a decision about what is the best treatment for HGD.

Two very divergent studies have assessed the risk of HGD in BE patients turning into adenocarcinoma.[54,55] In the Hines VA study, Schnell *et al.* noted 16% of patients evolving to adenocarcinoma over a follow-up interval of seven years and three months of surveillance endoscopies.[55] On the other hand, Reid's group at the University of Washington noted that 59% of their HGD patients had developed adenocarcinoma at the five-year time interval.[54] This marked divergence in the evolution of HGD to adenocarcinoma leads to significant doubt about the reproducibility of the diagnosis of HGD as supported by Maru's observations above.[53] What should be done for patients with HGD that has been verified by at least two experienced pathologists? The most effective and least harmful therapy should be recommended. Esophagectomy has traditionally been associated with significant morbidity and mortality. It is currently reserved for patients who are not considered candidates for less invasive, but potentially curative therapies, such as photodynamic therapy, endoscopic mucosal resection, and/or radiofrequency ablation.[56,57] Photodynamic therapy's relatively high rate of stricture formation and photosensitivity have limited its role now that other modalities are available.

Ell *et al.* pointed out the feasibility of endoscopic mucosal resection for HGD and early cancer in 64 BE patients with early esophageal cancer or HGD.[56] The best evidence for cure available at present is the use of endoscopic mucosal resection.[56] Another excellent endotherapy is radiofrequency ablation. The results reported in the 2009 *New England Journal of Medicine* paper from Shaheen *et al.* showed that the radiofrequency ablation method has its greatest benefit in patients with HGD. Patients were randomly assigned to receive the actual treatment or a sham procedure. Eradication of HGD was found in 81% of the group receiving the therapy.[57] Compared to historical reports of the natural history of BE, ablation may be associated with a reduction in cancer incidence. But heterogeneous studies limit the comparison. A frequently asked question is whether radiofrequency ablation should be added to endoscopic mucosal resection to improve follow-up results. The answer is not known at present. Also, the role of laparoscopic or traditional surgery to cure an EA has not been compared to endoscopic mucosal resection or radiofrequency ablation to date in a randomized controlled trial. These prospective studies are needed.

In summary, the wise management of HGD is based on understanding that there is variability in the diagnosis of HGD by pathologists. At present, endoscopic mucosal resection therapy with or without radiofrequency ablation appears to be reasonable therapy for HGD or early esophageal carcinoma. Research data also favor the use of radiofrequency ablation compared to photodynamic therapy because of fewer complications and better efficacy. However, neither endoscopic mucosal resection nor radiofrequency ablation has been studied in randomized controlled trials and compared to surgical therapy. Long-term follow-up data are needed for all forms of therapy.

Conflicts of Interest

The authors declare no conflicts of interest.

References

1. Kahrilas, P.J. & J.E. Pandolfino. 2002. Gastroesophageal reflux disease and its complications, including Barrett's metaplasia. In *Sleisenger and Fordtran's Gastrointestinal and Liver Disease: Pathophysiology/Diagnosis/Management.* Chapter 33. M. Feldman, L.S. Friedman & M.H. Sleisenter, Eds.: 616. Saunders. Philadelphia.
2. Spechler, S.J., R.C. Fitzgerald, G.A. Prasad & K.K. Wang. 2010. History, molecular mechanisms, and endoscopic treatment of Barrett's esophagus. *Gastroenterol* **138:** 854–859.
3. Society of Thoracic Surgeons, website, http://www.sts. org/.2010.
4. Blot, W.J. & J.F. Fraumeni, Jr. 1987. Trends in esophageal cancer mortality among US blacks and whites. *Am. J. Public Health* **77:** 296–298.
5. Polednak, A.P. 2003. Trends in survival for both histologic types of esophageal cancer in US surveillance, epidemiology and end results areas. *Int. J. Cancer* **105:** 98–100.
6. Camilleri, M., D. Dubois, B. Coulie, *et al.* 2005. Prevalence and socioeconomic impact of upper gastrointestinal disorders in the United States: results of the US Upper Gastrointestinal Study. *Clin. Gastroenterol. Hepatol.* **3:** 543–552.
7. Hayeck, T.J., C.Y. Kong, S.J. Spechler, *et al.* The prevalence of Barrett's esophagus in the US: estimates from a simulation model confirmed by SEER data. *Dis. Esophagus,* **23:** 451–457.
8. Gerson, L.B., R. Edson, P.W. Lavori & G. Triadafilopoulos. 2001. Use of a simple symptom questionnaire to predict Barrett's esophagus in patients with symptoms of gastroesophageal reflux. *Am. J. Gastroenterol.* **96:** 2005–2012.
9. Ronkainen, J., P. Aro, T. Storskrubb, *et al.* 2005. Prevalence of Barrett's esophagus in the general population: an endoscopic study. *Gastroenterology* **129:** 1825–1831.
10. Oberg, S., J. Johansson, J. Wenner & B. Walther. 2002. Meta-

11. Su, Y., X. Chen, M. Klein, *et al.* 2004. Phenotype of columnar-lined esophagus in rats with esophagogastroduodenal anastomosis: similarity to human Barrett's esophagus. *Lab. Invest.* **84:** 753–765.
12. Souza, R.F., K. Krishnan & S.T. Spechler. 2008. Acid, bile, and CDX: the ABCs of making Barrett's metaplasia. *Am. J. Physiol. Gastrointest. Liver Physiol.* **295:** G211–G218.
13. Alvaro-Villegas, J.C., S. Sobrino-Cossio, A. Hernandez-Guerrero, *et al.* Dilated intercellular spaces in subtypes of gastroesophagic reflux disease. *Rev. Esp. Enferm. Dig.* **102:** 302–307.
14. Abela, J.-E., J.J. Going, J.F. Mackenzie, *et al.* 2008. Systematic four-quadrant biopsy detects Barrett's dysplasia in more patients than nonsystematic biopsy. *Am. J. Gastroenterol.* **103:** 850–855.
15. Ajumobi, A., K. Bahjri, C. Jackson & R. Griffin. 2010. Surveillance in Barrett's esophagus: an audit of practice. *Dig. Dis. Sci.* **55:** 1615–1621.
16. Komanduri, S., G. Swanson, L. Keefer & S. Jakate. 2009. Use of a new jumbo forceps improves tissue acquisition of Barrett's esophagus surveillance biopsies. *Gastrointest. Endosc.* **70:** 1072–1078.
17. Reid, B.J., P.L. Blount, Z. Feng & D.S. Levine. 2000. Optimizing endoscopic biopsy detection of early cancer in Barrett's high-grade dysplasia. *Am. J. Gastroenterol.* **95:** 3089–3096.
18. Manath, J., V. Subramanian, J. Hawkey & K. Ragunath. 2010. Narrow band imaging for characterization of high-grade dysplasia and specialized intestinal metaplasia in Barrett's esophagus: a meta analysis. *Endoscopy* **42:** 351–359.
19. Blaser, M.J. 1999. Hypothesis: the changing relationships of *Helicobacter pylori* and humans: implications for health and disease. *J Infect Dis.* **179:** 1523–1530.
20. Abe, Y., K. Iijima, T. Koike, *et al.* 2009. Barrett's esophagus is characterized by the absence of *Helicobacter pylori* infection and high levels of serum pepsinogen I concentration in Japan. *J. Gastroenterol. Hepatol.* **24:** 129–134.
21. Kimura, K. 1973. Chronological changes of atrophic gastritis. *Nippon Shokakibyo Gakkai Zasshi.* **70:** 307–315.
22. Kim, D.H., G.H. Kim, J.Y. Kim, *et al.* 2007. Endoscopic grading of atrophic gastritis is inversely associated with gastroesophageal reflux and gastropharyngeal reflux. *Korean J. Intern. Med.* **22:** 231–236.
23. El-Zimaity, H.M., H. Ota, D.Y. Graham, *et al.* 2002. Patterns of gastric atrophy in intestinal type gastric carcinoma. *Cancer* **94:** 1428–1436.
24. Rokkas T., D. Pistiolas, P. Sechopoulos, *et al.* 2007. Relationship between *Helicobacter pylori* infection and esophageal neoplasia: a meta-analysis. *Clin Gastroenterol. Hepatol.* **5:** 1413–1417.
25. Wang, C., Y. Yuan & R.H. Hunt. 2009. *Helicobacter pylori* infection and Barrett's esophagus: a systematic review and meta-analysis. *Am. J. Gastroenterol.* **104:** 492–500.
26. Mccoll, K.E. 2007. *Helicobacter pylori* and oesophageal cancer–not always protective. *Gut.* **56:** 457–459.
27. Axon, A.T. 2004. Personal view: to treat or not to treat? *Helicobacter pylori* and gastro-oesophageal reflux disease—an alternative hypothesis. *Aliment. Pharmacol. Ther.* **19:** 253–261.

plastic columnar mucosa in the cervical esophagus after esophagectomy. *Ann. Surg.* **235:** 338–345.

28. Holtmann, G., C. Cain & P. Malfertheiner. 1999. Gastric *Helicobacter pylori* infection accelerates healing of reflux esophagitis during treatment with the proton pump inhibitor pantoprazole. *Gastroenterology* **117:** 11–16.

29. Yachida, S., D. Saito, T. Kozu, *et al.* 2001. Endoscopically demonstrable esophageal changes after *Helicobacter pylori* eradication in patients with gastric disease. *J. Gastroenterol. Hepatol.* **16:** 1346–1352.

30. Peters, F.T., E.J. Kuipers, S. Ganesh, *et al.* 1999. The influence of *Helicobacter pylori* on oesophageal acid exposure in GERD during acid suppressive therapy. *Aliment. Pharmacol. Ther.* **13:** 921–926.

31. Raghunath, A.S., A.P. Hungin, D. Wooff & S. Childs. 2004. Systematic review: the effect of *Helicobacter pylori* and its eradication on gastro-oesophageal reflux disease in patients with duodenal ulcers or reflux oesophagitis. *Aliment. Pharmacol. Ther.* **20:** 733–744.

32. Kuipers, E.J., G.F. Nelis, E.C. Klinkenberg-Knol, *et al.* 2004. Cure of *Helicobacter pylori* infection in patients with reflux oesophagitis treated with long term omeprazole reverses gastritis without exacerbation of reflux disease: results of a randomised controlled trial. *Gut.* **53:** 12–20.

33. Wang, K.K. & R.E. Sampliner. 2008. Updated guidelines 2008 for the diagnosis, surveillance and therapy of Barrett's esophagus. *Am. J. Gastroenterol.* **103:** 788–797.

34. Spechler, S.J., A.H. Robbins, *et al.* 1984. Adenocarcinoma and Barrett'esophagus: an overrated risk? *Gastroenterology* **87:** 927–933.

35. Cameron, A.J., B.J. Ott, *et al.* 1985. The incidence of adenocarcinoma in columnar-lined (Barrett's) esophagus. *N. Engl. J. Med.* **313:** 857–859.

36. Weston, A.P., A.S. Badr, *et al.* 1999. Prospective multivariate analysis of clinical, endoscopic, and histological factors predictive of the development of Barrett's multifocal high-grade dysplasia or adenocarcinoma. *Am. J. Gastroenterol.* **94:** 3413–3419.

37. Hage, M., D. Siersema, *et al.* 2004. Oesophageal cancer incidence and mortality in patients with long-segment Barrett's oesophagus after a mean follow-up of 12,7 years. *Scand. J. Gastroenterol.* **12:** 1175–1179.

38. Peters, F.T., S. Ganesh, *et al.* 1999. Endoscopic regression of Barrett's esophagus during omeprazole treatment: a randomized double-blind study. *Gut.* **45:** 489–494.

39. Gurski, R., J.H. Peters, *et al.* 2003. Barrett's esophagus can and does regress after antireflux surgery: a study of prevalence and predictive features. *J. Am. Coll. Surg.* **196:** 706–712.

40. Csendes, A., I. Braghetto, *et al.* 2009. Late results of surgical treatments of 125 patients with short-segment Barrett's esophagus. *Arch. Surg.* **144:** 921–927.

41. Hofstetter, W.L., J.H. Peters, *et al.* 2001. Long-term outcome of anti-reflux surgery in patients with Barrett's esophagus. *Ann. Surg.* **234:** 532–539.

42. Parrilla, P., L.F. Martinez de Haro, *et al.* 2003. Long-term results of a randomized prospective study comparing medical and surgical treatment of Barrett's esophagus. *Ann. Surg.* **237:** 291–298.

43. Rossi, M., M. Barreca, *et al.* 2006. Efficacy of Nissen fundoplication versus medical therapy in the regression of low-grade dysplasia in patients with Barrett esophagus. A prospective study. *Ann. Surg.* **243:** 58–63.

44. Martinez de Haro, L., A. Ortiz, *et al.* 2001. Intestinal metaplasia in patients with columnar lined esophagus is associated with high levels of duodenogastroesophageal reflux. *Ann. Surg.* **233:** 34–38.

45. Todd, J.A., K.K. Basu, *et al.* 2005. Normalisation of oesophageal pH does not guatantee control of duodenogastro-esophageal reflux in Barrett's esophagus. *Aliment. Pharmacol. Ther.* **21:** 969–975.

46. Chang, E.Y., C.D. Morris, *et al.* 2007. The effect of antireflux surgery on esophageal carcinogenesis in patients with Barrett's esophagus. *Ann. Surg.* **246:** 11–21.

47. Corey, K.E., S.M. Schmitz, *et al.* 2003. Does a surgical antireflux procedure decrease the incidence of esophageal adenocarcinoma in Barrett's esophagus? A meta-analysis. *Am. J. Gastroenterol.* **98:** 2390–2394.

48. Lambert, R. & P. Hainaut. 2007. Esophageal cancer: the precursors (Part II). *Endoscopy* **39:** 659–664.

49. Singh, R., G.K. Anagnostopoulos, K. Yao, *et al.* 2008. Narrow-band imaging with magnification in Barrett's esophagus: validation of a simplified grading system of mucosal morphology patterns against histology. *Endoscopy* **40:** 457–463.

50. Mannath, J., V. Subramanian, C.J. Hawkey, *et al.* 2010. Narrow band imaging for characterization of high-grade dysplasia and specialized intestinal metaplasia in Barrett's esophagus: a meta-analysis. *Endoscopy* **42:** 351–359.

51. Kara, M.A., F.P. Peters, P. Fockens, *et al.* 2006. Endoscopic video-autofluorescence imaging followed by narrow band imaging for detecting early neoplasia in Barrett's esophagus. *Gastrointest. Endosc.* **64:** 176–185.

52. Curvers, W.L., L.A. Herrero, M.B. Wallace, *et al.* 2010. Endoscopic tri-modal imaging is more effective than standard endoscopy in targeting early-stage neoplasia in Barrett's esophagus. *Gastroenterology* [Epub ahead of print].

53. Maru, D.M. 2009. Barrett's esophagus: diagnostic challenges and recent developments. *Ann. Diag. Path.* **13:** 212–221.

54. Reid, B.J., D.S. Levine, G. Longton, *et al.* 2000. Predictors of progression to cancer in Barrett's esophagus: baseline histology and flow cytometry identify low- and high-risk patient subsets. *Am. J. Gastroenterol.* **95:** 1669–1676.

55. Schnell, T.G., S.J. Sontag, G. Chejfec, *et al.* 2001. Long-term nonsurgical management of Barrett's esophagus with high-grade dysplasia. *Gastroenterology* **120:** 1607–1619.

56. Ell, C., A. May, L. Grossner, *et al.* 2000. Endoscopic mucosal resection for early cancer and high-grade dysplasia in Barrett's esophagus. *Gastroenterology* **118:** 670–677.

57. Shaheen, N.J., P. Sharma, B.F. Overholt, *et al.* 2009. Radiofrequency ablation in Barrett's esophagus with dysplasia. *N. Engl. J. Med.* **360:** 2277–2288.

Ann. N.Y. Acad. Sci. ISSN 0077-8923

ANNALS OF THE NEW YORK ACADEMY OF SCIENCES

Issue: *Barrett's Esophagus: The 10th OESO World Congress Proceedings*

Molecular aspects of esophageal development

Mark Rishniw,[1] Pavel Rodriguez,[2] Jianwen Que,[2,3] Zoe D. Burke,[4] David Tosh,[4] Hao Chen,[5] and Xiaoxin Chen[5]

[1]College of Veterinary Medicine, Department of Biomedical Sciences, Cornell University, Ithaca, New York. [2]Department of Cell Biology, Duke University Medical Center, Durham, North Carolina. [3]Department of Biomedical Genetics, University of Rochester, Rochester, New York. [4]Centre for Regenerative Medicine, Department of Biology and Biochemistry, University of Bath, Bath, United Kingdom. [5]Julius L. Chambers Biomedical/Biotechnology Research Institute, North Carolina Central University, Durham, North Carolina.

The following on molecular aspects of esophageal development contains commentaries on esophageal striated myogenesis and transdifferentiation; conversion from columnar into stratified squamous epithelium in the mouse esophagus; the roles for BMP signaling in the developing esophagus and forestomach; and evidence of a direct conversion from columnar to stratified squamous cells in the developing esophagus.

Keywords: BMP signaling; esophagus; forestomach; stratification; differentiation; myogenesis; transdifferentiation; fate mapping; embryonic esophageal culture model; columnar epithelium; stratified squamous epithelium

Concise summaries

- Embryologically, the esophageal musculature begins as a smooth muscle-lined tube in all species, with subsequent conversion to varying proportions of striated muscle in a craniocaudal direction.
- Using mice as a model of esophageal myogenesis, where the conversion from one cell type to the other is virtually 100%, coexpression of smooth muscle and striated muscle markers in *muscularis externae* myocytes has been shown by immunohistochemical labeling, suggesting that smooth muscle cells were able to switch phenotype well after commitment and differentiation. Esophageal striated myogenesis does not occur via a process of transdifferentiation; rather, striated and smooth muscle cells arise from distinct precursor populations.

- In the early embryo, when the esophagus is separated from the anterior foregut tube, the epithelium is simple columnar. Using several genetically engineered mouse lines, it has been shown that bone morphogenetic protein (BMP) signaling plays important roles in the early molecular mechanisms underlying the conversion of the epithelium foregut development.
- Immunostaining for the proliferation marker Ki-67 was made to determine whether the switch from columnar to stratified squamous epithelium was due to selective overgrowth of the squamous epithelium.
- The possibility that the cells of the basal layer arise directly from the columnar epithelium has also been investigated.
- The embryonic esophageal culture model has provided evidence of a direct conversion from columnar to stratified squamous cells in the developing esophagus.

1. Esophageal striated myogenesis: transdifferentiation or not?

Mark Rishniw
mr89@cornell.edu

The adult esophagus is composed of several muscle layers—a smooth muscle *muscularis mucosae* layer and two *muscularis externae* layers (longitudinal and circumferential). The *muscularis externae* layers are variably composed of striated and smooth muscle elements, with substantial differences existing between species, for example, they are composed almost entirely of striated muscle in the adult mouse and are completely smooth muscled in birds.

doi: 10.1111/j.1749-6632.2011.06071.x
Ann. N.Y. Acad. Sci. 1232 (2011) 309–315 © 2011 New York Academy of Sciences.

Embryologically, however, the esophageal musculature begins as a smooth muscle-lined tube in all species, with subsequent conversion to varying proportions of striated muscle in a craniocaudal direction.

This conversion process has been the focus of several studies over the past 15 years, beginning with an observation by Patapoutian *et al.* that smooth muscle cells directly transdifferentiated into striated muscle cells.[1] Using mice as a model of esophageal myogenesis, where the conversion from one cell type to the other is virtually 100%, these authors showed coexpression of smooth muscle and striated muscle markers in *muscularis externae* myocytes by immunohistochemical labeling, and suggested that smooth muscle cells were able to switch phenotype well after commitment and differentiation. These findings were both supported by other investigators and challenged by other investigators.[2] Thus, the mechanism of esophageal striated myogenesis remained unresolved. We performed a series of experiments to determine whether transdifferentiation accounts for esophageal muscle phenotype switching.[3–5]

In the first experiment, we fate mapped smooth muscle cells by crossing a mouse expressing eGFP and Cre-recombinase under the control of the smooth muscle myosin heavy chain (SmMHC) promoter (so-called SMCG2 mice) with R26R mice.[3] The expression of eGFP and Cre-recombinase is strictly confined to smooth muscle cells in the SMCG2 mouse. R26R mice (also known as Rosa26R mice) have a constitutively expressed β-lactamase gene (under the control of the Rosa promoter), which is inhibited from expression by a lox-P flanked stop codon. Removal of the stop codon by Cre-recombinase results in constitutive β-lactamase expression. Thus, by crossing the SMCG2 and R26R mice, we could selectively activate β-lactamase expression in any cell that has expressed SmMHC (i.e., smooth muscle cells). Examination of E15 mouse embryos showed robust eGFP and Cre-recombinase expression (and β-lactamase expression) along the full length of the esophagus. However, P1 and P15 esophagi showed expression of these smooth muscle elements to more caudal portions of the esophagus. Importantly, no striated muscles in the *muscularis externae* showed β-lactamase expression (as evidenced by X-gal staining). This would suggest that these cells had never activated the SmMHC pro-

moter to express Cre-recombinase and, therefore, did not derive from a smooth muscle cell precursor cell.

We then used the SMCG2 mouse to examine coexpression of eGFP or Cre-recombinase (which is localized to nuclei in smooth muscle cells) and the striated muscle transcription factor, myogenin.[4] We could find no instances of coexpression of these two markers (one smooth, one striated) in any cells within the developing *muscularis externae*.

Finally, we used a selective deletion strategy to determine whether smooth muscle cells transdifferentiate into striated muscles.[5] We used the SMCG2 mouse to selectively delete the myogenin gene from smooth muscle cells by crossing it with a mouse that had a lox-P-flanked myogenin gene. Since myogenin is essential for striated myogenesis, we hypothesized that, if smooth muscle cells transdifferentiated into striated muscle cells within the esophagus, deletion of myogenin in these cells prior to the transdifferentiation process would prevent this event, resulting in a myodysplasia, characterized by persistence of smooth muscle along the length of the esophagus. However, despite robust Cre-recombinase expression (and, presumably, efficient myogenin deletion), esophageal myogenesis progressed in these mice in a normal manner.

Taken together, our data convincingly suggest that esophageal striated myogenesis does not occur via a process of transdifferentiation, but that striated and smooth muscle cells arise from distinct precursor populations.

2. Conversion from simple columnar into stratified squamous epithelium in the mouse esophagus and forestomach is regulated by BMP signaling

Pavel Rodriguez and Jianwen Que
jianwen_Que@urmc.rochester.edu

The epithelium lining of the adult esophagus is squamous and stratified. However, in the early embryo when the esophagus is separated from the anterior foregut tube the epithelium is simple columnar.[6,7] Our laboratory is interested in molecular mechanisms underlying the conversion of the epithelium using the mouse as a model organism. We include the forestomach in our studies as the epithelium lining this tissue also goes through similar

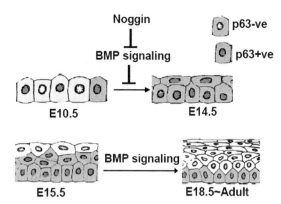

Figure 1. Model proposing that between E10.5 and E13.5, the inhibition of BMP signaling, as mediated by an inhibitor such as Noggin, is necessary to allow the stratification of simple columnar to multilayered epithelium. Then, after E14.5-15.5, active BMP signaling is required for suprabasal differentiation of the epithelium.

morphological and histological transitions. We previously showed that BMP signaling plays important roles in the early foregut development,[8] and here we further explored its role in the development of the esophagus and forestomach using several genetically engineered mouse lines.

We first used a BMP reporter mouse line harboring a *BRE-lacZ* allele along with *in situ* hybridization to localize transcripts for BMP signaling components, including different antagonists. We demonstrated that when epithelium stratifies between embryonic day (E) 10.5 and E14.5, BMP signaling is not activated in the epithelium of the esophagus and forestomach, correlating with the presence of the BMP antagonist Noggin. However, activation of BMP signaling after E14.5 at the top layers of the epithelium is correlated with differentiation of the epithelium (Fig. 1). We further showed that deletion of the *Noggin* gene stalls the conversion of simple columnar into stratified epithelium. We then exploited a *Shh-Cre* allele that drives recombination in the embryonic foregut epithelium to generate either gain-or-loss-of-function models for the Bmpr1a (Alk3) receptor.

In gain-of-function embryos (*Shh-Cre; Rosa26$^{CAG-loxstoploxp-caBmpRIa}$*), high levels of ectopic BMP signaling also prevents the transition from simple columnar to multilayered undifferentiated epithelium in the esophagus and forestomach. In loss-of-function experiments, conditional deletion of the BMP receptor in *Shh-Cre;Bmpr1a$^{flox/flox}$* embryos allows the formation of a multilayered

squamous epithelium, but which fails to differentiate, as shown by the absence of expression of the suprabasal markers, loricrin, and involucrin.

Together, these findings suggest multiple roles for BMP signaling in the developing esophagus and forestomach.[9]

3. Conversion of columnar to stratified squamous epithelium in the developing esophagus

Zoe D. Burke and David Tosh
d.tosh@bath.ac.uk

The mammalian esophagus exhibits a remarkable change in epithelial organization during the transition from embryonic to adult tissue. Initially, the esophagus is lined by a simple columnar epithelial layer, which is gradually replaced by a stratified squamous tissue comprised a clearly distinct basal layer surrounded by the spinous, granulated, and cornified suprabasal layers.

The replacement of one epithelium with another during esophageal development has been documented in both mouse and human, and in 1993, Thorey *et al.* proposed that the basal layer of the stratified squamous epithelium is derived from the columnar epithelium.[10–12] However, direct evidence for this conversion was lacking due to the availability of suitable model systems.

We have developed an *in vitro* model for studying esophageal development based on the culture of esophageal explants from embryonic day 11.5 (E11.5) mouse embryos. This culture model recapitulates the *in vivo* development of the esophagus.[7] Using immunohistochemical analysis of sections from developing mouse embryos, we initially demonstrated that the transition from columnar to stratified squamous epithelium is accompanied by a change in expression of the intermediate filament proteins cytokeratin 8 (K8, a marker of columnar epithelium) and 14 (K14, a marker for the basal epithelial layer). At E11.5 all the cells of the esophageal epithelium express K8 but not K14. Gradually, between E15.5 and E17.5, K8 expression is lost in the basal layer but is retained in the suprabasal layers until postnatal day 3 when it is completely lost. In contrast, K14 is absent in the esophageal epithelium at E11.5 but begins to be expressed

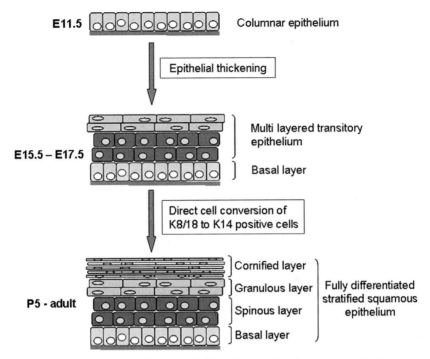

Figure 2. Summary of the conversion of esophageal epithelium from simple columnar to stratified squamous tissue during development. At E11.5 the esophageal epithelium consists of a single layer of K8-expressing cells. Between E15.5 and E17.5, the epithelium starts to become multilayered and the loss of columnar K8 expression from the basal layer coincides with the onset of K14 expression. In postnatal/adult esophagus, K8 expression is not detectable, the basal layer cells express only K14, and the esophagus is fully differentiated as a stratified squamous tissue.

around E17.5 in the basal cells, which are no longer expressing K8.

The explant culture model was established by placing esophageal tissue dissected from E11.5 embryos onto fibronectin-coated glass coverslips. Within 24 h, the explants attached and flattened onto the fibronectin substratum at which stage they are composed of a tube of epithelium surrounded by mesenchyme. The explants remain viable in culture for up to 20 days and differentiate as stratified squamous epithelium, exhibiting the same switch in expression of K8 to K14 as observed *in vivo*.

To determine the origin of the stratified squamous epithelium, we used our explant model to explore the possibility that basal cells arise through programmed cell death of the columnar cells, selective overgrowth of the squamous epithelium, or though a direct conversion of one cell type to another.

To distinguish the first of these possibilities, we separated the cells after 7, 11, or 15 days of culture by flow cytometry and then immunostained for either K8 or K14 and propidium iodide to iden-

tify dead cells. If the switch in cell type was due to a preferential death of the columnar cell population, the number of dead cells would be higher in the K8-expressing population. However, there was no observable difference in the proportion of dead cells in the K8- and K14-positive populations indicating that programmed cell death does not play a role in the conversion from columnar to stratified squamous epithelium.

To determine whether the switch from columnar to stratified squamous epithelium was due to selective overgrowth of the squamous epithelium we immunostained for the proliferation marker Ki-67. The embryonic esophageal epithelium in culture is highly proliferative up until the culture differentiates into multilayers after which time the majority of the proliferating cells become localized to the K14-positive cells of the basal layer. In order to determine whether cell division was required for conversion, we treated esophageal explants with mitomycin C, a DNA crosslinking agent that prevents the cells from entering the cell cycle. If the cell conversion is dependent on cell division, then we predicted it would not be able to occur in the presence of a cell cycle inhibitor. However, the transition from K8-positive columnar layer to the K14-expressing cells continued to occur in the presence of mitomycin C indicating that cell proliferation does not play a role in the epithelial cell conversion.

The possibility that the cells of the basal layer arise directly from the columnar epithelium was also investigated. Upon costaining for K8 and K14, we found some cells coexpressing both markers suggesting that K14-positive cells arose directly from K8-positive cells. To trace the lineage of the stratified squamous basal cells, we electroporated a reporter plasmid, the K14 promoter driving GFP expression, into esophageal explants obtained from E15.5 embryos. This timepoint was chosen since the basal phenotype starts to appear between E15.5 and E17.5. Costaining for GFP and K8 revealed that at least some of the cells that have an activate K14 promoter (GFP-positive) also express K8, indicating that the basal cells of the squamous epithelium arise through a direct conversion from K8-positive columnar cells.

The embryonic esophageal culture model has provided evidence of a direct conversion from columnar to stratified squamous cells in the developing esophagus (Fig. 2). Further analysis of the mechanisms involved in this conversion may also provide important insights underlying the mechanism(s) involved in Barrett's metaplasia in which the reverse conversion from stratified squamous epithelium to columnar epithelium occurs.[13]

4. Understanding Barrett's esophagus from the perspective of development

Hao Chen and Xiaoxin Chen
lchen@nccu.edu

The developmental process by which a single fertilized egg becomes a complex organism has fascinated people for many years, and continues to interest biologists today. Discoveries in developmental biology constantly generate insights on the molecular basis of many human diseases. Indeed, many disease-related genes and pathways were identified first as critical ones in embryonic development, such as BMP, WNT, Hedgehog.

Barrett's esophagus (BE) is a premalignant lesion of esophageal adenocarcinoma in which the nor-mal squamous epithelium is replaced by intestinalized columnar epithelium. Although it is known to develop as a consequence of chronic gastroesophageal reflux, its molecular aspect is not fully understood. Two lines of evidence suggested that research on esophageal development may shed light on the molecular mechanism of BE. (a) BE may originate from stem cells residing in the esophagus (e.g., interpapillary basal cells, ductal cells of submucosal glands). (b) Human embryonic esophagus is initially lined with a ciliated pseudostratified columnar epithelium containing goblet cells, which is later replaced by a stratified non-keratinized squamous epithelium containing submucosal glands. A question becomes obvious, Is BE an adaptive reversal of embryonic development?

Current status
Human esophagus begins to form during the 4th week of embryonic development, with the formation of the foregut. Up to the 8th week, the esophageal epithelium appears as a pseudostratified columnar epithelium which then becomes ciliated. Starting from the 4th month of gestation, the ciliated epithelium is gradually replaced by a squamous epithelium until a non-keratinized stratified squamous epithelium is fully developed. Residual islands of columnar epithelium remain and downgrow to generate submucosal glands. The ducts are therefore lined partly by squamous epithelial cells. Keratinization does not normally occur in humans, nor in carnivores, although it is normally seen in rodents and ruminants. At about the 6th or 7th week of gestation, the circular muscle coat, ganglion cells of the myenteric plexus, and blood vessels start to develop.[14]

However, molecular mechanism of esophageal development is poorly understood. Only several genes and molecular pathways have been reported to be involved in esophageal development. Among them, P63 and Sox2 play key roles in epithelial development, as well as the pathways, such as BMP, Hedgehog, NGF/NGFR and Nrf2/Keap1. As for neural development, SULF1/SULF2 regulate heparan sulfate-mediated GDNF signaling for esophageal innervation.[15] Rassf1a was also found to be involved in development of esophageal nerve, both ganglia and nerve fibres. As for the muscle and blood vessels, FOXM1 was required. Gene methylation also participates in modulating gene

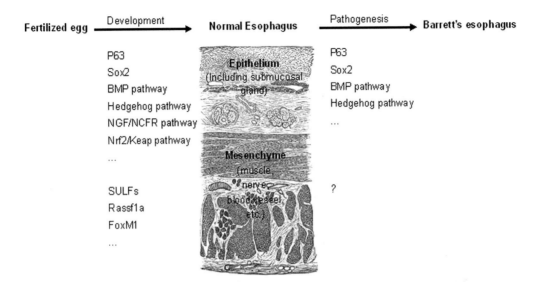

Figure 3. Understanding Barrett's esophagus from the perspective of development. Several developmental genes and pathways are known to play important roles in the development of Barrett's esophagus. Others remain to be identified and studied for their potential contribution to Barrett's esophagus.

expression during esophageal development.[16] A recent microarray study found a group of transcriptional factors exclusively expressed in esophageal progenitor cells, Foxe1, Dlx3, Erf, Nfix, Nrl, Otx1, Pitx1, Tcfab2c, Twist1 and Zfpn1a2, and therefore provided clues to further demonstrate their functions in esophageal development.

Future perspectives

It is obvious that we need more research on esophageal development for the sake of understanding BE and other esophageal diseases as well. Both the epithelium and the mesenchyme may be equally important because of epithelium-mesenchymal interactions in development and the involvement of mesenchymal structures in BE. For example, it is not known how lower esophageal sphincter muscle develop; how motor nerves develop and regulate the function of muscles; how sensory nerves develop and respond to reflux; how submucosal glands develop and whether we may stimulate glandular secretion for antacid therapy;[17] how the epithelium develop and keratinize (in rodents) and whether we may manipulate this process to enhance epithelial resistance to reflux.

Although most work on the molecular aspect of esophageal development was performed in mice,[18] selection of proper animal species in this research area is always a critical issue. Non-keratinization

of the esophageal squamous epithelium, presence of submucosal glands, availability of proper transgenic and knockout techniques and tools, cost of maintenance, are all important factors for consideration. Each animal species has its advantages and limitations. Mice remain the first choice in most labs, although they do not have submucosal glands and their epithelium is keratinized. In case a genetic modification is lethal, *ex vivo* and *in vivo* organ culture of embryonic esophagus may still generate useful information. Pig esophagus is very similar to human esophagus in anatomy and physiology. However, cost of maintenance is a major limitation. Recently we have identified a short piece of non-keratinized stratified squamous epithelium in zebrafish pharynx similar to human esophageal epithelium. An obvious advantage of the zebrafish system is that genetic manipulation is more convenient and economic in zebrafish than in other larger animals.

In summary, we believe developmental research can make great contributions to our understanding of the molecular mechanism of BE. Those critical genes and molecular pathways for development may play important roles in BE as well (Figure 3). Take P63 as an example, a translational approach may be adopted for future studies. P63 was first demonstrated as a critical gene in the development of esophageal epithelium in knockout mice. Loss of P63 resulted in a simple columnar epithelium which failed to develop into stratified squamous epithelium in the esophagus. P63 expression was then found to be negative in most cases of human BE. Moreover it was already lost in some cases of multi-layered epithelium, a transitional stage before normal esophagus and BE. Recent *in vitro* cell culture studies confirmed that exposure of esophageal squamous epithelial cells to gastroesophageal refluxate down-regulated P63 expression. Now, there is an obvious need to generate an esophagus-specific conditional P63 knockout model to demonstrate whether loss of P63, either alone or in combination with other genetic factors, may lead to BE *in vivo*. Supported by NIH grants U56 A092077 and P20 MD000175.

Conflicts of interest

The authors declare no conflicts of interest.

References

1. Patapoutian, A., B.J. Wold & R.A. Wagner. 1995. Evidence for developmentally programmed transdifferentiation in mouse esophageal muscle. *Science* **270:** 1818–1821.
2. Stratton, C.J., Y. Bayguinov, K.M. Sanders & S.M. Ward. 2000. Ultrastructural analysis of the transdifferentiation of smooth muscle to skeletal muscle in the murine esophagus. *Cell Tissue Res.* **301:** 283–298.
3. Rishniw, M., H.B. Xin, K.Y. Deng & M.I. Kotlikoff. Skeletal myogenesis in the mouse esophagus does not occur through transdifferentiation. *Genesis* **36:** 81–82.
4. Rishniw, M., P.W. Fisher, R.M. Doran, *et al.* 2007. Smooth muscle persists in the muscularis externa of developing and adult mouse esophagus. *J. Muscle. Res. Cell Motil.* **28:** 153–165.
5. Rishniw, M., P.J. Fisher, R.M. Doran, *et al.* 2009. Striated myogenesis and peristalsis in the fetal murine esophagus occur without cell migration or interstitial cells of Cajal. *Cells Tissues Organs* **189:** 410–419.
6. Que, J., T. Okubo, J.R. Goldenring, *et al.* 2007. Multiple dose-dependent roles for Sox2 in the patterning and differentiation of anterior foregut endoderm. *Development* **134:** 2521–2531.
7. Yu, W.Y., J.M. Slack & D. Tosh. 2005. Conversion of columnar to stratified squamous epithelium in the developing mouse oesophagus. *Dev. Biol.* **284:** 157–170.
8. Que, J., M. Choi, J.W. Ziel, *et al.* 2006. Morphogenesis of the trachea and esophagus: current players and new roles for noggin and BMPs. *Differentiation* **74:** 422–437.
9. Rodriguez, R., S. Da Silva, L. Oxburgh, *et al.* 2010. BMP signaling in the development of the mouse esophagus and forestomach. *Development* **137:** 4171–4176.
10. Raymond, C., V. Anne & G. Millane. 1991. Development of esophageal epithelium on the fetal and neonatal mouse. *Anat. Rec.* **230:** 225–234.
11. Johns, B.A. 1952. Developmental changes in the oesophageal epithelium in man. *J. Anat.* **86:** 431–442.
12. Thorey, I.S., J.J. Menses, N. Neznanov, *et al.* 1993. Embryonic expression of human keratin 18 and K18-beta-galactosidase fusion genes in transgenic mice. *Dev. Biol.* **160:** 519–534.
13. Jankowski, J.A. *et al.* 1999. Molecular evolution of the metaplasia-dysplasia-adenocarcinoma sequence in the esophagus. *Am. J. Pathol.* **154:** 965–973.
14. Enterline, H. & J. Thompon, *et al.* 1984. Pathology of the Esophagus. Springer-Verlag New York, pp. 1–21.
15. Ai, X. *et al.* 2007. SULF1 and SULF2 regulate heparin sulfate-mediated GDNF signaling for esophageal innervation. *Development* **134:** 3327–3338.
16. Rishniw, M. *et al.* 2007. Smooth muscle persists in the muscularis externa of developing and adult mouse esophagus. *J Muscle Res Cell Motil.* **28:** 153–165.
17. Long, J.D. *et al.* 1999. Esophageal submucosal glands: structure and function. *Am J Gastroenterol* **94:** 2818–2824.
18. Wu, W.-Y. *et al.* 2005. Conversion of columnar to stratified squamous epithelium in the developing mouse oesophagus. *Dev Biol* **284:** 157–170.

Ann. N.Y. Acad. Sci. ISSN 0077-8923

ANNALS OF THE NEW YORK ACADEMY OF SCIENCES
Issue: *Barrett's Esophagus: The 10th OESO World Congress Proceedings*

Esophageal stem cells and 3D-cell culture models

Rhonda F. Souza,[1] Robert E. Schwartz,[2,3] and Hiroshi Mashimo[4,5]

[1]Division of Gastroenterology, University of Texas Southwestern Medical Center and the VA North Texas Health Care System, Dallas, Texas. [2]Harvard-MIT Health Science and Technology, MIT, Cambridge, Massachusetts. [3]Division of Gastroenterology, Hepatology, and Endoscopy, Department of Medicine, Brigham and Women's Hospital, Boston, Massachusetts. [4]Gastroenterology Section, VA Boston Healthcare System, Boston, Massachusetts. [5]Division of Gastroenterology, Hepatology and Endoscopy, Brigham and Women's Hospital, Boston, Massachusetts

The following on esophageal stem cells and 3D-cell culture models contains commentaries on metaplasia through transdifferentiation and through stem cells; transcription factors that may determine an intestinal-like phenotype; the *in vitro*, organotypic cell culture models; and the role of stem cells in Barrett's esophagus and its dysplastic progression.

Keywords: stem cells; transdifferentiation; bile reflux; acid reflux; Barrett's esophagus; metaplasia; neoplastic progression; 3D-cell culture models

Concise summaries

- Metaplasia may arise by changing the differentiation pattern of stem cells or by changing already fully differentiated cells, a process termed transdifferentiation. However, the transdifferentiation hypothesis does not account for the processes of epithelial cell maintenance and self-renewal that are required for the persistence of the metaplastic Barrett's epithelium. Such physiologic properties are characteristic of stem cells.

- Using staining to detect either a Y chromosome or the expression of β-galactosidase, it has been shown that bone marrow-derived cells contribute to the formation of columnar metaplasia in animal models, suggesting that stem cells may contribute to esophageal metaplasia, and a stem cell origin might explain their predisposition to malignancy.

- It is likely that acid and bile, the components of reflux and/or the reflux-induced inflammation, trip the metaplastic switch, by inducing transcription factors directly in the esophageal epithelial cells, or by activating developmental signaling pathways.

- Several groups have attempted to develop and create both *in vitro* and *in vivo* models of Barrett's esophagus (BE). Currently, there are no models of BE that capture the complete dynamics of metaplasia and neoplastic progression; however, there are several *in vitro* and *in vivo* models that do recapitulate parts of the natural history of BE.

- Although esophageal adenocarcinoma (EAC) may contain cells with stem cell characteristics, the identity of normal cells that acquire the early genetic hits triggering carcinogesis remains unknown.

- EAC lines represent a definitive endpoint in the progression of BE and have been studied extensively both to better understand esophageal carcinogenesis and, from a therapeutic standpoint, an organotypic-cell culture model has been developed, leading to the hypothesis that a potentiator is required for metaplasia along with a transcription factor. One downside to the current organotypic model is that there is no integration of a stem cell compartment into the model.

- The appreciation of migrant bone marrow-derived stem cell (BMSCs) in the injured esophagus raises questions whether aberrant signaling, genetic aberrations and/or fusion of these stem cells with esophageal cells could play a role in the "field cancerization," as marked by reduced apoptosis, aberrant proliferation, and genomic instability.

doi: 10.1111/j.1749-6632.2011.06070.x

Ann. N.Y. Acad. Sci. 1232 (2011) 316–322 © 2011 New York Academy of Sciences.

- Taken together, the identification of different pockets of stem cells in skin and esophagus allows a new appreciation of the complex cellular biology underlying the maintenance of BE and its dysplastic progression to adenocarcinoma.

- Recent discoveries, including the isolation and culture of stem cells as well as micropatterning techniques in two and three dimensions, may help better mimic the *in vivo* disease process and help enable a better understanding of BE pathogenesis, neoplasia, and treatment.

---

1. A phenotypic switch turns on BE

Rhonda F. Souza
rhonda.souza@utsouthwestern.edu

Metaplasia is the replacement of one adult cell type by another. In the formation of Barrett's metaplasia, the normal stratified squamous epithelium is replaced by specialized intestinal epithelium. In general, metaplasia may arise by changing the differentiation pattern of stem cells or by changing already fully differentiated cells, a process termed transdifferentiation.

Metaplasia through transdifferentiation
In general, metaplasias arise between tissue types present in the same organ during embryological development. In the embryonic esophagus, the initial lining is of a columnar phenotype presumable due to high-expression levels of a number of morphogenic stimuli. As maturation ensues, the morphogenic stimuli decrease, genes are turned off, and a stratified, squamous epithelium replaces the columnar one. Therefore, by turning on and off the expression of certain genes, it is possible for the lining of the esophagus to change between a squamous and columnar phenotype.

Thus, Barrett's metaplasia may simply be a reversal of this normal, developmental process. However, the transdifferentiation hypothesis does not account for the processes of epithelial cell maintenance and self-renewal that are required for the persistence of the metaplastic Barrett's epithelium. Rather, such physiologic properties are characteristic of stem cells.

Metaplasia through stem cells
In general, stem cells give rise to daughter stem cells, a process termed self-renewal, as well as to transit amplifying cells, which in the esophagus can undergo a limited number of cell divisions before becoming fully differentiated squamous cells. The reflux of acid and bile acids, the components of gastric reflux, and/or the resulting esophageal inflammation (reflux esophagitis) could conceivably interfere at any point during this process such that cells do not differentiate normally into squamous cells but rather into metaplastic cells. The stem cell that gives rise to the metaplasia may come from either the esophagus itself or from the bone marrow.

We and others have investigated the possibility of BMSCs giving rise to metaplastic Barrett's cells.[1,2] In both of these studies, rodents (rats or mice) were lethally irradiated to destroy their bone marrow cells after which their bone marrow was reconstituted with the bone marrow of donor mice. The transplanted cells were either from a male bone marrow donor (female rats were used for the irradiation experiments), or from that of a mouse whose bone marrow cells were genetically engineered to express the β-galactosidase enzyme.

The animals then underwent an esophago-jejunostomy, which results in severe, ulcerative esophagitis, and intestinal metaplasia. Using staining to detect either a Y chromosome or the expression of β-galactosidase, both groups identified bone marrow-derived cells contributing to the formation of columnar metaplasia in these animal models, suggesting that BMSCs may contribute to esophageal metaplasia, and a stem cell origin might explain their predisposition to malignancy.

Reflux may "trip" the metaplastic switch
Regardless of where the stem cell originates, it is likely that acid and bile, the, components of reflux, and/or the reflux-induced inflammation, trip the metaplastic switch. There are at least two ways in which reflux might contribute to esophageal metaplasia. The components of refluxed gastric juice

(e.g., acid and bile acids) or the resulting esophageal inflammation (reflux esophagitis) may (1) induce transcription factors, like Cdx-2 or SOX9, which determine an intestinal-like phenotype, directly in the esophageal epithelial cells, or (2) activate developmental signaling pathways like sonic hedgehog/bone morphogenic protein-4 that, in turn, induce transcription factors that determine an intestinal-like phenotype.[3,4]

Data from esophageal squamous and metaplastic Barrett's epithelial cells cultured *in vitro*, animal models, and human biopsy specimens of esophageal squamous and Barrett's mucosa suggest that either proposed mechanism is possible (reviewed in Ref. 5).

2. The hidden dimension in *in vitro* cell culture

Robert E. Schwartz
reschwartz@partners.org

The esophageal squamous epithelium is similar to other epithelial cell types in that it is continually renewed with differentiated cells slowly migrating from the basal layer to the surface before being sloughed off into the lumen due to apoptosis, injury, or senescence.

Normally, the epithelial layer is turned over regularly, however injury caused by a variety of insults including infection, toxins, or acid and bile exposure can also stimulate esophageal renewal and turnover. However, prolonged acid exposure, instead of causing normal or increased turnover, has been shown to cause metaplasia, the process in which one adult cell type replaces another and is also known as BE. In BE, the normal stratified squamous epithelium is replaced by specialized intestinal epithelium as demonstrated by the presence of columnar enterocytes and goblet cells.

Although many different studies demonstrate and examine the process of metaplasia, there are several different hypotheses as to the origin of the cells that contribute to BE. Different possibilities include changing the differentiation pattern of stem cells or by directly altering the differentiated state of already differentiated cells. In either case, BE is clinically important because it increases the chance of progression to EAC by 30–125-fold. And although acid exposure through gastrointestinal reflux is be-

lieved to be the causative stimulus, use of proton pump inhibitors to suppress acid production has not eliminated the formation of BE or its progression to dysplasia.

As the epithelium goes through a metaplastic process to become replaced with a specialized intestinal epithelium with goblet cells, it can also undergo a neoplastic process acquiring defects in p16, p53, and CDKN2A, developing low- and high-grade dysplasia, ultimately resulting in EAC.

Given this neoplastic risk, several groups have attempted to develop and create both *in vitro* and *in vivo* models of BE. Currently, there are no models of BE that capture the complete dynamics of metaplasia and neoplastic progression. Existing models range from computer simulations to two-dimensional cultures, which lack many of the details of the human disease to animal models that are not physiologically similar to the human disease. With that said, there are several *in vitro* and *in vivo* models that do recapitulate parts of the natural history of BE and will be reviewed here.

The *in vitro* models of BE include esophageal squamous cell lines, BE cell lines, EAC cell lines, and organotypic esophageal models. There are multiple *in vivo* models in the mouse, rat and, canine. These models have advantages over *in vitro* models, in particular the canine model, which is believed to most closely mimic the human disease, however, given the difficulty and expense of this model, its use has fallen into disfavor.

Since BE is hypothesized to originate from the squamous esophageal epithelium, several groups have worked with squamous esophageal cell lines with the aim to transdifferentiate the squamous epithelium to columnar epithelium and columnar epithelium with intestinal specification. Kong *et al.* demonstrated columnar and intestinal specification from a immortalized esophageal cell line treated with Cdx-2 and 5-AZA cytidine.[6]

They demonstrate that Cdx-2 and 5-AZA cytidine causes the squamous epithelial cells to increase their expression of villin, KRT 20 on the mRNA level as well as on the protein level. There are many problems with this approach, as it is not clear which cells are expressing these markers and if such expression is contained within one cell or distributed among many cells.

To address this issue directly, several groups attempted in the late 1990s to isolate Barrett's esophageal cell lines from biopsies, and the Rabinovitch group reported the isolation of several lines using h-TERT immortalization. They found that these cell lines spontaneously gave rise to LOH with the ultimate loss of p16 and CDKN2 both markers associated *in vivo* with the natural development of dysplasia.[7] However, these lines often developed markedly abnormal cytogenetics, thereby decreasing the overall utility of these lines. More recently, several lines were developed in a similar manner, but unlike prior cell lines they allow for long-term culture, maintain a diploid chromosome number, contact inhibition, and anchorage-dependent growth.[8] Moreover, under the appropriate condition they express markers including villin, cytokeratins 4, 8, and 18 and during the course of culture lose p16 expression, all consistent with the natural history of BE.

EAC lines represent a definitive endpoint in the progression of BE and have been studied extensively both to better understand esophageal carcinogenesis and well as from a therapeutic standpoint. Several problems with this approach exist, as most cell lines turned out not to be derived from the esophageal carcinoma itself but from contamination of other cell types or cell lines. In addition, given the process that cells must go through in order to become cancer, it is unclear how those findings would apply to the earliest changes in metaplasia and intestinalization. As we have described, two-dimensional *in vitro* systems do not adequately recapitulate *in vivo* environment, do not take into account the presence of multiple cell types and are missing the three-dimensional environment.

With this in mind, the Rustgi group has developed an organotypic cell culture model.[9] They culture fibroblasts on the bottom of a collagen/matrigel matrix mixture and plate primary esophageal keratinocytes on top, and over several days a layered structure forms. Over several papers they have shown that this system remains viable over a several week period, allowing for the study of various chemical and genetic insults to take their course. Though this system better mimics aspects of Barrett's initiation and progression, it does not incorporate inflammatory or endothelial cells and does not form crypts or contain a stem cell compartment, thereby missing some of the important dynamics of the human disease. In one paper EPC2, an esophageal keratinocyte line was immortalized using TERT and

either Myc or Myc + Cdx-1 was added. Esophageal cells exposed to Myc and Cdx-1 have Muc5AC staining demontrating mucin expression.[9]

Moreover, evaluation of keratin expression showed normal cytokeratin expression in the TERT immortalized and c-myc-treated cells in contrast to the TERT immortalized and c-myc and Cdx-1-treated cells with aberrant cytokeratin 8 and 19 expression along with the loss of cytokeratin 13 expression. This led the Rustgi group to the hypothesis that a potentiator such as Myc is required for metaplasia along with a transcription factor such as Cdx-1 an effector. This confirms what has been shown *in vivo* as well, and although similar findings have been shown in 2D systems, more complex studies can be completed such as varying support fibroblast cells, matrix, or esophageal cells, adding a complexity to the system that cannot be easily performed in two dimensions. Consequently, Grugan *et al.* worked with fetal esophageal fibroblasts, fibroblasts isolated from patients with esophageal cancer (now referred to as esophageal CAFs or cancer associated fibroblasts) and fetal skin fibroblasts that were embedded in a collagen/matrigel mixture with either two established esophageal squamous cell lines or a genetically transformed esophageal primary cell line plated on top to form this organotypic culture.[9]

Fetal esophageal fibroblasts and esophageal CAFs were found to promote matrix invasion of the squamous cell lines. After thorough analysis, it was determined that fetal esophageal fibroblasts lines and esophageal CAFs that promote invasion both produce HGF at high levels. MET, the HGF receptor has been shown to be overexpressed in esophageal cancer tissues. The authors then show that both HGF production from esophageal fibroblasts and MET receptor expression activity on squamous epithelial cells may promote squamous cell invasion. This elegant study could not have been completed in two-dimensions and demonstrates the importance of the three-dimensional system.

As stated earlier, one downside to the current organotypic model is that there is no integration of a stem cell compartment into the model. One possibility to integrate stem cells into this model is a recent discovery by Hans Clevers' lab that after the isolation of Lgr5+/EPCAM+ cells from the small intestine one can culture these cells in matrigel and that crypts with a native stem cell compartment will develop.[10] Further analysis of these structures after sectioning demonstrates that they express the markers villin, muc2, lysozyme, and chromogranin, demonstrating that the initial stem cells form all the structural units normally found in the small intestine.

In conclusion, no model of BE captures the dynamics of metaplasia and neoplastic progression, however organotypic models better capture the dynamics of this disease process due to their prolonged viability, their incorporation of relevant cells of interest, and the three-dimensional environment. Despite these benefits, this culture system does not integrate inflammatory, endothelial, or stem cells and does not develop crypts. However recent discoveries including the isolation and culture of stem cells as well as micropatterning techniques in two- and three-dimensions may help better mimic the *in vivo* disease process and help enable a better understanding of BE pathogenesis, neoplasia, and treatment.

3. Role of stem cells in BE and its dysplastic progression: lessons from analogy to the skin

Hiroshi Mashimo

Hiroshi˙mashimo@hms.harvard.edu

The normal squamous epithelium lining the esophagus can be considered a type of "skin," with what appears to be multiple distinct pockets of cells harboring regenerative stem cell characteristics. Cells in the deep esophageal glands, submucosal glands, basal layer, and even swirls of cells within the squamous epithelium, stain for proliferative markers such as Ki-67 and may represent cells that could give rise to reparative cells during acute and chronic injury.

BE is presently considered a consequence of such injuries and is histologically defined as a metaplastic change from this seemingly uniform squamous epithelium to specialized intestinal phenotype containing goblet cells. While this evolving definition requiring the presence of goblet cells remains controversial, this lining is not clearly "intestine," but a unique and more variable lining, akin to reparative skin after superficial burn. Little is known about the specific stem cells that give rise to and maintain BE, or those that give rise to dysplastic cells that are thought to eventuate in EAC.

However, recent advances in uncovering stem cells involved in skin regeneration may shed light on the biology of the analogous esophageal lining. As in the esophagus, the skin also harbors multiple pockets of proliferative cells. These can be found in the basal layer, bromo-deoxyuridine label-retaining cells (LRC) in the bulge region of hair follicles, in the neck of sebaceous glands, and within sweat glands, for examples. Besides proliferation and self-renewal, stem cells must also exhibit the property of multipotency. Various cells expressing distinct markers such as Lgr6, Blimp1, Lrig1, and Lgr5 are not only responsible for the homeostatic maintenance of these appendages, but after injury may regenerate the full diversity of cells of the skin.

By analogy, BE is also a regenerative covering. Unlike the normal intestine, where there are only a few LRCs per crypt, in BE the proliferative compartment is expanded, with upregulation of both the proliferative WNT signaling as well as the repressive BMP signaling pathways. Many of the potential stem cell markers described in skin and intestine are also found in BE, including Musashi-1 and Lgr5. The latter marker, for example, which is involved in WNT signaling, is normally restricted to just a few cells near the crypt base in the intestine. However in BE, we demonstrated that Lgr5-expressing cells are markedly expanded in number, and are found diffusely and higher up along the crypts in BE.

Such aberrant Lgr5 expression can also be found in other gut pathologies harboring malignant potential such as gastric, duodenal, and colonic adenomas.[11] This marker also may have clinical significance since its expression correlates with poor survival from EAC, consistent with the notion that such stem cells are less sensitive to adjuvant therapy.[12] The complacency that BE represents a stable, benign response to injury is also shaken by evidence of genetic instability, manifest as aneuploidy on image cytometry, and particularly within the basal crypt cells, in 37% of patients with nondysplastic BE.[13]

Despite such aberrant regulation, there is still cellular hierarchy that regulates the balance between cell renewal and cell death in BE. However, unlike the normal intestine, there is variable extent of differentiation. There can be patchy areas within any BE segment devoid of goblet cells and Paneth cells— cells that are assuredly and regularly present in the normal intestine. In fact, in one series, only 31% of

BE patients showed Paneth cells, and their presence correlated with glands containing goblet cells.[14] This may reflect that the degree of differentiative capability of BE cells varies among individuals as well as within an individual.

Presently, superficial Barrett's glands are thought to be mainly responsible for the maintenance of BE, and are the target of recently popularized radiofrequency ablations. However, it is possible that similar to the skin, diverse pockets of stem cells are involved, including ducts from deep esophageal glands that are noted in 10% of BE.[14] Besides the variant regulatory mechanisms controlling proliferation, apoptosis, and differentiation including WNT, BMP, and AKT pathways, the potential varying sources of stem cells could also help explain the cellular heterogeneity within a BE segment.

The role of BMSCs in repopulating areas of injury has gained increasing attention. Animal models and human recipients of bone marrow transplants have demonstrated homing and even recruitment of these cells to areas of injury in many parts of the body, including BE. This plasticity of BMSCs has been explained by some to arise from the ability of these cells to fuse with cells at the sites of injury. Nonetheless, the stem cell niche (microenvironment) plays a critical role in regulating the balance of self-renewal and differentiation, and is likely to be important in the phenotypic switch from predominantly squamous epithelium to BE and to EAC. Besides direct reconstitution of the epithelium, the BMSCs can have paracrine effect to promote healing through collagen synthesis and through elaborating growth and proangiogenic factors.

Some studies suggest that their ability to modify the tissue microenvironment by secreting soluble factors may contribute more significantly to tissue repair than their multipotential differentiation. Moreover, BMSCs may modulate the immune and inflammatory responses to promote healing. These cells can express high levels of IL-1 receptor antagonist and inhibit inflammatory responses. Some BMSCs that integrate into areas of wound are also noted to play a role as antigen-presenting cells.

As with the pathogenesis of BE, the exact origin and role of stem cells in the pathogenesis of EAC is unknown. The cancer stem cell theory states that tumor-forming cells in the cancer can self-renew and generate cells that differentiate. Although

EAC may contain cells with such stem cell characteristics, the identity of cells that acquire the early genetic hits triggering carcinogesis remains unknown. Moreover, a given segment of BE can contain independently-arising and divergent foci of dysplasia or EAC, as suggested by mutational analysis, implicating that different pockets of cells could be involved. The appreciation of migrant BMSCs in the injured esophagus raises questions whether aberrant signaling, genetic aberrations, and/or fusion of these BMSCs with esophageal cells could play a role in the "field cancerization," as marked by reduced apoptosis, aberrant proliferation, and genomic instability. Indeed, the noted plasticity of various stem cells may be a double-edged sword, and instability of cellular phenotypes may lead to corruption of the BE architecture and eventually give rise to malignant cells.

Taken together, the identification of different pockets of stem cells in skin and esophagus is giving a new appreciation of the complex cellular biology underlying the maintenance of BE and its dysplastic progression to EAC.

Conflicts of interest

The authors declare no conflicts of interest.

References

1. Sarosi, G., G. Brown, K. Jaiswal, *et al.* 2008. Bone marrow progenitor cells contribute to esophageal regeneration and metaplasia in a rat model of Barrett's esophagus. *Dis. Esophagus* **21:** 43–50.
2. Hutchinson, L., B. Stenstrom, D. Chen, *et al.* 2010. Human Barrett's adenocarcinoma of the esophagus, associated myofibroblasts, and endothelium can arise from bone marrow-derived cells after allogeneic stem cell. *Transplant. Stem. Cell Dev.*
3. Milano, F., J.W. Van Baal, Ns. Buttar, *et al.* 2007. Bone morphogenetic protein 4 expressed in esophagitis induces a columnar phenotype in esophageal squamous cell. *Gastroenterology* **132:** 2412–2421.
4. Wang, D.H., N.J. Clemons, T. Miyashita, *et al.* 2010. Aberrant epithelial-mesenchymal Hedgehog signaling characterizes Barrett's metaplasia. *Gastroenterology* **138:** 1810–1822.
5. Wang, D.H., & R.F. Souza. 2011. Biology of Barrett's esophagus and esophageal adenocarcinoma. *Gastrointest. Endosc. Clin. N. Am.* **21:** 25–38.
6. Kong, J., H. Nakagawa, B.K. Isariyawongse, *et al.* 2009. Induction of intestinalization in human esophageal keratinocytes is a multistep process. *Carcinogenesis* **30:** 122–130.
7. Palanca-Wessels, M.C., M.T. Barrett, P.C. Galipeau, *et.al.* 1998. Geneticanalysis of Barrett's esophagus Epithelial cultures exhibiting cytogenetic and ploidy abnormalities. *Gastroenterology* **114:** 295–304.

8. Okawa, T., C.Z. Michaylira, J. Kalabis, *et al.* 2007. The functional interplay between EGFR overexpression, hTERT activation, and p53 mutation in esophageal epithelial cells with activation of stromal fibroblasts induces tumor development, invasion, and differentiation. *Genes Dev.* **21:** 2788–2803.

9. Grugan, K.D., C.G. Miller, Y. Yao, *et.al.* 2010. Fibroblast-secreted hepatocyte growth factor plays a functional role in esophageal squamous cell carcinoma invasion. *Proc. Natl. Acad. Sci. USA* **107:** 11026–11031.

10. Sato, T., R.G. Vries, H.J. Snippert, *et al.* 2009. Single Lgr5 stem cells build crypt–villus structures *in vitro* without a mesenchymal niche. *Nature* **459:** 262–265.

11. Becker L., Q. Huang, & H. Mashimo. 2008. Immunostaining of Lgr5, an intestinal stem cell marker, in normal and premalignant human gastrointestinal Tissue. *Sci. World J.* **8:** 1168–1176.

12. Becker, L., Q. Huang & H. Mashimo. 2009. Lgr5, an intestinal stem cell marker, is abnormally expressed in Barrett's esophagus and esophageal adenocarcinoma. *Dis. Esophagus* **23:** 168–174.

13. Zhang, X., Q. Huang R.K. Goyal & R.D. Odze. 2008. DNA Ploidy abnormalities in basal and superficial regions of the crypts in Barrett's esophagus and associated neoplastic lesions. *Am. J. Surg. Pathol.* **32:** 1327–1335.

14. Takubo, K., J.M. Nixon & J.R. Jass. 1995. Ducts of esophageal glands proper and paneth cells in Barrett's esophagus: frequency in biopsy specimens. *Pathology* **27:** 315–317.

Ann. N.Y. Acad. Sci. ISSN 0077-8923

ANNALS OF THE NEW YORK ACADEMY OF SCIENCES

Issue: *Barrett's Esophagus: The 10th OESO World Congress Proceedings*

The esophagogastric junction

Larry S. Miller,[1] Anil K. Vegesna,[1] James G. Brasseur,[2] Alan S. Braverman,[3] and Michael R. Ruggieri[3]

[1]Department of Medicine, Temple University, Philadelphia, Pennsylvania. [2]Department of Mechanical Engineering, Bioengineering and Mathematics, Pennsylvania State University, University Park, Pennsylvania. [3] Departments of Urology and Pharmacology, Temple University, School of Medicine, Philadelphia, Pennsylvania

The following discussion of the esophagogastric junctions includes commentaries on the three component structures of the sphincteric segment between the stomach and the esophagus; the pressure contributions from the three sphincteric components in normal subjects and in gastroesophageal reflux (GERD) patients; the mechanism of action of endoscopic plication to determine the underlying pathophysiology of GERD; and *in vitro* muscle strip studies of defects within the gastroesophageal sphincteric segment potentially leading to GERD.

Keywords: clasp muscle fibers; sling muscle fibers; gastroesophageal junction; lower esophageal sphincter; upper gastric sphincter defects in GERD; missing sphincter; Endocinch; muscarinic receptors; *in vitro* muscle strips; stretch-induced tone; nicotine-induced relaxations

Concise summaries

- The relative alignments and contributions of the different sphincteric components have recently been quantified in the normal gastroesophageal junction high-pressure zone (HPZ).[5]
- By carrying out intraluminal manometric pull-throughs concurrently with high-frequency ultrasound in normal subjects during breath-hold at full inspiration (FI) and full expiration (FE), it has been shown that the HPZ is axially broader in FE. However, the atropine-suppressed pressure profile was independent of diaphragmatic position and was correlated with the anatomic crus.
- The high pressure zone of the distal esophagus consists of three individual components. The first component is the skeletal muscle crural diaphragm. The smooth-muscle sphincter has two components. The proximal smooth-muscle component (lower esophageal circular muscle, LEC) moves with the crural sphincter. The distal smooth muscle appears to be associated with sling/clasp muscle fibers at the esophagocardiac junction (upper gastric sphincter). This third sphincteric component could be considered the first line of defense against the reflux of gastric contents and may have a significant role

in preventing gastroesophageal reflux disease (GERD).
- Comparison of the pressure contributions from the three sphincteric components in normal subjects to those in GERD patients has shown that the subtraction curve in the GERD patients contained only a single pressure peak that moved with the crural diaphragm, while the distal pressure peak of the intrinsic smooth-muscle component (the upper gastric sphincter), which was previously observed in normal subjects, was absent.
- Endoscopic plication in GERD patients reestablishes this distal pressure profile, apparently by correcting a structural anatomic abnormality of the gastric clasp and sling muscle fibers. The observation that atropine attenuates this newly established pressure profile implies that the neural innervations to this area remain intact and functioning.
- It has been known for at least 50 years that administration of the muscarinic receptor antagonist atropine reduces the pressure of the lower esophageal HPZ in humans. Several studies have shown that stretch-induced tone of *in vitro* muscle strips from the lower esophageal high-pressure zone is unaffected by atropine

doi: 10.1111/j.1749-6632.2011.06073.x
Ann. N.Y. Acad. Sci. 1232 (2011) 323–330 © 2011 New York Academy of Sciences.

and thus is not the major mechanism of *in vivo* sphincteric tone.

- In an investigation using relaxation of muscarinic receptor precontracted muscle strips as an *in vitro* model of *in vivo* sphincteric relaxation, cumulative concentration response curves to the mixed muscarinic and nicotinic receptor agonist carbachol produced greater

tension in sling fibers than clasp fibers, confirming the results of previous studies.

- The *in vitro* contractility and muscarinic receptor density of the gastric sling/clasp muscle fibers is abnormal in GERD patients, which may help explain the missing sling-clasp fiber contribution to the upper gastric sphincter HPZ that is observed in GERD patients.

1. Structure of the gastroesophageal junction HPZ

Larry Miller, Anil Vegesna, and James G. Brasseur
vivi@temple.edu

Background
Relaxation and phasic tone of the crural sphincter and its contribution in the gastroesophageal junction have been studied by Ingelfinger and Boyle *et al.*[1,2] Code *et al.* were early reporters of an intraluminal HPZ in the segment separating the esophageal body from the gastric cardia, and suggested that intrinsic smooth muscles of the distal esophagus may be responsible for maintaining a high-pressure barrier to reflux.[3] Liebermann-Meffert *et al.*[4] measured, in cadavers a thickened wall of smooth muscle at the junction that coincides with the gastric sling-clasp muscle groups. Relative alignments and contributions of all the different sphincteric components have recently been quantified in the normal gastroesophageal junction HPZ.[5]

Aim
To quantitate skeletal and smooth-muscle contributions to the normal gastroesophageal junction HPZ. To identify the relative position of various components of the HPZ, and their changes with respect to respiration.

Methods
Intraluminal manometric pull-throughs were carried out concurrently with high-frequency ultrasound in 15 normal subjects during breath-hold at FI and FE. Pull-throughs were repeated after intravenous atropine to suppress smooth-muscle pressure. Postatropine pressures were subtracted from full pressure after referencing to the anatomical right crus (from ultrasound), which indirectly mea-

sures the smooth-muscle contribution to the gastroesophageal junction HPZ. In a separate study, seven patients undergoing general anesthesia for nonesophageal pathology were administered cisatrcurium to paralyze the crural sphincter and directly measure the smooth-muscle contribution to the gastroesophageal junction HPZ. Displacements of the anatomical versus physiological crural sphincter were determined from the initial position of the catheter at initiation of pull-through.

All subjects gave institutional review board approved informed consent to take part in this study. Exclusion criteria included subjects on any medication that could affect the gastroesophageal HPZ including prokinetic agents, erythromycin type antibiotics, and anticholinergics. Other exclusion criteria were patients with GERD, hiatal hernia, abdominal surgery involving the stomach or esophagus, diabetes, scleroderma, achalasia, hypertension, cardiac disease, and current pregnancy.

Results
The HPZ was axially broader in FE. However, the atropine-suppressed (striated) pressure profile was independent of diaphragmatic position and was correlated with the location of the anatomic crus ($R^2 = 0.83$) while displacing $\sim$2 cm between FI-FE diaphragmatic positions. The subtracted (smooth muscle contribution) pressure profile was double peaked, with one peak proximal that moved in lockstep with the diaphragm, while the other pressure peak is distal to the diaphragm (Fig. 1). The FI-subtracted profile matched closely the direct smooth-muscle profile with cisatrcurium during breath holding in the inspiratory phase (Fig. 2). The proximal peak moved with the crus and the two peaks separated $\sim$1 cm as the crural diaphragm moved superiorly from FI to FE.

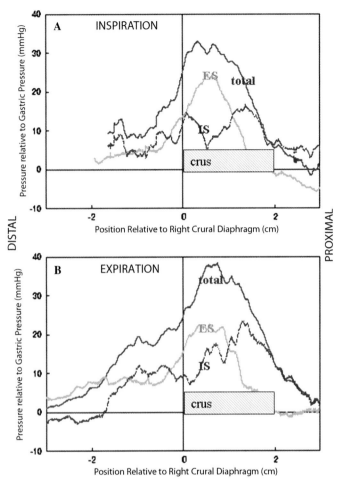

Figure 1. Panels A and B show average pressure curves from the same group of 15 normal subjects, referenced to distal margin of the right crus muscles Panel A is for full inspiration and Panel B for full expiration. The red curves are averaged pressure before administering atropine, the green curves are post atropine pressure and the blue curve is the average of the difference between pre and post atropine pressures (effectively the red curve minus the green curve). The vertical line at zero is the lower margin of the right crural diaphragm.

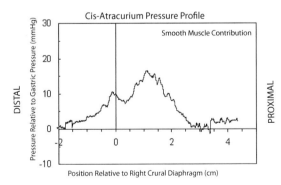

Figure 2. Average pressure curve in full inspiration, referenced to the lower margin of the right crus muscles, from seven subjects undergoing surgery for nongastric or esophageal pathology after giving Cis-atracurium to paralyze the skeletal muscle.

Conclusions

The atropine-ablated and subtracted esophagogastric segment (EGS) pressure profiles approximated the striated and smooth-muscle sphincteric contributions, indicating that the smooth-muscle sphincter has two components. The proximal smooth-muscle component, the lower esophageal circular muscle, moves with the crural sphincter, implying rigid attachment by phrenoesophageal ligaments. The distal smooth-muscle component is distal to the diaphragm, approximately at the location of the sling-clasp muscle fibers at the esophagocardiac junction. We propose that this third sphincteric component is associated with the sling-clasp muscle groups, may be the first line of defense against the reflux of gastric contents into the esophagus, and may have a significant role in protecting against GERD. Grant support from NIH.

2. Defects in gastroesophageal junction HPZ leading to GERD

Anil Vegesna, Larry Miller, and James G. Brasseur
vivi@temple.edu

We have summarized research[5] showing that the tonic pressure contribution to the HPZ of the EGS contains contributions from a skeletal muscle crural diaphragmatic component[1,2] and two distinct components of the smooth-muscle intrinsic sphincter, a proximal physiological component associated with the lower esophageal circular muscle,[12] and a distal component associated with the sling-clasp muscle fibers.[5]

Aims

(1) To report on research in which the pressure contributions from the three sphincteric components in normal subjects were compared with those in GERD patients.[11]
(2) To define the mechanism of action of endoscopic plication and to determine the underlying pathophysiology of GERD.

Methods

A simultaneous endoluminal ultrasound (EUS) and manometry catheter was used to study 15 healthy volunteers (age 34 ± 8.5 years) and seven patients (age 45 ± 10.7 years) with symptomatic GERD. Endoscopic plication was performed in GERD patients using the Bard Endocinch device. The catheter was pulled through the EGS before and after administration of atropine.[6] Preatropine (complete muscle tone), postatropine (nonmuscarinic muscle tone plus residual muscarinic tone), and subtracted

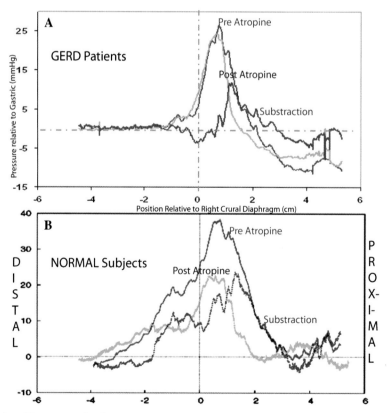

Figure 3. Similarly to Figure 1, Panel A shows average pressure curves in full expiration from seven GERD patients, referenced to right crural diaphragm. Panel B shows the average pressure curves in full expiration from 15 normal control subjects from Figure 1. The red curve shows average pressure preatropine pressure and the green curve post atropine.The blue curve is the subtraction curve (red curve minus green curve). The vertical line at zero is the lower margin of the right crus muscles.

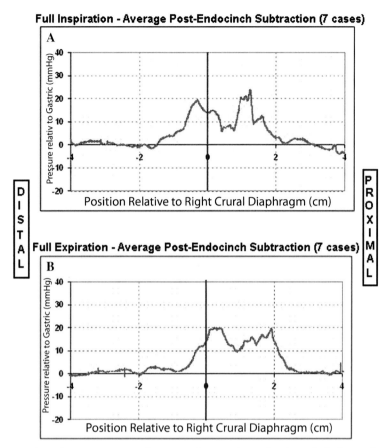

Figure 4. The average subtraction pressure curves from seven GERD patients after the Endocinch procedure in full inspiration (Panel A) and full expiration (Panel B) procedure.

(pure muscarinic muscle tone) pressure contributions to the sphincter were averaged after referencing spatially to the lower margin of the right crural diaphragm and the pull-through start position. In patients who had undergone endoscopic plication, evaluation with simultaneous ultrasound and manometry was performed before and one month after the Endocinch procedure. All subjects gave institutional review board approved informed consent to take part in this study. Exclusion criteria included subjects on any medication which could affect the gastroesophageal HPZ including prokinetic agents, erythromycin type antibiotics, and anticholinergics. Other exclusion criteria were abdominal surgery involving the stomach or esophagus, diabetes, scleroderma, achalasia, and current pregnancy.

Results

In the normal group the atropine-resistant and atropine-attenuated pressures identified the crural and smooth-muscle sphincteric components, respectively. The subtraction curve in normal subjects contained proximal and distal pressure components. The proximal component moved with the crural diaphragm between FI and FE and represents the lower esophageal circular sphincter. The distal component coincided with the gastric sling-clasp muscle fiber complex. The subtraction curve in the GERD patients contained only a single pressure component, representing the lower esophageal circular muscle, that moved with the crural diaphragm, while the distal pressure peak of the intrinsic smooth-muscle component, which was previously recognized in the normal subjects, was absent (Fig. 3B).

In GERD patients after the Endocinch procedure, the distal pressure peak, which was previously absent (Fig. 3A), was reestablished at the same axial location as the distal pressure peak in normal volunteers (Fig. 4). The newly established distal pressure in GERD patients was attenuated by the application of atropine. Using high-resolution ultrasound we localized all sutures within the plications to the submucosal space. Eighty percent of the patients in this study experienced either an improvement or elimination of their reflux symptoms in the short term.

Conclusions

We hypothesize that the lower muscarinic smooth-muscle pressure component is the gastric sling/clasp muscle fiber (upper gastric sphincter) component. The absence of this lower smooth-muscle pressure component suggests that the gastric sling/clasp muscle fiber component is defective in GERD patients. The distal muscarinic pressure peak normally constitutes one-third of the gastroesophageal junction HPZ pressure profile as measured by the area under the curve in normal subjects. This distal pressure profile may be important to the antireflux barrier, since it is the most distal component at the esophagogastric junction and therefore the first line of defense against reflux of gastric contents into the esophagus in the resting state.

Endoscopic plication in GERD patients reestablishes this distal pressure profile by correcting a structural anatomic abnormality of the gastric clasp and sling muscle fibers. The observation that atropine attenuates this newly established pressure profile implies that the neural innervations to this area remain intact and functioning. Hence the underlying abnormality might be due to an anatomic structural abnormality of the gastric clasp and sling muscle fibers. Endoscopic plication has fallen out of favor for the treatment of GERD, because of limited long-term efficacy, which might be due to the tension in the sutures pulling out through the flimsy submucosal tissue over time, leading to breakdown of the plications. [Grant support from NIH, BARD].

3. Defects within the gastroesophageal sphincteric segment potentially leading to GERD: *in vitro* muscle strip studies

Michael R. Ruggieri, Anil K. Vegesna, Alan S. Braverman, and Larry S. Miller
rugg@temple.edu

The major neurotransmitter controlling most smooth-muscle contraction, including gastrointestinal smooth muscle, is acetylcholine. Cholinergic receptors are classified into two major classes: muscarinic and nicotinic. Muscarinic receptors are G-protein coupled receptors that consist of a single polypeptide chain that spans the plasma membrane seven times. There are five subtypes of muscarinic receptors. Nicotinic receptors are ligand-gated ion channel receptors that consist of five polypeptide subunits that surround the central ion channel. Because there are many different isoforms of these five subunits that can form functional receptors, the potential diversity of subunit composition for nicotinic receptors far exceeds the capacity of the currently available ligands to distinguish subtypes on the basis of selectivity of ligands.

It has been known for at least 50 years that administration of the muscarinic receptor antagonist atropine reduces the pressure of the lower esophageal HPZ in humans.[7] A considerable amount of work has been carried out on stretch-induced tone in smooth-muscle strips from the lower esophageal HPZ that demonstrates that this tone is calcium sensitive but is not reduced by atropine.[8,9]

Therefore, stretch-induced tone of *in vitro* muscle strips from the lower esophageal HPZ is not the major mechanism of *in vivo* sphincteric tone because it is unaffected by atropine. In this investigation we used relaxation of muscarinic receptor precontracted muscle strips as an *in vitro* model of *in vivo* sphincteric relaxation. Whole human stomach and esophagus specimens were obtained by third-party organizations (National Disease Research Interchange and the International Institute for the advancement of Medicine) from brain dead patients on life support after harvesting organs to be used for organ transplant.

Very limited medical history is available for these patients and no medical diagnosis of GERD is available. Medical history is limited to interviews with the next of kin including reports of the use of acid suppressive medication and heartburn, which was classified as probable GERD. Definitive diagnosis of GERD is based on histologic diagnosis of Barrett's esophagus by a board-certified histopathologist. Because our previous *in vivo* studies using ultrasonography combined with high-resolution manometry demonstrated that the sling-clasp fiber contribution to the pressure profile is missing in GERD patients, this study focused on muscle strips dissected from the clasp and sling fibers in these human specimens.

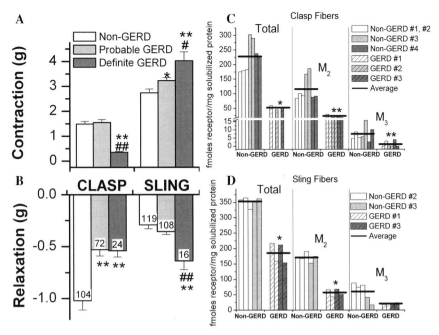

Figure 5. (A) and (B) show that clasp fibers from two definite GERD donors contracted less in response to maximally effective carbachol concentrations than 11 non-GERD and four probable GERD donors, whereas clasp fibers from both probable and definite GERD donors relaxed less than non-GERD donors. Sling fibers of both probable and definite GERD donors contracted greater than non-GERD donors, and sling fibers from definite GERD donors relaxed more than non-GERD donors. The density of M_2 and M_3 muscarinic receptors, determined by immunoprecipitation, was lower in clasp fibers of GERD donors (C) and M_2 density was lower in sling fibers of GERD donors (D).

Cumulative concentration response curves to the mixed muscarinic and nicotinic receptor agonist carbachol produced greater tension in sling fibers than clasp fibers, confirming previous studies.[10] Increasing intensity of contraction continued to be produced by carbachol concentrations up to 30 μM but higher concentrations (100 μM, 300 μM, and 1mM) produced abrupt relaxations. The muscarinic receptor selective agonist bethanechol (0.01 μM–1mM) also produced greater contractions in sling than clasp fibers and these muscarinic contractions were relaxed in a dose-dependent fashion by nicotine (30 μM–1mM). Both high-concentration carbachol-induced relaxations and nicotine-induced relaxations in bethanechol precontracted strips were greater in clasp than sling fibers. In both sling and clasp fibers, the nicotine-induced relaxations of bethanechol precontracted strips were prevented in a dose-dependent fashion by the nitric oxide synthase inhibitor L-nitro arginine methyl ester, and the β adrenergic receptor antagonist propranolol, whereas the glycine receptor antagonist ginkgolide B was inefective in both

and the $GABA_A$ antagonist SR95531 inhibited relaxations in sling fibers only.[13]

Figure 5A and 5B shows that clasp fibers from two definite GERD donors contracted less in response to maximally effective carbachol concentrations compared with 11 non-GERD and four probable GERD donors, whereas clasp fibers from both probable and definite GERD donors relaxed less than non-GERD donors. Sling fibers of both probable and definite GERD donors contracted greater than non-GERD donors and sling fibers from definite GERD donors relaxed more than non-GERD donors. The density of M_2 and M_3 muscarinic receptors, determined by immunoprecipitation, was lower in clasp fibers of GERD donors (Fig. 5C) and M_2 density was lower in sling fibers of GERD donors (Fig. 5D).

These results demonstrate that the *in vitro* contractility and muscarinic receptor density of the gastric sling-clasp muscle fibers is abnormal in GERD patients, which may help explain the missing sling-clasp fiber pressure contribution to the upper gastric sphincter HPZ that we observed in GERD patients.

Conflicts of interest

The authors declare no conflicts of interest.

References

1. Ingelfinger, F.J. 1958. Esophageal motility. *Physiol. Rev.* **38:** 533–584

2. Boyle, J.T, S.M. Altschuler, T.E. Nixon, *et al.* 1985. Role of the diaphragm in the genesis of the lower esophageal sphincter pressure in the cat. *Gastroenterology.* **88:** 723–730.

3. Code, C.F, F.E. Fyke Jr., J.F. Schlegel, *et al.* 1956. The gastroesophageal sphincter in healthy human beings. *Gastroenterologia* **86:** 135–150.

4. Liebermann-Meffert, D, M. AllgÖwer, P. Schmid & A.L. Blum. 1979. Muscular equivalent of the lower esophageal sphincter. *Gastroenterology* **76:** 31–38.

5. Brasseur, J.G, R. Ulerich, Q. Dai, *et al.* 2007. Pharmacological dissection of the human gastroesophageal segment into three sphincteric components *J. Physiol.* **3:** 961–975.

6. Dodds, W.J., J. Dent, W.J. Hogan, *et al.* 1981. Effect of atropine on esophageal motor function in humans. *Am. J. Physiol.* **240:** G290–G296.

7. Bettarello, A., S. G. Tuttle, M. I. Grossman, *et al.* 1960. Effects of autonomic drugs on gastroesophageal reflux. *Gastroenterology* **39:** 340–346.

8. Farre, R. *et al.* 2007. Mechanisms controlling function in the clasp and sling regions of porcine lower oesophageal sphincter. *Br. J. Surg.* **94:** 1427–1436.

9. Farre, R. *et al.* 2006. Pharmacologic characterization of intrinsic mechanisms controlling tone and relaxation of porcine lower esophageal sphincter. *J. Pharmacol. Exp. Ther.* **316:** 1238–1248.

10. Tian, Z.Q. *et al.* 2004. Responses of human clasp and sling fibers to neuromimetics. *J. Gastroenterol. Hepatol.* **19:** 440–447.

11. Miller, L.S., Q. Dai, A. Vegesna, A. Korimilli, R. Ulerich, B. Schiffner, J.G. Brasseur. 2009. A Missing Sphincteric Component of the Gastro-Esophageal Junction in Patients with GERD. *Neurogastroentero Motil* **20:** 813–821.

12. Kahrilas, P.J. 1997. Anatomy and physiology of the gastroesophageal junction. *Gastroenterol Clin North Am* **26:** 467–486.

13. Braverman, A.S., A.K. Vegesna, L.S. Miller, M.F. Barbe, M.I. Tiwana, K. Hussain & M.R. Ruggieri Sr. 2011. Pharmacologic specificity of nicotinic receptor mediated relaxation of muscarinic receptor pre-contracted human gastric clasp and sling muscle fibers. *J. Pharmacol. Exp. Ther.* **338:** 39–46.

Ann. N.Y. Acad. Sci. ISSN 0077-8923

ANNALS OF THE NEW YORK ACADEMY OF SCIENCES
Issue: *Barrett's Esophagus: The 10th OESO World Congress Proceedings*

Distensibility testing of the esophagus

Barry P. McMahon,[1] Satish S.C. Rao,[2] Hans Gregersen,[3,4] Monika A. Kwiatek,[5] John E. Pandolfino,[5] Asbjørn Mohr Drewes,[4] Anne Lund Krarup,[4] Christian Lottrup,[4] and Jens Brøndum Frøkjær[4]

[1]Department of Medical Physics & Clinical Engineering and Trinity College, Adelaide & Meath Hospital, Dublin, Ireland. [2]Division of Gastroenterology/Hepatology University of Iowa Hospitals and Clinics, Iowa City, Iowa. [3]Sino-Danish Center for Education and Research, Aarhus University, Denmark. [4]Mech-Sense, Department of Gastroenterology, Aalborg Hospital, Science and Innovation Center (AHSIC), Aalborg, Denmark. [5]Division of Gastroenterology, Northwestern University, Feinberg School of Medicine, Chicago, Illinois

The following contains commentaries on distensibility testing using the functional lumen imaging probe (FLIP); the use of the distention test of the esophageal body in the clinic diagnosis of noncardiac chest pain; the functional lumen imaging in gastroesophageal reflux disease-impaired esophagogastric junction; a multimodal pain model for the esophagus; the rationale for distensibility testing; and further developments in standardized distension protocols.

Keywords: esophagogastric junction; motility; distensibility; esophageal balloon distention test; noncardiac chest pain; functional luminal imaging probe; fundoplication

1. The functional lumen imaging probe (FLIP) technology: basis and development

Barry P. McMahon and Hans Gregersen
barry.mcmahon@tcd.ie

The principal role of the esophagus is in the transport of ingested materials from the oral cavity to the stomach and the release of gases and solids from the stomach at appropriate intervals.

This mechanical action happens through the complex neuromuscular activity that occurs during peristalsis. Although peristalsis involves a particular sequence of muscle relaxation and contraction, primarily in a radial direction, the principle direction of bolus movement is in the longitudinal direction. Despite this, manometry, the main measurement tool for motility in the esophagus, focuses on measurement of the contraction, or squeeze, and can tell us very little about relaxation and only infers longitudinal movement from the radial squeeze patterns observed. Historically, against this context, manometry has also been used to assess competence in the area of the esophagogastric junction (EGJ), and in particular the lower esophageal sphincter (LES), but it has long been know that this is not a reliable measure of the role of valvular function at the junction in disease.

EGJ competence involves a complex interaction between the LES tone, diaphragmatic movement during the respiratory cycle, and the valvular effect caused by the sling fibers or what is sometimes known as the cardiac notch. Manometric techniques, such as vector volume and the dent sleeve, have only marginally improved our understanding of the EGJ and have never made there way into routine clinical use. Even high-resolution manometry (HRM), while providing excellent visual data on motility patterns in the esophagus, cannot directly measure EGJ competence or function.

More than 40 years ago, Harris *et al.* identified that sphincters do not necessarily need to contract tightly to be competent, and their work suggested that resistance to distension by measurement of radial force should be the prime determinant of sphincteric strength.[1]

Until recently, very little work has focused on the relationship between distension and competence. In Figure 1, a simple animated drawing from dashed

doi: 10.1111/j.1749-6632.2011.06069.x

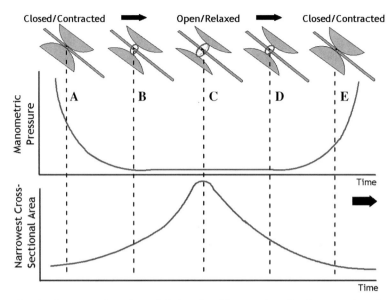

Figure 1. Diagram showing the pattern of opening and closing of a sphincter region. Also shown are plots of manometric pressure profiles and a plot of changes in the narrowest cross-sectional area.

lines A to E illustrates the cycle of opening and closing in a simple representation of how a sphincter in the body might open and close. At A, the valve is closed, toned, or competent, and with manometry, this is demonstrated by high pressure, but a plot of radial cross-sectional area at this point reads zero. The opening process cannot commence until the sphincter region relaxes, which is signified by a drop in pressure observed manometrically. So, by the time we reach point B, pressure is at baseline and telling us nothing about the opening process. However the cross-sectional area in the sphincter has increased from zero to some greater value indicating that the opening process has commenced. By the time the sphincter is fully open at C, pressure measurements remain of no significance, but the cross-sectional area (CSA) has increased to represent the maximum value of valve opening. As the sphincter heads toward closing again at points D and E the reverse process occurs until CSA is zero again and pressure has increased.[2]

More recently, some researchers have investigated the idea of using distensibility techniques to measure the EGJ. While these techniques, such as the one by Pandolfino *et al.*, have shown that measuring opening patterns can be an indicator of the status of the junction in health or disease, these early techniques are cumbersome and not suitable for clinical practice.[3]

Impedance planimetry represents a method of exciting saline in a bag fitted on the distal end of a catheter by electrical current across two outer external excitation electrodes. This allows a voltage to be detected across central electrodes that is inversely proportional to the cross-section of the saline at that point. Our research has involved making multiple measurements of CSAs at fixed intervals along a catheter in a saline bag. This allows for the detection of the CSA profiles through a sphincter region. Monitoring these changes dynamically presents a challenge as EGJ function involves continuous change. To simplify data presentation and review, we looked at reconstructing the CSA geometries through the sphincter region to provide a functional representation of this valvular region.

Hence the concept of the FLIP was created. This visualization of sphincter dynamics during distension can distinguish between normal sphincters, patients with reflux disease, and patients with achalasia.[4] The narrowest region during distension can be plotted against bag pressure to provide a graph of compliance. This idea has been used intraoperatively.

To demonstrate that this measurement technique is accurate, we undertook to construct a simple sphincter phantom out of a block of nylon. Measurements of the sphincter-shaped block

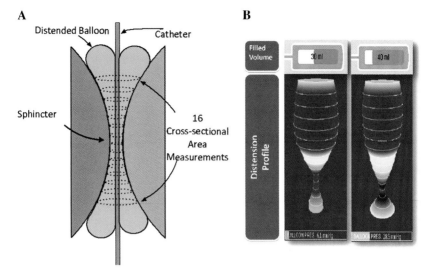

Figure 2. (A) Impression of the FLIP probe distended in the region of the esophagogastric junction. (B) Profile of the probe when distended in the esophagogastric junction of a patient with achalasia. Profiles at fill volumes of 30 mL and 40 mL are shown.

were then made by using a radial scanning ultrasound probe and were compared with the measurements made by FLIP. This work indicated that the FLIP could measure geometries in the sphincter just as well as the ultrasound probe. More recently, a commercial version of the system known as EndoFLIP (Crospon, Galway, Ireland) was developed, which can measure 16 CSAs over a 7.5 cm length (Fig. 2a).

Figure 2b shows how EndoFLIP was used to confirm achalasia in a patient. It can be seen that even though the bag on the probe is inflated to a volume of 40 mL and a pressure of 28.5 mmHg, the CSA shapes shown indicate that the sphincter still remains closed. More recent work by Pandolfino *et al.* suggests that compliance of the OGJ at set volumes can be shown on a distensibililty plot where the minimum CSA is plotted against pressure.[5] FLIP may also have a role in measuring the upper esophageal sphincter (UES). We have demonstrated UES opening patterns using FLIP in pilot experiments.

In conclusion, transport is a major role of the esophagus, current motility testing methods are limited in what they can tell us about the EGJ. A practical method to measure resistance to distension in the esophagus and in particular to measure valvular function is needed. Distensibility testing using FLIP has the potential to provide this role.

2. Distention test of the esophageal body: use in clinic diagnosis of non-cardiac chest pain

Satish S.C. Rao
satish-rao@uiowa.edu

Esophageal chest pain or non cardiac chest pain or functional chest pain are synonyms that describe a condition characterized by recurrent and often incapacitating chest pain without demonstrable cardiac abnormality.[6] It is common and affects up to 25% of the general population, however, it is rarely persistent. In USA, annual costs exceed $8 billion for ruling out coronary artery disease in patients with unexplained chest pain.[6]

Why should one test esophageal sensation?
Tests of esophageal sensory function can provide, (a) a better understanding of the pathophysiological mechanisms that cause heart burn or chest pain; (b) A more accurate diagnosis of visceral hypersensitivity; (c) Facilitate the evaluation of response to treatment(s) and (d) they can be used for mapping gut-brain sensory pathways.[6]

Unlike somatic pain that is usually more localized, sensation and pain that arises from the esophagus is usually diffuse in nature and is poorly localized.[7] Many times, it is not possible to link a source of injury to the genesis of pain. At other times, the pain may be referred to various locations, such as

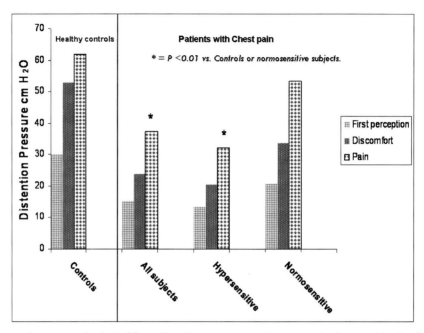

Figure 3. *Top*: a color contour plot derived from 16 serial measurements of a cross-sectional area inside a bag being gradually distended in the esophagogastric junction. The blue color shows the narrow zone becoming narrower at a higher degree of distension (also observed in the bottom right plot). The bag fills first and mostly in the stomach (the red area). The white tracing is the bag pressure. *Bottom*: the pressure and narrow band width as function of time and the pressure as function of the narrow band width.

the neck, across the chest or sometimes even into the abdomen. Visceral pain may be accompanied by autonomic or emotional changes. Thus, visceral pain defers significantly from somatic pain.[2]

In the esophagus, there are at least three different forms of sensory receptors that mediate pain or cause nociception.[7] *Chemoreceptors* that are sensitive to acid or alkaline reflex have been described. These receptors sub serve sensations of heartburn and chest pain that can be induced by acid reflux. Similarly, *thermoreceptors* that are sensitive to either heat or cold are also present which typically provide sensations such as a warm or cold feeling in the esophagus as food travels down this tube. Finally, there are in-series or in-parallel *mechanical or tension receptors* that respond to stretch and are activated by distention;[7] these noriceptors are usually used as surrogates to identify the underlying mechanism of visceral hyperalgesia.

Esophageal hypersensitivity can be tested with the Bernstein test where acid or saline is infused in a blinded manner or with edrophonium, a drug that is infused and esophageal motor and pain responses are quantified. Other tests that have been used to study esophageal pain include 24 hour ambulatory

pH study, combined manometry and pH study, electrical stimulation, evoked potential and multimodal esophageal stimulation using a probe that incorporates balloon distention, as well as chemical and electrical stimulation.[6] Here, I focus on esophageal balloon distention test.

How useful is esophageal balloon distention test?

Richter *et al.*[8] showed that a higher proportion of patients reported chest pain during syringe assisted balloon distention when compared to healthy controls.[6] Although some studies agreed with this concept, other studies found that many healthy controls reported discomfort at or about the same thresholds.[6]

We undertook a comprehensive evaluation of esophageal sensory function, motor function and biomechanical properties using a novel balloon distention technique called impedance planimetry. In this technique an impedance probe that comprises of four ring electrodes housed inside a latex balloon was used to perform balloon distention.[9] The balloon was distended stepwise by raising or lowering a leveling container and infusing a dilute electrolyte solution into a balloon placed 10 cm above the lower esophageal sphincter. Esophageal biomechanical properties, sensory properties and peristaltic properties were simultaneously assessed.[9]

A series of studies over the last decade has characterized the effects of gender, age and balloon location inside the esophagus.[6] The proximal esophagus was significantly more sensitive than the distal esophagus and the lower esophageal sphincter was least sensitive.[6] Also esophageal sensory thresholds were similar between men and women whereas older individuals had higher sensory thresholds than younger individuals,[6] indicating that aging decreases esophageal perception. In one study of 24 patients with unexplained chest pain with normal cardiac evaluation, normal endoscopy, and normal manometry and either normal 24 hour pH study or failed to respond to PPI therapy, balloon distention using impedance planimetry showed that the sensory thresholds for first sensation, discomfort and pain were significantly lower in patients with non-cardiac chest pain when compared to healthy controls.[6] Additionally, the esophagus was hyper reactive and poorly compliant.[9]

A further study revealed that the esophagus was more sensitive in the striated than smooth muscle portion and that in one third of individuals the hyper sensitivity was only confined to one esophageal segment. In order to identify if the hypersensitivity or the hyperreactivity is a key mechanism for chest pain, we performed balloon distention following atropine infusion.[1] It revealed that the hypersensitivity persisted, showing that this is a key dysfunction in these individuals and if anything, patients became more sensitive after atropine.

In a most recent study of 189 subjects with esophageal chest pain, 75% of subjects had a hypersensitive esophagus and 25% has normosensitive esophagus.[10] In the hypersensitive group, typical chest pain was reproduced in 74% during esophageal balloon distention test. The patients with hypersensitivity have significantly lower thresholds for first sensation, discomfort and pain when compared to healthy controls. (Fig. 1).

In a another prospective study of 342 patients with unexplained chest pain, the diagnostic yield of esophageal balloon distention was assessed.[11] This study revealed that endoscopy revealed a source of chest pain in 14%, a 24 hour pH study was abnormal in 28% of individuals, esophageal manometry was abnormal in 6 percent with 2% showing achalasia esophageal balloon distention was abnormal and revealed a source of chest pain in 37% of subjects; 13% of subjects showed normal esophageal function. Thus, a source of chest pain could be identified in the vast majority of patients and over one third of subjects had esophageal hypersensitivity as an important source of chest pain confirming the role of Balloon Distention Test in the diagnosis of esophageal chest pain.

What are the performance characteristics of esophageal balloon distention test?

Several techniques have been used for performing esophageal balloon distention test including a hand held syringe-assisted balloon distention method, barostat-assisted balloon distention, and the dynamic balloon distention using impedance planimetry. The hand-held technique is fraught with technical problems such as the rate and volume of balloon distention and the lack of objective control. In a study that compared barostat-assisted balloon distention with dynamic balloon distention technique in healthy controls, it was noted that although sensory thresholds were reproduced at similar pressure distentions, only 50% of subjects tolerated barostat-assisted balloon distention compared to nearly 90% of subjects with dynamic balloon distention.[6] Thus, the barostat method appears to be less suitable technique for performing esophageal balloon distention test.

The balloon distention test also appears to demonstrate pharmaco-therapeutic responsiveness as shown in a study where there was minimal or no change with placebo infusion whereas there was a significant increase in sensory thresholds with theophylline.[6] Similarly, in a study of balloon distention during adenosine infusion, a 22% change from base line was observed for first sensory threshold, a 25% change for discomfort threshold and a 33% change for pain threshold.[1] Thus, the balloon distention technique can demonstrate therapeutic responsiveness for sensory thresholds and that it is reliable.

What is an ideal balloon distention test?

Based on current studies, it is recommended that a balloon that is 4–5 cm long, highly compliant, and placed 10 cm above the lower esophageal sphincter should provide the best characteristics for performing the esophageal balloon distention test.[6]

Ideally, an intermittent balloon distention protocol with increments in pressure of 3–5 mm Hg is preferred. Most recently a multi-modal esophageal probe has become available through which it be possible to assess esophageal sensation with balloon distention and simultaneously assess other esophageal function.

In summary, the esophageal balloon distention test is the simplest and most practical method of assessing esophageal hypersensitivity and for providing an accurate diagnosis of esophageal/non cardiac chest pain. It has very good performance characteristics. There is a lack of commercially available esophageal balloon device, but this can be overcome by adapting the balloon devices in a clinic motility laboratory as shown by a recent study of simplified balloon distention technique.

3. Functional luminal imaging and EGJ disease

Monika A. Kwiatek and John E. Pandolfino
monika.kwiatek@gmail.com

Excessive EGJ compliance is a primary pathophysiological abnormality in many cases of GERD. Increased EGJ compliance allows greater volumes of gastric content to reflux into the esophagus, increases the frequency with which transient LES relaxations are elicited by proximal gastric distension, and allows gastric juice to track within the contracted sphincter. These physiological aberrations result in an increased number of reflux events, increased spatial distribution of refluxate within the esophagus, and increased esophageal acid exposure, all of which increase the likelihood of esophageal mucosal injury and reflux-related symptoms.

However, current clinical assessment of EGJ function is typically limited to endoscopic imaging, reflux testing with pH-metry, or manometric measures. Although these techniques can confirm excessive reflux, contractile defects in the LES pressure or crural diaphragm, and misalignment between the two that is common in GERD, they do not quantify EGJ compliance. Despite the recent evolution of manometric technology, it still fundamentally measures intraluminal pressure, while by definition (change in volume when subject to an applied force), measuring EGJ compliance requires both a measure of intraluminal pressure and intra-

luminal geometry. Physiologic studies pioneering the measurement of EGJ compliance used a barostat and subsequently a hydrostat;[3,12,13] however, both techniques were cumbersome, requiring bulky instrumentation, fluoroscopy, and poststudy image processing making them clinically impractical.

A recently developed method, the FLIP uses the principles of the hydrostat but substitutes high-resolution impedance planimetry for fluoroscopy. FLIP recordings allow dynamic imaging of EGJ distention as a cylinder of varying diameter based on instantaneous CSA measurements with a concurrent intrabag pressure measurement, thereby facilitating measurement of EGJ distensibility. In its most recent iteration, the FLIP equipment comprises a smaller probe designed to either fit through the instrumentation channel of an endoscope or allow transnasal/oral placement, moving the measure of EGJ compliance closer to being a part of diagnostic evaluation. Initial studies using FLIP technology in GERD[14] and fundoplication (FP)[5] patients confirm this possibility.

FLIP, passed through the endoscopic instrumentation channel and positioned across the EGJ during routine upper endoscopy, was used to assess EGJ distensibility in 20 GERD patients (without overt hiatus hernia) and 20 controls.[14] The stepwise distensions showed the hiatus to be the least distensible locus at the EGJ in both groups. The distending pressure was consistently 6–15 mmHg less in GERD patients and at any given distensile pressure the extent of EGJ opening in GERD patients was greater. These results validated the FLIP against the earlier barostat technique and confirmed previously described differences in EGJ distensibility between GERD patients and controls.[13] The resultant distensibility index (hiatal CSA/intrabag pressure) was on average 2–3 fold greater in GERD patients and correlated poorly with the endoscopic estimation of EGJ distensibility, the flap valve grade. However, the index also varied substantially among GERD patients confirming the inherent heterogeneity of this patient group.

FP aims to correct impaired EGJ function in GERD. Its effect on EGJ distensibility was assessed with FLIP in 10 controls and 12 patients who have had laproscopic Nissen FP surgery with satisfactory to good functional outcome.[5] Once again, FLIP isolated the hiatus as the least distensible locus within the EGJ in both groups. The balloon pressure at each stepwise distension was significantly higher in the FP patients than in the controls, but the EGJ dimensions were comparable, suggesting that a post-FP higher pressure is required to initiate and maintain luminal opening. Interestingly, FLIP measure of EGJ distensibility did not correlate with the manometric measures of respiratory EGJ pressure morphology, emphasizing the difference between assessing contractility in a closed lumen and distensibility (opening dimensions) in the setting of EGJ relaxation. These FLIP findings indicate that even in patients with satisfactory-to-good outcome post-FP surgery, although the FP may counter poor EGJ distensibility of GERD, it does not normalize EGJ function.

The FLIP data verify the EGJ function dichotomy between GERD and FP patients. GERD patients exhibit a more distensible EGJ, while FP patients exhibit a less distensible EGJ. Although the hiatal geometry is comparable to that of controls, the distensibility is altered by either a decrease or an increase in intraluminal pressure at the EGJ in GERD or FP patients, respectively. This verification of previous results, together with recent commercialization of the FLIP technology, provides us with a method for a clinical setting to potentially differentiate patients within the heterogeneous GERD group with a highly distensible EGJ and to show the altered mechanics post-FP not discerned by manometry, and thus aid clinical management.

4. Multimodal testing of esophageal sensory disorders

Asbjørn Mohr Drewes, Anne Lund Krarup, Christian Lottrup, and Jens Brøndum Frøkjær
amd@mech-sense.com

Stimulation of the esophagus

Basic mechanisms in pain perception, transduction, and processing can be explored by means of human-experimental pain models. These models, when applied to healthy volunteers or to patients, provide an important translational link between animal studies and human clinical trials. In clear contrast to clinical pain, experimental pain models allow the possibility for controlling the duration, the intensity and the nature of the pain stimulus. However, as pain is a multidimensional perception, it is obvious that the reaction to a single stimulus of a certain modality only represents a limited part of the pain experience

and therefore, a variety of stimulus modalities are required.

The multimodal model

Another approach of mimicking the clinical situation is the use of a *multimodal test*, where different receptor types and mechanisms are activated as in the disease state. The multimodal model has shown its value in *somatic* pain testing, where single stimuli have been inadequate to test for example pathophysiological changes and effects of specific drugs. Hence, it has been reported that a tricyclic antidepressant increased the somatic pain threshold to electrical stimuli, but did not reduce pain after immersion of the hand in cold water.[15]

These considerations were the rationale for development of the multimodal pain model for the esophagus.[16] The main advantage of the model is that it allows a differentiated assessment of the superficial and deep structures of the gut wall, activation of different nerve fibers, and peripheral as well as central pain mechanisms (Fig. 4). The model has been widely used to understand basic sensory mechanisms in the esophagus as well as mechanical properties. The validity of the model was confirmed in studies where the model was used to explore the pathophysiology of esophageal disorders such as erosive and nonerosive reflux disease, Barrett's esophagus and noncardiac chest pain.

Evaluation of drugs with esophagus as a visceral target

In evaluation of different drugs—especially analgesics—most models have used the skin, but *deep pain* having another organization of the nervous system (and hence response to analgesics) is of outmost clinical importance. Using the multimodal model with activation of different nerve fibers and pain mechanisms, the researcher is able to increase the likelihood for detecting an analgesic effect of drugs with various effects on receptors and nerve pathways.

However, in drugs studies reproducibility of the model is an important factor in the testing of analgesics, as it is necessary to repeat the pain stimulation several times during active and placebo treatment. If the reproducibility is low, then the change in the evoked pain needs to be large for the model to detect it. Many experimental models are not sufficiently robust over time and data on reproducibility are lacking. However, reproducibility has

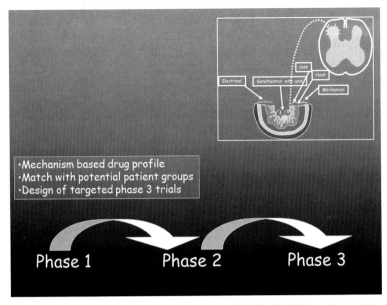

Figure 4. The multimodal model is able to activate and sensitize nerves localized in different layers of the esophageal mucosa. Using this model in drug research–especially when hyperalgesia is evoked–the clinical situation is mimicked and phase II trials in healthy volunteers can be used to identify drug mechanisms and optimize further phase III trials in large patient groups.

been proven for the multimodal model in esophagus.[17] *Assessment* of pain can be done with either psychophysiological methods (typically different visual analog scales) or objective methods such as nociceptive reflexes, imaging, and evoked brain potentials. These methods give different information on the pain system, but most importantly they have to prove their reliability and robustness. We have developed a visual analog scale with anchor words[16] and have shown its sensitivity and reliability in a series of trials in different diseases drug studies (see www.mech-sense.com).

The multimodal model has major *sensitivity* to differentiated effects of analgesics such as oxycodone, morphine, and different preclinical drugs. Recently we have used the model in translational studies, where it was shown that sensitization of the esophagus with a combination of hydrochloric acid and capsaicin resulted in generalized hyperalgesia of the sensory system like that seen in patients.[18]

Using the model we were able to show a differentiated effect of oxycodone and morphine in healthy volunteers, similar to what has previously been found in patients with a sensitized pain system due to chronic pancreatitis.[19] The model has also been used in several preclinical (phase IIa) studies where mechanisms of early drugs have been shown.

In this way the model can be used as a bridge from studies in healthy volunteers to patients with a sensitized pain system. Using the model we are able to optimize the design of targeted phase III trials with a sufficient match to potential patient groups (Fig. 4). In this way, time and money can be saved and in the end it will result in better identification and treatment of the patients.

5. Future perspectives of distensibility testing

Hans Gregersen and Barry P. McMahon
hag@adm.au.dk

Esophageal function can be studied with a number of different techniques. Among the most well known are manometry, endoscopy, fluoroscopy, and endoscopic ultrasonography. The standard manometric techniques with 3–6 recordings along the length of esophagus was several years ago further developed into high-resolution manometry and high density manometry, both techniques with a much better spatial resolution.

New techniques are needed to obtain more knowledge about dysfunction of the esophagus and the EGJ in organic or functional diseases, especially

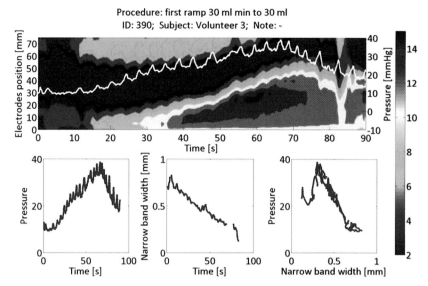

Figure 5. The multimodal model is able to activate and sensitize nerves localized in different layers of the esophageal mucosa. Using this model in drug research—especially when hyperalgesia is evoked—the clinical situation is mimicked and phase II trials in healthy volunteers can be used to identify drug mechanisms and optimize further phase III trials in large patient groups.

distension technologies, as the multimodal probe and the FLIP have gained interest in recent years. The multimodal probe is very useful for studying symptom mechanisms and for differentiation of drug effects in clinical trials. The multimodal probe has been described in other reviews from the 10th OESO World Conference. Here, we focus on the FLIP technology and the future perspectives for distension techniques.

The rationale for distensibility testing is that we need to study the lumen geometry and the wall distensibility when a force is applied internally. By doing so, it is possible to study the mechanical function of the organ under study, the geometric and mechanical remodeling due to diseases, and for monitoring endoscopic and surgical treatments. Distensibility testing is also useful for studying the motor and sensory responses to distension such as excitatory motor reflexes and distension-evoked pain.

When considering mechanical properties of the esophageal wall, it is important to use valid and useful measures. Previously used parameters such as compliance is not of much use and conclusions may be based on erroneous interpretation of the data. Solid mechanical measures of mechanical deformation in terms of strains are necessary. Strain dependents on the geometric loaded and no-load states. The strain varies as function of location and

direction and therefore it is important to have serial measurements. Strain is often evaluated together with the mechanical stress from which the tissue stiffness can be derived. Another reason for conducting serial measurements is that tissue segments like the EGJ varies considerably along its length in terms of geometry and pressure profiles.[20]

FLIP is based on the impedance planimetric technique that makes it possible to measure the CSA of a distending bag in the lumen of the esophagus. In impedance planimetry, the CSA is derived from calibrated electrical impedance recordings between electrodes in the middle of the bag. Current FLIP probes have enough electrodes to make 16 CSA recordings in the bag, for example over an 8 cm length of the probe (half centimeter between measurements). It is hereby possible to profile the lumen of the organ under study. Several studies have been done on the esophagogastric junction;[4,21] it has demonstrated variations in the properties along the junction and differences between patients with GERD and healthy volunteers.[5]

It has recently also become possible to show the data as color contour plots with the distance along the electrodes on the *y*-axis and time on the *x*-axis (Fig. 5)

FLIP was originally developed for studying mechanical and physiological properties of the FGJ in healthy volunteers and GERD patients but recently it is being tested for other applications. Key in these applications is the use of FLIP as a sizing tool during endoscopic antireflux procedures or bariatric surgery for obesity. In the future, we hope to experience further developments in terms of even better spatial resolution than today. This will be combined with optimized analysis for deriving mechanical parameters, including advanced muscle mechanics and with optimized and standardized distension protocols.

Conflicts of interest

Barry McMahon and Hans Gregersen invented the FLIP technology and hold a royalty agreement with Crospon Ltd. The other authors declare no conflicts of interest.

References

1. Harris, L.D. & C.E. Pope. 1964. "Squeeze" versus resistance: an evaluation of the mechanism of sphincter competence. *J. Clin. Invest*. **43:** 2272–2278.
2. McMahon, B.P., B.A. Jobe, J.E. Pandolfino & H. Gregersen. 2009. Do we really understand the role of the oesophagogastric junction in disease? *World J. Gastroenterol.* **15:** 144–150.
3. Pandolfino, J.E., G Shi, J. Curry, *et al.* 2002. Esophagogastric junction distensibility: a factor contributing to sphincter incompetence. *Am. J. Physiol. Gastrointest. Liver Physiol.* **282:** G1052–G1058.
4. McMahon, B.P., J.B. Frokjaer, P. Kunwald, *et al.* 2007. The functional lumen imaging probe (FLIP) for evaluation of the esophagogastric junction. *Am. J. Physiol. Gastrointest. Liver Physiol.* **292:** G377–G384.
5. Kwiatek, M.A., P.J. Kahrilas, N.J. Soper, *et al.* 2010. Esophagogastric junction distensibility after fundoplication assessed with a novel functional luminal imaging probe. *J. Gastrointest. Surg.* **14:** 268–276.
6. Chahal, P.S. & S.S. Rao. 2005. Functional chest pain. Nociception and visceral hyperalgesia. *J. Clin. Gastroenterol.* **39:** S204–S209.
7. Cervero, F. & W. Janig. 1992. Visceral nociceptors: a new world order? *Trends Neurosci.* **15:** 374–378.
8. Richter, J.E., C.F. Barish & D.O. Castell. 1986. Abnormal sensory perception in patients with esophageal chest pain. *Gastroenterology* **91:** 845–852.
9. Rao, S.S., H. Gregersen, B. Hayek, *et al.* 1996. Unexplained chest pain: the hypersensitive, hyperreactive, and poorly compliant esophagus. *Ann. Intern. Med.* **124:** 950–958.
10. Nasr, I., A. Attaluri, S. Hashmi, *et al.* 2010. Investigation of esophageal sensation and biomechanical properties in functional chest pain. *Neurogastroenterol. Motil.* **22:** 520–527.
11. Nasr, I. & S.S. Rao. 2007. How useful is esophageal sensory (Balloon distention) testing in evaluation of functional chest pain. *Gastroenterology* **135:** A26.
12. Pandolfino, J.E. *et al.* 2005. Restoration of normal distensive characteristics of the esophagogastric junction after fundoplication. *Ann. Surg.* **242:** 43–48.
13. Pandolfino, J.E. *et al.* 2003. Esophagogastric junction opening during relaxation distinguishes nonhernia reflux patients, hernia patients, and normal subjects. *Gastroenterology* **125:** 1018–1024.
14. Kwiatek, M.A. *et al.* 2010. Esophagogastric junction distensibility assessed with an endoscopic functional luminal imaging probe (EndoFLIP). *Gastrointest. Endosc.* **72:** 272–278.
15. Enggaard, T.P., L. Poulsen, L. Arendt-Nielsen, *et al.* 2001. The analgesic effect of codeine as compared to imipramine in different human pain models. *Pain* **922:** 277–282.
16. Drewes, A.M., K.-S. Schipper, G. Dimcevski, *et al.* 2002. Multimodal assessment of pain in the oesophagus: a new experimental model. *Am. J. Physiol. Gastrointest. Liver Physiol.* **283:** G95–G103.
17. Olesen, A.E., C. Staahl, C. Brock, *et al.* 2009. Evoked human oesophageal hyperalgesia—a potential tool for analgesic evaluation? *Basic Clin. Pharmacol. Toxicol.* **105:** 126–136.
18. Olesen, A.E., C. Staahl, L. Arendt-Nielsen & A.M. Drewes. 2010. Different effects of morphine and oxycodone in experimentally evoked hyperalgesia—a human translational study. *Br. J. Clin. Pharmacol.* **70:** 189–200.
19. Staahl, C., G. Dimcevski, S.D. Andersen, *et al.* 2007. Differential effect of opioids in patients with chronic pancreatitis. An experimental pain study. *Scand. J. Gastroenterol.* **42:** 383–390.
20. Brasseur, J.G., R. Ulerich, Q. Dai, *et al.* 2007. Pharmacological dissection of the human gastro-oesophageal segment into three sphincteric components. *J. Physiol.* **580:** 961–975.
21. McMahon, B.P., A.M. Drewes & H. Gregersen. 2006. Functional oesophago-gastric junction imaging. *World J. Gastroenterol.* **12:** 2818–2824.

Ann. N.Y. Acad. Sci. ISSN 0077-8923

ANNALS OF THE NEW YORK ACADEMY OF SCIENCES

Issue: *Barrett's Esophagus: The 10th OESO World Congress Proceedings*

Mechanism-based evaluation and treatment of esophageal disorders

Hans Gregersen,[1] Asbjørn Mohr Drewes,[1,2] Jens Brøndum Frøkjær,[2] Anne Lund Krarup,[2] Christian Lottrup,[2] Adam D. Farmer,[3] Qasim Aziz,[3] and Anthony R. Hobson[4]

[1]Sino-Danish Center for Education and Research, Aarhus, Denmark. [2]Mech-Sense, Department of Gastroenterology, Aalborg Hospital, Denmark. [3]Wingate Institute of Neurogastroenterology, Centre for Gastroenterology, Blizard Centre for Cell and Molecular Science, Barts and the London School of Medicine and Dentistry, Queen Mary University of London, London, United Kingdom. [4]Neurogastroenterology Diagnostic Centre, The Princess Grace Hospital, London, United Kingdom

The following on mechanism-based evaluation and treatment of esophageal disordered contains commentaries on multimodal stimulation to study esophageal function, the neurophysiological and autonomous assessment of sensory abnormalities, and the clinical value of the novel diagnostic combinations to propose a mechanically targeted treatment.

Keywords: esophageal function; mechanical stimulation; functional gastrointestinal disorders; endophenotyping; high resolution manometry; esophageal cortical evoked potentials

Concise summaries

- New technology can provide objective mechanistic evidence to aid clinicians in making crucial management decisions for patients that often present with very similar clinical and symptomatic profiles.

- The sensory properties of the esophagus can be assessed in many different ways: psychophysical assessments of pain response using visual analog scales (VASs), assessment of the autonomic response to pain using changes in heart rate, blood pressure, autonomic reflexes, etc., and neurophysiological assessment at the spinal cord and brain level.

- Multimodal stimulation is based on the concept that symptom and pain mechanisms are multifactorial and mediated through different pathways from the periphery to the brain. Thermal and chemical stimuli primarily stimulate receptors in the inner esophageal layers (mucosa–submucosa), whereas mechanical stimuli stimulate receptors in the muscle layers. Electrical stimuli affect the nerve endings throughout the wall. The currently available multimodal systems allow mechanical, thermal, chemical and electrical stimulation combined with measurements of bag size, pressure, and temperature, along with pressures proximal and distal to the bag.

- The model allows a differentiated assessment of the superficial and deep structures of the esophageal wall, activation of different nerve fibers and peripheral, as well as central pain mechanisms, and has been widely used to understand basic sensory mechanisms in the oesophagus as well as mechanical properties.

- The multimodal probe has been used to differentiate between noncardiac chest pain patients, gastroesophageal reflux disease (GERD) patients and nonerosive reflux disease (NERD) patients. In addition to being a potential diagnostic tool, the multimodal probe has also gained interest as a testing tool for new drugs.

- Functional esophageal disorders are a group of prevalent disorders whose incidence is considered to be increasing, comprising functional heartburn, functional chest pain of presumed esophageal origin, functional dysphagia, and globus. Their pathophysiology remains incompletely understood but abnormalities within the

doi: 10.1111/j.1749-6632.2011.06068.x

stress responsive physiological systems, such as the autonomic nervous system (ANS), is considered by many authorities to be of central importance.

- The use of esophageal cortical evoked potentials (CEPs) to measure extrinsic afferent pathway sensitivity in patients with suspected esophageal hypersensitivity has revealed that cohorts of patients with clinical homogenous symptoms can be subgrouped based on the presence or absence of enhanced primary afferent signaling.
- A novel concept and approach to investigating the pathophysiology of these disorders is that of endophenotyping subjects' psychophysiological susceptibility to pain through genetic, personality traits, and physiological responses to a sensory stressor, allowing the clinicians to tailor their management of these disorders and thereby improve outcome.
- The next phase of clinical research in GI physiology will be to further validate diagnostic algorithms that utilize appropriate combinations of tests to help drive mechanistic based treatment strategies for patients with upper gastrointestinal (GI) disorders.

---

1. New technologies for individualized diagnosis of esophageal diseases

Hans Gregersen and Asbjørn Mohr Drewes
hag@adm.au.dk

Many techniques have been developed in the past for studying esophageal function. Conventional methods include among the most important: manometry, endoscopy, fluoroscopy, and endoscopic ultrasonography. Several years ago, the standard manometric techniques with 3–6 recordings along the length of esophagus developed into high-resolution manometry and high-density manometry, both techniques with a much better spatial resolution.

However, new techniques are needed to obtain more knowledge about esophageal dysfunction in organic or functional diseases. Requirements for new diagnostic tools are that they are accurate, reliable, repeatable, safe, validated against existing tools, needed, and FDA approved for use in the United States and Conformité Européenne (CE) marked for use in Europe. Distension technology has especially gained interest in recent years with the multimodal probe, the functional luminal imaging probe (FLIP) and ultrasonography, combined with bag distension.

Since the latter two technologies are described in detail in other responses stemming from the 10th OESO World Conference, here we focus on the multimodal technology.

Multimodal stimulation is based on two important concepts. First, mechanical stimulation had proven its usefulness in a large number of studies. For example, Rao *et al.*[1] used the technique to demonstrate clear differences between healthy volunteers and patients with noncardiac chest pain. Furthermore, they managed to differentiate groups of chest pain patients (hypersensitive and hyperreactive). This finding obviously had implications for treatment of the two patient subgroups. Second, multimodal stimulation is based on the concept that symptom and pain mechanisms are multifactorial and mediated through different pathways from the periphery to the brain. Thermal and chemical stimuli primarily stimulate receptors in the inner esophageal layers (mucosa–submucosa), whereas mechanical stimuli stimulate receptors in the muscle layers. Electrical stimuli affect the nerve endings throughout the wall.

The currently available multimodal systems allow mechanical, thermal (cold and heat), chemical, and electrical stimulation combined with measurements of bag size, pressure, and temperature, along with pressures proximal and distal to the bag (Fig. 1). Sensory data are obtained by means of visual analog scales, referred pain areas, evoked potentials, etc. The stimulation battery is a very strong tool when combined with the sensory testing. The stimuli can be combined with developing a state of local hyperalgesia in multiple ways, for example, mechanical stimulation followed by acid infusion can be used

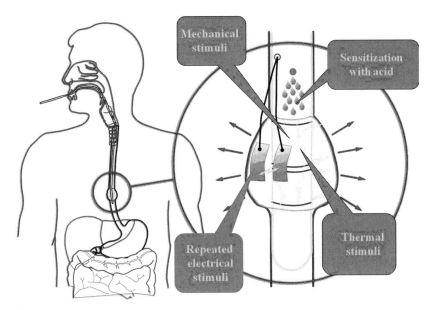

Figure 1. Multimodal system.

to evaluate whether sensitization to acid is exhibited after repeated mechanical stimulation.

The multimodal probe has been used to differentiate between noncardiac chest pain patients, GERD patients, and NERD patients.[2,3] Hoff *et al.* used a modified version with embedded ultrasound transducers and laser Doppler flow measurements to evaluate mucosal perfusion.[4] Hereby, it was possible to differentiate whether solid mechanical (strain) and blood flow (mucosal perfusion) mechanisms were the cause of distension-induced pain in normal volunteers and patients with noncardiac chest pain.

In addition to being a potential diagnostic tool, the multimodal probe has also gained interest as a testing tool for new drugs. The multimodal probe was used in a drug study in healthy volunteers for the first time in 2005–2006. It was used to explore the differential effects of the two well-known opioids morphine and oxycodone (strong analgesics). Among other findings, it was shown during heat stimulation of the esophagus that the effect of morphine was equal to that of placebo, while oxycodone attenuated pain better. Both morphine and oxycodone were more effective than placebo in attenuating mechanical pain in the esophagus.[5] Currently other drugs are being tested using the multimodal concept.

2. Neurophysiological assessment of sensory abnormalities

Jens Brøndum Frøkjær, Anne Lund Krarup, Christian Lottrup, and Asbjørn Mohr Drewes
jf@mech-sense.com

Assessment of esophageal sensory properties

The sensory properties of the esophagus can be assessed in many different ways:

(1) *psychophysical assessments* of pain response using (VASs) and different kinds of pain questionnaires;
(2) assessment of the *autonomic response* to pain using changes in heart rate, blood pressure, autonomic reflexes, etc.; and
(3) *neurophysiological assessment* at the *spinal cord* level (the nociceptive reflex and measurement of referred pain areas) and at the *brain level*. The latter is based on functional magnetic resonance imaging (fMRI), positron emission tomography (PET), electroencephalography (EEG)/CEPs, magnetoencephalography (MEG), single photon emission computed tomography (SPECT), and the multimodal combinations of these techniques. The use of these techniques has brought new insight into the

complex brain processes underlying pain perception and paved new ways in our understanding of visceral pain. However, the methods give different information on the pain system, but most importantly the methods shall have proven their reliability and robustness.

VAS

Sensory assessments on a VAS can be problematical in visceral pain, as pain is multidimensional, diffuse, and often difficult to characterize. To assess pain in a simple and efficient way, we used an electronic VAS with anchor words for evaluation of the perception. The usefulness and robustness of this instrument has been demonstrated to assess painful visceral stimuli in the esophagus, small and large intestine in healthy subjects, and in patients with visceral hyperalgesia, and in a series of trials in different drug studies[6] (see also www.mech-sense.com).

Referred pain area measurements

The simplified referred pain area is considered to be due to the convergence of visceral and somatic afferents and is used as a proxy for the central/spinal pain mechanisms. As an example, esophagitis patients had larger and more widespread referred pain areas to esophageal distension than controls, indicating that central pain mechanisms may also explain some of the symptoms in these patients.[7]

Evoked brain potentials after esophageal stimulation

CEPs are the recordings of electrical activity on the scalp induced by activation of centers in the brain to esophageal stimulations and can be used to study the nociceptive pain response including the sequential brain activation. A number of studies have examined differences in amplitudes/latencies of CEPs to electrical stimulation in various patient groups. As an example, diabetes patients with autonomic neuropathy and GI symptoms had increased latencies and reduced amplitudes of CEPs in response to esophageal stimulation.[8] This indicates changes in the pain processing, which could be due to a possible functional reorganization of the central nervous pathways. The location of brain centers underlying CEPs can be determined by multichannel EEG recordings combined with *inverse modeling*. This method possesses the opportunity to study pain-specific cortical activation dynamically, as it reflects

the sequential activation of neuronal pain networks underlying the CEPs. As an example, experimental acid sensitization of the esophagus in healthy volunteers induced a posterior shift and latency reduction of the anterior cingulate dipole,[9] which may translate to the clinic where patients with NERD often have unpleasant chest sensations and pain despite normal endoscopy.[9] Hence, we have shown that the symptoms in some esophageal disorders, such as erosive and nonerosive reflux disease and noncardiac chest pain, may be partly explained by alterations in the central processing of visceral pain.

Experimental pain models

The methods above can be integrated into experimental pain models (Fig. 2). These models, when applied to healthy volunteers or to patients, can provide important information on sensory processing in health and disease, and evaluate the effect of drug treatment. In clear contrast to clinical pain, experimental pain models allow the possibility for controlling the duration, the intensity, and the nature of the pain stimulus.

Furthermore, the advanced sensory assessments can be combined with the multimodal pain model, which mimic the clinical situation by applying different stimulus types, such as mechanical distension, heat, cold, electrical, and chemical, where different receptor types and mechanisms are activated as in the disease state.[10] The model allows a differentiated assessment of the superficial and deep structures of the gut wall, activation of different nerve fibers and peripheral, as well as central, pain mechanisms, and has been widely used to understand basic sensory mechanisms in the esophagus.

3. Mechanism-based evaluation and treatment of esophageal disorders: autonomous assessment of sensory abnormalities

Adam D. Farmer and Qasim Aziz
q.aziz@qmul.ac.uk

Pain is a complex phenomenon with sensory discriminative, affective motivational, and cognitive evaluative components. There is considerable intra- and interindividual variability in pain responsiveness in both health and disease. The factors that

Experimental sensory models

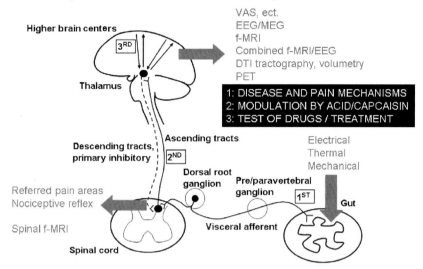

Figure 2. Concept of the experimental pain model: the advanced sensory assessments at both the spinal and supraspinal level can be combined with the multimodal pain model. Hence, investigation of different disease and pain mechanisms in both health and disease is possible, including the evaluation of drug treatment.

underlie this variability have been proposed to be (among others) genetic, psychological, physiological, and neuroanatomical in nature.[11] Of note, chronic unexplained visceral pain exerts a considerable burden on society through direct and indirect healthcare costs, loss of productivity through absenteeism and presenteeism, and through an individual's failure to fulfill their potential.

Functional gastrointestinal disorders (FGID), a group of medically unexplained syndromes whose defining feature is chronic unexplained visceral pain, are a group of prevalent disorders whose incidence is considered to be increasing. Contained under the umbrella term of FGID are the functional esophageal disorders comprising the disorders of functional heartburn, functional chest pain of presumed esophageal origin, functional dysphagia, and globus.[12]

Despite considerable academic endeavor, their pathophysiology remains incompletely understood, and their treatment is generally empirical and is of limited efficacy in many patients. Susceptibility factors for the development of these disorders have not been well studied, but abnormalities within the stress responsive physiological systems, such as the

ANS, are considered by many authorities to be of central importance.[12]

The ANS

The ANS is a bidirectional, hierarchically controlled, brain–body interface that integrates the external environment with the internal milieu. The ANS is considered to be a stress responsive system, and aberrant stress responsiveness has been considered to be a risk factor for the development of FGID. Not surprisingly, this autonomous effector of sensory GI function has been extensively investigated across a number of FGID.

However, results have been disappointingly inconsistent particularly with respect to functional esophageal disorders. This is most likely due to inconsistent research methodologies, changes in the definition of these disorders, and limitations in autonomic neuroscience technology. The most widely used proxy for measuring autonomic tone is heart rate variability (HRV). HRV has considerable limitations particularly with respect to its limited temporal resolution. However, recent advances in autonomic neuroscience technology have facilitated the measurement of real time, beat-to-beat indices of autonomic tone. For instance, the validated parameter of parasympathetic efferent tone, known as cardiac vagal tone (CVT), has facilitated a fascinating insight into the changes in parasympathetic tone to pain in health and disease. Such a technological advance may prove to be the prerequisite step in improving our understanding of the role of the ANS in the pathophysiology of these disorders.

This is of particular pertinence considering a recent meta-analysis has suggested the central abnormality in FGID may lie in the parasympathetic nervous system.[13] A recent study by Paine *et al.* using the novel measure of CVT, examined the hitherto poorly characterized relationship between personality and autonomic tone to pain.[14] In healthy controls, it was demonstrated that pain evoked novel parasympathetic/sympathetic coactivation, and that the personality trait of neuroticism predicted an increase in CVT to esophageal pain. This latter observation may prove to be of particular relevance to FGID. The personality trait of neuroticism is considered to be a risk factor for increased pain sensitivity, yet an increase in parasympathetic tone has been postulated to be analgesic.

This raises the possibility that the increase in parasympathetic tone in neurotic individuals "offsets" the increase in pain sensitivity that the personality trait is thought to confer. Similarly, preliminary data in a cohort of subjects with functional chest pain of presumed esophageal origin are more neurotic than age, sex, and ethnicity matched healthy controls, and that in response to esophageal distension they too increased in parasympathetic tone.[15] These data provide an interesting insight into nociceptive physiology in health and disease and may allow the identification of specific abnormalities in the stress responsive physiology. These preliminary findings warrant further investigation in a larger cohort of patients with other chronic pain disorders, especially FGID.

The concept of endophenotyping nociceptive responses in FGID

A novel concept and approach to investigating the pathophysiology of these disorders is that of endophenotyping subjects' psychophysiological susceptibility to pain. An endophenotype can be defined as measurable subclinical trait, and adopting such an approach in FGID may prove to be the paradigm shift that is needed to elucidate the phys-

iological mechanisms that may act as susceptibility factors. As these disorders are defined in terms of their symptom complexes, attempting to endophenotype sufferers, for instance through genetics, personality traits, or physiological responses to a sensory stressor, may allow the clinicians to tailor their management of these disorders and thereby, hopefully, to improve outcome.

Conclusion

The recent past has heralded some important advances in increasing our understanding of nociceptive physiology in health and disease. The future is extremely exciting, and further work is now urgently needed, particularly with respect to endophenotyping psychophysiological responses to stressors in patients with functional esophageal disorders and FGID.

4. Clinical utility of using novel diagnostic combinations to guide mechanistically targeted esophageal therapeutics

Anthony R. Hobson
anthonyhobson@hotmail.com

In the late 1990s, there was a period of relative stagnation in the development of clinical tools to evaluate patients with upper GI disorders. Many of the techniques commonly applied in GI laboratories had been in use for decades, and researchers were left examining the minutia of the limited information provided by these techniques in order to extract novel insights into pathological mechanisms. We had the proton pump inhibitors to apparently solve most of our clinical problems and, to most people outside of the field, there was not a lot left to do.

However, for those of us working with complex neurogastroenterology patients on a day-to-day basis, there were many unmet needs that could not be addressed with the diagnostic tools at our disposal. In addition, the tools that we did have were prone to technical limitations, artifacts, and were certainly insensitive to detecting a host of potential pathophysiological mechanisms.

In the last five years, there has been a tremendous development in new technologies available to assess many aspects of GI physiology. Esophageal manometry has morphed into high-resolution manometry and impedance (HRMI), esophageal pH-metry

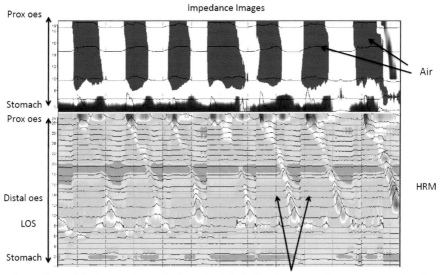

Image shows air in the oesophageal body moving in both directions generating a common cavity effect

Patient had normal pH study

Figure 3. A representative image taken from a combined high-resolution manometry and impedance study. This patient had previously been diagnosed with a nonspecific motility disorder and reflux disease on conventional testing and was being considered for antireflux surgery. During the test, it was observed that the patient had repeated aerophagia episodes (air is seen as blue regions of high impedance on the top level image) and subsequent supragastric belching. Aerophagia was associated with esophageal pressurization as seen with HRM and reproduced the patient's typical symptomatic sensations. This patient was referred for behavioral therapy to try and reduce air swallowing episodes and did not require antireflux surgery.

has evolved into multichannel intraluminal pH and impedance (MII), esophageal CEPs have allowed the first objective evaluation of extrinsic afferent sensitivity, and the wireless motility capsule has been developed as a potential alternative to gastric emptying scintigraphy. Suddenly, the arsenal of diagnostic tools of the GI scientist has been replenished, and the opportunities to provide new insights into the pathophysiology of a range of GI disorders are manifold.[16,17] The following section briefly summarizes some of the developments that have been made.

High-resolution manometry and impedance

The work of Clouse *et al.* to develop esophageal manometric catheters with many more channels than the 4–8 used by most laboratories and the novel software algorithms to analyze these data, have provided many benefits. The first and most pragmatic benefit has been that the coverage of the entire length of the area under study from cricopharynx to stomach prevents the need of the catheter being moved during the study, speeding up the procedure for both clinician and patient. In addition, artifacts such

as "pseudo-relaxations" sometimes seen in patients with achalasia due to esophageal shortening, previously undetectable with standard manometry, can now be easily observed with HRM.

The Chicago classification of 2009 has done a tremendous amount to provide an agreed upon framework for clinicians and researchers to move forward and to validate this new technology in large populations of patients.[16] The recent advent of combined impedance has added a new dimension to HRM as a diagnostic technique, not only evaluating the patterns of peristalsis but also the effectiveness of peristalsis in clearing liquid, viscous, and solid boli. In addition, esophageal "gas" handling can also be readily observed, allowing the detection of antegrade and retrograde passage of air in patients with undiagnosed aerophagia, for example. Figure 3 shows an example of tracing using combined HRMI in a young, female patient that was referred following conventional manometry and pH-metry had revealed a nonspecific motility disorder with significant gastroesophageal reflux. The referring doctor was considering antireflux surgery, but because the patient had responded poorly to PPIs, wanted to further evaluate her esophageal physiology. From the onset of the study, it could be clearly seen that the patient had severe aerophagia, with air being swallowed and then being expelled via supragastric belching. This was associated with esophageal body pressurization associated with subtle changes in esophageal motility. MII/pH confirmed hundreds of episodes of aerophagia and very little gastroesophageal reflux, and this patient was referred for behavioral therapy rather than for antireflux surgery. This offers a stark example of how this new technology can provide objective mechanistic evidence to aid clinicians in making crucial management decisions for patients that often present with very similar clinical and symptomatic profiles.

Similarly, the use of esophageal cortical evoked potentials to measure extrinsic afferent pathway sensitivity in patients with suspected esophageal hypersensitivity has also revealed that cohorts of patients with clinical homogenous symptoms can be subgrouped based on the presence or absence of enhanced primary afferent signaling. In a study by Hobson *et al.* it was shown that patients may either "over report" the intensity of esophageal stimuli or have genuine afferent nerve sensitization. As the treatment for these two conditions would be different (psychotherapy versus visceral analgesic therapy, for example), then the utility of such sensitive tools is obvious.[18]

In summary, the next phase of clinical research in GI physiology will be to further validate diagnostic algorithms that use appropriate combinations of tests to help drive mechanistic based treatment strategies for patients with upper GI disorders.

Conflicts of interest

The authors declare no conflicts of interest.

References

1. Rao, S.S., H. Gregersen, B. Hayek, *et al.* 1996. Unexplained chest pain: the hypersensitive, hyperreactive, and poorly compliant esophagus. *Ann. Intern. Med.* **124:** 950–958.

2. Drewes, A.M., J. Pedersen, H. Reddy, *et al.* 2006. Central sensitization in patients with non-cardiac chest pain: a clinical experimental study. *Scand. J. Gastroenterol.* **41:** 640–649.

3. Reddy, H., C. Staahl, L. Arendt-Nielsen, *et al.* 2007. Sensory and biomechanical properties of the esophagus in non-erosive reflux disease. *Scand. J. Gastroenterol.* **42:** 432–440.

4. Hoff, D.A., H. Gregersen, S. Odegaard, *et al.* 2010. Sensation evoked by esophageal distension in functional chest pain patients depends on mechanical stress rather than on ischemia. *Neurogastroenterol. Motil.* [Epub ahead of print]

5. Staahl, C., L.L. Christrup, S.D. Andersen, *et al.* 2006. A comparative study of oxycodone and morphine in a multi-modal, tissue-differentiated experimental pain model. *Pain* **123:** 28–36.

6. Drewes, A.M., H. Gregersen & L. Arendt-Nielsen. 2003. Experimental pain in gastroenterology: a reappraisal of human studies. *Scand. J. Gastroenterol.* **38:** 1115–1130.

7. Drewes, A.M., H. Reddy, J. Pedersen, *et al.* 2006. Multimodal pain stimulations in patients with grade B oesophagitis. *Gut* **55:** 926-932.

8. Frokjaer, J.B., E. Softeland, C. Graversen, *et al.* 2009. Central processing of gut pain in diabetic patients with gastrointestinal symptoms. *Diabetes Care* **32:** 1274–1277.

9. Sami, S.A., P. Rossel, G. Dimcevski, *et al.* 2006. Cortical changes to experimental sensitization of the human esophagus. *Neuroscience* **140:** 269–279.

10. Drewes, A.M., K.P. Schipper, G. Dimcevski, *et al.* 2002. Multimodal assessment of pain in the esophagus: a new experimental model. *Am. J. Physiol. Gastrointest. Liver Physiol.* **283:** G95–103.

11. Nielsen, C.S., R. Staud & D.D. Price. 2009. Individual differences in pain sensitivity: measurement, causation, and consequences. *J. Pain* **10:** 231–237.

12. Galmiche, J.P., R.E. Clouse, A. Balint, *et al.* 2006. Functional esophageal disorders. *Gastroenterology* **130:** 1459–1465.

13. Tak, L.M., H. Riese, G.H. De Bock, *et al.* 2009. As good as it gets? A meta-analysis and systematic review of methodological quality of heart rate variability studies in functional somatic disorders. *Biol. Psychol.* **82:** 101–110.

14. Paine, P., J. Kishor, S.F. Worthen, *et al.* 2009. Exploring relationships for visceral and somatic pain with autonomic control and personality. *Pain* **144:** 236–244.

15. Farmer, A.D., H. Havqi, S. Coen & Q. Aziz. 2010. Phenotyping pain in disease–psychophysiological responses to visceral and somatic pain in functional chest pain–A case control study. *Neurogastroenterol. Motil.* **22** (suppl 1): A46.

16. Kahrilas, P.J. & D. Sifrim. 2008. High-resolution manometry and impedance-pH/manometry: valuable tools in clinical and investigational esophagology. *Gastroenterology* **135:** 756–769.

17. Sifrim, D., K. Blondeau & L. Mantillla. 2009. Utility of non-endoscopic investigations in the practical management of oesophageal disorders. *Best Pract. Res. Clin. Gastroenterol.* **23:** 369–386.

18. Hobson, A.R., P.L. Furlong, S. Sarkar, *et al.* 2006. Neurophysiologic assessment of esophageal sensory processing in noncardiac chest pain. *Gastroenterology* **130:** 80–88.

ANNALS OF THE NEW YORK ACADEMY OF SCIENCES
Issue: *Barrett's Esophagus: The 10th OESO World Congress Proceedings*

High-resolution manometry

John O. Clarke,[1] C. Prakash Gyawali,[2] and Roger P. Tatum[3]

[1]Division of Gastroenterology, The Johns Hopkins University Hospital, Baltimore, Maryland. [2]Division of Gastroenterology, Washington University, St. Louis, Missouri. [3]Department of Veterans Affairs Medical Center, University of Washington, VA Puget Sound Health Care System, Seattle, Washington

The following presents commentaries on the interest of high-resolution manometry for understanding the anatomy and physiology of the esophagogastric junction; the subtypes of achalasia, as diagnosed by high-resolution manometry; the interest of high-resolution manometry in the evaluation of dysphagia following fundoplication; and the appropriate clinical protocol for high-resolution manometry.

Keywords: manometry; GERD; fundoplication; dysphagia; Clouse plots

Concise summaries

- Using high-resolution manometry (HRM), it is possible to clearly distinguish separate contributions from the LES and crural diaphragm in a manner not achieved with conventional manometry.

- There are several proposed means by which relaxation of the esophagogastric junction (EGJ) can be assessed: nadir pressure, e-sleeve pressure, 3-sec nadir e-sleeve relaxation pressure, and integrative relaxation pressure.

- When evaluating patterns of activity, several discrete manometric profiles can be appreciated by high-resolution manometry. HRM has particularly high sensitivity and positive predictive value for the diagnosis of lower esophageal sphincter (LES) relaxation errors, with very low false positive rates. The gain in sensitivity in the diagnosis of achalasia is significant. With this tool, the nadir residual pressure can be assessed above the gastric baseline prior to the arrival of the esophageal peristaltic contraction at the LES.

- Three distinct subtypes of achalasia have been described, with varying management implications: classic achalasia, achalasia with esophageal compression, and achalasia with spasm. In all patterns, LES postdeglutitive residual pressures and intrabolus pressure proximal to the LES are elevated above that expected in the absence of obstruction.

- Inspection of the HRM Clouse plots and use of newer tools of LES interrogation may help differentiate the etiology of LES obstruction. Incomplete forms of LES relaxation, especially with preserved esophageal body peristalsis, may benefit from botulinum toxin injections.

- Fundoplication results in increased resistance at the esophagogastric junction, which in turn is readily demonstrable on HRM by the presence of an elevated intrabolus pressure in comparison to that seen in healthy controls. Further, intrabolus pressures appear to be much higher in patients who specifically report postfundoplication dysphagia. Other than this, no characteristic HRM pattern corresponding to postfundoplication dysphagia has been identified, but this technique has the potential to reveal physiologic and anatomic abnormalities that are known to result in fundoplication failure.

- Techniques and protocols learnt from conventional manometry continue to be applied to HRM, but a major difference is that the stationary pull through maneuver is no longer required with HRM.

- The standard HRM clinical protocol uses 10 wet swallows in the supine position in the fasting

doi: 10.1111/j.1749-6632.2011.06067.x

patient. The addition of multiple rapid swallows may be of value, and needs to be added to the standard protocol. Use of bolus consistencies other than liquid need to be further studied, and diagnostic value may be augmented with the use of high-resolution impedance manometry.

---

1. The esophagogastric junction: anatomy and physiology on high-resolution manometry

John O. Clarke
john.clarke@jhu.edu

The EGJ consists of two components: the LES and the crural diaphragm (CD). The esophageal musculature is composed of circular and longitudinal muscle layers; however, only the circular layer is clearly interpretable with manometry.

Using HRM, it is possible to clearly distinguish separate contributions from the LES and CD in a manner not achieved with conventional manometry. When interpreting a HRM study, the following parameters should be established for optimal interpretation of EGJ function: mean basal pressure, proximal EGJ margin, distal EGJ margin, presence or absence of a hiatal hernia, the respiratory inversion point (RIP), and appropriateness of relaxation.

Normative data for EGJ pressure during expiration are 23.9 mmHg (SD 9.3) and during inspiration are 40.9 mmHg (SD 12.3) when compared to atmospheric pressure. Relative to gastric pressure, the mean EGJ expiratory pressure in normal subjects is 18.4 mmHg (2 SD range of normal 4.0–32.0 mmHg) and the mean EGJ inspiratory pressure in normal subjects is 32.3 mmHg (2 SD range of normal 12.3–52.3 mmHg).[1] Hiatal hernias can be subdivided into three categories based on the location of the LES, CD, and RIP.[2]

If the EGJ is not easily localized during placement of the catheter, one can ask the patient to breathe—which serves to highlight crural contractions and accentuate the differences between negative intrathoracic pressure and positive intragastric pressure. A second option is to ask the patient to swallow—which serves to mark the EGJ due to postdeglutitive LES contraction and can also be useful in unmasking a subtle sliding hiatal hernia.

There are several proposed means by which EGJ relaxation can be assessed: nadir pressure, e-sleeve pressure, 3-sec nadir e-sleeve relaxation pressure, and integrative relaxation pressure (IRP). When these parameters were compared in 75 asymptomatic controls, criteria for abnormal relaxation were defined as follows:

(1) single-sensor nadir ≥ 7 mmHg,
(2) HRM nadir ≥ 10 mmHg,
(3) three-sec nadir e-sleeve relaxation pressure ≥ 15 mmHg, and
(4) four-sec IRP ≥ 15 mmHg.[3]

When these methods were compared in patients with a clinical diagnosis of achalasia, the sensitivity was greatest using the 4-sec IRP with a sensitivity of 97% (as compared to the nadir pressure that had a sensitivity of only 52%).[3] For this reason, the 4-sec IRP is the preferred method for analysis of EGJ relaxation with a normative cutoff of 15 mmHg.

When one evaluates patterns of EGJ activity, several discrete manometric profiles can be appreciated. Normal EGJ relaxation has parameters detailed above. Achalasia is characterized by impaired EGJ relaxation (defined as a 4-sec IRP > 15 mmHg) in combination with aperistalsis. Functional EGJ obstruction refers to a 4-sec IRP > 15 mmHg with clear peristalsis in the esophageal body and elevated intrabolus pressure.

A fundoplication can be appreciated by persistent pressure at the EGJ, often (but not always) with impaired relaxation. Finally, a hiatal hernia can be appreciated due to separation between the CD and LES components of the EGJ.

2. Achalasia subtypes on high resolution manometry: does it predict outcome?

C. Prakash Gyawali
cprakash@im.wustl.edu

High-resolution manometry (HRM) allows detailed interrogation of esophageal motor phenomena. Achalasia is diagnosed by identification of absent esophageal body peristalsis in the presence of abnormal lower esophageal sphincter (LES) relaxation. Isobaric pressure increases can be noted in the esophageal body, ending in a dam effect at the level of a non- or poorly relaxing LES.[4]

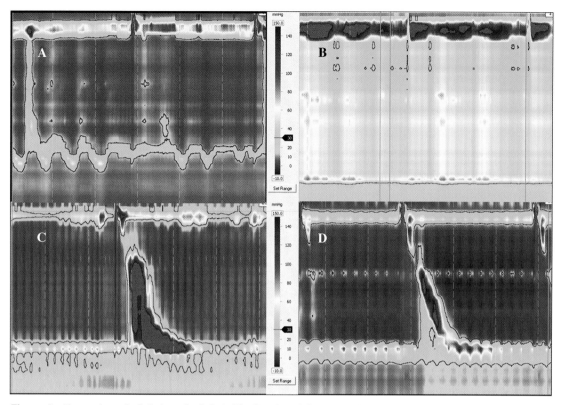

Figure 1. Clouse plots of achalasia and achalasia-like disorders. (A) Type I achalasia. Absent peristalsis and abnormal LES relaxation, but without esophageal compartmentalization of pressure. (B) Type II achalasia. Absent peristalsis with no LES relaxation, with compartmentalization of pressure. Panesophageal isobaric pressure increases exceed 30 mmHg in this instance. (C) Type III achalasia. Simultaneous high amplitude contractions are noted in the smooth muscle esophagus, with absent LES relaxation. Note the elevated intrabolus pressures preceding the contraction sequence. (D) Incomplete LES relaxation with preserved esophageal body peristalsis. This pattern may respond to intermittent botulinum toxin injections into the LES high-pressure zone.

HRM has particularly high sensitivity and positive predictive value for the diagnosis of LES relaxation errors, with very low false positive rates. The gain in sensitivity in the diagnosis of achalasia is significant, from 52–69% using point pressure sensors, to 93–97% using an electronic sleeve tool that allows interrogation of a specified segment of the LES high pressure zone.[5,6] With this tool, the nadir residual pressure can be assessed above the gastric baseline prior to the arrival of the esophageal peristaltic contraction at the LES, using either the 3-sec nadir pressure method or the 4-sec integrated relaxation pressure (IRP) that assesses a 4-sec flow permissive period during postdeglutitive LES relaxation.

Using these new tools for assessment of LES relaxation, and upon evaluating pressure patterns in the esophageal body, three distinct subtypes of achalasia have been described, with varying management implications.[4] In all instances, abnormal LES relaxation is defined by elevated postswallow residual pressures of ≥15 mm Hg.

(A) Type I: classic achalasia, with the esophagus dilated and boggy, results in very little compartmentalization of pressure within the esophageal body (Fig. 1A). This pattern is associated with a suboptimal response of transit symptoms to all forms of LES intervention, pharmacologic or mechanical. Heller myotomy provided a 67% response, while pneumatic dilation resulted in only 38% response in one report, while botulinum toxin injection was unsuccessful in improving symptoms (Table 1). This indicates the presence of significant stasis within a dilated esophageal body.

Table 1. Response of achalasia and achalasia-like disorders to therapy

	Type I achalasia	Type II achalasia	Type III achalasia	Preserved peristalsis, incomplete LES relaxation*
Botulinum toxin	0	86%	22%	0 − 55%
Pneumatic dilation	38%	73%	0%	0%
Surgical myotomy	67%	100%	0%	100%
First intervention	44%	83%	9%	55%
Final intervention	56%	96%	29%	33 − 58%

*Only limited data exists, with small patient numbers. Data obtained from Refs. 4, 7, and 8.

(B) Type II: achalasia with esophageal compression is associated with compartmentalization of pressure within a nondilated esophagus, typically with panesophageal pressurization and high intrabolus pressures ≥ 30 mmHg (Fig. 1B). This pattern is associated with the best response to any form of therapy (Heller myotomy, 100%, pneumatic dilation, 73%, botulinum toxin injection, 86%, Table 1). It is likely that this represents some of the older designation of "vigorous achalasia." Compartmentalization of pressure has been associated with esophageal longitudinal muscle contraction using high frequency ultrasound.

(C) Type III: achalasia with spasm is associated with spastic features in the esophageal body in $\geq 20\%$ of sequences, usually in the form of simultaneous high amplitude contractions in the distal esophagus (Fig. 1C). This pattern is associated with the poorest response to therapy (overall symptomatic response 9%, Table 1), with persisting perceptive symptoms such as chest pain persisting despite therapy. Multiple interventions are more common compared to the other patterns, and a final response rate of 29% has been reported.

Several incomplete forms of LES abnormalities have been observed with HRM.[7,8] A distinct syndrome of LES obstruction with preserved peristalsis has been described (Fig. 1D). This can result from both abnormal LES relaxation (variant or incomplete achalasia, true isolated LES relaxation errors) and from structural or restrictive abnormalities at the esophagogastric junction (strictures, infiltrating disorders such as eosinophilic esophagitis and cancer, postfundoplication, old peptic injury).

In all patterns, LES postdeglutitive residual pressures and intrabolus pressure proximal to the LES are elevated above that expected in the absence of obstruction.[7] Inspection of the HRM Clouse plots and use of newer tools of LES interrogation may help differentiate the etiology of LES obstruction. For instance, the second contraction segment (proximal of the two smooth muscle contraction segments in the esophageal body) may be most prominent in mechanical or restrictive abnormalities at the esophagogastric junction, while the third contraction segment (distal of the two smooth muscle contraction segments) demonstrates exaggerated contraction with LES relaxation errors. The latter can be seen as an overlap feature with spastic motor disorders of the esophageal body, which are believed to result for abnormal esophageal inhibitory nerve function.

Management to affect LES tone, including botulinum toxin injection into the LES may have value;[8] in another small series, no benefit was observed with nonsurgical approaches.[7] On the contrary, in restrictive disorders, disruption or dilation may be necessary for symptom relief.

In summary, three distinct subtypes of achalasia have been described, with implications on outcome of management. Incomplete forms of LES relaxation, especially with preserved esophageal body peristalsis, may benefit from botulinum toxin injections, and can be distinguished from inspection of HRM Clouse plots and use of newer tools of LES interrogation.

3. Has high-resolution manometry helped in the evaluation of postfundoplication dysphagia?

Roger P. Tatum
rtatum@u.washington.edu

Dysphagia in one form or another is a commonly reported symptom after Nissen fundoplication, seen in up to 100% of patients within the first three months after surgery and chronically, to some degree, in anywhere from 3 to 24% of fundoplication patients.[9]

Outcomes of revisional antireflux surgery, when performed for the primary symptom of dysphagia in particular, are reportedly not as good as those for other indications; therefore, it has been suggested that HRM may be of benefit in identifying underlying physiologic factors responsible for this symptom after fundoplication.[10,11]

To date, there are relatively few reports in the literature detailing the use of HRM in patients after fundoplication. A recent randomized controled trial comparing conventional (open) Nissen fundoplication to the laparoscopic technique specifically reports the evaluation of 20 patients (10 open, 10 laparoscopic) with recurrent symptoms using HRM; eight of these were found to have ineffective esophageal motility, and three had hypertensive LES. There was no correlation between any of the HRM findings and the symptom of dysphagia, however.[12]

The manometric characteristics of postfundoplication dysphagia were specifically addressed by Scheffer *et al.* in a 2005 study using HRM to examine the pressure characteristics of the esophagogastric junction both before and after laparoscopic Nissen fundoplication in 12 patients.[13] Postfundoplication HRM studies reveal significantly increased intrabolus pressures in the distal esophagus when compared to preoperative tracings (from 4 mmHg to 9 mmHg). This likely occurs as a result of increased resistance at the esophagogastric junction; increased intrabolus pressure is necessary to overcome the restriction of hiatal opening, and impaired esophagogastric relaxation observed after antireflux surgery. Interestingly, postoperative dysphagia scores in this group of patients did not correlate with either intrabolus pressures or EGJ nadir relaxation pressures.

Scherer *et al.* used HRM to evaluate eight patients who had presented with severe dysphagia following Nissen fundoplication, using this group as a comparator group to 16 patients with functional EGJ obstruction.[14] The distal esophageal intrabolus pressure was 40 mmHg (normal <15 mmHg), which was significantly higher than that of the functional obstruction group, as well as impaired EGJ relaxation (mean IRP = 25 mmHg). They interpreted these findings as evidence of EGJ outflow obstruction.

The relationship between EGJ distensibility and HRM characteristics of the LES was later examined in detail by this same group, using functional luminal impedance planimetry (FLIP) technology to evaluate the compliance of the EGJ and HRM to assess pressure parameters in 10 patients after fundoplication and 10 healthy controls.[15]

Finding that intrabolus pressures were related to the amplitude of the distal contractile integral (DCI), they proposed that this was likely explained as a response to overcome the outflow resistance at the EGJ. Interestingly, however, unlike the study involving postfundoplication dysphagia patients, they found that intrabolus pressures, as measured on HRM, were not significantly different between controls and fundoplication patients, and that there were no correlates between the decreased distensibility of the EGJ observed in the fundoplication group and pressure characteristics measured by HRM. Further, they found that the length of the high-pressure zone (HPZ) in the fundoplication group was shorter than that of the controls, while fundoplication patients had a longer zone of constriction as measured by FLIP. They concluded that FLIP may be a better method for evaluating the physiologic outcome of fundoplication than HRM. Of note, none of the patients from this study reported significant levels of dysphagia. Another recent study specifically examined the use of HRM in the evaluation of 18 patients considered to have fundoplication failure.[11] This study included four patients with significant dysphagia. The most significant finding was a correlation between the presence of a dual high pressure zone and objective evidence of abnormal esophageal acid exposure by 24-h pH monitoring; though there were no particular manometric predictors of dysphagia, it was also concluded that HRM was clinically useful in ruling out a new motility abnormality as a cause of this symptom.

In conclusion, there are very few studies thus far that have focused on the evaluation of patients after fundoplication using high-resolution manometry, and fewer still that shed much light on the causes or manometric correlates of postfundoplication dysphagia. From the current HRM literature, it is known that fundoplication results in increased resistance at the esophagogastric junction, which, in turn, is readily demonstrable on HRM by the presence of an elevated intrabolus pressure in comparison to that seen in healthy controls. Further, intrabolus pressures appear to be much higher in patients who specifically report postfundoplication dysphagia. Other than this, no characteristic HRM pattern corresponding to postfundoplication dysphagia has been identified.

Given the wealth of data that are available from HRM tracings, however, this technique has the potential to reveal physiologic and anatomic abnormalities that are known to result in fundoplication failure, including recurrent hiatus hernia, slipped fundoplication, wrap dehiscence, and others. Future studies on fundoplication patients, particularly involving those patients who report recurrent or new symptoms after surgery, are needed at this time in order to better define those characteristics on HRM that can both aid diagnosis and guide further treatment.

4. The optimal high resolution manometry clinical protocol

C. Prakash Gyawali
cprakash@im.wustl.edu

HRM allows detailed interrogation of esophageal motor phenomena with the use of multiple circumferential high fidelity solid state sensors on an esophageal manometry catheter, dedicated software for filling in data points between recording sites with best fit data, and computerized topographic contour plots, wherein preassigned colors reflect contraction amplitudes and pressure phenomena in the esophagus. The entire esophagus can be simultaneously interrogated with the creation of vivid images that are now termed "Clouse plots" in honor of Ray Clouse, who conceived HRM in the 1990s.

Techniques and protocols learned from conventional manometry continue to be applied to HRM. For instance, the HRM catheter is introduced through the nostril, and positioned with the last three sensors in the stomach. A major difference is that the stationary pull-through maneuver is no longer required with HRM. The topographic image visualized on the initial screen is anchored by the upper esophageal sphincter (UES) and the lower esophageal sphincter (LES) (Fig. 2A). After a brief period of acclimatization, basal pressures are assessed over a 10–20 sec swallow free interval, termed the landmark ID. It is important for the technician or nurse performing the procedure to recognize if the LES and diaphragmatic crura have been traversed. This can easily be achieved by observing the intrathoracic and intra-abdominal pressure changes with breathing, the directionality of which reverse at the level of the diaphragmatic crura (Fig. 2B). Sometimes, in the presence of a large hiatus hernia, the LES may be traversed but not the diaphragmatic crura (Fig. 2C).

The HRM procedure is typically performed after an overnight (at least six hours) fast.[16] As with conventional manometry, patients are asked to discontinue use of medications that could affect esophageal motor patterns (e.g., prokinetic agents, smooth muscle relaxants, anticholinergics, caffeine). Conscious sedation is not used for manometry, but topical anesthetics to the nostril are acceptable. The catheter is introduced with the patient sitting upright, and sips of water through a straw help the catheter advance through the esophageal sphincters.[16]

There are limited studies comparing the sitting and supine positions for data collection with HRM. In a study of 100 patients, Roman *et al.* demonstrated insignificant differences in basal and postswallow residual LES pressures.[17] While the likelihood of low contraction amplitudes and shorter wave duration were significantly higher while sitting, contraction front velocity was not different. The likelihood of finding a hiatus hernia was less while sitting (Table 2). Other studies using conventional manometry have documented similar findings. There is a small increase in the proportion of ineffective contraction sequences, as well as simultaneous sequences in the upright position, potentially related to the fact that gravity affects bolus transit while upright. However, the diagnosis rates of

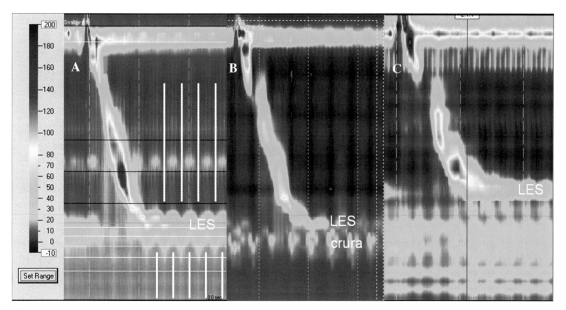

Figure 2. Clouse plots from high-resolution manometry demonstrating the lower esophageal sphincter (LES) and gastroesophageal junction. (A) The LES and diaphragmatic crura are at the same level. The respiratory inversion point (RIP) or pressure inversion point (PIP) is within the LES high-pressure zone, as indicated by reversal of the directionality of respiratory pressure change at this level (the white bars indicate nadir pressures, which occur during inspiration superior to the diaphragm, and during expiration below the diaphragm). (B) A short separation of the LES from crural diaphragm, indicating the presence of a 2-cm axial hiatus hernia. (C) The LES is traversed by the motility catheter, but the pressure signature of the crural diaphragm is not seen. This indicates the likely presence of a sizeable axial hiatus hernia.

named motor disorders including achalasia, aperistalsis from severe hypomotility, diffuse esophageal spasm, or other forms of hypertensive peristalsis are no different between supine and upright positions.[17,18]

Therefore, while research needs to continue in the more physiologic upright position for swallowing, available data continues to support performing water swallows in the supine position. Turning the patient slightly to the left aids administration of the liquid bolus (with a syringe or straw) and is more comfortable for the patient.

Conventionally, 10 wet swallows using 5 mL water boluses have been utilized for esophageal

Table 2. High-resolution manometric parameters compared between supine and sitting positions

	Supine position	Sitting position	P value
Basal LESP (mmHg)	8.1 ± 1.1	7.1 ± 1.2	0.31
Residual LESP (mmHg)	4.4 ± 0.6	4.8 ± 0.6	0.92
Esophageal body			
Contraction amplitude (mmHg)	71 ± 4	60 ± 4	<0.01
Wave duration (s)	3.4 ± 0.1	3.2 ± 0.1	<0.01
Wave velocity (cm/s)	5.5 ± 0.4	6.0 ± 0.7	0.32
DCI* (mmHg/cm/s)	1639 ± 194	1126 ± 130	<0.01

*DCI, distal contractile integral. Changes in LES parameters were nonsignificant between supine and sitting positions. While esophageal body contraction amplitude, wave duration, and DCI were significantly more prominent in the supine position, the difference did not translate into a change in diagnosis or clinical impression. Additionally, hiatus hernias were better characterized in the supine position. Adapted from Ref. 17.

manometry—the same protocol continues to be applied for HRM. Boluses of alternated consistencies have been studied. Normative values have been established for viscous swallows, which are only minimally different from liquid swallows. Semisolid (viscous) and solid (bread) swallows may result in a higher proportion of patients diagnosed with weak peristalsis (ineffective esophageal motility) and spastic processes such as diffuse esophageal spasm. However, early studies using barium-impregnated bread and fluoroscopy suggest that it may take more than one peristaltic sequence to clear bread, especially unchewed bread, even in normal individuals.[19] The use of semisolid and solid boluses needs further research to determine if altering bolus consistencies can help identify abnormal motor patterns in symptomatic patients. However, the 10 water swallow protocol continues to be the standard even with HRM. The use of high-resolution impedance manometry, which superimposes bolus clearance data using impedance on HRM plots, may provide additional data on bolus clearance. Using liquid, viscous, and yogurt swallows, no difference was noted in peristaltic performance and bolus clearance in normal adults, but failed sequences uniformly resulted in bolus escape. This technique shows promise in assessing bolus clearance, especially in symptomatic states.

Multiple rapid swallows (MRS) can be potentially used to assess peristaltic reserve in patients with weak peristalsis. When five swallows are administered 2–3 sec apart, esophageal body peristalsis is inhibited with profound LES relaxation during the swallows, followed by a robust esophageal body contraction sequence, and LES after contraction in normal individuals. Perstaltic performance during MRS generally follows that observed during standard wet swallows. However, normalization of peristalsis has been noted after MRS in as many as 48% of subjects with low distal esophageal body contraction amplitudes (ineffective esophageal motility) after MRS.[20] This may prove to be a useful tool in predicting postoperative improvement in postoperative manometric function, but outcome data are not available yet and research is ongoing.

In conclusion, the standard HRM clinical protocol utilizes 10 wet swallows in the supine position in the fasting patient. The addition of MRS may be of value; because, however, this is a simple procedure, it needs to be added to the standard protocol. Use of bolus consistencies other than liquid need to be further studied, and diagnostic value may be augmented with the use of high-resolution impedance manometry.

Conflicts of interest

The authors declare no conflicts of interest.

References

1. Pandolfino, J.E., S.K. Ghosh, Q. Zhang, *et al.* 2006. Quantifying EGJ morphology and relaxation with high-resolution manometry: a study of 75 asymptomatic volunteers. *Am. J. Physiol. Gastrointest. Liver Physiol.* **290:** G1033–G1040.
2. Pandolfino, J.E., M.R. Fox, A.J. Bredenoord, *et al.* 2009. High-resolution manometry in clinical practice: utilizing pressure topography to classify oesophageal motility abnormalities. *Neurogastroenterol. Motil.* **21:** 796–806.
3. Ghosh, S.K., J.E. Pandolfino, J. Rice, *et al.* 2007. Impaired deglutitive EGJ relaxation in clinical esophageal manometry: a quantitative analysis of 400 patients and 75 controls. *Am. J. Physiol. Gastrointest. Liver Physiol.* **293:** G878–G885.
4. Pandolfino, J.E., M.A. Kwiatek, T. Nealis, *et al.* 2008. Achalasia: a new clinically relevant classification by high-resolution manometry. *Gastroenterology* **135:** 1526–1533.
5. Ghosh, S.K., J.E. Pandolfino, J. Rice, *et al.* 2007. Impaired deglutitive EGJ relaxation in clinical esophageal manometry: a quantitative analysis of 400 patients and 75 controls. *Am. J. Physiol.* **293:** G878–G885.
6. Staiano, A. & R.E. Clouse. 2001. Detection of incomplete lower esophageal sphincter relaxation with conventional point-pressure sensors. *Am. J. Gastroenterol.* **96:** 3258–3267.
7. Scherer, J.R., M.A. Kwiatek, N.J. Soper, *et al.* 2009. Functional esophagogastric drome sometimes akin to achalasia. *J. Gastrointest. Surg.* **12:** 2219–2225.
8. Porter, R. & C.P. Gyawali. 2011. Botulinum toxin injection in dysphagia syndromes with preserved esophageal peristalsis and incomplete lower esophageal sphincter relaxation. *Neurogastroenterol. Motil.* **23:** 139–144.
9. Tatum, R.P., G. Shi, M.A. Manka, *et al.* 2000. Bolus transit assessed by an esophageal stress test in postfundoplication dysphagia. *J. Surg. Res.* **91:** 56–60.
10. Lamb, P.J., J.C. Myers, G.G. Jamieson, *et al.* 2009. Long-term outcomes of revisional surgery following laparoscopic fundoplication. *Br. J. Surg.* **96:** 391–397.
11. Tatum, R.P., R.V. Soares, E. Figueredo, *et al.* High-resolution manometry in evaluation of factors responsible for fundoplication failure. *J. Am. Coll. Surg.* **210:** 611–619.
12. Broeders, J.A., H.G. Rijnhart-De Jong, W.A. Draaisma, *et al.* 2009. Ten-year outcome of laparoscopic and conventional nissen fundoplication: randomized clinical trial. *Ann. Surg.* **250:** 698–706.
13. Scheffer, R.C., M. Samsom, A. Haverkamp, *et al.* 2005. Impaired bolus transit across the esophagogastric junction in postfundoplication dysphagia. *Am. J. Gastroenterol.* **100:** 1677–1684.
14. Scherer, J.R., M.A. Kwiatek, N.J. Soper, *et al.* 2009. Functional esophagogastric junction obstruction with intact

peristalsis: a heterogeneous syndrome sometimes akin to achalasia. *J. Gastrointest. Surg.* **13:** 2219–2225.

15. Kwiatek, M.A., K. Kahrilas, N.J. Soper, *et al.* Esophagogastric junction distensibility after fundoplication assessed with a novel functional luminal imaging probe. *J. Gastrointest. Surg.* **14:** 268–276.

16. Murray, J.A., R.E. Clouse, J.L. Conklin, *et al.* 2003. Components of the standard oesophageal manometry. *Neurogastroenterol. Motil.* **15:** 591–606.

17. Roman, S., H. Damon, P E. Pellissier, *et al.* 2010. Does body position modify the results of oesophageal high resolution manometry? *Neurogastroenterol. Motil.* **22:** 271–275.

18. Bernhard, A., D. Pohl, M. Fried, *et al.* 2008. Influence of bolus consistency and position on esophageal high-resolution manometry findings. *Dig. Dis. Sci.* **53:** 1198–1205.

19. Pouderoux, P., G. Shi, R.P. Tatum, *et al.* 1999. Esophageal solid bolus transit: studies using concurrent videofluoroscopy and manometry. *Am. J. Gastroenterol.* **94:** 1457–1463.

20. Fornari, F., I. Bravi, R. Penagini, *et al.* 2009. Multiple rapid swallowing: a complementary test during standard oesophageal manometry. *Neurogastroenterol. Motil.* **21:** 718–725.

Ann. N.Y. Acad. Sci. ISSN 0077-8923

ANNALS OF THE NEW YORK ACADEMY OF SCIENCES

Issue: *Barrett's Esophagus: The 10th OESO World Congress Proceedings*

Testing for gastroesophageal reflux in the 21st century

Sabine Roman,[1,2] John E. Pandolfino,[1] Philip Woodland,[3] Daniel Sifrim,[3] and Johannes Lenglinger [4]

[1]Department of Medicine, The Feinberg School of Medicine, Northwestern University, Chicago, Illinois. [2]Digestive Physiology, Lyon 1 University and Hospices Civils de Lyon, Lyon, France. [3]Barts and The London School of Medicine and Dentistry Queen Mary, University of London, London, United Kingdom. [4]Department of Surgery, Medical University of Vienna, Vienna, Austria

The following on testing for gastroesophageal reflux in the 21st century contains commentaries on wireless pH monitoring; extension of pH recording duration to 48 or 96 h; extraesophageal GERD syndromes, diagnosis paradigms, and related investigating tools; off- or on-PPI reflux monitoring in the preoperative setting; and the potential influence of PPIs on reflux parameters.

Keywords: wireless pH monitoring; gastroesophageal reflux disease; extraesophageal GERD syndromes; acid exposure time; symptom associated probability; laryngitis; asthma; PPI

Concise summaries

- The typical duration for clinical catheter-based reflux monitoring is 24 h. In contrast, the wireless pH monitoring system allows one to extend monitoring beyond 24 h to up to 96 h, allowing for testing off- and on-medication in a single examination.
- The reproducibility of the wireless capsule is good between the two first days of recordings, and increasing the recording duration may also enhance the sensitivity to detect pathological gastroesophogeal reflux disease (GERD). The prolongation of esophageal pH recordings may also predict the severity of the disease according to the number of days with elevated acid esophageal exposure, but no study stratifying the occurrence of mucosal lesions or patient's outcomes according to the number of days with abnormal esophageal acid exposure have been published.
- The wireless system has not yet been validated with any symptom association with predict clinical outcome.
- There is a high prevalence of gastroesophageal reflux (GER) and/or an increased sensitivity to GER in subgroups of patients with laryngeal and respiratory disorders. Extraesophageal GER syndromes are becoming increasingly apparent in clinical practice, although may be difficult to diagnose. Within this group, there are established associations with GER, namely reflux cough syndrome; reflux laryngitis syndrome; reflux asthma syndrome; and reflux dental erosion syndrome. Within these syndromes it has been demonstrated that a proportion of patients with extraesophageal symptoms responds well to antireflux therapy, and represent a clear example of the potential relationship between GER and extraesophageal symptoms. In contrast to heartburn, the symptoms of extraesophageal manifestations of GER are often more nebulous, and the temporal relationship between reflux events and these symptoms may be less obvious and more difficult to demonstrate.
- Current standards of diagnosis are important to specify, and prediction of therapy response in the major extraesophageal reflux syndromes is challenging.
- A high proportion of symptomatic patients are endoscopy negative, including those with true nonerosive reflux disease (NERD) and subjects with healed esophagitis. Multichannel impedance and pH monitoring have the advantage of detecting reflux independent of

doi: 10.1111/j.1749-6632.2011.06066.x

intraluminal pH. In patients nonresponsive to proton pump inhibitor PPI medication, reflux monitoring on therapy allows a differentiation of symptoms related to acid or nonacid reflux versus symptoms not associated with reflux. In patients undergoing antireflux surgery, present data do not clearly favor either off- or on-PPI reflux monitoring by multichannel impedance and pH monitoring in the preoperative setting.

---

1. Quantifying distal esophageal acid exposure: 24, 48, or even 96 h

Sabine Roman and John E. Pandolfino
roman.sabine@gmail.com

Different techniques are available to quantify esophageal acid exposure: the conventional pH monitoring with a transnasal catheter, the wireless pH catheter, and the pH impedance monitoring system.[1] No consensus regarding the optimal technique or methodology exists, in part, because there are no randomized controlled trials that compare pH monitoring alone or combined with pH impedance to predict clinical outcomes. However, extending the recording duration may be an argument to choose one technique over another. The typical duration for clinical catheter-based reflux monitoring is 24 h. In contrast, the wireless pH monitoring system allows one to extend monitoring beyond 24 h up to 96 h. Secondary to improved tolerance of the catheter-free wireless system, the prolongation of pH studies reduces the potential for false negative studies due to day to day variability. It also allows for testing off and on medication in a single examination. Finally, it may stratify the severity of the disease according to the number of days with pathological acid exposure.

Different studies have shown the feasibility of increasing the recording duration to 48, 72, or 96 h using the wireless pH capsule. Because of spontaneous capsule detachment, recordings were available in 89–100% of patients for 48 h, in 48–100% for 72 h, and in 41–100% for 96 h.[2–4] The reproducibility of the wireless capsule is good between the two first days of recordings. Pandolfino noted that the median percentage of time with esophageal pH below 4 was similar between the first and the second days in controls and in patients with GERD.[3] Nevertheless, using 5.3% as the upper limit of normal for total percent time with the pH below 4, 16% of controls, and 29% of GERD patients exhibited a pathological acid exposure based on having one day abnormal highlighting the importance of considering day to day variability.

Increasing the recording duration may also enhance the sensitivity to detect pathological GERD. Prakash showed that extending recording to 48 h increased the detection of pathological GERD based on elevated acid esophageal exposure in 12% of patients.[5] He also reported that extending the duration to two days increased the number of symptoms reported and the number of patients reporting symptoms. Thus, the significance of symptom association changed in 20% of patients. Taking into account the esophageal acid exposure and the symptom association, the overall diagnostic yield was 33% for the patients off PPI. The best criteria to define a pathological study might be the results of the worst day of recording.

Using a pathological result on both days, Pandolfino noted that the sensitivity to predict esophagitis was only 78%, whereas the sensitivity and negative predictive values were 100% using the worst day.[3] The caveat was that the specificity was not perfect and the rate of false positives was quite high (18%).

Another advantage of pH monitoring prolongation is the ability to investigate patients off and on PPI therapy in a single examination. Hirano proposed to test patients off therapy the first two days and on medication the following two days.[2] This represented an efficient approach to address the controversy regarding pH assessment on or off therapy in refractory GERD.

Finally, the prolongation of esophageal pH recordings may predict the severity of the disease according to the number of days with elevated acid esophageal exposure. Pandolfino noted that the esophageal acid exposure was elevated during both days in 78% of patients with esophagitis compared to 36% of patients with NERD.[3] However, no study stratifying the occurrence of mucosal lesions or patients outcomes according to the number of days with abnormal esophageal acid exposure has been published.

Using the wireless capsule to extend recordings duration has some limitations:

(1) the early capsule detachment,
(2) the requirement of additional endoscopic procedures for the capsule insertion,
(3) the requirement of removal in some rare case of severe chest pain, and
(4) the possibility to overestimate reflux events number by including swallow events.

In conclusion, extending the pH recording duration is feasible. It increases the sensitivity of pathological esophageal acid exposure detection and positive symptom-reflux association. Nevertheless the wireless system has not yet been validated with any symptom association with predict clinical outcome. Further studies are also required to test the propensity to stratify disease severity based on the number of days with positive acid esophageal exposure.

2. Reflux monitoring standards in patients with atypical GERD symptoms

Philip Woodl and Daniel Sifrim
d.sifrim@qmul.ac.uk

To most people, GERD is easily recognized as a condition in which heartburn is caused by reflux of acidic stomach contents into the esophagus. The Montreal classification (2006) recognizes this as an example of a typical esophageal symptomatic syndrome in GERD.[6] Of course we now appreciate that the spectrum of disease is much broader, with regard to both the nature of the refluxate causing the symptoms, and to the symptom complexes that result. Of note, there is a high prevalence of GER and/or an increased sensitivity to GER in subgroups of patients with laryngeal and respiratory disorders. This is reflected by the additional category of extraesophageal GERD syndromes.

Within this group, there are established associations with GER, namely reflux cough syndrome; reflux laryngitis syndrome; reflux asthma syndrome; and reflux dental erosion syndrome. Within these syndromes, it has been demonstrated that a proportion of patients with extraesophageal symptoms respond well to antireflux therapy and represent a clear example of the potential relationship between GER and extraesophageal symptoms.

Unfortunately, while typical GERD symptoms can be challenging to diagnose and treat on occasion, this is even truer of extraesophageal GER manifestations, and an individual's response to antireflux therapy is very difficult to predict. The appropriate diagnostic tools and techniques are often less established or are beset by technical difficulties. In contrast to heartburn, the symptoms of extraesophageal manifestations of GER are often more nebulous, and the temporal relationship between reflux events and these symptoms may be less obvious and more difficult to demonstrate. The result of this is that, historically, our ability to diagnose these conditions and predict their response to treatment has been poor.

Below, we discuss current standards of diagnosis and prediction of therapy response in the major extraesophageal reflux syndromes.

GER and cough

GERD has been reported as the third most common cause of chronic cough. The potential for reflux to induce cough has been long realized, and indeed acid perfusion into the distal oesophagus has been shown to induce or increase cough. Since there may be more sinister or more obvious causes of chronic cough (e.g., malignancy, allergy, drugs, asthma, postnasal drip) these should first be excluded. But rather than as a diagnosis of exclusion, how can GER-related cough be positively diagnosed? The patient's clinical history may suggest some clues (e.g., cough occurs mostly during the day, in the upright position, upon rising from bed, during phonation or during eating) but the sensitivity and specificity for this is low. Unfortunately, suggestive typical reflux symptoms such as heartburn and regurgitation are rarely present in GER-related cough ("silent" GER occurs in over 70% of these cases).

What of the investigative tools at our disposal for diagnosis of GERD in cough?

Many patients will have endoscopic evaluation as a first line. Macroscopic abnormality may be expected in only 15% of patients with reflux-induced cough. A common diagnostic method used is an empirical trial of PPI therapy. Unfortunately studies have failed to demonstrate PPIs as a successful treatment. A Cochrane meta-analysis of the outcome of acid suppressive therapy in chronic cough failed to show a significant difference between PPI treatment and placebo for total resolution of cough.[7]

We have become increasingly aware that not only acid, but also weakly acidic reflux events (such as are found in patients "on" PPI therapy) can be important in triggering cough. A recent study of 100 chronic cough patients using combined pH multichannel intraluminal impedance (pH-MII) monitoring showed that weakly acidic GER was a potential cause for cough events in 24%.[8] A further problem with PPI therapy is that, if used, there is uncertainty as to what dose should be used, and for how long. A study by Baldi *et al.* has shed some light on the answer to this problem. They found that a four-week trial of double-dose PPI therapy appeared to be an effective criterion for selecting those patients who will respond well to standard PPI therapy. More than 80% of those patients who responded to PPI therapy had a positive response to the initial trial, compared to approximately 20% of those who failed the trial.[9] More objective reflux measurement techniques are often used in the diagnosis of typical GERD.

For reflux–cough syndrome, standard 24 h pH monitoring is limited again by the ability of weak-acid reflux events to trigger cough. It is also compounded by the high level of GERD in the background population. Increased 24 h esophageal acid exposure has a 90% sensitivity for GER-related cough, but only a 66% specificity. Only 35% of patients with a positive test respond well to PPI therapy. A more sophisticated method of investigation is likely to be required in order to effectively diagnose GER-related cough. First, there is a need to establish a temporal relationship between reflux events and cough. Integral to this is a need to be able to accurately identify cough episodes by the recording equipment. Objective cough monitoring equipment using manometric or acoustic detection has been developed and is an important step toward identifying any true relationship.

Second, more refined methods of detecting reflux should be used. Combined pH-MII monitoring is able to detect not just acid reflux events, but also reflux events that are weakly-acidic. As such, this is likely to be the current gold standard test for reflux in this situation. Third, we need to establish a method for demonstrating a relationship between reflux events and cough. It may be that we need to use an altered version of a currently used algo-

rithm, or perhaps a combination of algorithms for better prediction of treatment response. Statistical algorithms can evaluate the likelihood of a chance association between cough and reflux and may be used to identify patients who are more likely to respond to antireflux therapy.

Studies have looked at reflux–cough associations using symptom index (SI) and symptom associated probability (SAP) with time windows of five minutes and two minutes respectively. These time windows were initially used to establish reflux–heartburn associations, and reflux–cough associations may need a different analysis. A recent study by Hersh *et al.* considered a hierarchical approach of several analyses in order to predict response to PPI therapy in those with chronic cough. In this retrospective study, an increased 24 h esophageal acid exposure time (AET) was very poor in determining response to PPI therapy. If a high AET was combined with a positive SAP *and* an SI of >25% on 24 h pH monitoring, then there was an 85.7% prediction of response to PPI therapy.[10] This high specificity was at the expense of a poor sensitivity (32%).

Perhaps the sensitivity can be increased by using a more sensitive test for GER (i.e., pH impedance) and by changes in the SAP algorithm? It has been shown that the extension of the time-window of interest to the SAP calculation to four minutes (when used in conjunction with a manometric cough detector) can increase the sensitivity of 24 h pH-MII monitoring (to detect acid and nonacid reflux events) for detecting GER-related cough to 85%, while maintaining a negative predictive value of 84%.[11]

The temporal relationship between cough and reflux may be further complicated by the fact that in some circumstances reflux can *follow* cough, as well as vice versa. A study using acoustic cough detection and pH impedance monitoring in patients with chronic cough showed that there was a temporal relationship between cough and reflux events (defined by SAP with a two minute window) in 70% of cases.[12] In 48% of cases, the relationship was for reflux followed by cough, however in 56% of patients this relationship was for cough followed by reflux. It appears that cough can provoke reflux episodes in some patients. In 32% of patients in the study the SAP was positive for both relationships, suggesting that reflux–cough–reflux can be a self-perpetuating cycle. This study suggests the important possibility that reflux may induce a hypersensitivity of the cough reflex, perhaps in people who are already predisposed to coughing.

Reflux–laryngitis syndrome

A total of 10% of visits to ear, nose, and throat specialists are due to chronic laryngitis. A total of 50–60% of chronic laryngitis are suggested to be related to GER. The first line investigation performed is usually direct laryngoscopy, and on this the most suggestive finding for reflux–laryngitis are posterior cricoid wall erythema, true vocal folds erythema, or arytenoid medial wall erythema. Unfortunately, these findings are neither sensitive nor specific for reflux–laryngitis syndrome. As for reflux–cough syndrome, 24 h pH monitoring is often used as a diagnostic tool, but again, this unfortunately has important limitations. Only half of suspected cases of reflux–laryngitis syndrome have increased AET. To confound matters, up to 40% of healthy, asymptomatic subjects may have pharyngeal acid reflux. A recent meta-analysis demonstrated that treatment of *suspected* GER-related laryngitis with PPIs has been shown to be ineffective.[13]

As with reflux–cough syndrome, reflux–laryngitis syndrome may be more accurately assessed (and perhaps treatment-responders more accurately predicted) using combined pH impedance monitoring. However supraesophageal reflux can still be difficult to detect with significant false-negative rates. This is because reflux is often aerosolized at this level and not detected by standard pH-MII catheters.

A new catheter (Dx-pH Measurement system, Restech) is under investigation and may increase diagnostic yield for supraesophageal reflux. This catheter sits in the oropharynx and is designed to detect the pH of aerosolized reflux.

Reflux–asthma syndrome

GER and asthma commonly coexist, with GER being present in 30–80% of asthmatic patients.[14]

Acid reflux is "clinically silent" (i.e., not associated with typical reflux symptoms) in 25–60% of asthmatic patients. However on endoscopic evaluation, esophagitis will be present in 37% of such patients, and esophageal pH monitoring will reveal an increased AET in 51%. Hence there is a definite need to identify GERD and treat accordingly in a subset of recurrent wheezers. It would follow (as for all extraesophageal reflux syndromes) that those with concurrent typical reflux symptoms should be treated with PPI therapy, and indeed, asthma sufferers *with* typical GER symptoms have been shown to reduce exacerbations and improve asthma quality of life.[15] In those without typical GERD symptoms, identification of those who will respond to therapy is more difficult. Again, use of more sensitive reflux detection techniques (i.e., pH-MII) and better objective wheeze detection (such as with the recent development of computerized wheeze detectors) may help identify those with a GER–asthma association.

Summary

Extraesophageal GER syndromes are becoming increasingly apparent in clinical practice, although may be difficult to diagnose. Despite the clear response of some patients to antireflux therapy, predicting which patients will respond is challenging. The diagnostic paradigms and tools used for classical reflux symptoms need to be revised to meet this challenge, and in recent years much progress has been made on these fronts as our understanding of the pathophysiology and diagnostic technologies have advanced.

3. Reflux monitoring in the preoperative session: on or off therapy?

Johannes Lenglinger
johannes.lenglinger@meduniwien.ac.at

Proton pump inhibitor (PPI) medication has become the standard first line therapy for symptoms suggestive of GERD. Most patients are or have been on a PPI before endoscopy. As a consequence, a high proportion of symptomatic patients are endoscopy-negative, including those with true NERD and subjects with healed esophagitis. Multichannel impedance and pH monitoring (MII-pH) have the advantage of detecting reflux independent of intraluminal pH. In patients non responsive to PPI medication, reflux monitoring on therapy allows a differentiation of symptoms related to acid or nonacid reflux versus symptoms not associated with reflux. Mainie *et al.* performed MII-pH on standard dose PPI in 168 patients with a history of PPI refractory symptoms. 144 (86%) subjects reported symptoms during the monitoring period and a positive SI was found in 69 (48%), predominantly with nonacid reflux (53 [37%]).[16]

Apart from the temporal association of reflux events with symptoms, other parameters such as acid exposure (% recording time with pH <4) and the number of reflux events obtained are used to classify results as normal or outside the range found in healthy volunteers, especially when no symptoms are provided by the patients, or symptom count is too low to calculate a meaningful symptom association.

Data whether PPI medication confounds these parameters are scarce and conflicting. Hemmink *et al.* studied 30 patients with heartburn, chest pain, or regurgitation on PPI bid first after seven days of PPI abstinence and after an interval of 1–4 weeks on double dose PPI.[17] The total number or reflux events did not differ significantly between the two measurements (73 ± 33 off versus 69 ± 35 on PPI, not significant). Symptom analysis using SAP was discordant. Four (off PPI) versus eight (on PPI) patients had either a negative SAP or reported no symptoms. This difference was not statistically significant, but the authors recommended to perform MII-pH preferably off PPI. In contrast, Bajbouj *et al.* reported a reduction of the number of reflux events with increasing the dose of esomeprazole from 40 to 80 mg (118.3 ± 44.8 versus 66.6 ± 35.6, $P < 0.0001$) in 45 patients.[18]

Two uncontrolled studies reported on good outcome of fundoplication when patients were selected for surgery according to the results of MII-pH on therapy: Mainie *et al.* reported 14-month follow-up of 17 out of 19 patients.[19] Sixteen of 17 patients with a positive SI preoperatively were asymptomatic or markedly improved. Del Genio *et al.* compared pre- and postoperative reflux symptoms and satisfaction rates in 62 patients stratified by outcome of pre-operative MII-pH results.[20] Thirty-three had increased acid exposure, 17 had an abnormally high number of reflux events, and 12 had a positive SI with normal acid exposure. The overall satisfaction rate was 98%, and no significant differences in postoperative reflux symptoms between the three groups occurred.

In conclusion, present data do not clearly favor either off- or on-PPI reflux monitoring by MII-pH in the preoperative setting. Two studies, with low patient numbers included, report a satisfactory outcome of antireflux surgery in patients with positive SI either on or off PPI medication. The potential influence of PPIs on reflux parameters requires further study. MII-pH on antisecretories may, however, have lower sensitivity.

Conflicts of interest

The authors declare no conflicts of interest.

References

1. Hirano, I., & J.E. Richter. 2007. ACG practice guidelines: esophageal reflux testing. *Am. J. Gastroenterol.* **102:** 668–685.
2. Hirano, I., Q. Zhang, J.E. Pandolfino, & P.J. Kahrilas. 2005. Four-day Bravo pH capsule monitoring with and without proton pump inhibitor therapy. *Clin. Gastroenterol. Hepatol.* **3:** 1083–1088.
3. Pandolfino, J.E., J.E. Richter, T. Ours, *et al.* 2003. Ambulatory esophageal pH monitoring using a wireless system. *Am. J. Gastroenterol.* **98:** 740–749.
4. Scarpulla, G., S. Camilleri, P. Galante, *et al.* 2007. The impact of prolonged pH measurements on the diagnosis of gastroesophageal reflux disease: 4-day wireless pH studies. *Am. J. Gastroenterol.* **102:** 2642–2647.
5. Prakash, C., R.E. Clouse 2005. Value of extended recording time with wireless pH monitoring in evaluating gastroesophageal reflux disease. *Clin. Gastroenterol. Hepatol.* **3:** 329–334.
6. Vakil, N., S.V. Van Zanten, P. Kahrilas, *et al.* 2006. The Montreal definition and classification of gastroesophageal reflux disease: a global evidence-based consensus. *Am. J. Gastroenterol.* **101:** 1900–1920; quiz 43.
7. Chang, A.B., T.J. Lasserson, J. Gaffney, *et al.* 2006. Gastro-oesophageal reflux treatment for prolonged non-specific cough in children and adults. Cochrane Database of Systematic Reviews.
8. Sifrim, D., L. Dupont, K. Blondeau, *et al.* 2005. Weakly acidic reflux in patients with chronic unexplained cough during 24 hour pressure, pH, and impedance monitoring. *Gut* **54:** 449–454.
9. Baldi, F., R. Cappiello, C. Cavoli, *et al.* 2006. Proton pump inhibitor treatment of patients with gastroesophageal reflux-related chronic cough: a comparison between two different daily doses of lansoprazole. *World J. Gastroenterol.* **12:** 82–88.
10. Hersh, M.J., G.S. Sayuk, & C.P. Gyawali. 2010. Long-term therapeutic outcome of patients undergoing ambulatory pH monitoring for chronic unexplained cough. *J. Clin. Gastroenterol.* **44:** 254–260.
11. Blondeau, K., L.J. Dupont, V. Mertens, *et al.* 2007. Improved diagnosis of gastro-oesophageal reflux in patients with unexplained chronic cough. *Aliment Pharmacol. Ther.* **25:** 723–732.
12. Smith, J.A., S. Decalmer, A. Kelsall, *et al* 2010. Acoustic cough-reflux associations in chronic cough: potential triggers and mechanisms. *Gastroenterology* **139:** 754–762.
13. Qadeer, M.A., C.O. Phillips, A.R. Lopez, *et al.* 2006. Proton pump inhibitor therapy for suspected GERD-related chronic laryngitis: a meta-analysis of randomized controlled trials. *Am. J. Gastroenterol.* **101:** 2646–2654.
14. Harding, S.M. 2004. Pulmonary complications of gastroesophageal reflux. In: *The Esophagus.* 4th ed. D. Castell & J.E. Richter, eds.: 530–545. Lippincott Williams and Wilkins. Philadelphia.

15. Littner, M.R., F.W. Leung, E.D. Ballard, *et al.* 2005. Effects of 24 weeks of lansoprazole therapy on asthma symptoms, exacerbations, quality of life, and pulmonary function in adult asthmatic patients with acid reflux symptoms. *Chest* **128:** 1128–1135.

16. Mainie, I., R. Tutuian, S. Shay, *et al.* 2006. Acid and non-acid reflux in patients with persistent symptoms despite acid suppressive therapy: a multicentre study using combined ambulatory impedance-pH monitoring. *Gut* **55:** 1398–1402.

17. Hemmink, G.J., A.J. Bredenoord, B.L. Weusten, *et al.* 2008. Esophageal pH-impedance monitoring in patients with therapy-resistant reflux symptoms: 'on' or 'off' proton pump inhibitor? *Am. J. Gastroenterol.* **103:** 2446–2453.

18. Bajbouj, M., V. Becker, V. Phillip, *et al.* 2009. High-dose esomeprazole for treatment of symptomatic refractory gastroesophageal reflux disease-a prospective pH- metry/impedance-controlled study. *Digestion* **80:** 112–118.

19. Mainie, I., R. Tutuian, A Agrawal, *et al.* 2006. Combined multichannel intraluminal impedance-pH monitoring to select patients with persistent gastro-oesophageal reflux for laparoscopic Nissen fundoplication. *Br. J. Surg.* **93:** 1483–1487.

20. Del Genio, G., S. Tolone, F. Del Genio, *et al.* 2008. Prospective assessment of patient selection for antireflux surgery by combined multichannel intraluminal impedance pH monitoring. *J. Gastrointest. Surg.* **12:** 1491–1496.

Ann. N.Y. Acad. Sci. ISSN 0077-8923

ANNALS OF THE NEW YORK ACADEMY OF SCIENCES
Issue: *Barrett's Esophagus: The 10th OESO World Congress Proceedings*

The new requirements of endoscopy

Peter Heeg[1] and Ingo F. Herrmann[2]
[1]Institute of Medical Microbiology and Hygiene, Eberhard-Karls-University, Tübingen, Germany. [2]Department of Otorhinolaryngology, European Hospital, Rome, Italy

The following on new requirements of endoscopy contains commentaries on the risk of infection in endoscopy, the need to eliminate contamination, and the use of a disposable system in transnasal endoscopy.

Keywords: endoscopy; infection; contamination

Concise summaries

A great number of outbreaks of exogenous endoscopy-related infection have been published.

- Outbreaks reported in the literature and newspapers probably cover only a small part of the infections that have really taken place. The inner surface of gastroscopes, colonscopes, and bronchoscopes shows indentations and irregularities especially at and near the distal opening and the proximal entrance of the working channel as well as at the bifurcation (working channel and suctioning channel), and the presence of visible deposits in the working channel is the indicator for contamination.

- Although existing data related to current endoscopic methods are not sufficient to describe the risk of the patient, improvement of reprocessing measures will reduce contamination risks and enhance patient safety. Relevant sources of infections associated with endoscope reprocessing are faulty practices for processing including storage of scopes and accessory devices, noncompliance with state-of-the-art policies and, very likely, design of endoscopes. Effective cleaning is difficult when dealing with endoscopes equipped with channels for air, water, or instruments, and there is no general agreement on methods and reference values for the validation of cleaning.

- The safety level of disposable sheaths is not acceptable due to the possibility of breaks or tears during use.

- Reprocessing of the scope and accessory devices using a standardized, validated format according to acknowledged standards may therefore be necessary. Endoscopes should be designed allowing easy access for cleaning and disinfecting agents to all external and internal surfaces including antiadhesive materials for working channels.

- A disposable tube system (DTS) has been developed. It is attached to the endoscope and has a suctioning rinsing and working channel. The use of nose-drops for decongestion and local anesthesia (e.g., drops of oxybuprocain 2–4%) especially in allergic subjects is useful. The endoscopy is performed without sedation and with the patient in sitting position in order to analyze the function.

- The advantages of this method are numerous: no sedation, no risk of contamination, cost-effectiveness. The question is how far will the disposable system go to improve the future of the endoscopic procedures.

doi: 10.1111/j.1749-6632.2011.06065.x
Ann. N.Y. Acad. Sci. 1232 (2011) 365–368 © 2011 New York Academy of Sciences.

1. Standard and/or flexibility in upper gastrointestinal tract endoscopy: avoiding contamination risks

Peter Heeg
Peter.Heeg@med.uni-tuebingen.de

Medline analysis for the years 1966–2005 reveals no less than 70 outbreaks of exogenous endoscopy-related infection; more than 50% were associated with bronchoscopy. However, the number of unreported outbreaks and single cases of infection is presumed to be high. As the leading cause of inadequate processing practices have been identified, it is clear that the great majority of infections could have been prevented by implementation of adequate processes and controls.[1] Although existing data—related to current endoscopic methods—are not sufficient to describe the risk of the patient, improvement of reprocessing measures will reduce contamination risks and enhance patient safety.

Relevant sources of infections associated with endoscope reprocessing are faulty practices for processing including storage of scopes and accessory devices, noncompliance with state-of-the-art policies and—very likely—reprocessing given the "unfriendly" design of endoscopes. European directives[2] require that all processes (cleaning, disinfection, and where necessary, sterilization) must be standardized, validated, and reproducible, including documentation of results. Endoscopy staff requires special education, training, and experience. Furthermore appropriate technical equipment has to be provided, thus questioning the notion of "simple" manual processing.

The essential prerequisite for successful disinfection/sterilization is effective cleaning, which, in particular, is difficult when dealing with endoscopes equipped with channels for air, water, or instruments. Since the performance of automatic washer disinfectors currently on the market is not satisfying, additional manual cleaning following a standardized policy is required. There is, unfortunately, no general agreement on methods and reference values for the validation of cleaning. As far as disinfection is concerned, a reduction between four and six log steps, depending on the type of pathogen, has to be achieved. The use of transparent disposable sheaths has been suggested to avoid laborious cleaning and disinfection procedures. However, the safety level of the sheaths is not acceptable due to the possibility of breaks or tears during use. Therefore, disposable sheaths are not appropriate to replace complete reprocessing of the endoscope after each use.

Good clinical practice (GCP) in endoscopy of the aerodigestive tract provides a general set-up of measures to reduce contamination:

- Hand hygiene—hygienic hand disinfection using alcoholic rubs (instead of antimicrobial soaps), use of gloves whenever hand contact with body fluids or secretions is likely or expected.
- Protective equipment for the patient and staff—disposable barrier drapes for the patient, protective gown, and, in the case of aerosol or droplet releasing procedures—face protection (mask and goggles or face protection shield).
- Reprocessing of the scope and accessory devices using a standardized, validated format according to acknowledged standards.[3]

What we primarily need is greater knowledge for endoscopists and assistant staff concerning patients' and staff safety requirements in line with internationally accepted standards. Technical equipment should include washer disinfectors of appropriate size with short (chemo-thermal) cycles for reprocessing of endoscopes. Endoscopes should be designed allowing easy access for cleaning and disinfecting agents to all external and internal surfaces including antiadhesive materials for working channels.

2. The transnasal endoscopy and the advantage to combine a videoendoscope with a disposable tube system (DTS)

Ingo F. Herrmann
herrmann@ingoscope.com

In the last few years, the communications about infections using flexible endoscopes with integrated channel systems became more frequent. Outbreaks reported in the literature and newspapers probably cover only a small part of the infections that really have taken place. The difficulty of cleaning the outer, and especially the inner, surface of the flexible endoscopes with integrated channel systems has been demonstrated.

The outer surfaces of the endoscopes were evaluated with the OPMI 11 Microscope (Zeiss), the proximal and distal entrances of the working and rinsing channels included. The surface of the integrated channels was analyzed with a 0.77 mm flexible fiber optic (10,000 pixel). Two bronchoscopes (new and used for four years), two gastroscopes (used for six and nine years), and two colonscopes (used for seven and nine years) were investigated.

Relatively new endoscopes with a smooth coating on the outer surface are less sensitive to the attachment of contaminated material. The outer surface of the frequently used and/or aged endoscopes becomes rough over the years. Finally, more defects of the coating are exhibited.

After manual cleaning followed by reprocessing, deposits of tissue or other material are visible at these locations under microscopic view. More frequently, the contaminated material is attached to coating defects.

The inner surface of gastroscopes, colonscopes, and bronchoscopes show indentations and irregularities especially at and near the distal opening and the proximal entrance of the working channel as well as at the bifurcation (working channel and suctioning channel). All these "irregularities" cause obstacles, on which contaminated material may get stuck. The most dangerous region is the bifurcation of the suctioning and working channel. At this place we have regularly seen remaining material suspicious of contamination.

The technical challenge is to take calculated samples under endoscopic view to analyze, if bacteria or viruses, etc., are present in the deposits as a consequence of contamination. It was not possible to take samples from the working channel under sterile conditions at small costs. The origin and location—where the sample was taken exactly—could also not be defined. The necessary financial investment for the development of a technique to prove the presence of viruses at certain places inside the channel was too high. We abandoned this goal, which from a technical point of view, was too difficult and too expensive to reach.

The presence of visible deposits in the working channel was an indicator of contamination. Visible material or deposits in the channel, compared with the submicroscopic dimension of viruses, are like an elephant compared with an ant. If deposits in the channel system are not visible during endoscopy, it does not mean, however, that there is no contamination risk.

The consequence of this experiment was the need to eliminate the contamination and the resulting infection risk. To this end, we developed a DTS. Following our analysis, the possibility to connect a DTS with a solid endoscope (i.e., without an integrated working and rinsing channel) is the main option for the prevention of the infection risks. The width of the nasal passage of an adult is sufficient to allow the passage of two tubes up to 3.8 mm diameter. They would be positioned one above the other (7.6 mm endoscope + disposable tube). Endoscopes without an integrated channel system are smooth and easy to clean. The DTS is attached to the endoscope and has a suctioning–rinsing and working channel. The use of nose drops for decongestion and local anesthesia (e.g., drops of oxybuprocain 2–4%) especially in allergic subjects is useful. The endoscopy is performed without sedation and with the patient in sitting position in order to analyze the function. The endoscope passes the upper sphincter while the patient is drinking a sip of clear water with a straw. For air insufflation, the patient changes to recumbent position. Biopsies can be taken from the duodenum, the stomach, and the esophagus as usual. The advantages of this method are:

- there is no risk of drug associated, intravenous infection, because no sedation is used;
- there is no risk of contamination with disposable channel systems;
- the endoscopic technique allows examination of the function of the digestive tract and provides an opportunity to take reflux (gas and liquid) samples under visual control;
- the inversion of the endoscope in the esophagus and duodenum and the measurement of size and shape of a pathologic change are now possible;
- this new technique permits intervention procedures to be performed at the same time;
- it is more cost-effective: the patient is able to function normally immediately after endoscopy (e.g., he can drive his car or can return to work);
- less assistance is required, because the patient is able to collaborate;
- there is a reduction in cost for public health care, for the economy, and for patients due to resulting decrease of the cost/efficiency index with the reduction of the infection risks.

The disadvantages are:

- the endoscopist must be flexible enough to change his/her traditional method to use a new technique;

- there may be a possible change of current target markets for the companies who manufacture endoscopes. The more desirable route would be to start with countries that have a high incidence of AIDS and hepatitis C. This would allow us to specify the adaptation without commercial bias;
- the disposable system has no Albarran lever; the endoscopy of the ductus choledochus and ductus pancreaticus has not been possible up till now.

The question is how far can the disposable system go to improve the future of the endoscopic procedures. Is reprocessing of the outer surface of the endoscope with a wash-disinfector necessary? Are there other possibilities to clean the smooth outer surface of the endoscopes?

Conflicts of interest

The authors declare no conflicts of interest.

References

1. Seoane-Vazquez, E., R. Rodriguez-Monguio, J. Visaria & A. Carlson. 2006. Exogenous endoscopy-related infections, pseudo-infections and toxic reactions: clinical and economic burden. *Curr. Med. Res. Opin.* **22:** 2007–2021.
2. Council Directive 93/42 EEC of 14 June 1993 concerning medical devices. http://eur-lex.europa.eu
3. ISO 15883-4:2008. Washer disinfectors: part 4. Requirements and tests for washer disinfectors employing chemical disinfection for thermolabile endoscopes.
4. Allan, M. 2008. http://www.lasvegassun.com/news/2008/feb/29/clinic-cut-corners-profit-critics-say/ (accessed February 29, 2008)
5. Bader, L., G. Blumenstock, B. Birkner, *et al.* 2002. Hygea (hygiene in gastroenterology—endoscope reprocessing): study on quality of reprocessing flexible endoscopes in hospitals and in the practice setting. *Z. Gastroenterol.* **40:** 157–170.
6. Herrmann, I.F., S. Arce Recio, F. Cirillo & P. Bechi. 2008. The role of functional endoscopy in understanding upper GI functioning. *Acta Endosc.* **3:** 247–261.
7. Herrmann, I.F., P. Heeg, B. Matteja, *et al.* 2008. Silent risks and hidden dangers in endoscopy: what to do? *Acta Endosc.* **5:** 493–502.

Ann. N.Y. Acad. Sci. ISSN 0077-8923

ANNALS OF THE NEW YORK ACADEMY OF SCIENCES

Issue: *Barrett's Esophagus: The 10th OESO World Congress Proceedings*

Esophageal disease: updated information on inflammation

Roy C. Orlando,[1] William G. Paterson,[2] Karen M. Harnett,[3] Jie Ma, Jose Behar,[3] Piero Biancani,[3] Michele Pier Luca Guarino,[4] Annamaria Altomare,[4] Michele Cicala,[4] and Weibiao Cao[5]

[1]Gastroenterology, Cell, and Molecular Physiology, University of North Carolina School of Medicine at Chapel Hill, Chapel Hill, North Carolina. [2]Gastrointestinal Diseases Research Unit and Department of Medicine Queen's University, Hotel Dieu Hospital, Kingston, Ontario, Canada. [3]Gastrointestinal Motor Function Research Laboratory, Rhode Island Hospital and Brown University, Providence, Rhode Island. [4]Department of Digestive Diseases, Campus Bio-Medico University, Rome, Italy. [5]Department of Medicine and Pathology, Brown Medical School and Rhode Island Hospital, Providence, Rhode Island

The following on esophageal disease provides updated information the mucosal defense against acid and acid–pepsin injury; the roles of platelet activating factor, mast cells, proinflammatory cytokines, and chemokines in inflammation; differences and similarities in erosive and nonerosive esophagitis; acid and vanilloid receptors in esophageal mucosa; and bile acid receptors in esophageal epithelium.

Keywords: tight junction; adherens junction; claudins; e-cadherin; paracellular permeability; dilated intercellular spaces; esophagitis; gastro-esophageal reflux; squamous cells; TRPV-1 receptor; platelet activating factor; substance P; cytokines; inflammatory mediators; nonerosive reflux disease; chemosensitive nociceptors; inflammatory mediators; adenocarcinoma; NOX5-S; TGR5

Concise summaries

- The first component of the mucosal defense against acid and acid–pepsin injury is its barrier capability. This is comprised of the apical cell membrane and apical junctional complex, the latter comprised of the tight junction, adherens junction, and to a lesser extent the desmosomes.

- The initial change that occurs in the apical junctional complex in acute acid-injured esophageal epithelium is the cleavage of the adherens junction protein, e-cadherin. Under conditions of gastroesophageal reflux disease (GERD), there are notable changes in claudins, which are the bridging proteins for the tight junction.

- Such changes to the proteins involved with junctional barrier function can account for the observed increase in paracellular permeability and dilated intercellular spaces in human esophageal epithelium of patients with GERD. They also provide a notable "leak" pathway for luminal hydrogen ions (H^+) to diffuse into the tissue where it can access the sensory nociceptors and trigger the symptom of heartburn.

- Inflammation of the esophagus begins with activation of the transient receptor potential channel vanilloid subfamily member-1 (TRPV1) in the mucosa, and production of interleukin 8 (IL-8), substance P (SP), calcitonin gene-related peptide (CGRP), and platelet activating factor (PAF). Production of SP and CGRP, but not PAF, is abolished by the neural blocker tetrodotoxin (TTX), suggesting that SP and CGRP are neurally released and that PAF arises from nonneural pathways.

- PAF is known to be released from mast cells, but also appears to be secreted by esophageal squamous epithelial cells, and plays a significant role in mucosal injury. It may be a major mediator of acid-induced esophagitis. Whether this is related to attenuation of mast cell release from the lamina propria, squamous epithelium, or both is uncertain at this time.

- Esophageal keratinocytes, that constitute the first barrier to the refluxate, may also serve as the initiating cell type in esophageal inflammation, secreting inflammatory mediators, proinflammatory cytokines and chemokines, affecting leukocyte recruitment, and activity.

- In the absence of visible mucosal breaks, heartburn would develop due to an impaired junctional complex and increased paracellular permeability (to water, electrolytes such as H^+, and small molecules). Probably, the crossing of H^+ into the intercellular space would lead to activation of chemosensitive nociceptors and the transmission of the signal to the brain via the spinal cord.

- Nonerosive reflux disease (NERD) patients represent a distinct group of the GERD population, characterized by enhanced sensitivity to chemical and mechanical stimulation, and acid-sensing TRPV1 receptors may be involved in esophageal hypersensitivity. The role of these acid-sensing receptors, in patients with NERD exhibiting mucosal integrity and normal acid exposure, remains to be elucidated.

- It is reasonable to hypothesize that differences in chemoattractants, in NERD versus erosive reflux disease (ERD) patients, may account for the differences in the granulocyte infiltrate and, ultimately, the mucosal damage.

- Mechanisms of the progression from Barrett's esophagus (BE) to esophageal adenocarcinoma (EAC) are not fully understood. Reactive oxygen species (ROS) may play an important role in the development of EA since their levels are increased in BE and adenocarcinoma.

- Bile acids may also play an important role in the progression from BE to adenocarcinoma.

- A novel cell membrane receptor of bile acid, TGR5, has been shown to be important in bile acid-regulated lipid metabolism, and is present in an adenocarcinoma cell line, FLO, and a Barrett's cell line, BAR-T. Taurodeoxycholic acid-induced increase in cell proliferation depends on upregulation of NOX5-S expression in FLO cells. It is possible that bile acid reflux present in BE patients may increase ROS production and cell proliferation via activation of TGR5, thereby contributing to the development of EA.

---

1. Acid and acid–pepsin-induced changes in the barrier properties of esophageal epithelium

Roy C. Orlando
rorlando@med.unc.edu

The esophagus is lined by a moist, nonkeritinized stratified squamous epithelium. This epithelium has three functional layers: stratum corneum, which contains the barrier layers; stratum spinosum, which is larger and involved with ion transport; and stratum basalis, which is the replicating layer. Squamous epithelium secretes no mucus and no bicarbonate and, though both are secreted by esophageal subcosal glands, the mucin (MUC 5B) is soluble, leaving the epithelium without a well-defined mucus coat and little effective surface buffering defense.[1] This leaves the epithelium proper as the major mucosal defense against refluxed acid and acid-pepsin.

The first component of the mucosal defense against acid and acid–pepsin injury is its barrier capability. This comprises the apical cell membrane and apical junctional complex, the latter comprises the tight junction, adherens junction, and to a lesser extent, the desmosomes.[2] The earliest sign that this barrier is breached when esophageal epithelium is in contact with acid is a fall in its transmural electrical potential difference. This fall is due to an increase in paracellular permeability that is subsequently reflected in the development within the epithelium of dilated intercellular spaces.[1]

The initial change that occurs in the apical junctional complex in acute acid-injured esophageal epithelium is the cleavage of the adherens junction protein, e-cadherin.[4] E-cadherin is important because it serves as the protein that bridges the intercellular space, resulting in adhesion of adjacent cells. Moreover, the strength of this adhesion is important for the creation and maintenance of the tight junction, the latter being the structure that largely governs the types and rate of movement of ions and uncharged molecules that can traverse the paracellular pathway. The cause for this cleavage of e-cadherin appears to be acid activation of a membrane metalloproteinase in esophageal epithelial cells. Under conditions of more chronic acid injury as is indicative of gastroesophageal reflux disease, there are other changes noted in the structures representing the apical junctional complex. For instance, there are notable changes in claudins, which are the bridging proteins for the tight junction.

In a rat model of reflux esophagitis, Asaoka *et al.* has shown that expression of claudin-1 decreased, claudin-3 increased, and both occludin and claudin-4 shifted protein from the cell membrane to cell cytoplasm.[3] In humans, to date, the major change noted in the claudins is that claudin-4 expression is substantially reduced, while claudin-1, occludin, and other claudins were unchanged.[4] GERD occurs when acid contact with SqE is sufficient to alter the junctional permeability barrier.

Such changes to the proteins involved with junctional barrier function are important since they can account for the observed increase in paracellular permeability and dilated intercellular spaces in human esophageal epithelium in patients with GERD. They also provide a notable "leak" pathway for luminal hydrogen ions (H^+) to diffuse into the tissue where it can access the sensory nociceptors and trigger the symptom of heartburn.[5] Moreover, this leak pathway allows H^+ (and chloride ions) access to the basolateral membranes of squamous cells. The exposure of the basolateral membrane to acidic media is significant since it enables acid absorption into the squamous cell on an ion transporter known as the sodium-independent, chloride–bicarbonate exchanger.[1] Absorption of acid, in turn, results in cell acidification and cell necrosis. Cell acidification and necrosis are a trigger for inflammation, a phenomenon that further extends the damaging process leading ultimately to erosive eosphagitis.

2. The role of platelet activating factor and mast cells in acid-induced esophageal inflammation

William G. Paterson

patersow@hdh.kary.net

The majority of research on the pathophysiology of gastroesophageal reflux disease has focused on the associated motor abnormalities. Until recently, relatively little attention has been paid to the mechanisms whereby luminal acid induces mucosal injury and esophagitis.

It is clear from the work of Orlando and colleagues[6] that acid *per se* can induce epithelial cell necrosis by interfering with the volume regulatory mechanisms of the squamous epithelial cell. In addition, there is increasing evidence that the epithelial cells themselves can play an active role in inflammation by secreting proinflammatory cytokines in response to acid activation of the TRPV-1 receptor.[7]

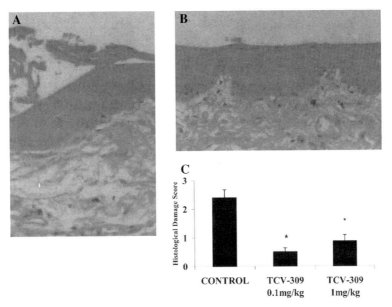

Figure 1. In control opossums, luminal acid perfusion induces acute epithelial injury characterized by cell sloughing and cleft formation between layers of cells (A). This is completely prevented by pretreatment with the selective PAF antagonists TCV-309 (B). Quantitative data on the effect of PAF antagonism on acid-induced injury scores are depicted in C. Adapted from Ref. 9.

Another factor that appears to contribute to acid-induced esophagitis is the mast cell, which resides primarily in the lamina propria of the esophageal mucosa, ideally positioned to respond to molecules that permeate the squamous epithelium. Indeed, relative brief periods of intraluminal acid perfusion in an animal model will lead to mast cell degranulation and histamine release.[8] However, stabilizing mast cells pharmacologically does not appear to prevent acute acid-induced esophageal mucosal injury.[9] This may be because mediators released from mast cells have both a damaging and protective effect. For instance, mast cell derived histamine leads to reactive vasodilation and increased mucosal blood flow in response to luminal acid via an NO-dependent mechanism.[10] This increased blood flow likely has a protective effect that would be abrogated by mast cell stabilizers.

PAF is a molecule that plays a significant role in mucosal injury in other regions of the gastrointestinal tract. PAF is known to be released from mast cells, but also appears to be secreted by esophageal squamous epithelial cells.[7] A recent study in the opossum model[9] revealed that luminal acid induced PAF release. Furthermore, pretreating the animals with the selective PAF antagonist TCV-309 completely prevented the acute epithelial injury induced by luminal acid perfusion (Fig. 1).

These data suggest that PAF may be a major mediator of acid-induced esophagitis. Whether this is related to attenuation of mast cell release from the lamina propria, squamous epithelium, or both is uncertain at this time.

3. Acid and vanilloid receptors in esophageal mucosa

Karen M. Harnett, Jie Ma, Jose Behar, and Piero Biancani
karen˙harnett@brown.edu

We have focused on understanding the onset of GERD gastroesophageal reflux disease (GERD) by examining the mucosal response to the presence of acid in the esophageal lumen. Upon exposure to HCl, inflammation of the esophagus begins with activation of the transient receptor potential channel vanilloid subfamily member-1 (TRPV1) in the mucosa, and production of interleukin 8 (IL-8), substance P (SP), calcitonin gene-related peptide (CGRP), and platelet activating factor (PAF). Pro-duction of SP and CGRP, but not PAF, is abolished by the neural blocker tetrodotoxin (TTX), suggesting that SP and CGRP are neurally released and that PAF arises from nonneural pathways.[11] Epithelial cells contain TRPV1 receptor mRNA and protein and respond to HCl and to the TRPV1 agonist capsaicin with production of PAF.[12]

PAF, SP, and IL-8 act as chemokines, inducing migration of peripheral blood leukocytes (PBL). PAF and SP activate PBL inducing the production of H_2O_2.[13] Exposure of the epithelial cells to HCl, similarly upregulates other chemokines such as eotaxins, macrophage inflammatory protein 1 α, and monocyte chemoattractant protein- 1, but their effect on the esophageal mucosa has not yet been examined.

Thus, esophageal keratinocytes, that constitute the first barrier to the refluxate, may also serve as the initiating cell type in esophageal inflammation, secreting inflammatory mediators, proinflammatory cytokines and chemokines, and affecting leukocyte recruitment and activity.

This work was supported by NIH Grant: R01 DK057030.

4. Erosive esophagitis and nonerosive esophagitis: differences and similarities

Michele Pier Luca Guarino, Annamaria Altomare, and Michele Cicala
m.guarino@unicampus.it

GERD develops when the reflux of gastric contents into the esophagus leads to troublesome symptoms, with or without mucosal damage, and/or complications. The majority of patients with typical reflux symptoms show no evidence of erosive esophagitis at endoscopy; these patients, when the pH-impedance test and/or symptom response to proton pump inhibitors (PPIs) are positive, are considered to have NERD.[14] ERD patients and NERD patients present a similar frequency of heartburn and regurgitation, as well as a similar symptom severity score, but patients with ERD have a higher average esophageal acid exposure, in terms of total number of refluxes and also acid exposure time (AET); moreover, the number of mixed liquid-gas refluxes increases with the severity of esophagitis.[14,15]

These findings have led NERD to be considered as a mild form of GERD that might progress with time to ERD. However, this classical view can be challenged by longitudinal observations and studies demonstrating different epidemiological features, different responses to comparable treatments, and enhanced esophageal sensitivity to gastric refluxate. When comparing the two groups of patients, no differences were found in terms of gender, mean age, body mass index, alcohol consumption, smoking habit, and presence of *Helicobacter pylori* infection, except for the presence of hiatal hernia, which appears to be more frequent in patients with ERD.[14]

The most relevant difference is that patients with NERD often also present functional gastrointestinal symptoms such as functional dyspepsia and irritable bowel syndrome; a common denominator for this association could be visceral hypersensitivity. Furthermore, NERD patients, presenting physiological acid exposure may exhibit a positive symptom index (hypersensitive esophagus), with an even higher percentage than ERD patients and Barrett's patients and, moreover, the perception of mixed refluxes is higher in NERD than in ERD.[14,15]

The histological features of GERD are based on a combination of findings, including basal cell hyperplasia, *papillae* elongation, and inflammation. However, these abnormalities can also be found in healthy subjects. The only clear difference is that the combined presence of intraepithelial neutrophils and erosion/necrosis is found only in patients with ERD.[14]

It would be reasonable to expect that the esophageal mucosa in NERD patients, that gives rise to such troublesome reflux symptoms, even if apparently normal, should at least display some microscopic evidence of damage.

Various research groups have reported the presence of dilated intracellular space (DIS) in NERD patients, the values observed being similar to those in ERD patients.[14]

On the other hand, in the attempt to better understand the relationship between the ultrastructural changes, typical symptoms, and esophageal acid exposure, Caviglia *et al.* carried out investigations on NERD patients, all of whom were clear responders to PPI treatment, whether or not they presented normal or abnormal acid exposure. Irrespective of the acid exposure, all patients had intercellular space values at least twice those in controls, and DIS appeared to be a sensitive and objective marker of NERD.[16]

In the absence of visible mucosal breaks, heartburn would develop due to an impaired junctional complex and increased paracellular permeability (to water, electrolytes such as H^+, and small molecules). Probably, the crossing of H^+ into the intercellular space would lead to activation of chemosensitive nociceptors and the transmission of the signal to the brain via the spinal cord.

This hypothesis is supported by recent evidence, such as the detection of TRPV1 in the esophageal mucosa of NERD and ERD patients, and is able to restore the visceral, chemical, and mechanical hypersensitivity reported in NERD, as well as the possible involvement of TRPV1 in the pathogenesis of heartburn in these patients.[17]

In a recent study, biopsies obtained from the distal esophagus of NERD and ERD patients, as well as healthy controls, were used for conventional histology, for Western blot analysis, and/or quantitative real-time polymerase chain reaction.[17] Controls also underwent ambulatory pH-testing in order to assess esophageal acid exposure. TRPV1, mRNA, and protein expression are significantly increased in all NERD and ERD patients. The only difference between NERD and ERD patients was the presence of neutrophils/eosinophils observed in mucosal esophageal biopsies only from ERD patients. Furthermore, no correlation with acid exposure was found.[17]

The role of these acid-sensing receptors, in patients with NERD-exhibiting mucosal integrity and normal acid exposure, remains to be elucidated. Indeed, NERD patients may require higher doses of PPIs than ERD patients in order to control symptoms.[14] Resistance to acid suppressive drugs, in NERD patients, may be due to a more sensitive esophagus resulting from enhanced excitability of visceral sensory neurons on account of over expression of TRPV1 in the epithelial layer and in afferent fibers of the lamina propria.

Besides their role in visceral hypersensitivity, TRPV1 have been hypothesized to contribute to inflammation by releasing sensory neurotransmitters, such as substance P (SP) and CGRP and other inflammatory mediators including platelet-activating factor (PAF), which has been shown to cause histological damage in the acid-perfused opossum esophagus. Moreover, it has been shown that transgenic mice, lacking TRPV1 receptors, are less likely to develop esophagitis in response to acid exposure than wild type mice.

All of these results suggest that NERD patients represent a distinct group of the GERD population, characterized by enhanced sensitivity to chemical and mechanical stimulation, and that acid-sensing TRPV1 receptors may be involved in esophageal hypersensitivity. It is reasonable to hypothesize that differences in chemoattractants, in NERD versus ERD patients, may account for the differences in the granulocyte infiltrate and, ultimately, the mucosal damage.

5. Role of a novel bile acid receptor TGR5 in the progression from Barrett's esophagus to esophageal adenocarcinoma

Weibiao Cao
wcao@hotmail.com

Mechanisms of the progression from BE to EAC are not fully understood. Reactive oxygen species (ROS) may play an important role in the development of esophageal adenocarcinoma since levels of ROS are increased in BE and adenocarcinoma. ROS may cause damage to DNA, RNA, lipids, and proteins, which may result in increased mutation and altered functions of enzymes and proteins (e.g., activation of oncogene products and/or inhibition of tumor suppressor proteins). However, the sources of ROS in these conditions have not been well defined. We have shown that the NADPH oxidase isoform NOX5-S is present in FLO EAC cells[18] and that levels of NOX5-S are significantly increased in EAC cells and in Barrett's esophageal mucosa with high-grade dysplasia.[19]

Bile acids may also play an important role in the progression from BE to EAC,[20] because:

(1) in animal models, diversion of duodenal contents into the lower esophagus leads to EAC; and

(2) reflux of bile acids into the esophagus not only causes short-term damage to the mucosa but also induces long-term oxidative stress and cellular DNA damage.

Recently, a novel cell membrane receptor of bile acid, TGR5 (a G-protein-coupled receptor) has been shown to be important in bile acid-regulated lipid metabolism, energy homeostasis, and glucose metabolism. We have shown that this receptor is present in an EAC cell line FLO and a Barrett's cell line BAR-T. TGR5 mRNA and protein levels are significantly higher in EAC tissues than in normal esophageal mucosa or Barrett's mucosa.[21] We have also reported that taurodeoxycholic acid (TDCA, one of the major bile acids in the refluxate) significantly increased NOX5-S expression, H_2O_2 production, and cell proliferation in FLO EAC cells. This increase in cell proliferation (as evidenced by increased thymidine incorporation) was significantly reduced by knockdown of NOX5-S. Knockdown of TGR5 markedly inhibits TDCA-induced increase in NOX5-S expression, H_2O_2 production, and thymidine incorporation in FLO cells. Overexpression of TGR5 significantly enhances TDCA's effects in FLO cells.[21] TGR5 receptors are coupled with $G\alpha q$ and $G\alpha i$-3 proteins, but only $G\alpha q$-mediated–TDCA-induced increase in NOX5-S expression, H_2O_2 production and thymidine incorporation in FLO cells.

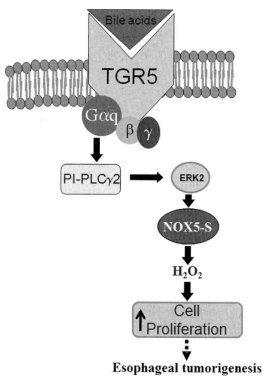

Figure 2. TDCA-induced NOX5-S expression may be mediated by sequential activation of the TGR5 receptor, $G\alpha q$ protein, PI-PLCγ2, and ERK-2 MAP kinase in FLO cells. It is possible that bile acid reflux present in BE patients may increase reactive oxygen species production and cell proliferation via activation of TGR5, $G\alpha q$, PI-PLCγ2, ERK-2 MAP kinase, and NOX5-S, thereby contributing to the development of esophageal adenocarcinoma.

In addition, the TDCA-induced increase in cell proliferation was significantly reduced by U73122, an inhibitor of phosphatidylinositol-specific phospholipase C (PI-PLC). PI-PLC β1, β3, β4, γ1, and γ2, but not β2 and δ1, were detectable in FLO cells by Western blot analysis. Knockdown of PI-PLC-γ2 or ERK-2 MAP kinase with small interfering RNAs significantly decreases TDCA-induced NOX5-S expression, H_2O_2 production and cell proliferation. In contrast, knockdown of PI-PLC β1, β3, β4, γ1, or ERK-1 MAP kinase has no significant effect. TDCA significantly increases ERK-2 phosphorylation, an increase which is reduced by U73122 or PI-PLC-γ2 siRNA.[22]

These data indicate that TDCA-induced increase in cell proliferation depends on upregulation of NOX5-S expression in FLO cells. TDCA-induced NOX5-S expression may be mediated by sequential activation of the TGR5 receptor, Gαq protein, PI-PLCγ2, and ERK-2 MAP kinase in FLO cells (Fig. 2). It is possible that bile acid reflux present in BE patients may increase ROS production and cell proliferation via activation of TGR5, Gaq, PI-PLCγ2, ERK-2 MAP kinase, and NADPH oxidase NOX5-S, thereby contributing to the development of EAC. Thus, our data may provide potential targets to prevent and/or treat Barrett's EAC.

[These studies are supported by NIDDK R01 DK080703].

References

1. Orlando, R.C. 2004. Pathophysiology of gastroesophageal reflux disease: esophageal epithelial resistance. In: *The Esophagus*, D.O. Castell & J.E. Richter, Eds.: 421–433. Lippincott Williams & Wilkins. Philadelphia.

2. Tobey, N.A., Z. Djukic, L.E. Brighton, *et al.* Lateral cell membranes and shunt resistance in rabbit esophageal epithelium. *Dig. Dis. Sci.* **55:** 1856–1865.

3. Asaoka, D., H. Miwa, S. Hirai, *et al.* 2005. Altered localization and expression of tight-junction proteins in a rat model with chronic acid reflux esophagitis. *J. Gastroenterol.* **40:** 781–790.

4. Jovov, B.J., Z. Djukic, N.J. Shaheen, & R.C. Orlando. 2009. E-cadherin cleavage in GERD. *Gastroenterology* **136:** M1834.

5. Barlow, W.J. & R.C. Orlando. 2005. The pathogenesis of heartburn in nonerosive reflux disease: a unifying hypothesis. *Gastroenterology* **128:** 771–778.

6. Orlando, R.C. 2003. Pathogenesis of gastroesophageal reflux disease. *Am. J. Med. Sci.* **326:** 274–278.

7. Ma, J., K.M. Harnett, J. Behar, *et al.* 2010. Signaling in TRPV1-induced platelet activating factor (PAF) in human esophageal epithelial cells. *Am. J. Physiol. Gastrointest. Liver Physiol.* **298:** G233–G240.

8. Barclay, R.L., P.K. Dinda, G.P. Morris & W.G. Paterson. 1995. Morphological evidence of mast cell degranulation in an animal model of acid-induced esophageal mucosal injury. *Dig. Dis. Sci.* **40:** 1651–1658.

9. Paterson, W.G., C.A. Kieffer, M.J. Feldman, *et al.* 2007. Role of platelet-activating factor in acid-induced esophageal mucosal injury. *Dig. Dis. Sci.* **52:** 1861–1866.

10. Feldman, M.J., G.P. Morris, P.K. Dinda, & W.G. Paterson. 1996. Mast cells mediate acid-induced augmentation of opossum esophageal blood flow through a Histamine- and Nitric Oxide-dependent mechanism. *Gastroenterology* **110:** 121–128.

11. Cheng, L., S. de la Monte, J. Ma, *et al.* 2009. HCl-activated neural and epithelial vanilloid receptors (TRPV1) in cat esophageal mucosa. *Am. J. Physiol. Gastrointest. Liver Physiol.* **297:** G135–G143.

12. Ma, J., K.M. Harnett, J. Behar, *et al.* 2010. Signaling in TRPV1-induced platelet activating factor (PAF) in human esophageal epithelial cells. *Am. J. Physiol. Gastrointest. Liver Physiol.* **298:** G233–G240.

13. Ma, J., A. Altomare, S. De la Monte, *et al.* 2010. HCl-induced inflammatory mediators in esophageal mucosa increase migration and production of H2O2 by peripheral blood leukocytes. *Am. J. Physiol. Gastrointest. Liver Physiol.* **299:** G791–G798.

14. Modlin, I.M., R.H. Hunt, P. Malfertheiner, *et al.* 2009. Diagnosis and management of non-erosive reflux disease – the Vevey NERD Consensus Group. *Digestion* **80:** 74–88.

15. Emerenziani, S., D. Sifrim, F.I. Habib, *et al.* 2008. Presence of gas in the refluxate enhances reflux perception in nonerosive patients with physiological acid exposure of the oesophagus. *Gut* **57:** 443–447.

16. Caviglia, R., M. Ribolsi, M. Gentile, *et al.* 2007. Dilated intercellular spaces and acid reflux at the distal and proximal oesophagus in patients with non-erosive gastro-oesophageal reflux disease. *Aliment Pharmacol. Ther.* **25:** 629–636.

17. Guarino, M.P., L. Cheng, J. Ma, *et al.* 2010. Increased TRPV1 gene expression in esophageal mucosa of patients with non-erosive and erosive reflux disease. *Neurogastroenterol Motil* **22:** 746–751.

18. Hong, J., M. Resnick, J. Behar, *et al.* Acid-induced p16 hypermethylation contributes to development of esophageal adenocarcinoma via activation of NADPH oxidase NOX5-S. *Am. J. Physiol. Gastrointest. Liver Physiol.* **299:** G697–G6706.

19. Fu, X., D.G. Beer, J. Behar, *et al.*, 2006. cAMP-response element-binding protein mediates acid-induced NADPH oxidase NOX5-S expression in Barrett esophageal adenocarcinoma cells. *J. Biol. Chem.* **281:** 20368–20382.

20. Bernstein, H., C. Bernstein, C.M. Payne, *et al.* 2005. Bile acids as carcinogens in human gastrointestinal cancers. *Mutat. Res.* **589:** 47–65.

21. Hong, J., J. Behar, J. Wands, *et al.* Role of a novel bile acid receptor TGR5 in the development of oesophageal adenocarcinoma. *Gut* **59:** 170–180.

22. Hong, J., J. Behar, J. Wands, *et al.* Bile acid reflux contributes to development of esophageal adenocarcinoma via activation of phosphatidylinositol-specific phospholipase Cgamma2 and NADPH oxidase NOX5-S. *Cancer Res.* **70:** 1247–1255.

Ann. N.Y. Acad. Sci. ISSN 0077-8923

ANNALS OF THE NEW YORK ACADEMY OF SCIENCES

Issue: *Barrett's Esophagus: The 10th OESO World Congress Proceedings*

Esophageal disease and pathology

Melissa P. Upton,[1] Rish K. Pai,[2] Michael Vieth,[3] Helmut Neumann,[4] and Cord Langner[5]

[1]Rodger C. Haggitt Gastrointestinal and Hepatic Pathology Service, University of Washington, Seattle, Washington. [2]Department of Anatomic Pathology, Cleveland Clinic Foundation, Cleveland, Ohio. [3]Institute of Pathology, Klinikum Bayreuth, Bayreuth, Germany. [4]Medical Clinic I, University of Erlangen, Erlangen, Germany. [5]Institute of Pathology, Medical University Graz, Graz, Austria

The following on esophageal disease and pathology contains commentaries on the varied definitions of Barrett's esophagus (BE); the optimal biopsy strategy in BE; reliable biomarkers for progression to neoplasia in BE; and the role of bone marrow stem cells in the morphogenesis of Barrett's esophagus.

Keywords: Barrett's esophagus; goblet cells; practice guidelines; stem cells; biopsy strategy; progression; dysplasia; early detection research network; aneuploidy; p53; metaplasia; bone marrow; cancer stimulating cells

Concise summaries

- Pathologists continue to struggle with inadequate or superficial biopsies, biopsies that may not be labeled as to location in esophagus, increased risk of progression to neoplasia in columnar metaplasia without histologic findings of goblet cells, diagnostic procedures that are ready for use in routine pathology practice to identify patients at increased risk for neoplasia, and the opportunities for pathologists in OESO to collaborate in developing new diagnostic strategies, new practice guidelines and new consensus approaches.
- Only two biomarkers, DNA content abnormalities and p53, have been evaluated in prospective studies and the Early Detection Research Network. While biomarkers may be helpful in risk-stratifying BE patients, no biomarker can entirely replace grade of dysplasia. In most studies, the grade of dysplasia, despite its interobserver variability, is still the most sensitive marker of neoplastic risk.
- It is widely accepted that stem cells play a central role in the development of Barrett's esophagus (BE). However, the cell of origin involved in the transition from normal squamous epithelium into intestinal metaplasia has not yet been identified. Stem cells are now widely accepted to play a central role in the morphogenesis of BE. They may well be located below the squamous epithelium and may be activated after ulceration of the mucosal surface, but the source of these cells is not clear.

1. Controversies regarding the definition and terminology of Barrett's esophagus

Melissa P. Upton
mupton@u.washington.edu

In the spirit of full disclosure, I would like to share my personal experiences that drive my needs for specific answers. First, I represent patients. I myself am a patient with short-segment BE, no dysplasia, with DNA flow cytometry studies negative for aneuploidy or increased synthetic fraction; however, after I first received my diagnosis of BE, my life insurance premium tripled in cost, and I entered the system of regular surveillance.

Second, I represent the community of diagnostic pathologists. I am a practicing surgical pathologist with a specialty focus in gastrointestinal pathology, and my practice includes lots and lots of BE and its

doi: 10.1111/j.1749-6632.2011.06063.x

complications. In this role I am an educator, directing the training of pathology residents and fellows in GI pathology, and I also teach gastroenterology fellows.

In addition, our GI pathology group serves as regional consultants. University of Washington is the only academic medical center for the WWAMI region—Washington, Wyoming, Alaska, Montana, and Idaho, and we are a major referral center for pathology consultations, for endoscopic therapeutic interventions, for surgical treatment of complicated esophageal pathology, and for oncologic management of esophageal cancers. From my vantage point in these various roles, I ask our speakers and the audience to contemplate the following questions.

How do we take good care of patients with Barrett's esophagus?

Pathologists and clinicians need to identify people with real disease, identify people with risk factors to develop cancer, identify early neoplastic disease, and intervene to prevent complications. We need to be sure that the intervention and its complications are not worse than the disease. Our diagnostic procedures and therapeutic interventions must be cost-effective.

How can our decisions be informed by the history of BE?

The original description by Mr. Norman Barrett was columnar lining in tubular esophagus, and this definition is still used in a number of countries, including England and Japan. During the 1990s, the definition shifted in the U.S. to an emphasis on the finding of goblet cells, or "specialized columnar epithelium," as the diagnostic marker of increased risk for neoplasia. This change was based on mapping studies of esophagectomy specimens for adenocarcinoma, in which the great majority of patients with carcinomas had goblet cells detected in the regions of columnar metaplasia of the esophagus.

Currently, there are proposed revisions to this concept based on evidence of neoplasia arising in columnar lined esophagus without identifiable goblet cells.[1,2] There is a preliminary report that the upcoming American Gastroenterological Association Institute's technical review on BE recommendation will include the following statement: "Barrett's esophagus should now be defined as 'the condition in which any extent of metaplastic columnar epithelium that predisposes to cancer development replaces the stratified squamous epithelium that normally lines the distal esophagus'."[3]

But, what is the role of goblet cells in the development of neoplasia in BE?

I hope to learn how we should report findings on biopsies and EMRs, how we should report and diagnose goblet cells at the GEJ, and whether we need new practice guidelines in pathology. How should our clinical colleagues act on or interpret our reports?

A suggestion for reporting

I propose the use of specific descriptors in our pathology reports. We should list the types of epithelium seen in biopsies: goblet cells, cardiac-type, cardio-fundic type, fundic type, squamous, multilayered epithelium, etc. If a biopsy or endoscopic mucosal resection specimen is clearly from the esophagus with any columnar type other than goblet cells, we should use the descriptor "columnar metaplasia of esophagus without goblet cells seen." Features that allow us to locate a specimen as esophageal include the presence of submucosal glands and/or their ducts, the presence of squamous mucosa, and the presence of duplicated muscularis mucosae.[4,5]

Changing horses in the middle of the road?

In North America, do we continue to use "BE" only when goblet cells are identified? If we shift to using "BE" to comprise any esophageal columnar metaplasia, how do we communicate the change in terminology to our clinicians and our colleagues?

What is the optimal biopsy strategy?

Some pathologists continue to struggle with inadequate or superficial biopsies, and biopsies may not be labeled as to location in esophagus. What clinical information do we need from clinicians to optimize our reports and to optimize care? How do we build more effective collaborations with our clinical colleagues to improve the quality of practice, with respect to biopsy quality, biopsy protocol, and clinical-pathologic correlation?

Other questions to be addressed by our community

Are there biomarkers that indicate increased risk of progression to neoplasia in columnar metaplasia without histologic findings of goblet cells? Are there stains or diagnostic procedures that are ready for use in routine pathology practice to identify patients at increased risk for neoplasia? What is known about the progenitor cells for BE? Can a stem cell population be defined?

Finally, are there opportunities for pathologists in OESO to collaborate in developing new diagnostic strategies, new practice guidelines, and new consensus approaches? This multidisciplinary international organization offers unique opportunities for discussion and for developing common approaches and practice guidelines. I hope that the questions raised form the basis for future collaborative approaches that can both advance knowledge and improve the care of our patients.

2. What is the role of nonmorphologic biomarkers in Barrett's esophagus?

Rish K. Pai

pair@ccf.org

BE affects approximately 1.5% of the developing world and significantly increases the risk of EAC. Current management of BE is governed primarily by the grade of dysplasia. However, many patients with nondysplastic BE and those with low-grade dysplasia (LGD) may never progress to high-grade dysplasia (HGD) or EAC. Screening these patients is endoscopically intensive and costly. Developing biomarkers that can predict those patients that progress to HGD and EAC is an attractive solution to this problem.

The Early Detection Research Network has proposed five phases of validation before a biomarker is ready for clinical use. The biomarker must be validated first in retrospective studies and then in prospective screening studies. The impact of the biomarker on reducing the burden of disease in a population must then be evaluated. So far only two biomarkers have been evaluated in prospective studies, DNA content abnormalities and p53.

In 2000, Reid *et al.* evaluated the ability of DNA content abnormalities (aneuploidy and increased tetraploidy) to predict progression in BE patients with varying grades of dysplasia.[6]

DNA content abnormalities were identified in 81 patients of whom 29 progressed to EAC. However, 12 of 241 patients without DNA content abnormalities also progressed to EAC. Furthermore, nine of 247 patients with LGD, indefinite for dysplasia, or nondysplastic BE progressed to EAC, and

a DNA content abnormality was only detected in six of nine. Thus, screening only those patients with DNA content abnormalities would miss a substantial percentage of progressors.

A follow-up study by Reid *et al.* evaluated 17p loss of heterozygosity (LOH), the chromosomal location of *TP53*, in a similar cohort of patients.[7] The relative risk of development of EAC in patients with 17p LOH was 16, indicating that this is a good marker of progression. However, of the 23 patients with either LGD, indefinite for dysplasia, or no dysplasia who progressed to HGD or EAC, only five had 17p LOH.

A prospective study by Weston *et al.* in 2004 screened 48 patients with LGD for abnormal p53 expression by immunohistochemistry in their baseline biopsies.[8] Although those with abnormal p53 expression were more likely to progress to multifocal HGD or EAC (3 of 10), 2 of 38 patients without abnormal p53 expression at baseline also progressed. The two patients with absent p53 expression who progressed did have abnormal p53 expression in subsequent biopsies; however, this raises the important question of when to test for the biomarker. If a biomarker needs to be tested frequently, then its utility in clinical practice will be limited as it will impose an extra cost burden without significantly decreasing screening.

More recently, Galipeau *et al.* demonstrated that the presence of multiple molecular abnormalities confers the greatest risk of progression to EAC; however, 3 of 85 patients with no molecular abnormality at baseline still progressed to EAC.[9] Maley *et al.* performed an exciting study in 2006 in which multiple biomarkers were measured along the length of a BE segment.[10] A map of clones along the BE segment was then generated. In this study, increased clonal diversity was associated with an increased risk of progression. Based on these studies, it is likely that a panel of biomarkers may be necessary to appropriately risk stratify patients.

Despite the significant advancement in biomarker research in BE, there are some limitations.

In most studies, grade of dysplasia, despite its interobserver variability, is still the most sensitive marker of neoplastic risk. Specificity of dysplasia as a marker of progression can be improved by consulting another pathologist with expertise in gastrointestinal pathology. New biomarkers such as those that measure epigenetic changes as well as a panel of biomarkers may improve sensitivity and specificity.

In summary, while biomarkers may be helpful in risk-stratifying BE patients, no biomarker can entirely replace grade of dysplasia.

3. The role of bone marrow-derived stem cells in Barrett's esophagus

Michael Vieth, Helmut Neumann, and Cord Langner
Vieth.LKPathol@uni-bayreuth.de

The morphogenesis of BE has not been fully elucidated until now. Several theories are available on the topic:

(1) BE derives from gastric epithelium.
(2) BE derives from cardiac epithelium.
(3) BE derives from esophageal glands.
(4) BE derives from esophageal stem cells.

It is now widely accepted that stem cells play a central role in the development of BE. Unfortunately, however, the cell of origin involved in the transition from normal squamous epithelium into intestinal metaplasia has not yet been identified.[11] For a long time it was believed that squamous cell epithelium cannot transdifferentiate into columnar epithelium based on the analysis of keratin patterns.[12] Recent publications, however, indicate that cultures of human esophageal squamous cells treated with bone morphogenic proteins (BMP4) express keratins characteristic for columnar cells.[13] Not necessarily all cultured cells need to be affected by this treatment. Consequently, there will be mechanisms to reverse maturation towards multipotential stem cells that can differentiate into various cell types or that stem cells harvested within the culture experiments can be activated through treatment of BMP4.

Even if it is now widely accepted that stem cells are involved, it is not clear where these stem cells can be found, for example:

(1) within the basal cell layer,
(2) within the ducts of proper esophageal glands, or
(3) directly from the bone marrow homing in the esophagus.

Several signaling pathways are involved: Wnt, Notch, sonic hedgehog, BMP, and TGFß. Moreover, it is known that there is a response to gastric acid, bile acid, or both, and that the activity within the

stem cell population leads to BE.[14] From the stomach we know that cancer may originate directly from multipotential bone marrow-derived stem cells, but also that so-called side populations play a role in the tumor-initiating sequence. Furthermore, it has been suggested that fusion cells between bone marrow-derived stem cells and intestinal epithelium may play a central role during tumor initiation and progression.[15]

Unlike the situation in many other tumors, it was not possible to demonstrate that surface antigens previously established as cancer stimulating cell markers enrich for tumor-initiating cells in esophageal adenocarcinoma.[11] Behind all these theories, it has to be realized why these stem cell concepts are so attractive for the development and progression of Barrett's epithelium:

(1) Bone marrow stem cells are self-renewing.
(2) They can differentiate into various types of (tumor) cells.
(3) They express markers indicating multipotent capacity.
(4) They can give rise to teratomas with all three germ layers.
(5) They may be related to multiple forms of cancer stem cells.

The role, however, of bone marrow-derived stem cells in the development and progression of BE is not fully understood.

In conclusion, stem cells are now widely accepted to play a central role in the morphogenesis of BE. They may well be located below the squamous epithelium and may be activated after ulceration of the mucosal surface. The source of these stem cells, however, is not clear: they may be dormant (local) cells or may be attracted directly from the bone marrow. Evidence for the latter hypothesis is, however, currently lacking and it does not appear justified to transfer data obtained from gastric and/or colon cell experiments to BE at the moment. The role of fusion cells between intestinal epithelium and bone marrow-derived cells remains speculative. Future experimental evidence is warranted.

Conflicts of interest

The authors declare no conflicts of interest.

References

1. Takubo, K., J. Aida, Y. Naomoto, *et al.* 2009. Cardiac rather than intestinal-type background in endoscopic resection

specimens of minute Barrett adenocarcinoma. *Hum. Pathol.* **40:** 65–74.

2. Maru, D. 2009. Barrett's esophagus: diagnostic challenges and recent developments. *Ann. Diagn. Pathol.* **13:** 212–221.

3. Spechler, J.S., R.C. Fitzgerald, G.A. Prasad, & K.K. Wang. 2010. History, molecular mechanisms, and endoscopic treatment of Barrett's Esophagus. *Gastroenterology* **138:** 854–869.

4. Takubo, K., K. Sasa, K. Yamashita, *et al.* 1991. Double muscularis mucosae in Barrett esophagus. *Hum. Pathol.* **22:** 1158–1161.

5. Srivastava, A., R.D. Odze , G.Y. Lauwers, *et al.* 2007. Morphologic features are useful in distinguishing Barrett esophagus from carditis with intestinal metaplasia. *Am. J. Surg. Pathol.* **31:** 1733–1741.

6. Reid, B.J., D.S. Levine, G. Longton, *et al.* 2000. Predictors of progression to cancer in Barrett's esophagus: baseline histology and flow cytometry identify low- and high-risk patient subsets. *Am. J. Gastroenterol.* **95:** 1669–1676.

7. Reid, B.J. *et al.* 2001. Predictors of progression in Barrett's esophagus II: baseline 17p (p53) loss of heterozygosity identifies a patient subset at increased risk for neoplastic progression. *Am. J. Gastroenterol.* **96:** 2839–2848.

8. Weston, A.P. *et al.* 2001. p53 protein overexpression in low grade dysplasia (LGD) in Barrett's esophagus: immunohistochemical marker predictive of progression. *Am. J. Gastroenterol.* **96:** 1355–1362.

9. Galipeau, P.C. *et al.* 2007. NSAIDs modulate CDKN2A, TP53, and DNA content risk for progression to esophageal adenocarcinoma. *PLoS Med* **4:** e67.

10. Maley, C.C. *et al.* 2006. Genetic clonal diversity predicts progression to esophageal adenocarcinoma. *Nat. Genet* **38:** 468–473.

11. Grotenhuis, B.A., W.N. Dinjens, B.P. Wijnhoven, *et al.* 2010. Barrett's oesophageal adenocarcinoma encompasses tumour-initiating cells that do not express common cancer stem cell markers. *J. Pathol.* **221:** 379–389.

12. Bechmann, S., M. Vieth, M. Stolte & R. Moll. 2003. Cytokeratins and cell-cell adhesion molecules in Barrett's esophagus: implications for its histogenesis. *Pathol. Res. Pract.* **199:** 268–269.

13. Milano, F., J.W. van Baal, N.S. Buttar, *et al.* 2007. Bone morphogenetic protein 4 expressed in esophagitis induces a columnar phenotype in esophageal squamous cells. *Gastroenterology* **132:** 2412–2421.

14. Peters, J.H. & N. Avisar. 2010. The molecular pathogenesis of Barrett's esophagus: common signaling pathways in embryogenesis metaplasia and neoplasia. *J. Gastrointest. Surg.* **14**(Suppl 1)**:** S81–S87.

15. Rizvi, A.Z., J.R. Swain, P.S. Davies, *et al.* 2006. Bone marrow-derived cells fuse with normal and transformed intestinal stem cells. *Proc. Natl. Acad. Sci. U S A* **103:** 6321–6325.

Ann. N.Y. Acad. Sci. ISSN 0077-8923

ANNALS OF THE NEW YORK ACADEMY OF SCIENCES

Issue: *Barrett's Esophagus: The 10th OESO World Congress Proceedings*

Molecular mechanisms of Barrett's esophagus and adenocarcinoma

Katerina Dvorak,[1,2] Aaron Goldman,[2] Jianping Kong,[3] John P. Lynch,[3] Lloyd Hutchinson,[4] Jean Marie Houghton,[4] Hao Chen,[5] Xiaoxin Chen,[5] Kausilia K. Krishnadath,[6] and Wytske M. Westra[6]

[1]Department of Cell Biology and Anatomy, College of Medicine, Tucson, Arizona. [2]Arizona Cancer Center, The University of Arizona, Tucson, Arizona. [3]Division of Gastroenterology, University of Pennsylvania, Philadelphia, Pennsylvania. [4]Division of Gastroenterology, Department of Medicine, University of Massachusetts Medical School, Worcester, Massachusetts. [5]Julius L. Chambers Biomedical/Biotechnology Research Institute, North Carolina Central University, Durham, North Carolina. [6]Department of Gastroenterology and Hepatology, Academic Medical Center, Amsterdam, The Netherlands

The following on molecular mechanisms of Barrett's esophagus and adenocarcinoma contains commentaries on the mechanism of bile and gastric acid induced damage; the roles of BMP-4 and CDX-2 in the development of intestinal metaplasia; the transcription factors driving intestinalization in Barrett's esophagus; the contribution of bone marrow to metaplasia and adenocarcinoma; activation and inactivation of transcription factors; and a novel study design targeting molecular pathways in Barrett's esophagus.

Keywords: ablation; Barrett's esophagus; incomplete ablation; DNA damage; CDX-2 transcription factor; *Helicobacter felis*; adenocarcinoma; signaling pathways; BMP-4; metaplasia; sonic hedgehog; noggin

Concise summaries

- In response to increased acidification and the associated DNA damage, normal esophageal cells may overexpress proteins that regulate pH to manage the chronic acid overload. Metaplastic change of the normal epithelium to Barrett's esophagus (BE) may be an adaptive process to regulate intracellular pH after exposure to acid and bile acids, which activate isoforms of nitric oxide synthase (NOS), leading to an increased nitric oxide production and partial inhibition of Na^+/H^+ exchangers (NHE). This consequently results in increased acidification and DNA damage, which may lead to mutations and cancer progression.

- Recent microarray studies have focused on the possibility that BE emerges from stem cells for the squamous epithelium, showing that the BE profile was as similar to the normal esophagus as it was to the small intestine, suggesting possibly a keratinocyte origin and possible relation of metaplasia to ectopic expression of the CDX-2

transcription factor in the esophageal keratinocytes. However, CDX-2 expression alone is not sufficient to induce the development of BE when ectopically expressed in the squamous esophagus; it likely requires the cooperation of other genetic factors and epigenetic alterations for the induction of complete BE identity.

- Studies using both a mouse surgical model of disease and human specimens have shown that bone marrow-derived cells have the ability to repopulate epithelial structures, raising the possibility of their contribution to mucosal disease. Bone marrow-derived cells can generate cancer-associated fibroblasts as well as contribute directly to epithelial cells in cancer of the esophagus and may shed light on signaling pathways essential for growth and survival of esophageal tumor cells, and may identify new targets for therapy.

- Organotypic cell culture is a promising method for investigating how transcription factors may modulate cellular behaviors, morphology, and gene expression. Nevertheless, the most critical

doi: 10.1111/j.1749-6632.2011.06062.x

evidence should come from *in vivo* models. Although mice remain the first choice in most labs, other animals, such as pigs, zebrafish may have certain unique features that may be used to address specific research questions and genetic manipulation of multiple transcription factors.

- Recent studies have shown that multilayered epithelium is a transitional stage in the metaplastic conversion of squamous to columnar epithelium in BE, but also suggested that loss of squamous transcription factors preceded gain of intestinal transcription factors in this process.

- Multiple molecular pathways and factors are known to contribute to BE, and trans-differentiation or metaplasia is mediated by activation or inactivation of transcription factors, which further regulate their target genes specific for certain cellular functions.

- Transcription of several intestine specific genes, such as Mucin 2, Villin, which are found in BE, are mediated by the caudal related homeobox gene CDX-2 and this factor is highly expressed in SIE/BE. The development of BE should be considered a multistep process, in which there may be an initial dedifferentiation of squamous epithelial cells into nonspecialized type of columnar epithelium that is BMP-4 mediated, subsequently followed by dedifferentiation into BE induced through a collaborative interaction of BMP4, a member of the TGF-β family, with CDX-2.

- An important observation in *ex vivo* studies is that the effect of BMP-4 could be inhibited by its natural antagonist Noggin, and the key aim of experimental studies has been to investigate whether Noggin can reverse the development of intestinal metaplasia.

- Noggin is a highly promising candidate as an inhibitor for the BMP-pathway, thus giving sense to the study of its effect on eradication of experimental intestinal metaplasia.

1. Novel mechanism of bile acid-induced DNA damage in Barrett's esophagus

Aaron Goldman and Katerina Dvorak
kdvorak@email.arizona.edu

Although the exact pathogenesis of BE is unclear, this lesion appears to be associated with chronic reflux of gastric acid and bile. It has been proposed that metaplastic intestinal tissue that replaces normal esophageal squamous epithelium is better adapted to noxious components of refluxate.[1] Gastric acid alone causes intracellular acidification, DNA hydrolysis and loss of purines and pyrimidines. These apurinic/apyrimidinic sites cause genomic instability by imperfect base excision repair, which is linked to carcinogenesis.

One of many protective measures evolved by cells to regulate intracellular pH is the extrusion of protons from the cytoplasm, mediated by the family of NHE. This transporter is a ubiquitously expressed protein found in multiple isoforms to regulate the intracellular pH (pH_i) and other physiological processes in mammalian cells including the gastrointestinal tract.[2] In addition, NHE expression in patients with gastroesophageal reflux disease (GERD) is higher compared to normal individuals

and is likely involved in the ability of BE to tolerate repeated exposure to acid.

The other major component of gastroesophageal reflux, bile acids, elicit carcinogenic effects by inducing proliferation through activation of different receptors and pathways, such as the epidermal growth factor receptor (EGFR), p38 and MAP kinase pathway, and repeated exposure to sublethal concentrations of hydrophobic bile acids, leads to apoptosis resistance. In addition, hydrophobic bile acids induce the production of reactive oxygen species (ROS) and nitric oxide (NO), which is associated with DNA damage.[3] Indeed, NOS, an enzyme responsible for NO production, is increased as BE tissue progresses from nondysplastic lesions to EAC. All isoforms of this enzyme can be hyperactivated following phosphorylation. Interestingly, previous reports show that NO has the ability to inhibit NHE activity via an unclear mechanism resulting in increased acidification.

Our recent *in vitro* studies elucidated the effects of bile acids and acid on intracellular pH and DNA damage, which is mediated by NO and NHE inhibition. Studies have elucidated that bile acids increase the protein levels of NOS and NO, which is responsible for DNA damage. It was speculated that

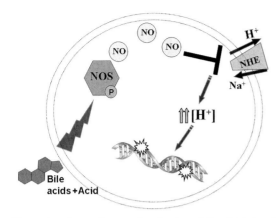

Figure 1. Scheme of proposed mechanism of bile acid–induced acidification.

inducible NOS (iNOS) is activated by transcription factor NF-κB hours after exposure to bile acids.[3] However, only recently has it been shown that bile acids induce an immediate phosphorylation and hyperactivation of all three isoforms of NOS, and the cell immediately experiences an increase in nitric oxide levels.[4] Concurrently, bile acids induce bicarbonate excretion and cell acidification. Furthermore, as a consequence, nitric oxide partially shuts down acid extrusion via NHE inhibition. This results in sequestration of intracellular acid. This effect is amplified when bile acids are combined with an acidic environment, mimicking reflux. Accordingly, with a precipitous drop in intracellular pH, there is a directly proportional increase in acid-mediated DNA damage—150% increase compared to acid alone[4] (Fig. 1 depicts this proposed mechanism).

In response to increased acidification and the associated DNA damage, normal esophageal cells may overexpress proteins that regulate pH to manage the chronic acid overload. In fact, it was identified that the NHE isoform 1 (NHE1) is an important NHE isoform expressed in BE tissues and BE-derived cells.[4] This finding strengthens the notion that metaplastic change of the normal epithelium to BE may be an adaptive process to regulate intracellular pH after exposure to acid and bile acids.

In summary, the results of this study identify a new mechanism of bile acid induced DNA damage. Our data suggest that bile acids present in the refluxate activate immediately all three isoforms of NOS, which leads to an increased NO production and partial NHE inhibition. This consequently re-

sults in increased acidification and DNA damage, which may lead to mutations and cancer progression. Therefore, we propose that in addition to gastric reflux, bile reflux should also be controlled in BE patients.

2. Ectopic expression of transcription factors drive intestinalization in Barrett's esophagus

Jianping Kong and John P. Lynch
lynchj@mail.med.upenn.edu

BE is the replacement of normal squamous mucosa of the esophagus with a specialized intestinal metaplasia. It typically arises in the setting of chronic GERD. BE is endoscopically recognizable as a patch of salmon-colored mucosa located at the gastroesophageal junction, and the diagnosis is confirmed by biopsy.[5] BE not only adopts an intestinal cell morphology, the gene expression pattern is similar to intestinal epithelium as well.

The molecular mechanisms underlying BE's pathogenesis are not well understood, nor is the cell of origin for BE known. Presently, there are four candidate cells of origin for BE:

(1) migration of cells from the gastric cardia or at the squamo-columnar junction;

(2) altered differentiation and lineage selection of esophageal squamous cells and stem cells;

(3) migration of cells from esophageal submucosal glands; and

(4) cells are of bone marrow origin.[1]

Although there are published reports with experimental data in support of each of the four candidates, our studies have focused on the possibility that BE emerges from stem cells for the squamous epithelium. Microarray studies comparing gene expression profiles from BE, normal esophagus, and normal intestinal epithelium determined, surprisingly, that the BE profile was as similar to the normal esophagus as it was to the small intestine, suggesting possibly a keratinocyte origin.[6]

Moreover, early during embryogenesis, the gut is lined by ciliated columnar cells that later differentiate into the multilayered squamous epithelium. Studies have demonstrated that this early ciliated epithelium can adopt alternative cell fates if co-cultured with mesenchyme from other regions or with the altered expression of certain transcription factors including Sox2 and p63.[1] This early plasticity is observed rarely in adult human tissues, when islands of squamous metaplasia are found in resected adenomatous polyps.[7]

We therefore sought to model BE metaplasia by ectopic expression of the Cdx2 (CDX-2) transcription factor in the esophageal keratinocytes. Cdx2 is an intestine-specific transcription factor that is ectopically expressed in BE but its role in this process is unclear. In previously reported work, we established retroviral-mediated Cdx2 expression in immortalized human esophageal keratinocytes.[8] We noted a profound repression of cell proliferation that could be rescued by cylin D1 but not a mutant p53. Cdx2 expression alone did not induce intestinalization. However, treatment with 5-aza-2-deoxycytidine (5-AzaC) to demethylate epigenetically silenced genes did lead to the expression of multiple Cdx2 target genes, including markers of intestinal differentiation and markers of BE. We concluded that ectopic proliferation signals and alterations in epigenetic gene regulation are required for Cdx2-mediated intestinalization of human esophageal keratinocytes in BE.

More recently, we have developed a novel murine transgenic model that ectopically expresses Cdx2 in esophageal basal keratinocytes using the cytokeratin-14 (K14) promoter. RT-PCR and Western blotting showed ectopic expression of Cdx2 in the epithelium of the esophagus, squamous forestomach, and other squamous tissues including the tongue. The morphology of the basal layer cells was significantly altered with Cdx2 expression. Cells became elongated in appearance. Moreover, there appeared to be more cells along the basal layer in the transgenic mice when compared to the wild-type littermate controls. Basal keratinocyte proliferation was diminished by 50% in the Cdx2 transgenic mice. By transmission electron microscopy, we observed diminished cell–cell adhesion, and the induction of a secretory cell ultrastructure marked by reduced keratin bundles and increased numbers of intracellular vesicles. This was confirmed by immunofluorescence and immunohistochemical studies demonstrating severely reduced DSC3 protein levels and increased endoplasmic reticulum proteins.

Finally, injection of these mice with 5-AzaC lead to the induction of Cdx2 target genes in the esophagus of the K14–Cdx2 mice and not controls. We conclude Cdx2 expression alone is not sufficient to induce the development of BE when ectopically expressed in the squamous esophagus. Cdx2 likely requires the cooperation of other genetic factors and epigenetic alterations for the induction of complete BE identity.

3. Bone marrow contribution to Barrett's metaplasia and cancer

Lloyd Hutchinson and Jean Marie Houghton
jeanmarie.houghton@umassmed.edu

The notion that bone marrow-derived cells (BMDC) could contribute to peripheral tissues began about 10 years ago and was rapidly followed by substantial controversy and skepticism. At that time, it was observed that cells originating from the bone marrow could be found within solid organs as epithelial, fibroblast, endothelial, and fat cells.[9,10]

It was debated initially (and to some degree is still debated) if the bone marrow cells responsible for this phenotype were various lineage-specific progenitor cells or a more pluripotent stem cell. The contribution that BMDCs make under physiologic conditions is minimal, and indeed several reports fail to find any contribution at all.[11]

For the most part, BMDC can be seen at increased numbers when there is concomitant injury and inflammation. It is thought the influx of these cells into injured tissues may be a reparative attempt by the body, however, if this is the case, it represents a short-term healing attempt, because cells are usually found as terminally differentiated cells and as such are short lived within the tissue. However, in some situations, BMDC may be found within the stem cell niche of peripheral tissues and function as peripheral stem cells. In this capacity, these BMDC have the potential to clonally repopulate tissue. This ability to repopulate epithelial structures raises the possibility of BMDC contributing to mucosal disease.

There is a strong association between inflammation, chronic tissue injury/repair, and cancer. It therefore seemed logical to pursue a role for BMDC and cancer. Previous studies from our laboratory using a mouse model of *H. felis*-induced gastric cancer has demonstrated that gastric cancer is derived from bone marrow cells.[12] Our laboratory has a broad interest in GI malignancies, and we have expanded our initial studies to include other areas of the

E-Cadherin	Alpha -SMA	CD31	CD45

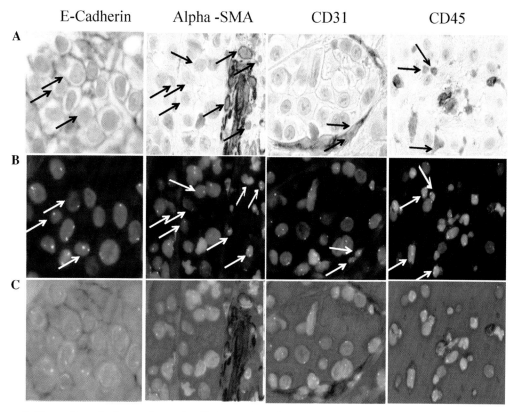

Figure 2. Human Barrett's adenocarcinoma. Specific immunohistochemistry and X/Y FISH analysis performed in tandem on the same slide. Immunohistochemistry as indicated, X (green) and Y (red) FISH followed by an overlay for each grouping. Epithelial cells stained with anti-E cadherin antibody, fibroblast cells within the stroma are stained with antibody against alpha smooth muscle actin, endothelial cells are stained with antibody directed against CD31, and leukocytes are stained with anti-CD45. Arrows point out 1×0Y and 2×0Y cells (from Ref. 13).

luminal digestive tract including adenocarcinoma of the esophagus.

The aim of this study[13] was to examine the contribution of BMDC to the stroma and the epithelium of Barrett's associated adenocarcinoma of the esophagus using both a mouse surgical model of disease and human specimens. Transplantation of bone marrow expressing β-galactosidase into a wild-type mouse, followed by surgical esophago-jejunostomy, allowed tracking of BMDCs into the surgical anastomosis and into resulting Barrett's metaplasia. Mice developed hard fixed and nonul-cerated exophytic lesions at the anastomotic site. Microscopically, these lesions were composed of columnar epithelium with markedly distorted gland structures, loss of nuclear polarity, and altered nu-clear to cytoplasmic ratio. These areas of columnar metaplasia were surrounded by stratified squamous epithelium, consistent with Barrett's metaplasia in

the mouse model. Immunohistochemistry (IHC) directed against bacterial β-galactosidase revealed donor-derived inflammatory cells within the esophagus, directly underlying metaplastic tissue and donor derived adipose cells within periglan-dular stroma. Interestingly, roughly half of the Barrett's glands contained β-galactosidase express-ing epithelial cells found in groups of three to four cells within glands, and never comprising entire glands. β-galactosidase and E-cadherin IHC were colocalized, thus confirming the epithelial pheno-type of the beta galactosidase positive cells. BMDC were found in clumps of two to three contiguous cells within the mouse Barrett's metaplastic glands rather than entire glands derived from a BM source.

This is consistent with the recent finding from human studies that demonstrate glands within Bar-rett's metaplasia contain more than one stem cell giving rise to "ribbons" of daughter cells up the length of the gland, and over time, presumably one dominant stem cell prevails. Human tissue from a male patient who had been transplanted with female bone marrow and later developed esophageal adenocarcinoma (EAC) allowed us to tract donor-derived cells into the tumor. X/Y FISH combined with specific lineage staining directed against epithelial, fibroblast, endothelial, and leukocyte markers confirm that, similar to the animal model, bone marrow cells contribute to both the epithelial and stromal component of EAC in humans (Fig. 2).

These findings demonstrate that BMDCs can generate cancer-associated fibroblasts as well as contribute directly to epithelial cells in cancer of the esophagus and may shed light on signaling pathways essential for growth and survival of esophageal tumor cells, and may identify new targets for therapy.

4. Inactivation of squamous transcription factors and activation of intestinal transcription factors in Barrett's esophagus

Hao Chen and Xiaoxin Chen
lchen@nccu.edu

In theory, metaplastic conversion of esophageal squamous epithelium into intestinalized columnar epithelium may develop in two distinct mechanisms. One possibility is direct conversion of differentiated cells, a process called *transdifferentiation.* Alternatively, it may develop from altered differentiation of esophageal *stem cells.* In general, the stem cell theory is favored by most researchers, although up to now there is no solid experimental evidence to exclude the possibility of transdifferentiation.

There are four potential cellular origins of BE in humans, each supported by experimental evidence:[14]

(a) *Stem cells of squamous epithelium* in the basal cell layer may undergo *de novo* metaplasia. The resulting metaplastic change produces stem cells for future BE.

(b) *Stem cells at the gastroesophageal junction* or transitional zone may colonize the gastric cardia or distal esophagus in response to noxious luminal contents.

(c) *Stem cells in the neck of the esophageal submucosal gland duct* may colonize the esophagus

after mucosal damage of the squamous epithelium takes place.

(d) *Bone marrow–derived stem cells* may migrate to the esophagus when there is inflammation or damage, and undergo metaplasia.

To understand the potential molecular mechanism of BE, we have recently analyzed three microarray data sets and one SAGE data set with SAM and SAGE(Poisson) to identify individual genes differentially expressed in BE. GSEA was used to identify *a priori* defined sets of genes that were differentially expressed. These gene sets were either grouped according to certain signaling pathways (GSEA curated), or the presence of consensus binding sequences of known transcription factors (GSEA motif). Immunostaining was then used to validate differential gene expression.

Both SAM and SAGE(Poisson) identified 68 differentially expressed genes with an arbitrary cutoff ratio ($\geq$4-fold). Besides individual genes, the TGF-β pathway and several transcription factors (Cdx2, HNF1, and HNF4) were identified by GSEA as enriched pathways and motifs in BE. Apart from nine target genes known to be upregulated in BE, immunostaining confirmed upregulation of 19 additional Cdx1/Cdx2 target genes in BE. These data suggested an important role of Cdx2 in the development of BE. The list of differentially expressed genes may serve as leads for elucidation of the molecular mechanism of BE.[15] In addition, using a cutoff ratio of twofold, we found upregulation of a group of intestinal transcription factors (e.g., HNF1α, HNF3α, HNF3β, HNF3γ, HNF4α, GATA4, GATA6, Sox9, Math1, POU5F1, TCF7L2, KLF4, SPDEF, Gfi1) and downregulation of a group of squamous transcription factors (e.g., P63, Sox2, Pax9) (unpublished data).

In another study[16] on the multilayered epithelium in a surgical rat model and humans, tissue sections were immunostained for transcription factors and differentiation markers of esophageal squamous epithelium and intestinal columnar epithelium. As expected, both rat and human squamous epithelium, but not intestinal metaplasia, expressed squamous transcription factors and differentiation markers (P63, Sox2, CK14, and CK4). Rat and human intestinal metaplasia, but not squamous epithelium, expressed intestinal transcription factors and differentiation markers (Cdx2, GATA4, HNF1α, villin, and Muc2). Our data not only supported the

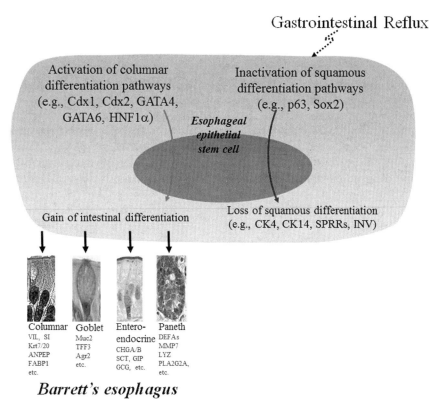

Figure 3. Inactivation of squamous transcription factors and activation of intestinal transcription factors in the development of Barrett's esophagus. Representative differentiation markers are listed under each cell lineage.

concept that multilayered epithelium is a transitional stage in the metaplastic conversion of squamous to columnar epithelium in BE, but also suggested that loss of squamous transcription factors preceded gain of intestinal transcription factors in this process.[16]

Based on these data, we propose the following mechanism of BE: when esophageal epithelial stem cells are stimulated by gastroesophageal reflux, the squamous differentiation pathway may be inactivated through inactivation of squamous transcription factors. Meanwhile, the columnar differentiation pathway may be activated through activation of intestinal transcription factors. These molecular events may lead to loss of squamous differentiation and gain of columnar differentiation. As a result, four major cell lineages of BE (columnar, Paneth, enteroendocrine, goblet) appear in the esophagus as BE (Fig. 3).[17]

This idea is consistent with a well-accepted theory that transdifferentiation or metaplasia is mediated by activation or inactivation of transcription factors, which further regulate their target genes specific for certain cellular functions.[18] We emphasize both the squamous and the intestinal aspects in the development of BE. Recent unpublished data of Cdx2 transgenic models (John Lynch's group and our group) provided additional support for this idea, because overexpression of Cdx2 alone failed to produce intestinal metaplasia in both mice and zebrafish.

Because multiple molecular pathways and factors are known to contribute to BE, it is quite challenging to assemble all pieces of this puzzle. We believe these pathways may act through the previously mentioned transcription factors. Indeed, it is known that TGF-β/BMP pathway interacts with Cdx1 and Cdx2 through SMADs and modulates expression of Sox9. WNT pathway regulates expression of Cdx1, Cdx2, Math1, and Sox9. NF-κB pathway, when activated, upregulates expression of Cdx1 and Cdx2. Notch pathway regulates expression of Math1 and interacts with Cdx2. The Hedgehog pathway induces expression of stromal Bmp4 and epithelial Sox9 in mouse esophagus. Retinoic acid alone or in synergy with the WNT pathway activates Cdx1, HNF1α, HNF4α, GATA4, and Sox9.

To elucidate how transcription factors, either alone or in combination, may contribute to BE, several model systems can be utilized. Organotypic cell culture is a promising method for investigating how transcription factors may modulate cellular behaviors, morphology, and gene expression. *Ex vivo* organ culture may allow development of metaplastic cell lineages in the esophagus through genetic manipulations. Nevertheless, the most critical evidence should come from *in vivo* models. Nonkeratinization of the esophageal squamous epithelium, presence of submucosal glands, availability of proper transgenic and knockout techniques and tools, and cost of maintenance, are all important issues for consideration.

Although mice remain the first choice in most labs, other animals may have certain unique features that may be used to address specific research questions. For example, pig esophagus is very similar to human esophagus in anatomy. Disease progression in pigs can be monitored by endoscopy and biopsy for pathological and molecular analyses. Recent development of a cystic fibrosis model in pigs suggested that pig models may better mimic human diseases than mouse models. In zebrafish pharynx, there is a short piece of nonkeratinized stratified squamous epithelium, which is very similar to human esophageal squamous epithelium. Genetic manipulation is more convenient and economic in zebrafish than in mice. This feature would be very significant if we consider genetic manipulation of multiple transcription factors in the same animals.

5. Novel insights in the development of intestinal type of epithelium or Barrett's esophagus: the collaborative roles of BMP-4 and CDX-2 in the development of intestinal metaplasia

Kausilia K. Krishnadath
k.k.krishnadath@amc.uva.nl

The role of BMP-4

We earlier demonstrated that BMP-4 is involved in the process of dedifferentiation of squamous epithelial cells into a nonspecialized type of columnar epithelium (NSCE), but not into the specialized intestinal type of epithelium that is more typical for BE.[19] It is known that transcription of several intestine specific genes, such as Mucin 2 (MUC-2), Villin, and many others, which are found in BE,[20] are mediated by the caudal-related homeobox gene CDX-2, and that this factor is highly expressed in SIE/BE.[21–24]

Whether CDX-2 mediates dedifferentiation into BE is however unclear.[25] Here, we hypothesized that NSCE that is induced by BMP-4 may further dedifferentiate into SIE/BE through a cooperative interaction of the BMP-4/Smad pathway and CDX-2.

Our aim was to conduct a preliminary study to test the synergistic cooperative transcriptional activity of BMP-4/Smad and CDX-2 on the activation of intestine-specific genes and further establish the role of this interaction in the development of intestinal metaplasia. A normal squamous esophageal cell line, HET-1A, was stably transfected with a CDX-2 expressing construct, and studied with and without costimulation by BMP-4. Nuclear expression of CDX-2 after transfection was observed by IHC. After stimulation with BMP-4, upregulation of the BMP-4–Smad pathway in the CDX-2 transfected HET-1A cell line was confirmed by expression of PSMAD 1,5,8. Western Blot demonstrated that a time-course incubation with BMP-4 of the CDX-2–transfected cells HET-1A cells significantly increased the expression of intestine specific genes such as MUC-2 and Villin (unpublished data). Confocal microscopy showed colocalization of the PSMAD protein and CDX-2 protein in the BMP-4–treated CDX-2–transfected HET-1A cells (unpublished data). An importantly co-immuno-precipitation assay of the BMP-4–treated and CDX-2–transfected HET-1A cell line demonstrated the direct cooperation of PSMAD and CDX-2. Further analysis by scanning and transmission electron microscopy revealed typical intestinal type of phenotypical changes, such as the formation of microvilli and gap junctions in the BMP-4–stimulated and CDX-2–transfected HET-1A cells (unpublished data). None of the above observations were seen in nontreated, or only BMP-4–stimulated, or only CDX-2–transfected HET-1A cells.

From these preliminary data, we can conclude that the development of BE is a multistep process, in which there may be an initial dedifferentiation of squamous epithelial cells into NSCE that is BMP-4-mediated, and subsequently this may be followed by dedifferentiation into BE that is induced through a collaborative interaction of BMP4 with CDX-2. Our results correspond with the clinical observation that during development of BE, NSCE overtime may be followed by development of BE. Importantly, our observations give us novel opportunities for preventing development of the premalignant BE by developing molecular strategies targeting the BMP-4/CDX-2 interaction.

6. Targeting molecular pathways in BE, a study design

Wytske M. Westra and K.K. Krishnadath
W.M.Westra@amc.uva.nl

BE is a metaplastic condition in which the normal squamous mucosa of the distal esophagus is substituted by a (specialized) columnar epithelium. This process is assumed to be the result of GERD in which bile and acidic reflux cause inflammation and induce transformation of squamous epithelium into a columnar type of epithelium.[26] On estimation at least 1% of males above the age of 50 have BE,[27] but an even higher incidence has been noted in a recent Swedish endoscopic screening study.[28] Patients with BE have a 40–125 times increased risk for developing EAC.[29–34]

EAC is a cancer with a very poor prognosis, with a five-year survival rate of less than 15%.[10] According to the central registry of causes of death, in the Netherlands, over 1,000 patients died from EAC in 2005. Even after surgical intervention, EAC patients have a cumulative two-year survival chance of less than 20%, while treatment at an early stage may improve survival rates to over 90%.[35] An important issue remains that only a small group of Barrett patients are currently included in surveillance programs.[36] Periodic surveillance enables treatment in early stages of cancer with overall good prognosis. Gaining insight into the biological events giving rise to BE, is of paramount importance for developing novel curative strategies for BE and, as such, prevention of EAC.

It is generally assumed that in esophageal metaplasia, the normal squamous epithelium transdifferentiates toward an epithelium that resembles that of the intestines, and is therefore referred to as specialized intestinal type of columnar epithelium. Previously, our group demonstrated[37,38] that BMP-4, a member of the TGF-β family, is a key player in the process of this metaplastic transformation. During embryogenesis, BMP-4, together with sonic hedgehog (Shh) and other morphogens such as Notch and Wnts, is involved in transforming the primordial gut epithelium into intestinal-type mucosae.[39,40] Shh and BMP-4 are also involved in the development of the esophagus from the primordial foregut.[41,42] Yet, here, the effect of BMP-4 is closely balanced through simultaneous expression of Noggin,[43] a natural antagonist of BMPs, whose action prevents development of columnar epithelium in the esophagus. In the normal adult esophagus, Shh and BMPs are no longer expressed. Our studies however showed that BMP-4 is reexpressed in esophagitis and BE.[37]

An important observation in these *ex vivo* studies is that the effect of BMP-4 could be inhibited by its natural antagonist Noggin. We therefore hypothesized that inhibition of the BMP/PSmad pathway may induce regression of intestinal metaplasia in the esophagus. The key aim of these studies is to investigate whether Noggin can reverse the development of intestinal metaplasia in a rat BE model.

Noggin is one of the most well-known and potent antagonists of BMPs, and has high affinity for BMP-4, BMP-2, and BMP-7.[44] We previously demonstrated that the BMP-4/PSmad pathway is also upregulated in the surgical rat esophagitis–BE model[37] 20–22 weeks postsurgery. In several *in vitro* and animal models, it has been demonstrated that Noggin can inhibit the BMP pathway and, for instance, prevent bone formation.[45] For these reasons, Noggin is a highly promising candidate as an inhibitor for the BMP pathway. However, BMPs have an important role in the homeostasis of the normal intestinal type of epithelia, as found in small bowel and colon, and are essential for bone development. Systemic administration of Noggin could have unwanted side effects on these organs. We will take advantage of the fact that Noggin exerts its action in the extracellular space, by exploring the possibility of oral application of Noggin. By using a carrier substance to target the distal esophagus, Noggin will be allowed to exert its action on the damaged, inflamed, and metaplastic esophageal mucosa.

The BE rat model that has now been established at the Academic Medical Center, is adapted from the Mayo Foundation (Rochester, MN, USA).[46] Briefly, general anesthesia is induced and maintained. Subsequently, a midline laparatomy is performed, and the gastroesophageal junction is localized and mobilized while preserving vascular structures and the vagal nerve. The junction is ligated and transected and a 5 mm jejunostomy is made just distal to the ligament of Treitz using electrocautery. An end-to-side esophagojejunostomy is created and the anastomosis is placed between the two liver lobes. The abdominal wall is closed in two layers using 5-0 monofilament. Typically, the animals develop severe reflux esophagitis three to four weeks postoperative, whereas intestinal metaplasia develops after 20–22 weeks at the anastomotic site and EAC approximately one year postsurgery.

First, in a proof of principle study, a total of 15 male Sprague–Dawley rats were operated on as described. We previously demonstrated that activation of the BMP-4 pathway can already be seen in the case of esophagitis. Therefore, after a minimal period of four weeks, once esophagitis and inflammation have developed in the animals,[46] rats ($n = 5$) were orally treated with recombinant Noggin in the carrier substance twice a day, in a dosage of 25 μg Noggin in 75 μL ($n = 15$ mg) for at least four days. Control groups consisted of a carrier substance only group ($n = 5$), and an only operated but not treated group ($n = 5$). An additional five rats were kept under control conditions to obtain normal tissues. In the dosing study, we have evaluated the effect of Noggin on the inhibition of the BMP/PSmad pathway as performed by Western blot and IHC of the inflamed esophagus at the anastomotic site and of the neighboring control tissues (i.e., normal esophagus and small and large bowel as controls). Blood draws were performed to monitor systemic Noggin levels.

To evaluate whether Noggin can eradicate IM, another 105 rats were operated on, which have been divided in the different groups as described. These rats were orally administered Noggin/carrier substance but only after IM has developed, which normally is at the 20th week after the induction of reflux. The rats were administered Noggin/carrier substance from week 26 to week 29 and then sacrificed. As in the previous study, the anastomotic site will be studied to detect the effect of Noggin on the presence of esophageal metaplasia by histopathology and for the effect on the BMP/Smad pathway, but also for factors upstream of BMP-4, such as Wnts, Shh, Ptch, and Smo by IHC, Western blot,

RT-PCR, and QPCR. By taking periodic blood of the animals, we will also investigate systemic levels of Noggin by Western Blot.

Conflicts of interest

The authors declare no conflicts of interest.

References

1. Ostrowski, J., M. Mikula, J. Karczmarski, *et al.* 2007. Molecular defense mechanisms of Barrett's metaplasia estimated by an integrative genomics. *J. Mol. Med.* **85:** 733–743.
2. Zachos, N.C., M. Tse & M. Donowitz. 2005. Molecular physiology of intestinal Na+/H+ exchange. *Annu. Rev. Physiol.* **67:** 411–443.
3. Jolly, A.J., C.P. Wild & L.J. Hardie 2009. Sodium deoxycholate causes nitric oxide mediated DNA damage in oesophageal cells. *Free Radic. Res.* **43:** 234–240.
4. Goldman, A.S.M., D. Goldman, G. Watts, *et al.* 2010. A novel mechanism of acid and bile acid-induced DNA damage involving Na$^+$/H$^+$ exchanger: implication for Barrett's oesophagus. *GUT.* In press.
5. Stairs, D.B., J. Kong & J.P. Lynch. Cdx genes, inflammation, and the pathogenesis of intestinal metaplasias. In *Molecular Biology of Digestive Organs*, K. Kaestner, Ed. Elsevier. In press.
6. Stairs, D.B., H. Nakagawa, A. Klein-Szanto, *et al.* 2008. Cdx1 and c-myc foster the initiation of transdifferentiation of the normal esophageal squamous epithelium toward Barrett's Esophagus *PloS ONE* **3:** e3534.
7. Pantanowitz, L. 2009. Colonic adenoma with squamous metaplasia. *Int. J. Surg. Pathol.* **17:** 340–342.
8. Kong, J., B.K. Isariyawonse, T. Ezaki, *et al.* 2009. Induction of intestinalization in human esophageal keratinocytes is a multi-step process. *Carcinogenesis* **30:** 122–130
9. Jiang, Y., B.N. Jahagirdar, R.L. Reinhardt, *et al.* 2002. Pluripotency of mesenchymal stem cells derived from adult marrow. *Nature* **418:** 41–46.
10. Krause, D.S., N.D. Theise, M.I. Collector, *et al.* 2002. Multiorgan, multi-lineage engraftment by a single bone marrow-derived stem cell. *Cell* **105:** 369–377.
11. Wagers, A.J., R.I. Sherwood, J.L. Christensen & I.L. Weissman. 2002. Little evidence for developmental plasticity of adult hematopoietic stem cells. *Science* **297:** 2256–2259.
12. Houghton, J., C. Stoicov, S. Nomura, *et al.* 2004. Gastric cancer originating from bone marrow-derived cells. *Science* **306:** 1568–1571.
13. Hutchinson, L., B. Stenstrom, D. Chen, *et al.* 2011. Human Barrett's adenocarcinoma of the esophagus, associated myofibroblasts, and endothelium can arise from bone marrow-derived cells after allogeneic stem cell transplant. *Stem Cells Dev.* **20:** 11–17.
14. Jankowski, J.A. *et al.* 2000. Barrett's metaplasia. *Lancet* **356:** 2079–2085.
15. Wang, J. *et al.* 2009. Differential gene expression in normal esophagus and Barrett's esophagus. *J. Gastroenterol.* **44:** 897–911.

16. Chen, X. *et al.* 2008. Multilayered epithelium in a rat model and human Barrett's esophagus: expression patterns of transcription factors and differentiation markers. *BMC Gastroenterol.* **8:** 1.

17. Chen, X. & C.S. Yang. 2009. Barrett's esophagus – preclinical models for investigation. In *Esophageal Tumors: Principles and Practice.* B.A. Jobe, *et al.*, Eds.: 61–67. Demos Medical Publishing. New York.

18. Slack, J.M. & D. Tosh. 2001. Transdifferentiation and metaplasia-switching cell types. *Curr. Opin. Genet. Dev.* **11:** 581–586.

19. Milano, F., J.W.P.M. Van Baal, S.J. Buttar, *et al.* 2007. Bone morphogenetic protein 4 expressed in esophagitis induces a columnar phenotype in columnar metaplasia. *Gastroenterology* **132:** 2412–2421.

20. Van Baal, J.W., F. Milano, A.M. Rygiel, *et al.* 2005. A comparative analysis by SAGE of gene expression profiles of Barrett's esophagus, normal squamous esophagus, and gastric cardia. *Gastroenterology* **129:** 1274–1281.

21. Beck, F. 2004. The role of Cdx genes in the mammalian gut. *Gut* **53:** 1394–1396.

22. Groisman, G.M., M. Amar & A. Meir. 2004. Expression of the intestinal marker Cdx2 in the columnar-lined esophagus with and without intestinal (Barrett's) metaplasia. *Mod. Pathol.* **17:** 1282–1288.

23. Phillips, R.W., H.F. Jr. Frierson & C.A. Moskaluk. 2003. Cdx2 as a marker of epithelial intestinal differentiation in the esophagus. *Am. J. Surg. Pathol.* **27:** 1442–1447.

24. Eda, A., H. Osawa, K. Satoh, *et al.* 2003. Aberrant expression of CDX2 in Barrett's epithelium and inflammatory esophageal mucosa. *J. Gastroenterol.* **38:** 14–22.

25. Kong, J., H. Nakagawa, B.K. Isariyawongse, *et al.* 2009. Induction of intestinalization in human esophageal keratinocytes is a multistep process. *Carcinogenesis* **30:** 122–130.

26. Haggitt, R.C. 1994. Barrett's esophagus, dysplasia, and adenocarcinoma. *Hum. Pathol.* **25:** 982–993.

27. Cameron, A.J. 2002. Epidemiology of Barrett's esophagus and adenocarcinoma. *Dis. Esophagus* **15:** 106–108.

28. Ronkainen, J., P. Aro, T. Storskrubb, *et al.* 2005. Prevalence of Barrett's esophagus in the general population: an endoscopic study. *Gastroenterology* **129:** 1825–1831.

29. Conio, M., S. Blanchi, G. Lapertosa, *et al.* 2003. Long-term endoscopic surveillance of patients with Barrett's esophagus. Incidence of dysplasia and adenocarcinoma: a prospective study. *Am. J. Gastroenterol.* **98:** 1931–1939.

30. Haggitt, R.C. 2000. Pathology of Barrett's esophagus. *J Gastrointest. Surg.* **4:** 117–118.

31. Hameeteman, W., G.N. Tytgat, H.J. Houthoff & J.G. Van Den Tweel. 1989. Barrett's esophagus: development of dysplasia and adenocarcinoma. *Gastroenterology* **96:** 1249–1256.

32. Provenzale, D., C. Schmitt & J.B. Wong. 1999. Barrett's esophagus: a new look at surveillance based on emerging estimates of cancer risk. *Am. J. Gastroenterol.* **94:** 2043–2053.

33. Spechler, S.J. 2000. Barrett's esophagus: an overrated cancer risk factor. *Gastroenterology* **119:** 587–589.

34. Van Der Veen, A.H., J. Dees, J.D. Blankensteijn & M. van Blankenstein. 1989. Adenocarcinoma in Barrett's oesophagus: an overrated risk. *Gut* **30:** 14–18.

35. Peracchia, A., L. Bonavina, A. Via & R. Incarbone. 1999. Current trends in the surgical treatment of esophageal and cardia adenocarcinoma. *J. Exp. Clin. Cancer Res.* **18:** 289–294.

36. Reid, B.J., X. Li, P.C. Galipeau & T.L. Vaughan. 2010. Barrett's oesophagus and oesophageal adenocarcinoma: time for a new synthesis. *Nat. Rev. Cancer* **10:** 87–101.

37. Milano, F., J.W.P.M. van Baal, S.J. Buttar, *et al.* 2007. Bone morphogenetic protein 4 expressed in esophagitis induces a columnar phenotype in columnar metaplasia. *Gastroenterology* **132:** 2412–2421.

38. Van Baal, J.W., F. Milano, A.M. Rygiel, *et al.* 2005. A comparative analysis by SAGE of gene expression profiles of Barrett's esophagus, normal squamous esophagus, and gastric cardia. *Gastroenterology* **129:** 1274–1281.

39. Ishizuya-Oka, A., T. Hasebe, K. Shimizu, *et al.* 2006. Shh/BMP-4 signaling pathway is essential for intestinal epithelial development during Xenopus larval-to-adult remodeling. *Dev. Dyn.* **235:** 3240–3249.

40. Sancho, E., E. Batlle & H. Clevers. 2004. Signaling pathways in intestinal development and cancer. *Annu. Rev. Cell Dev. Biol.* **20:** 695–723.

41. Litingtung, Y., L. Lei, H. Westphal & C. Chiang. 1998. Sonic hedgehog is essential to foregut development. *Nat. Genet.* **20:** 58–61.

42. Narita, T., K. Saitoh, T. Kameda, *et al.* 2000. BMPs are necessary for stomach gland formation in the chicken embryo: a study using virally induced BMP-2 and Noggin expression. *Development* **127:** 981–988.

43. Que, J., M. Choi, J.W. Ziel, *et al.* 2006. Morphogenesis of the trachea and esophagus: current players and new roles for noggin and Bmps. *Differentiation* **74:** 422–437. Recent study that shows that noggin is essential in for normal development of the anterior foregut into esophagus and trachea.

44. Gazzerro, E. & C. Minetti. 2007. Potential drug targets within bone morphogenetic signaling pathways. *Curr. Opin. Pharmacol.* **7:** 325–333.

45. Canalis, E., E.N. Economides & E. Gazzero. 2003. Bone morphogenetic proteins, their antagonists, and the skeleton, *Endocr. Rev.* **24:** 218–235.

46. Buttar, N.S., K.K. Wang, M.A. Anderson, *et al.* 2002. The effect of selective cyclooxygenase-2 inhibition in Barrett's esophagus epithelium: an in vitro study. *J. Natl. Cancer Inst.* **94:** 422–429.

Ann. N.Y. Acad. Sci. ISSN 0077-8923

ANNALS OF THE NEW YORK ACADEMY OF SCIENCES

Issue: *Barrett's Esophagus: The 10th OESO World Congress Proceedings*

Barrett's esophagus and animal models

Ryan A. Macke,[1] Katie S. Nason,[1] Ken-ichi Mukaisho,[2] Takanori Hattori,[2] Takashi Fujimura,[3] Shozo Sasaki,[3] Katsunobu Oyama,[3] Tomoharu Miyashita,[3] Tetsuo Ohta,[3] Koichi Miwa,[4] Michael K. Gibson,[1] Ali Zaidi,[1] Usha Malhotra,[1] Ajlan Atasoy,[1] Tyler Foxwell,[1] and Blair Jobe[1]

[1]Esophageal Cancer Program, University of Pittsburgh and University of Pittsburgh Medical Center, Hillman Cancer Center, Pittsburgh, Pennsylvania. [2]Department of Pathology, Shiga University of Medical Science, Shiga, Japan. [3]Gastroenterologic Surgery, Kanazawa University Hospital, Kanazawa, Japan. [4]Toyama Rosai Hospital, Shiga University of Medical Science, Shiga, Japan.

The following on Barrett's esophagus (BE) and animal models contains commentaries on the factors of BE carcinogenesis; a duodenoesophageal reflux model; translation of targeted therapies for esophageal adenocarcinoma; and novel target regimens selected through a proteomics screen.

Keywords: esophageal neoplasm; Barrett's esophagus; duodenogastric reflux; bile reflux; carcinoma; histogenesis; gut regenerative cell lineage; pyloric–foveolar metaplasia; fat intake; DNA adducts; *N*-nitroso bile acids; chemoprevention; duodenoesophageal reflux; thioproline; cyclooxygenase-2 inhibitor

Concise summaries

- Significant progress has been made in the last few decades using animal models to recreate the esophagitis–metaplasia–carcinoma sequence similar to that seen in human Barrett's esophagus (BE) and EAC. More recent works focus on molecular pathways associated with intestinal metaplasia and carcinogenesis, as well as similarities between genetic mutations occurring in humans and animal models, mouse, rat, pig, rabbit, guinea pig, dog, cat, ferret, and possum.

- Despite the lack of a perfect model, there is still significant potential in using these models to clarify the contribution of different types of reflux (gastric, biliary, and pancreatic) to esophageal adenocarcinoma and to determine how the different types of refluxate interact.

- Refluxed duodenal contents cause gastric and esophageal carcinoma in rats without exposure to carcinogens, and several rat duodenal contents reflux models have been developed. BE in the animal models has well-developed gob-

let cells positive for MUC2, gastric pyloric-type mucins positive for MUC6, and sometimes intermingled with gastric foveolar-type mucins positive for MUC5AC.

- A gut regenerative cell lineage, characterized by pyloric–foveolar metaplasia followed by the appearance of goblet cells, occurs in the regenerative process in response to chronic inflammation.

- High animal-fat dietary intake causes severe obesity, resulting in the development of increased abdominal pressure and increased refluxate, particularly of the duodenal contents. The *N*-nitroso bile acid conjugates, which have mutagenecity, play an important role in Barrett's carcinogenesis, and are stabilized by gastric acid.

- Experiments have been made in a rodent duodeno-esophageal reflux model using thioproline or cyclooxygenase-2 inhibitor to prevent the inflammation–metaplasia–adenocarcinoma sequence. Thioproline is one of the nitrite scavengers, which reduce the production of carcinogenic nitroso-compounds. Celecoxib could postpone the sequence itself,

doi: 10.1111/j.1749-6632.2011.06061.x

whereas thioproline could only prevent the evolution of Barrett's esophagus to cancer.

- The Levrat's surgical model of esophagoduodenal anatomosis in rats has been shown to induce gastroduodenojejunal reflux. This *in vivo* model reproduces the sequence of histologic and molecular events that lead to the development of BE and esophageal adenocarcinoma in humans and, as such, provides a realistic and translatable model for development of therapeutics for EAC.

- A pilot study using proteomics to evaluate for differentially expressed markers in the progression from metaplasia to dysplasia and ultimately adenocarcinoma in human tissues has been conducted.

- Differential expression of cytokeratin 20 in specimens from human patients and the Levrat's model substantiated the hypothesis that the animal model is representative of human cancer and, hence, further supporting the basis for its utilization.

- Furthermore, if this data is confirmed, the Levrat's approach may serve as a model for preclinical drug development. Up to ten potential novel target regimens identified and selected through the proteomics screen will be tested in a multi-arm study in rats.

---

1. Barrett's esophagus and animal models: is Barrett's carcinogenesis related to increased acid level, bile reflux, or both?

Ryan A. Macke and Katie S. Nason
nasonks@upmc.edu

It is generally agreed that BE and esophageal adenocarcinoma (EAC) develop as a result of exposure of the distal esophagus to gastroesophageal reflux. However, there is significant debate regarding which components of the refluxate are necessary and/or sufficient to produce BE/EAC. Specifically, the question of whether Barrett's carcinogenesis is related to increased acid level, bile reflux, or both remains a topic of great interest. Although acid reflux has been widely accepted as playing a key role, the necessity and sufficiency of biliary and pancreatic reflux (duodenoesophageal reflux [DER]) in BE/EAC pathogenesis has remained controversial. As with other cancers, animal models have been critically important in efforts to further elucidate the role of DER in the pathophysiology.

The ideal animal model for BE/EAC pathogenesis would possess anatomic, physiologic, and genetic similarities to humans. It has been proposed that a model with a naturally occurring squamocolumnar junction (SCJ) at the gastroesophageal junction (GEJ) and deep esophageal submucosal glands would best mimic the human esophagus. However, only a handful of animals meet these requirements and none of the models, except primates, develop BE/EAC spontaneously.

Fortunately, successful induction of EAC has been accomplished in mice, rats, and dogs (Table 1). Surgical manipulation of the foregut is the primary method used to induce epithelial metaplasia and carcinogenesis of the esophagus in animal models.

To facilitate focused analysis of the potentially harmful effects of different degrees and types of reflux (gastric, duodenal, pancreatic, and combinations thereof), a variety of foregut operations have been developed. Li *et al.* provides a useful review of some of the procedures traditionally used and their applications to guide researchers in the creation of future models[1] (Table 2).

In the majority of studies, chemical carcinogens have been used to induce esophageal cancer in surgically manipulated animals models, most notably 2,6-dimethylnitrosamine and methyl-n-amylnitrosamine.[2] The results of these studies, however, have been largely contradictory and appear to be strongly influenced by the surgical manipulations used and the degree and types of reflux that are induced.[3] In studies using the nitrosamine carcinogens, EAC comprised half of the tumors in rats with DER, while only ESCC was induced in those with GER.[2,3]

In at least one study, an increasing prevalence of EAC was seen with a decreasing ratio of GER relative to DER (i.e., partial versus total gastrectomy). This

Table 1. Anatomic and physiologic similarities of the foregut in animal models as well as pathogenesis and histopathology of esophageal cancers in these animals

Animal Model	Does model have spontaneous…		Anatomic features of model		Cancer develops in model?	
	Barrett's?	Reflux or vomiting?	SCJ located at anatomic GEJ?	Submucosal esophageal glands?	Physiologically induced?	Cell Type
Human	Yes	Yes	Yes	Yes	Yes	SC/AC
Mouse	No	No	No	No	Yes	SC/AC
Rat	No	No	No	No	Yes	SC/AC
Rabbit	No	No	Yes	Yes	No	N/A
Guinea Pig	No	No	Yes	Yes	No	N/A
Dog	No	Yes	Yes	Yes	Yes	AC
Cat	No	Yes	Yes	No	No	N/A
Ferret	No	Yes	Yes	Yes	No	N/A
Possum	No	No	Yes	Yes	No	N/A

SCJ, squamocolumnar junction; GEJ, gastroesophageal junction; SC, squamous carcinoma; AC, adenocarcinoma
Adapted from Ref. 2.

finding suggests that GER may be protective in the face of DER. Interestingly, the highest prevalence of EAC in this study was in the group with only DER.[3]

These findings conflict with the results of other experiments, however, and further exploration is warranted. For example, Yamashita *et al.* used carcinogen with surgically created biliary, pancreatic, or pancreaticobiliary reflux in a rat model to induce esophageal carcinogenesis.[4]

GER was excluded in this model. In contrast to other studies, EAC was not induced, with all the carcinomas being ESCC. Also, biliary reflux alone did not induce a significantly higher prevalence of malignancies compared to controls, whereas pancreatic and pancreaticobiliary reflux did have a higher cancer prevalence. Finally, the necessity of an added carcinogen to induce cancer has been challenged.

Fein *et al.* successfully induced EAC in a rat model without the use of carcinogens in the late 1990s.[5] In their study, surgical manipulation of the gastroesophageal anatomy was performed, creating DGER, DER, and no reflux groups. All rats with reflux developed esophagitis, the majority developed BE, and roughly half developed EAC by 16 weeks. There were no significant differences in the prevalence of EAC in the DGER and DER groups. Other animal models

Table 2. Summary of surgical procedures in reflux esophageal injury models

Representative surgical procedures	Esophageal injury models
Ligation of the pylorus	Esophagitis
Wendel esophagogastroplasty	Esophagitis
Total gastrectomy	Esophagitis, BE
External esophageal perfusion	Esophagitis
Mucosal excision with hiatal hernia creation	Esophagitis, BE
Esophago-jejunostomy	Esophagitis, BE, ECA
Esophago-duodenal anastomosis	Esophagitis, BE, ECA
Esophago-gastroduodenal anastomosis	Esophagitis, BE, ECA

developed during this same period produced varying results, but many of them noted that EAC could not be induced in the absence of the duodenal components of DGER.

Significant progress has been made in the last few decades using animal models to recreate the esophagitis–metaplasia–carcinoma sequence similar to that seen in human BE and EAC. Despite the lack of a perfect model, there is still significant potential in using these models to clarify the contribution of different types of reflux (gastric, biliary, and pancreatic) to EAC carcinogenesis and to determine how the different types of refluxate interact, the toxicity of the components that make up each type of refluxate, and how the acid/base environment alters the effects of these components.

More recent works are focusing on molecular pathways associated with intestinal metaplasia and carcinogenesis, as well as similarities between genetic mutations occurring in humans and animal models. This work will eventual translate into the development of diagnostic and therapeutic strategies. There is already convincing evidence that both GER and DER play significant roles in the progression to BE and EAC based on these animal models, and we anticipate that further clarity will be provided by future studies that use this valuable resource.

2. Pathogenesis and causative factors of Barrett's carcinogenesis

Ken-ichi Mukaisho and Takanori Hattori
mukaisho@belle.shiga-med.ac.jp

Pathogenesis of Barrett's esophagus and esophageal adenocarcinoma

Early lesion of Barrett's esophagus. BE develops in 5–20% of patients with chronic GERD symptoms and predisposes patients to EAC. Several epidemiological cohort studies suggest that both gastric acid and duodeno-gastroesophageal reflux induce BE, leading to increased risk of developing EAC. It has also been reported that duodenal contents reflux has great potential for malignant initiation, and refluxed duodenal contents cause gastric and esophageal carcinoma in rats without exposure to carcinogens.

To study the histogenesis of BE and EAC, several rat duodenal contents reflux models have been developed. BE leading to EAC developed in all these animal models. BE in the animal models has well-developed goblet cells positive for MUC2. Typical BE also has gastric pyloric-type mucins positive for MUC6 at their base, sometimes intermingled with gastric foveolar-type mucins positive for MUC5AC. The early lesion of BE consists of columnar cells that develop in the basal layer of the regenerative esophageal squamous ep-

ithelium are positive for MUC6 and/or MUC5AC. The mucous glands consisting of pyloric glands and foveolar cells were referred to as "pyloric–foveolar metaplasia."[6]

Gut Regenerative Cell Lineage (GRCL) carcinogenesis. We proposed the concept of a GRCL, which occurs in the regenerative process in response to chronic inflammation.[6] This is characterized by pyloric–foveolar metaplasia followed by the appearance of goblet cells. In addition, we found that the expression of both the intestine-specific caudal-related homeobox transcription factors CDX1 and CDX2 play a crucial role in directing intestinal-type differentiation of the GRCL.[7]

The occurrence of such pyloric–foveolar metaplasia has been often reported in the gut, described as aberrant pyloric glands/pseudopyloric metaplasia in the case of Crohn's disease, pseudopyloric gland metaplasia of the fundic stomach with chronic gastritis, gallbladder with chronic cholecystitis, gastric metaplasia in duodenal ulcers, and colonic dysplasia following ulcerative colitis, etc. We realized that there is a basic principle in regeneration of the gut. As shown in Figure 1, pyloric–foveolar metaplasia occurs at the early step, and, hence, we called this cell lineage the "GRCL." We also suggest that GRCL is related to intestinal-type carcinogenesis.[6]

Causative factors of Barrett's carcinogenesis
Changing patterns in the incidence of esophageal carcinoma. More than 90% of esophageal cancers are either squamous cell carcinomas (ESCC) or EAC. In 1975, approximately 75% of esophageal cancer cases diagnosed, even in the United States, were ESCC, and the remaining 25% were EAC. Among white men, the incidence of adenocarcinoma of the esophagus has increased since the mid-1970s, surpassing that of ESCC by around 1990. It has been reported that diet is associated with GERD, and an interesting recent report showed that high dietary fat intake is associated with an increased risk of GERD symptoms and erosive esophagitis. The mechanism of this effect remains unknown, but it could at least partially explain the rising rates of GERD in the U.S. because the fat content of the food supply in the U.S. increased by 38% between 1909 and 1988.

A modified animal model. Recently, we modified a previously reported animal model and introduced

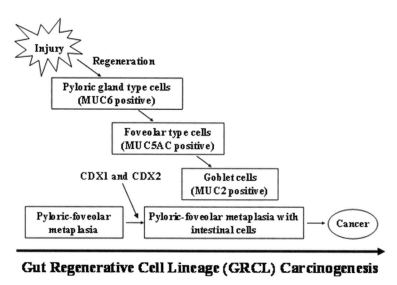

Figure 1. GRCL carcinogenesis. The GRCL is characterized by pyloric–foveolar metaplasia with goblet cell metaplasia, which occurs in the regenerative process in response to chronic inflammation. BE very likely develops through the GRCL, and Cdx1 and Cdx2 play a crucial role in directing intestinal-type differentiation of the GRCL. GRCL is related to intestinal-type carcinogenesis.

ligation through a serosal suture at the esophago–jejunal junction to increase the animals' survival rate and reduce the volume of reflux. Therefore, we successfully developed an animal model showing a higher ratio of squamous cell carcinoma compared to that of adenocarcinoma.[8]

High animal fat dietary intake as a causative factor of Barrett's carcinogenesis. Our hypothesis is as follows: high animal fat dietary intake causes severe obesity, resulting in the development of increased abdominal pressure and increased refluxate, particularly of the duodenal contents. Thus, this series of events raises the incidence of GERD, leading to Barrett's carcinogenesis.

To clarify our hypothesis that high animal fat intake plays an important role in the etiology of Barrett's carcinogenesis, the modified animal models were fed a high animal fat diet. Animals in the soybean oil group were fed the standard diet CE2 with 4.80% fat, mainly soybean oil, while animals in the high-fat group were fed a high-fat diet of Quick Fat, containing 13.9% fat, mainly beef fat. Sequential morphological changes in the animals from both groups were then studied for 30 weeks after surgery. At 30 weeks after surgery, the rats with duodenal

contents reflux in the high-fat group showed a significantly higher incidence of BE and Barrett's dysplasia than those in the soybean oil group. The incidence of EAC in the high-fat group also tended to be higher than that in the soybean oil group. We detected EAC of 16 animals in the soybean oil group, but EAC in these animals did not reach the adventitia. However, two of the six animals in the high-fat group who developed EAC, showed expansive invasion, and one animal exhibited invasion through the adventitia into the liver.[8]

Endogenous DNA adducts and *N*-nitroso bile acids. In our previous study to elucidate the factors underlying the development of EAC, thiazolidine-4-carboxylic acid (thioproline, TPRO) was applied to the reflux models as a nitrite scavenger.

Post-operatively, 31 animals were divided into two groups according to diet. Animals belonging to the control group were given a normal diet ($n = 18$), while the TPRO group was given food containing 0.5% TPRO ($n = 13$). All esophageal sections in both groups were histologically examined. EACs developed in 7 of 18 rats (38.9%) of the control group, whereas no EACs were detected in the TPRO group (Fisher's exact test, $P < 0.05$). Then, we suggested that nitroso compounds derived from reflux of duodenal contents play an important role in the development of EAC.[9]

In the recent study where we collaborated with National Cancer Center in Japan, Terasaki *et al.* studied the endogenous DNA adducts, which are produced from *N*-nitroso bile acid conjugates in the glandular stomach of duodenal contents reflux animals.[10] The *N*-nitroso bile acid conjugates, which have mutagenecity, play an important role in Barrett's carcinogenesis.

Gastric acid as a stabilizer of *N*-nitroso bile acids.
We must consider where *N*-nitroso-compounds are produced in our body. Because the esophagus and proximal cardia portion are located on the back side of the body, the esophagus is easily exposed to *N*-nitroso-compounds generated from refluxate in the stomach during sleep at night. We reported that one of the nitroso-compounds *N*-nitroso-glycocholate decomposed rapidly under alkaline conditions, but remained fairly stable under acidic condition. These findings suggest that, not only bile acids, but also gastric acid is important to retain *N*-nitroso-bile acids as a carcinogen.

Conclusions
(1) The pathogenesis of BE arises from GRCL.
(2) A high-fat diet plays an important role in the development of Barrett's adenocarcinoma.
(3) Endogenous DNA adducts produced from *N*-nitroso bile acid conjugates play a key role in the development of Barrett's adenocarcinoma.
(4) *N*-nitroso bile acids are stabilized by gastric acid.

3. Chemoprevention for esophageal adenocarcinoma using rat duodenoesophageal reflux model

Takashi Fujimura, Shozo Sasaki, Katsunobu Oyama, Tomoharu Miyashita, Tetsuo Ohta, Koichi Miwa, and Takanori Hattori
tphuji@staff.kanazawa-u.ac.jp

Introduction
A rapid increase in the incidence of esophageal adenocarcinoma (EAC) becomes a clinical problem among the Western countries. The sequence of several events progressing from gastroesophageal reflux disease to EAC is thought to involve the development of inflammation-stimulated hyperplasia and metaplasia such as Barrett's esophagus (BE), followed by multifocal dysplasia and adenocarcinoma (Fig. 2). Previously gastric juice was suggested to be an inducer of BE, dysplasia, and EAC. But recently duodenal juice was reported to be more responsible for this sequence than gastric juice.[11]

Chemoprevention for esophageal adenocarcinoma
We have established a rodent duodenoesophageal reflux model to induce BE and EAC.[12] Furthermore, we have reported chemopreventive effects of different chemicals such as thioproline, NSAIDs, and selective cyclooxygenase-2 inhibitors (COXIBs) on the metaplasia-dysplasia-adenocarcinoma (MDA) sequence using such models. In this paper, the outcomes of thiproline, celecoxib, and ursodeoxycholic acid (UDCA) are described.

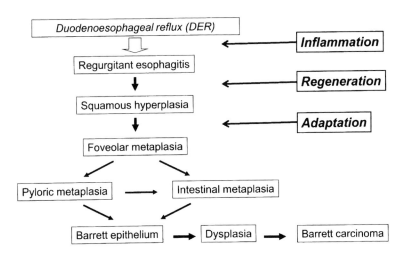

Figure 2.

Thioproline

Thioproline is one of the nitrite-trapping agents that reduce production of carcinogenic *N*-nitroso compounds. Rats receiving esophagojejunostomy, with sparing of the whole stomach, were fed with a thioproline-containing diet (TP group) or a regular diet (control group) for 45 weeks.[13] Incidences of BE and EAC in the TP group were 67% and 17%, respectively, while they were 94% and 69% in the control group. A significant reduction in the incidence of EAC was confirmed, but there was no difference in the incidence of BE between two groups. Urinary concentration of *N*-nitrosothioproline in the thioproline-treated group was much higher than in the control group; but in another experiment, nitrate concentration was not different between the two groups. These results strongly suggested that thioproline inhibited development of adenocarcinoma by blocking nitrosation.

Celecoxib

Cyclooxygenase-2 (COX-2) is strongly related with tumorigenesis in many cancers including esophageal adenocarcinoma.[14] Celecoxib, one of the COX-2 inhibitors (COXIBs), is prescribed in the United States for patients with familial adenomatous polyposis to prevent colorectal polyps. Rats receiving esophagojejunostomy after total gastrectomy were fed with a celecoxib-containing diet (CXB group) or control diet (control group) for 40 weeks.[16] Incidences of BE and EAC in the CXB group were 12% and 0%, respectively, while they were 89% and 47% in the control group (Table 3). There were significant differences between two groups in the incidence of BE and of EAC. The

Table 3.

Post-operative weeks	Group	No. of animals examined	Incidence of	
			Barrett's esophagus	Carcinoma
10 W	Control	10	10%	0%
	Celecoxib	5	0%	0%
20 W	Control	10	40%	0%
	Celecoxib	5	20%	0%
30 W	Control	10	50%	10%
	Celecoxib	5	40%	0%
40 W	Control	19	89%]**	47%]*
	Celecoxib	8	12%	0%

$**p < 0.01$ $*p < 0.05$.

expression of COX-2 mRNA was strongly increased during experiments in both groups comparing to the sham operation, especially during weeks 10 to 20. However, PGE2 production of the celecoxib-treated group was greatly decreased than of the control group. Ki-67 labeling index in the control group was greatly increased compared with sham operation but significantly decreased in the celecoxib group than in the control group. On the other hand, the apoptotic index of the celecoxib group greatly increased compared to that of the control group. These results demonstrated that celecoxib could inhibit or postpone MDA sequence by blocking COX-2 activity.

Ursodeoxycholic acid

Ursodeoxycholic acid (UDCA) is a unique hydrophilic bile acid possessing many physical functions, such as changing the proportion of bile acid, inhibiting inflammation, and reducing the NF-κB pathway. Rats receiving esophagojejunostomy after total gastrectomy were fed a UDCA-containing diet (UDCA group) or a regular diet (control group) for 40 weeks. Incidences of BE and EAC in the UDCA group were 20% and 10%, respectively, while they were 60% and 60% in the control group. Thus, the incidences of both BE and EAC were decreased by UDCA treatment.

While the amount of UDCA usually is very small in either rodent or human bile acid, the concentration of UDCA in the UDCA-treated group was significantly higher than in the control group; this altered the proportion of bile acids in the UDCA-treated group and thus the proportion of bile acids was very different between the two groups. Deoxycholic acid (DCA) and chenodeoxycholic (CDCA) acid strongly induce COX-2 through several pathways, such as NF-κB and AP-1 pathway; UDCA stimulates these pathways less and reduces the volume of DCA and CDCA by changing bile acid proportion.

Conclusions

Duodenal reflux plays an important role in the development of esophageal adenocarcinoma. We performed chemopreventive experiments using several chemicals in a rodent duodenal reflux model. These results demonstrated that both UDCA and celecoxib could inhibit, or postpone, MDA sequence itself (DBI), whereas thioproline could prevent only development of cancer from BE by blocking nitrosation.

4. Novel approach for rapid translation of targeted therapies for esophageal adenocarcinoma

Michael K. Gibson, Ali Zaidi, Usha Malhotra, Ajlan Atasoy, Katie S. Nason, Tyler Foxwell, and Blair A. Jobe

gibsonmk@upmc.edu

The incidence of esophageal adenocarcinoma (EAC) is on the rise in the United States.[16] Approximately 50% of patients present with advanced disease. With this in mind, the development of improved methods and models for prevention and treatment of EAC is paramount.

Barrett's esophagus (BE), the precursor of EAC, results from chronic injury to the esophagus from acid and bile.[17,18] The Levrat's surgical model of esophago-duodenal anatomosis in rats has been shown to induce gastroduodenojejunal reflux.[4,19,20] This *in vivo* model reproduces the sequence of histologic and molecular events that lead to the development of BE and EAC in humans and, as such, provides a realistic and translatable model for development of therapeutics for EAC.[21]

This translational research project aims to discover, validate, and test novel therapeutic drug targets in human EAC by:

(1) using proteomic technology to discover differentially expressed proteins in BE versus EAC in human samples that represent members of aberrant pathways that may be targeted by available drugs,

(2) using the Levrat's and primary heterotransplant animal models to screen for efficacy of these drugs against EAC, and

(3) bringing the most active agent to the clinic for testing of efficacy in phase II trial for patients with advanced EAC.

Aims

(1) To use proteomic technology to identify and characterize differentially expressed members of signaling pathways in human and rat BE and EAC.

(i) **Hypothesis.** Similarly differentially expressed proteins related to the malignant phenotype of EAC in the Levrat's model and human tissue will be identified, including members of pathways for which targeted therapies are available.

(ii) **Approach.** BE and EAC from the Levrat's model and from untreated human patients (primary surgical specimens) will be profiled by proteomics in the lab of Tom Conrads. Promising targets will be evaluated for efficacy in Aim 2.

(2) The primary heterotransplant (human) and Levrat's (rat) models will be used to assess the preclinical activity of agents directed against the differentially expressed protein or pathway target, as identified by proteomic profiling.

(i) **Hypothesis.** Inhibitor(s) of differentially expressed targets will be active against rat and human EAC in these animal models.

(ii) **Approach.** Primary heterotransplant and Levrat's models of EAC will be generated. Drugs of interest will be tested for efficacy in growth inhibition and dose response experiments.

(3) To evaluate the most active agent(s) in a single-agent, phase II prospective clinical trial in patients with refractory EAC.

(i) **Hypothesis.** Selected agents will show clinical efficacy in the trial.

(ii) **Approach.** Prospective, single-agent, phase II clinic trial to be carried out through the UPMC Esophageal Cancer Program.

Preliminary results

We conducted a pilot study using proteomics to evaluate for differentially expressed markers in the progression from metaplasia to dyplasia and ultimately adenocarcinoma in human tissues. Differences in protein abundance from BE-, HGD-, and EAC-derived cells were determined from their spectral count values. Those significant differentially distributed proteins were utilized for further hierarchical cluster analysis. A clear pattern was evident representing abundant level alterations of proteins that cluster with each stage of neoplastic progression.

In order to investigate shared expression of markers between human and rat tissues, we evaluated CK20 in both BE and EAC. Differential expression of this marker in specimens from human patients and the Levrat's model substantiated the hypothesis that the animal model is representative of human cancer and, hence, further support the basis for its use. We did not have paired normal tissue for both human and rat tumors, but they are being obtained. In addition, proteomic studies are ongoing.

This finding suggests that the rat model of esophageal carcinogenesis may be a representative surrogate for the same process in humans. Furthermore, if this data is confirmed, the Levrat's approach will serve as an excellent model for preclinical drug development.

Up to ten potential novel target regimens identified and selected through the proteomics screen will be tested in a multiarm study in Sprague–Dawley rats. Example agents include IGF-1R inhibitor (BMS), SMO inhibitor (BMS), SHH inhibitor (Infinity Pharmaceuticals), mTOR inhibitor (AZD and Novartis), VEGF inhibitor (Tactical Therapeutics and AZD), and an EGFR inhibitor (Amgen, BMS). Prior to testing in the animal models, dosages for each target agent shall be determined based on PK/PD work.

All drug treatment groups will be compared with a vehicle control group. During the course of the treatment, tumor volumes and weights shall be recorded routinely to determine efficacy. Active agents will be tested in human trials.

Conflicts of interest

The authors declare no conflicts of interest.

References

1. Li, Y. & R.C. Martin. 2007. Reflux injury of esophageal mucosa: experimental studies in animal models of esophagitis, Barrett's esophagus and esophageal adenocarcinoma. *Dis. esophagus* **20:** 372–378.

2. Attwood, S.E., T.C. Smyrk, T.R. Demeester, *et al.* 1992. Duodenoesophageal reflux and the development of esophageal adenocarcinoma in rats. *Surgery* **111:** 503–510.

3. Ireland, A.P., J.H. Peters, T.C. Smyrk, *et al.* 1996. Gastric juice protects against the development of esophageal adenocarcinoma in the rat. *Ann. Surg.* **224:** 358–370; Discussion 370–351.

4. Yamashita, Y., K. Homma, N. Kako, *et al.* 1998. Effect of duodenal components of the refluxate on development of esophageal neoplasia in rats. *J. Gastrointest. Surg.* **2:** 350–355.

5. Fein, M., J.H. Peters, P. Chandrasoma, *et al.* 1998. Duodenoesophageal reflux induces esophageal adenocarcinoma without exogenous carcinogen. *J. Gastrointest. Surg.* **2:** 260–268.

6. Mukaisho, K., K. Miwa, T. Hattori, *et al.* 2003. Gastric carcinogenesis by duodenal reflux through gut regenerative cell lineage. *Dig. Dis. Sci.* **48:** 2153–2158.

7. Tatsuta, T., K. Mukaisho, T. Hattori, *et al.* 2005. Expression of Cdx2 in early GRCL of Barrett's esophagus induced in rats by duodenal reflux. *Dig. Dis. Sci.* **50:** 425–431.

8. Chen, K.H., K. Mukaisho, T. Hattori, *et al.* 2007. High animal-fat intake changes the bile-acid composition of bile juice and enhances the development of Barrett's esophagus and esophageal adenocarcinoma in a rat duodenal-contents reflux model. *Cancer Sci.* **98:** 1683–1688.

9. Kumagai, H., K. Mukaisho, T. Hattori, *et al.* 2004. Thioproline inhibits development of esophageal adenocarcinoma induced by gastroduodenal reflux in rats. *Carcinogenesis* **25:** 723–727.

10. Terasaki, M., Y. Totsuka, K. Nishimura, *et al.* 2008. Detection of endogenous DNA adducts, O-carboxymethyl-2'-deoxyguanosine and 3-ethanesulfonic acid-2'-deoxycytidine, in the rat stomach after duodenal reflux. *Cancer Sci.* **99:** 1741–1746.

11. Kauer, W.K., J.H. Peters, T.R. DeMeester, *et al.* 1995. Mixed reflux of gastric and duodenal juice is more harmful to the esophagus than gastric juice alone. The need for surgical therapy re-emphasized. *Ann Surg* **222:** 525–533.

12. Miwa, K., M. Segawa, Y. Takano, *et al.* 1994. Induction of oesophageal and forestomach carcinomas in rats by reflux of duodenal contents. *Br J Cancer.* **70:** 185–189.

13. Sasaki, S., K. Miwa, T. Fujimura, *et al.* 2007. Ingestion of thioproline suppresses rat esophageal adenocarcinogenesis caused by duodenogastroesophageal reflux. *Oncol Rep* **18:** 1443–1449.

14. Fujimura, T., T. Ohta, K. Oyama, *et al.* 2006. Role of cyclooxygenase-2 in the carcinogenesis of gastrointestinal tract cancers: A review and report of personal experience. *World J Gastroenterol* **12:** 1336–1345.

15. Oyama, K., T. Fujimura, I. Ninomiya, *et al.* 2005. A COX-2 inhibitor prevents the esophageal inflammation-metaplasia-adenocarcinoma sequence in rats. *Carcinogenesis* **26:** 565–570.

16. Jemal, A., R. Siegel, E. Ward, *et al.* 2009. Cancer statistics, 2009. *CA Cancer J. Clin.* **59:** 225–249.

17. Paulson, T.G. & B.J. Reid. 2004. Focus on Barrett's esophagus and esophageal adenocarcinoma. *Cancer Cell* **6:** 11–16.

18. Lagergren, J., R. Bergstrom, A. Lindgren, *et al.* 1999. Symptomatic gastroesophageal reflux as a risk factor for esophageal adenocarcinoma. *N. Engl. J. Med.* **340:** 825–831.

19. Fein, M., K.H. Fuchs, H. Stopper, *et al.* 2000. Duodenogastric reflux and foregut carcinogenesis: analysis of duodenal juice in a rodent model of cancer. *Carcinogenesis* **21:** 2079–2084.

20. Levrat, M., R. Lambert, G. Kirshbaum. 1962. Esophagitis produced by reflux of duodenal contents in rats. *Am. J. Dig. Dis.* **7:** 564–573.

21. Bonde, P., G. Sui, S. Dhara, *et al.* 2007. Cytogenetic characterization and gene expression profiling in the rat reflux-induced esophageal tumor model. *J. Thorac. Cardiovasc. Surg.* **133:** 763–769.

Ann. N.Y. Acad. Sci. ISSN 0077-8923

Esophageal disease in pediatrics

Sudarshan R. Jadcherla[1] and Samuel Nurko[2]

[1]Department of Pediatrics, Sections of Neonatology, Pediatric Gastroenterology, and Nutrition, Nationwide Children's Hospital, and The Ohio State University College of Medicine, Columbus, Ohio. [2]Center for Motility and Functional Gastrointestinal Disorders, Children's Hospital Medical Center, Boston, Massachusetts

The following on esophageal disease in pediatrics contains commentaries on acquisition of neuromuscular maturation; physiology of esophageal peristaltic and sphincteric reflexes; implications for clinical practice; and conditions that predispose to severe gastroesophageal reflux disease (GERD) in children with potential risk for esophageal cancer.

Keywords: embryology; peristalsis; sphincteric reflexes; fetal swallowing; airway protection; Barrett's esophagus; GERD

Concise summaries

- Evidently, maturation plays a significant role in acquisition of neuromuscular maturation involved with safe oral feeding skills.
- Swallowing deficits result in those infants who have structural anomalies of gut, and polyhydramnios results as amniotic fluid fails to circulate. The lower esophageal sphincter is predominantly intrathoracic in neonates, and the intraabdominal part of the sphincter grows in infancy. Despite these maturational limitations, the human infant has to eat more volume per kilograms of body weight to sustain the growth phase.
- Development of safe swallowing skills is a process in continuum, modified during postnatal maturation and adaptation.
- The esophagus and airways share similar innervation by the vagus, and the interaction of afferent and efferent neuronal pathways modulate sensory–motor function to ensure safe swallowing and airway protection.
- Neuronal recruitment improves with maturation, as well as the magnitude and coordination of contractility. Neonatal maturational delays can result in motility disturbances and may form the basis for infant feeding problems.
- Most cases of esophageal adenocarcinoma in children have been described primarily in association with Barrett's esophagus (BE) and, in the pediatric population, the chief clinical concern is to detect those children with GERD that are at risk of developing BE. The exact role that genetic predisposition plays is not clear, but there are, however, well defined genetic syndromes, like Cornelia de Lange syndrome, that have been associated with severe GERD and its complications.
- There are certain underlying disorders that predispose pediatric patients to the most severe and chronic GERD, and its complications. Neurologic impairment is one of the common associated causes that predisposes to severe GERD.
- Another predisposing condition to severe GERD includes patients with congenital malformations, in particular esophageal atresia, in which most of the cases of esophageal adenocarcinoma have been described, thus rendering very close follow-up particularly important. Other inflammatory conditions, like eosinophilic esophagitis, also play a role in the development of BE.

doi: 10.1111/j.1749-6632.2011.06060.x

1. Development of esophageal peristaltic and defensive functions in infants: a synopsis

Sudarshan R. Jadcherla

Sudarshan.Jadcherla2@nationwidechildrens.org

Owing to the advances in obstetric and neonatal intensive care practices globally, more infants are now surviving but with aerodigestive concerns. As a result, prevalence of neonatal feeding and airway problems is increasing. Infants born at less than 28 weeks gestation have significant feeding delays, compared with infants born greater than 28 weeks gestation. Evidently, maturation plays a significant role in acquisition of neuromuscular maturation involved with safe oral feeding skills.

In this session, we discussed briefly: (1) embryology of the esophagus, and (2) the physiology of esophageal peristaltic and sphincteric reflexes and esophageal and airway interactions.

Developmental considerations

Fetal swallowing develops by 12 weeks, and development of safe swallowing skills is a process in continuum, modified during postnatal maturation and adaptation, as well as influenced by comorbidities. Swallowing deficits result in those infants that have structural anomalies of gut and polyhydramnios results as amniotic fluid fails to circulate.

Contrasting adult humans, the neonate has nasopharynx and hypopharynx and a relatively large tongue (no oropharynx), the hyoid larynx and epiglottis are in a higher position, and the pharyngeal phase of swallow triggers from the vallecula. Furthermore, the young infant has a shorter esophagus.

Postnatally, rapid development occurs in the first year of life with respect to structure and functions of the esophagus and feeding functions. The lower esophageal sphincter is predominantly intrathoracic in neonates, and the intraabdominal part of the sphincter grows in infancy. Despite these maturational limitations, the human infant has to eat more volume per kilograms of body weight to sustain the growth phase, and yet maintain a safe aerodigestive tract.

Physiology of esophageal peristaltic and sphincteric reflexes

Development of safe swallowing skills is a process in continuum, modified during postnatal maturation and adaptation. The functions of esophagus can be summarized as those involved with:

(1) aerodigestive safety, responsible for vigilance, coordination, and antireflux defenses;[1,4,5] and,
(2) deglutition, responsible for swallowing phases, coordination, and peristaltic propulsion.[1–3]

The esophagus and airways share similar innervation by the vagus, and interaction of afferent and efferent neuronal pathways modulate sensory–motor function ensuring safe swallowing and airway protection. These modulating mechanisms are aberrant in infants with dysphagia and airway problems.

In developing infants, we have characterized the sensory–motor basis for neonatal esophageal functions.[4,5] Abrupt bolus as a stimulus activates the esophageal receptors and afferents, resulting in activation of esophageal and airway efferents. Using this approach, we have defined the following reflexes during neonatal maturation: deglutition reflex, pharyngeal reflexive swallow, primary and secondary peristaltic reflexes, upper esophageal contractile reflex, lower esophageal sphincter relaxation reflex, pharyngoglottal closure reflex, and esophagoglottal closure reflex. Furthermore, volume-dependent increment in the recruitment of pharyngeal or esophageal and sphincteric reflexes has been noted, and that maturation improves the sensory–motor characteristics of such reflexes. Such findings suggest that neuronal recruitment improves with maturation, as well as the magnitude and coordination of contractility.

Implications for clinical practice

It is conceivable that deviation in esophageal motility defenses and peristaltic reflexes can occur in conditions such as extreme immaturity, maldevelopment of the foregut, neurological malfunction, or chronic lung disease. Neonatal maturational delays can result in motility disturbances and may form the basis for infant feeding problems. Important neonatal and infant problems related to the esophagus include dysphagia, gastroesophageal reflux disease and aggravation of airway injury due to malfunctions of the swallowing or airway protection mechanisms. Objective evaluation of esophageal motility may provide support for evidence-based management of feeding and airway protection strategies.

[This work was supported in part by grant funding from the National Institutes of Health RO1 068158 (Jadcherla)].

2. Pediatric esophageal conditions with a potential risk for esophageal cancer

Samuel Nurko

samuel.nurko@childrens.harvard.edu

Esophageal adenocarcinoma in children is extremely rare, but has been reported.[6] Most cases have been mainly described in association with BE, which is considered the precursor lesion of esophageal cancer.[6] BE occurs as a result of chronic and severe GERD. Therefore, in the pediatric population, the chief clinical concern is to prevent children with GERD from developing BE, and to detect those children with GERD that are at risk of developing BE.[6]

Certain underlying disorders that predispose pediatric patients to the most severe and chronic GERD, and its complications, include:

- otherwise healthy with chronic GERD,
- neurologic impairment,
- EA and other malformations,
- chronic lung disease: cystic fibrosis,
- family history and genetic predisposition,
- genetic syndromes: Cornelia de Lange syndrome,
- obesity, and
- other inflammatory problems.

The prevalence of BE in children seems to increase as the severity and chronicity of GERD increase. There are certain underlying disorders that predispose pediatric patients to the most severe and chronic GERD, and its complications. These are shown in Table 1. The exact incidence of BE in otherwise healthy children with GERD is not known. In a recent study that described 6,731 patients who underwent upper endoscopy in 12 pediatric facilities, they found biopsy proven intestinal metaplasia in nine patients (0.133%). Patients with suspected BE were older than patients without BE (median 14.7 vs. 10.1 years; $= 0.011$), and in logistic regression analyses, both hiatus hernia and older age were independent significant predictors of suspected BE. In another study of children with chronic GERD, esophageal metaplasia was present in some 10% of children with severe chronic GERD, half of whom had goblet cell metaplasia.[6] Looking at the population of children with GERD that is severe enough to require surgery, BE was found in 11 (7.3%) out of 150 children.

Neurologic impairment is one of the common associated causes that predisposes to severe GERD in children. Studies have mentioned that 10–25% of institutionalized intellectually disabled individuals have symptoms of vomiting, regurgitation, or rumination, and in a recent study of institutionalized individuals, it was found that GERD was more frequent and severe if patients had scoliosis, cerebral palsy, use of anticonvulsant drugs or other benzodiazepines, or who had an IQ < 3. Of those patients that had an endoscopy, BE was found in 18 (14.0%) and peptic strictures in five (3.9%).[6]

Another predisposing condition to severe GERD includes those patients with congenital malformations, in particular esophageal atresia (EA), in which most of the cases of esophageal adenocarcinoma have been described. A recent study that followed children for a mean of 36 years shows a prevalence of BE of 11%.[7] Therefore, children with EA need to have very close follow-up. Children with other malformations like diaphragmatic hernias are also at higher risk of developing severe GERD. Children with chronic lung disease, in particular patients with cystic fibrosis, have also been shown to have a higher prevalence of severe GERD and Barrett's BE. It has been suggested that the standardized incidence ration of esophageal adenocarcinoma in those patients is significantly higher.[8]

The exact role that genetic predisposition plays is not clear. Significant clusterings of reflux symptoms, HH, erosive esophagitis, BE, and esophageal adenocarcinoma occur in families, suggesting some heritability of GERD and its complications. There are, however, well defined genetic syndromes that have been associated with severe GERD and its complications. An example includes Cornelia de Lange syndrome in which BE seems to occur in 10% of those studied, and adenocarcinoma have been described.[9]

The recent obesity epidemic has been associated with an increased incidence of GERD both in adults and children. The impact that it will have in the incidence of BE in the pediatric population is not clear, but it has already been shown in pediatric cross-sectional studies that moderately and extremely obese children are more likely to have a diagnosis of GERD compared with normal weight children (OR 1.16, 95% CI: 1.02–1.32 and 1.32, 95% CI: 1.13–1.56, respectively).[10]

The role that other inflammatory conditions play in the development of BE is not clear. Eosinophilic esophagitis (EoE) is an allergy-mediated esophageal inflammation that produces severe esophagitis. BE has not been associated with EoE, but recently the first case reports of BE associated with EoE were published. Given that the incidence of EoE is increasing, long-term follow-up of these patients will be needed to establish if BE will occur more frequently in those patients. Supported by grant NIH K24 DK082792A.

Conflicts of interest

The authors declare no conflicts of interest.

References

1. Jadcherla, S.R., H.Q. Duong, C. Hofmann, *et al.* 2005. Characteristics of upper esophageal sphincter and esophageal body during maturation in healthy human neonates compared with adults. *Neurogastroenterol Motil* **17:** 663–670.
2. Omari, T.I., K. Miki, R. Fraser, *et al.* 1995. Esophageal body and lower esophageal sphincter function in healthy premature infants. *Gastroenterology* **109:** 1757–1764.
3. Staiano, A., G. Boccia, G. Salvia, *et al.* 2007. Development of esophageal peristalsis in preterm and term neonates. *Gastroenterology* **132:** 1718–1725.
4. Jadcherla, S.R., H.Q. Duong, R.G. Hoffmann, and R. Shaker. 2003. Esophageal body and upper esophageal sphincter motor responses to esophageal provocation during maturation in preterm newborns. *J. Pediatr.* **143:** 31–38.
5. Jadcherla, S.R., R.G. Hoffmann, and R. Shaker. 2006. Effect of maturation of the magnitude of mechanosensitive and chemosensitive reflexes in the premature human esophagus. *J. Pediatr.* **149:** 77–82.
6. Sherman, P.M., E. Hassall, U. Fagundes-Neto, *et al.* 2009. A global, evidence-based consensus on the definition of gastroesophageal reflux disease in the pediatric population. *Am. J. Gastroenterol.* **104:** 1278–1295.
7. Sistonen, S.J., A. Koivusalo, U. Nieminen, *et al.* 2010. Esophageal morbidity and function in adults with repaired esophageal atresia with tracheoesophageal fistula: a population-based long-term follow-up. *Ann. Surg.* **251:** 1167–1173.
8. Alexander, C.L., S.J. Urbanski, R. Hilsden, *et al.* 2008. The risk of gastrointestinal malignancies in cystic fibrosis: case report of a patient with a near obstructing villous adenoma found on colon cancer screening and Barrett's esophagus. *J. Cyst. Fibros.* **7:** 1–6.
9. Macchini, F., G. Fava, A. Selicorni, *et al.* 2010. Barrett's Esophagus and Cornelia de Lange Syndrome. *Acta Paediatr.* **99:** 1407–1410.
10. Koebnick, C., D. Getahun, N. Smith, *et al.* 2011. Extreme childhood obesity is associated with increased risk for gastroesophageal reflux disease in a large population-based study. *Int. J. Pediatr. Obes.* **6:** e257–e263.

Ann. N.Y. Acad. Sci. ISSN 0077-8923

ANNALS OF THE NEW YORK ACADEMY OF SCIENCES

Issue: *Barrett's Esophagus: The 10th OESO World Congress Proceedings*

Barrett's esophagus registries

Piers A.C. Gatenby,[1] Christine P.J. Caygill,[2] Anthony Watson,[2] Liam Murray,[3] and Yvonne Romero[4]

[1]Division of Surgery and Interventional Science, University College London, London, United Kingdom; NHS Medical Medical Directorate, Department of Health, London, United Kingdom & Academic Department of Surgery, Royal Marsden Hospital, London, United Kingdom. [2]Division of Surgery and Interventional Science, University College London, London, United Kingdom. [3]Epidemiology Research Group, Belfast, Northern Ireland. [4]Division of Gastroenterology and Hepatology, Department of Otolaryngology and GI Outcomes Unit, Mayo Clinic, Rochester, Minnesota

The following on Barrett's esophagus registries contains commentaries on the data sets to be included, organizational issues, and the demographic, lifestyle, and diagnostic differences between the United States and Europe. The importance of collaborative studies is also discussed.

Keywords: Barrett's registries; cancer risk; surveillance; esophageal cancer; tissue bank; quality of life

Concise summaries

- The crucial future role of registries is likely to involve further examination and refinement of surveillance strategies to assess risk, cost, and benefit with the result of targeting surveillance appropriately for individual patients. The associated symptoms of gastro-esophageal reflux are increasing, and it is expected that current trends in increased diagnosis of Barrett' esophagus and development of esophageal cancer are likely to continue.

- Registries have been set up to help to clarify the answers to some questions such as current trends in increased diagnosis of Barrett's esophagus and development of esophageal cancer, the natural history of the metaplastic segment, factors influencing cancer risk. They may be institution-based or population-based, and may provide infrastructure for central pathological confirmation, and coordination and recruitment of clinical studies.

- The method of data collection may be retrospective, which limits available information to patient identifiers, demographic data, date of diagnosis, and histological features, but allows a larger number of cases, where a long follow-up has already elapsed, to be collected in a short period of time at lower cost. They can be

prospective, allowing standardization of procedures with direct data collection from patients. The data collected vary depending on the organization of the registry and the purpose that it is intended to fulfill.

- Follow-up of registered patients is crucial as the registered cases then form a cohort, allowing study of outcomes.

- The common data set collected by existing registries includes patient identifiers, demographic data, and date of diagnosis. Further data include histological and endoscopic features, other clinical data and follow-up data. The registries differ in the subjects of interest, categorized by their specific disease phenotype at baseline, and the type of specimen collected.

- As an indirect consequence of registries, practice homogeneity and quality is improved with the introduction of standardization for the measurement of endoscopic landmarks and biopsy protocols at each site. The crucial future role of registries is likely to involve further examination and refinement of surveillance strategies to assess risk, cost, and benefit with the result of targeting surveillance appropriately for individual patients.

- There are a small number of Barrett's registries worldwide and collaboration is important for allowing comparison between different

doi: 10.1111/j.1749-6632.2011.06059.x

regions and pooling of data to improve study power. Collaboration among investigators, clinicians, patients, and registries may facilitate identification of translational discoveries that reduce the mortality rate of esophageal adenocarcinoma.

---

1. Do Barrett's registries have a role to play in research?

Piers A.C. Gatenby, Christine P.J. Caygill, and Anthony Watson
p.gatenby@ucl.ac.uk

The management of Barrett's esophagus presents a particular challenge in modern healthcare. This is an apparently new condition, or one whose presence has only been detected over recent decades. If the increasing rates of diagnosis have resulted from more than simply improvements in recognition of the metaplastic mucosa, the epidemiology of Barrett's esophagus is changing.

This hypothesis (that the observations represent a true increase in incidence of Barrett's esophagus) is supported by the rapid increase in esophageal adenocarcinoma. The rapid escalation in cases of esophageal adenocarcinoma is most marked in non-Hispanic white men in developed countries (with the highest global incidence being seen in Scotland and the highest in the U.S. in Massachusetts, where this conference has been held).[1] Furthermore, the associated symptoms of gastroesophageal reflux are increasing, and it is expected that current trends in increased diagnosis of Barrett's esophagus and development of esophageal cancer are likely to continue.

The natural history of the metaplastic segment is not fully documented. Overall, studies agree that the overall risk of progression to adenocarcinoma is around 0.6% per annum following diagnosis of Barrett's and exclusion of prevalent cancers, and 1% for development of high-grade dysplasia and adenocarcinoma.[2] While the risk of progression is relatively low, this means that typical surveillance centers will see a small number of cases of high-grade dysplasia or cancer and rely on larger studies, meta-analyses, and expert guidelines to direct their clinical practice.

Surveillance frequency and estimation of cancer risk are primarily based upon the detection of dysplasia at biopsy and although adjuncts to standard endoscopy and systematic biopsy are used in research and specialized centers, most patients' biopsies are not targeted by these techniques and adherence to biopsy protocols is variable. The reported rate of progression to high-grade dysplasia or cancer following a diagnosis of low grade dysplasia (which is further complicated by the difficulties with diagnosis in the center of the histological spectrum) is variable, and frequent resolution of findings of dysplasia at subsequent endoscopy make this a difficult area in Barrett's esophagus for clinicians to manage well.[3]

Other factors influencing cancer risk such as age, sex, metaplastic segment length, obesity, smoking, method of reflux control, and other medications have been examined, but overall, our ability to treat optimally, explain the associated risks clearly, and undertake targeted surveillance tailored to stratification of an individual patient's risk remain poor.

Registries have been set up to help to clarify the answers to some of these questions. They may be population-based (such as the Northern Ireland, Danish [reported at this conference], and Dutch registries), which usually register patients from histopathology databases or institution-based (such as the Mayo Clinic Barrett's Registry, Cleveland Clinic Barrett's Registry, Venice Region Barrett's Registry, and UK Barrett's Oesophagus Registry). The pathological databases are able to provide the appropriate population denominator and the institution-based registries can draw from multiple units to provide a large volume of Barrett's cases and may be able to access other clinical information for studies of associations. Barrett's registries may also provide infrastructure for central pathological confirmation, coordination, and recruitment of clinical studies such as the two large U.S. studies of radiofrequency ablation.[4,5]

The crucial future role of registries is likely to involve further examination and refinement of surveillance strategies to assess risk, cost, and benefit with the result of targeting surveillance appropriately for individual patients. Registries should also examine further for differences in geographical variation and variation in time. Further work should involve catalyzing collaboration and looking for opportunities to intervene earlier in the metaplasia–dysplasia–neoplasia sequence that can subsequently be tested by cohort and intervention studies.

2. Barrett's registries: what data set should be included?

Liam Murray

l.murray@qub.ac.uk

Defining a core data set for Barrett's registries is a complex question and perhaps the best way to approach it is by looking at the structure of existing Barrett's registries and the data set they include. Barrett's registries may be classified as those that are population-based or institution based. The method of data collection may be retrospective or prospective, and the data collected vary depending on the organization of the registry and the purpose that it is intended to fulfill.

Population-based registries

These may be further subdivided into those who have complete registration for a geographical area, which are usually based on national/regional histopathological databases and include the Dutch (PALGA) and Northern Irish nationwide pathology registries, the Rochester Epidemiology Project (U.S.), and the retrospective component of the Amsterdam Gastroenterological Association Barrett's Registry. Other registries such as the UK Barrett's Oesophagus Registry (UKBOR), the prospective component of the Amsterdam Gastroenterological Association Barrett's Registry, and Veneto Region Barrett's Registry (EBRA) are population representative.

These registries contain data from either all or a proportion of centers providing management of Barrett's esophagus in a region. They do not have the robust processes for identifying all cases from national data and, in examining their data, it is important to consider what reference population the cases are drawn from. Population-based registries allow the calculation of rates of Barrett's diagnosis and trends in these rates.

Hospital/Institution-based registries

Other registries may be hospital or institution-based such as the Mayo Clinic (EABE) and Cleveland Clinic Barrett's Register. Institutions may be able to specify data collection protocols more easily than multicenter registries, and those institutions with high expertise may have large numbers of Barrett's patients comparable to some of the regional population-based registries.

Retrospective data collection

Data collection may be prospective or retrospective. The Northern Irish Barrett's Registry and Dutch Pathology Registry collect data from pathology reports, which limits available information to patient identifiers, demographic data, date of diagnosis, and histological features (presence of specialized intestinal metaplasia and dysplasia).

Using these methods of data collection means that missing data are common, and these registries lack other important information such as the endoscopic features of the metaplastic segment. Diagnostic coding of the nonstandardized free text pathological reports can be difficult. These data can be enhanced by case note and endoscopy note review or histopathological review of biopsy specimens, but these are time consuming and expensive. The medical record review may still not be able to collect all missing data. Retrospective collection also allows little opportunity for standardization of diagnostic criteria and procedures (such as biopsy protocol and histopathological reporting). Furthermore, there may be difficulty in locating and retrieving records and specimens.

The advantages of retrospective data collection are that it allows a larger number of cases where a long follow-up has already elapsed to be collected in a short period of time at lower cost. The unselected cases may be more representative of the real life situation and analysis may be undertaken as soon as the data have been collected rather than having to wait for the accrual of cases prospectively.

Prospective data collection

This allows standardization of procedures with direct data collection from patients. Registries using prospective collection procedures have been able to collect data including identifiers, demographics, clinical data (indication for endoscopy, symptoms, lifestyle factors, anthropometry, comorbidities, medications, and treatment decisions), endoscopic data (segment length—often using the Prague classification,[6] presence of esophagitis, ulceration, and nodularity), specification of the biopsy protocol (e.g., quadrantic biopsies and biopsies from the stomach and squamous esophagus), pathology data (presence of specialist intestinal metaplasia, dysplasia, inflammation, and *Helicobacter Pylori*) and the collection of other biospecimens for storage and analysis (such as blood for genetic analysis).

Follow-up of registry cases

Follow-up of registered patients is crucial as the registered cases then form a cohort. This allows study of outcomes: disease progression (and regression), development of high-grade dysplasia and esophageal adenocarcinoma, extraesophageal malignancies, and mortality. The influence of management: antireflux surgery, acid suppression, entry into surveillance, NSAIDs, and statins can be examined.

Passive follow-up may involve death registration, links to cancer registration, identification of high-grade dysplasia, and surveillance biopsies, and following cessation of active surveillance or moving away from their surveillance center, patients may still be followed-up to a limited degree using these tools.

Active follow-up may be either opportunistic or at scheduled surveillance appointments and further samples may also be taken at this time.

Organizational issues

Running an effective registry requires good management and is a multidisciplinary task involving gastroenterology, gastrointestinal surgery, pathology, epidemiology, database management/IT, and specialist nurses. A steering committee is required, which generally includes representatives from the involved disciplines as well as funders and lay representatives. It will be involved in strategic decision making, acquisition of funding (which is often insecure), and govern access to data.

Registries will need to have ethical/IRB permission for the study from the appropriate board and are increasingly requiring informed consent from patients for use of their data (although this may not always be required for some population-based studies). The registry will also need to take steps to ensure data security and confidentiality.

Comparability and collaboration

There are a small number of Barrett's registries worldwide, and collaboration is important allowing comparison between different regions and pooling of data to improve study power. There are challenges with data harmonization in particular between those registering retrospectively and prospectively, but early steps have been taken and a workshop of European Barrett's Registries met in Venice in 2007.[7]

Conclusion

Ideally, registries will contain as much data as is practical. The common data set collected by existing registries includes patient identifiers, demographic data, and date of diagnosis. Further data include histological and endoscopic features, other clinical data, and follow-up data.

3. Barrett's esophagus registries: what are the demographic, lifestyle, and diagnostic differences between the United States and Europe, and can these be overcome for future collaborative studies?

Yvonne Romero and Christine P.J. Caygill
romero.yvonne@mayo.edu

As per the Centers for Disease Control, a registry is a "system for collecting and maintaining in a structured record, information on specific persons from a defined population with specified health characteristics." Although there are at least 20 registries of patients with Barrett's esophagus throughout Europe and the United States, for simplicity, comparisons will be made using four prominent registries: the Mayo Clinic Esophageal Adenocarcinoma and Barrett's Esophagus (EABE) Registry,[8] the Italian European Barrett's Registries Association (EBRA),[9] the Northern Ireland Barrett's Register (NIBR),[10] and the United Kingdom National Barrett's Oesophagus Registry (UKBOR).[11]

The registries differ in the subjects of interest, categorized by their specific disease phenotype at baseline (Table 1), the type of specimen (e.g., blood and tissue) collected, and how it is processed (e.g., fresh-frozen, formalin-fixed paraffin embedded). Three of the registries store formalin-fixed tissue, the exception being UKBOR. The EABE Registry additionally collects fresh-frozen tissue. Blood is only collected in the EABE Registry. The registries also differ in the manner in which clinical information (e.g., demographics, symptoms, risk factors, and quality of life) is collected (retrospective chart review,

Table 1. Phenotypes collected in each registry at baseline

	Phenotypes of Interest						
	Cancer			Barrett's esophagus (BE)			
	Adenocarcinoma		Esophageal squamous cell carcinoma	LSBE	SSBE	Endoscopic BE without biopsy confirmation
Registry	Esophageal	GEJ				
EABE	X	X	X	X		
EBRA				X	X	
NIBR				X	X	
UKBOR				X	X	X

Note: Endoscopic BE without biopsy confirmation = any endoscopic length of salmon-colored mucosa thought to be in the esophagus without confirmation of columnar cells, intestinal metaplasia, or goblet cells.
LSBE, long-segment ($\geq$ 3 cm) BE (specialized intestinal metaplasia); SSBE, short-segment (< 3 cm) BE (specialized intestinal metaplasia). EABE, Mayo Clinic Esophageal Adenocarcinoma and Barrett's Esophagus registry; EBRA, Italian European Barrett's Registries Association; NIBR, Northern Ireland Barrett's Register; UKBOR, United Kingdom National Barrett's Oesophagus Registry. This table is the work and intellectual property of Yvonne Romero.

prospective annual questionnaires) and annotated (Table 2). Another difference is in the diagnostic criteria used by registries. In UKBOR a patient is considered as having Barrett's esophagus if the diagnostic biopsy shows gastric type mucosa but no intestinal metaplasia.

There are advantages to each registry. Prospectively collected fresh-frozen tissue and blood may be particularly helpful in biomarker discovery, while formalin-fixed specimens serially collected over time will be helpful in confirming the utility of biomarker panels, especially on a population-wide basis. Registries help to define the natural history of disease.

As an indirect consequence of registries, practice homogeneity, and quality is improved with the introduction of standardization for the measurement of endoscopic landmarks and biopsy protocols at each site. Patients with nondysplastic Barrett's esophagus have a low (0.5%) annual risk of progression to esophageal adenocarcinoma.[12]

Due to the infrequent event rate, informal sample size calculations have suggested that 10,000 patients followed for 10 years would be required

Table 2. Method and type of clinical information collected in each registry

	Prospective self-report questionnaires								
	Baseline				Follow-up				Retrospective medical record abstraction
Registry	Sx	Risk factors	Dem/Life	QOL	Sx	Risk factors	Dem/Life	QOL	
EABE	X	X	X	X	X	X	X	X	
EBRA	X								X
NIBR									X
UKBOR									X

Sx, symptoms; dem/Life, demographic information and lifestyle factors; QOL, quality of life; EABE, Mayo Clinic Esophageal Adenocarcinoma and Barrett's Esophagus registry; EBRA, Italian European Barrett's Registries Association; NIBR, Northern Ireland Barrett's Register; UKBOR, United Kingdom National Barrett's Oesophagus Registry. This table was created by Yvonne Romero.

to discover and validate biomarkers of neoplastic transformation.

Thus, collaboration among investigators, clinicians, patients, and registries may facilitate identification of translational discoveries that reduce the mortality rate of esophageal adenocarcinoma.

Acknowledgments

We would like to thank Piers Gatenby, M.D., Liam Murray, M.D., and Giovanni Zaninotto, M.D., for their help writing and checking the accuracy of the data presented in this manuscript.

Conflicts of Interest

The authors declare no conflicts of interest.

References

1. Curado, M., B. Edwards, H. Shin, *et al.* 2007. *Cancer Incidence in Five Continents.* Volume **IX.** IARC Scientific Publications. Lyon.

2. Gatenby, P., C. Caygill, J. Ramus, *et al.* 2008. Barrett's columnar-lined esophagus: demographic associations and adenocarcinoma risk. *Dig. Dis. Sci.* **53:** 1175–1185.

3. Gatenby, P., J. Ramus, C. Caygill, *et al.* 2009. Routinely diagnosed low grade dysplasia in Barrett's esophagus: a population-based study of natural history. *Histopathology* **54:** 814–819.

4. Ganz, R., B. Overholt, V. Sharma, *et al.* 2008. Circumferential ablation of Barrett's esophagus that contains high-grade dysplasia: a U.S. Multicenter Registry. *Gastrointest. Endosc.* **68:** 35–40.

5. Lyday, W., F. Corbett, D. Kuperman, *et al.* 2010. Radiofrequency ablation of Barrett's esophagus: outcomes of 429 patients from a multicenter community practice registry. *Endoscopy* **42:** 272–278.

6. Sharma, P., J. Dent, D. Armstrong, *et al.* 2006. The development and validation of an endoscopic grading system for Barrett's esophagus: the Prague C & M criteria. *Gastroenterology* **131:** 1392–1399.

7. Caygill, C., G. Zaninotto, M. Rugge. 2008. Participants of International Workshop on Barrett's Registries in Europe. Barrett's Registries in Europe: report of an International Workshop. *Eur. J. Cancer Prev.* **17:** 426–429.

8. Miller, R.C., P.J. Atherton, B.F. Kabat, *et al.* 2010. Marital status and quality of life in patients with esophageal cancer or Barrett esophagus: a Mayo Clinic Esophageal Adenocarcinoma and Barrett's Esophagus Registry Study. *Dig. Dis. Sci.*

9. Murray, L., P. Watson, B. Johnston, *et al.* 2003. Risk of adenocarcinoma in Barrett's esophagus: population based study. *BMJ* **327:** 534–535.

10. Caygill, C.P., G. Zaninotto, & M. Rugge. 2008. Barrett's registries in Europe: report of an International Workshop. *Eur. J. Cancer Prev.* **17:** 426–429.

11. Caygill, C.P., P.I. Reed, A. Watson, & M.J. Hill. 2001. The UK National Barrett's Esophagus Registry (UKBOR): aims and progress. *Eur. J. Cancer Prev.* **10:** 97–99.

12. Shaheen, N. 2004. Endoscopy for Barrett's esophagus and esophageal adenocarcinoma. *Am. Fam. Physician* **69:** 2060–2061.

Ann. N.Y. Acad. Sci. ISSN 0077-8923

ANNALS OF THE NEW YORK ACADEMY OF SCIENCES

Issue: *Barrett's Esophagus: The 10th OESO World Congress Proceedings*

Interventional endoscopy and single incision surgery

Lee L. Swanström[1] and Silvana Perretta[2]

[1]Minimally Invasive Surgery Division, Oregon Health Sciences University, Portland, Oregon. [2]IRCAD, Department of Surgery and Endocrine Surgery, Hôpitaux Universitaires, Strasbourg, France

The following on interventional endoscopy and single incision surgery contains commentaries on transluminal endoscopic esophageal surgery, flexible endoscopy, triangulation, advanced flexible operating platforms, experimental transesophageal procedures, and para- and intra-esophageal endoscopic surgery.

Keywords: natural orifice; ergonomics; transluminal endoscopic surgery; myotomy; submucosal dissection; lymphnode mapping; sentinel node biopsy; flexible endoscopy; NOTES; esophagus; mediastinum; achalasia

Concise summaries

- A major hurdle to make natural orifice transluminal endoscopic surgery (NOTES) a clinical reality was instrumentation. One major requirement is an ergonomic operating platform that would convert the typical flexible endoscopic operating paradigm to a more laparoscopic one, allowing the surgeon to transfer control of the camera to an assistant and manipulate instruments directly, controlling two or more at the same time, with the ability of the end effectors to achieve triangulation: a 50% improvement in efficiency can already be documented with an early form of such an operating platform with a corresponding decrease in the operative workload.

- The other needed development for complex flexible endoscopic surgery is a full complement of endoscopic instruments, including robust graspers, multifunctional dissection devices and effective energy sources, with rapid, easy and effective closure technologies.

- Flexible endoscopy is rapidly adapting itself to a laparoscopic, surgical, paradigm. Not only will this permit the practice of flexible endoscopic laparoscopy including natural orifice access, but it will also radically affect interventional endoscopy and advance therapeutic options for treatment of early esophageal and gastric cancers.

- Clinical experience of submucosal endoscopic esophageal myotomy for esophageal achalasia by peroral endoscopic technique is quite recent. Comparison of open surgical and submucosal endoscopic approaches has been made to address the impact of the length of the myotomy on the physiological results: transesophageal endoscopic myotomy is safe, but not as effective as open surgery in reducing the high pressure zone at manometry. However, the EndoFLIP® demonstrates that both techniques achieve similar results and that for both the main change in distensibility and diameter is related to the division of circular fibers at the level of the EGJ. Using a flexible endoscopic approach for submucosal access and tunneling the "third space" down to the lower esophageal sphincter provides the possibility of dividing only the internal layer of circular muscle fibers—presumably the only affected LES component in achalasia, and may obviate the need of an otherwise necessary anti-reflux procedure.

- In at least experimental animal studies, the feasibility of breaching the intact esophageal wall has already been proven. Techniques such as creating a mucosal flap have been successfully described for secure access and allow easy

doi: 10.1111/j.1749-6632.2011.06058.x

subsequent closure with standard endoscopic clips or T-tag sutures.

- Facing the problem of accurately identifying patients without lymph node involvement due to limitations on the accuracy of endoscopic ultrasound and computed tomography or anatomical access difficulties, the feasibility of focused mediastinal explorative operations through the evolution of a transesophageal technique is currently evaluated for sentinel node mapping based on MRI lymphography.
- MRI imaging may provide a new tool for systematic sentinel node identification completely noninvasive, requiring no preliminary aggressive dissection and without ionizing radiation. Nonsurvival porcine models have been used to demonstrate how targeted mediastinal lymph node biopsy could be when performed transesophageally by a combination of endoscopic submucosal lymphatic mapping, MRI imaging and NOTES.
- In further experiments, following mapping, *en bloc* esophagogastrectomy was performed to confirm that the sentinel nodes basin distribution at MRI would match the blue dye lymphatic uptake.

- Less morbid resection and reconstruction techniques of the esophagus are currently warranted for patients ranging from neonates with long-gap esophageal atresia to adults after esophageal resection.
- Bilateral longitudinal endoscopic myotomies have the ability to significantly lengthen the esophagus with selective division of only the circular muscular fibers. Preservation of the longitudinal fibers may allow lengthening and native organ reconstruction with less long-term dilatation.
- Today, the availability of sophisticated endoscopic tools and techniques, in addition to physiology and imaging modalities, should allow truly minimally invasive and precise image-guided treatments to go further than laparoscopic or endoscopic replications of open surgical techniques.
- As technology advances, simplified techniques facilitated by a flexible endoscopic approach will allow improved access to the mediastinum for a multitude of diagnostic and therapeutic applications. It appears that fundamental surgical principles and traditional paradigms have to be adapted and surgical textbooks will have to be rewritten in the near future.

---

1. A new generation of flexible endoscopic instruments to facilitate NOTES

Lee L. Swanström
lswanstrom@orclinic.com

The initial concept of NOTES was to use standard flexible endoscopes to perform basic diagnostic and simple therapeutic procedures within the abdomen.[1] As the spectrum of possible procedures quickly expanded—from basic peritoneoscopy and appendectomy to more complex ones like cholecystectomy and gastrojejunostomy—it rapidly became apparent that a major hurdle to make NOTES a clinical reality was going to be instrumentation. The NOSCAR group published a consensus white paper in 2006 that spelled out the early projection of what such "NOTES specific" instrumentation would look like.[2] A major component detailed was an ergonomic operating platform that

would convert the typical flexible endoscopic operating paradigm to a more laparoscopic one.[3] This specifically involved maintaining full flexibility of the endoscope but allowing the surgeon to transition to a stable platform, typically by mounting the scope to the bed or a stand, when the scope was positioned at the target area. This permitted the surgeon to transfer control of the camera to an assistant and manipulate instruments directly, controlling two or more at the same time in a coordinated fashion typical of laparoscopic procedures.

Another element of this advanced flexible operating platform was the ability of the end effectors to achieve triangulation. This was considered essential to achieve fine operating maneuvers such as retraction for exposure, traction/counter traction for fine dissection and even that signature complex skill, suturing. Over the ensuing four years since the publication of this seminal document detailing

Table 1. Operating platforms in development which satisfy the original NOSCAR criteria

Device	Company	Status
DDES	Boston Scientific	In development
Transport	USGI Medical	Available
Endosamurai	Olympus	In development
Anubiscope	Storz	In development

such a platform, several such platforms have been designed and prototyped by industry though none have reached the stage of commercialization at this date (Table 1).

The importance of developing such an operating platform can't be stressed enough—the ergonomics of the standard endoscope make performance of team activities difficult and the bias created by having the endoscopist both directing the image and controlling multiple instruments means the mental workload of the surgeon is maxed out while that of the assist(s) is underutilized. This leads to a tremendous loss in efficiency for NOTES procedures.[4] Likewise, the efficiency gained by having even a small degree of triangulation is tremendous. Our group has quantified the efficiencies to be gained by having some form of triangulation, no matter how primitive. A 50% improvement in efficiency was documented with an early form of an operating platform with a corresponding decrease in the operative workload.[5]

The other needed development for complex flexible endoscopic surgery is a full complement of endoscopic instruments, including robust graspers, multifunctional dissection devices, and effective energy sources. These "laparoscopic like" instruments are very slowly becoming available; slow because the profit margin on such low tech devices is small making it less interesting for industry to develop. An additional and important element of NOTES instrument design is rapid, easy, and effective closure technologies. Currently there are several endoscopic suturing devices coming on to the market in addition to the surgical platforms that permit traditional intracorporeal suturing. Perhaps more significantly is the possibility of stabling devices that will facilitate full-thickness resections as well as anastomosis and closures.

Conclusion

Flexible endoscopy is rapidly adapting itself to a laparoscopic, surgical, paradigm. Not only will this permit the practice of flexible endoscopic laparoscopy including natural orifice access, but it will also radically affect interventional endoscopy and advance therapeutic options for treatment of early esophageal and gastric cancers.

2. Experimental studies with transesophageal procedures

Silvana Perretta, J. Wall and B. Dallemagne
silvana.perretta@ircad.fr

Once every few decades in science or medicine, an idea emerges that is so powerful that it changes forever how we think about that field. The idea of decreasing the morbidity of an operation by changing not only the way the surgery is delivered, but the surgical strategy itself is captivating. NOTES has the potential to do this by breaking the physical barrier between bodily trauma and surgery.

Minimally invasive esophageal surgery is still relatively new. It is an ideal field for improvement as it presents many unanswered questions. Endoluminal and transluminal esophageal endoscopic procedures for both diagnostic and therapeutic purposes have recently been explored. To date multiple transesophageal endoscopic procedures, such as mediastinal lymph-node resection,[6–8] vagotomy, sympatectomy thoracic duct ligation, thymectomy,[7] lung and pleura biopsy[6–9] epicardial coagulation, pericardial fenestration, and Heller myotomy have been described.[6]

Most impressively perhaps, Haruhiro Inoue[10] has recently reported the first clinical experience of submucosal endoscopic esophageal myotomy for esophageal achalasia with a Peroral Endoscopic Myotomy (POEM) technique in 17 patients. Revisitation of endoscopic myotomy was intitiated by Pasricha et al.[11] who, on the wave of NOTES, decribed submucosal endoscopic esophageal myoyomy in an experimental setting. The innovation brought by Inoue's technique lies in the in selective division of the circular muscular bundles while leaving the outer longitudinal esophageal musculature intact. The procedure reproduced the standard surgical myotomy including 6 cm of the esophagus and 2 cm of the stomach.

Our group has subsequently taken another step in Inoue's revisitation of the myotomy. We have compared open surgical and submucosal endoscopic approaches to address the impact of the length of the myotomy on the physiological results. We measured physiologic results with both standard manometry and a new method measuring the distensibility of the esophago-gastric junction (EGJ) the functional lumen imagining probe, EndoFLIP[TM].

Our data shows that transesophageal endoscopic myotomy is safe, but not as effective as open surgery in reducing the high pressure zone at manometry. The EndoFLIP demonstrates that both open and endoscopic techniques achieve similar results and that for both the main change in distensibility and diameter is related to the division of circular fibers at the level of the EGJ. Extending the myotomy proximally in the esophagus is not beneficial. Therefore, a selective (circular bundles) and short myotomy can achieve good functional outcome. This concept may have an impact on the occurrence of postoperative gastro-esophageal reflux and is currently under investigation. This could in turn open new frontiers in the understanding of esophageal physiology and suggests that we could be facing a change, not only in surgical technique, but in the preoperative and intraoperative evaluation of achalasia patients.

Having developed expertise in esophageal mural tunneling for the purposes of endoscopic Heller's myotomy, we are now exploring the feasibility of focused mediastinal explorative operations through the evolution of a transesophageal technique for sentinel node (SN) mapping based on MRI lymphography. The SN concept may allow less invasive operation with selective lymphadenectomy, or in node negative patients, organ-preserving cancer resection by totally endoscopic techniques (e.g., endoscopic mucosal and submucosal dissection). SN biopsy by natural orifice has already been described in the animal model for colon and gastric mapping.[12–14] Ideally, the sentinel node is confined to a single node or lymph node station such as in breast cancers and melanomas. Regarding upper gastrointestinal cancers, sentinel nodes mapping is feasible but complicated by multidirectional lymphatic drainage. This is particularly true in esophageal cancer where a wide distribution and an unpredictable pattern of lymph node spread with multiple nodal station in-

volved can be seen in up to 21% of patients.[15] As a result, the clinical relevance of sentinel concept in the current treatment of patients with esophageal cancer is limited and requires extensive dissection to accurately depict the entire node basin. Dye only guided mapping would, in fact, entail an operative mobilization of the esophagus for real time observation of the lymphatic route, and mobilization itself could interfere with the lymphatic flow from the primary tumor. Reducing the extent of dissection needed to detect the sentinel node is a key advantage of the combined MRI imaging technique. MRI imaging may provide a new tool for systematic sentinel node basin identification completely noninvasive requiring no preliminary aggressive dissection and without ionizing radiation. If proved sufficiently reliable, it may represent a step further towards an image guided solely endoscopic node harvest, diagnosis and resection of the primary tumor.

Nonsurvival porcine models were used to demonstrate how targeted mediastinal lymph node biopsy could be when performed transesophageally by a combination of endoscopic submucosal lymphatic mapping, MRI imaging and NOTES. First, lymphatic mapping of the area of interest is performed by endoscopic submucosal injection of 2 mL of the MRI contrast agent gadolinium combined with methylene blue into the distal esophagus. This suspension of small molecular size dye particles is rapidly taken up by the submucosal lymphatic efferents and transported to the primary draining lymph nodes which are then detectable by their blue discoloration. A transesophageal submucosal tunnel is used to exit into the mediastinum proper and search for blue dyed lymph nodes for selective lymphadenectomy. The salient nodes are then retrieved via the esophagotomy, and MRI scanned to confirm the presence of gadolinium in the colored nodes. In further experiments, mapping was repeated as described above but, instead of retrieving only the sentinel nodes, an en bloc esophagogastrectomy was performed to confirm that the sentinel nodes basin distribution at MRI would match the blue dye lymphatic uptake. The gadolinium combined with methylene blue was found in the sentinel nodes in all animals.

As emerging organ sparring techniques are established for early stage esophageal tumors, less morbid resection and reconstruction techniques are also warranted. Esophageal reconstruction presents a significant clinical challenge in patients ranging from neonates with long-gap oesophageal atresia to adults after esophageal resection. Both gastric and colonic replacement conduits carry significant morbidity. Beyond achalasia, highly selective endoscopic myotomy techniques described previously may play a future role in esophageal reconstruction. Open esophageal lengthening myotomies have been reported in multiple configurations, including circular and spiral. However, they have been generally abandoned due to long-term esophageal dilatation. Our group has performed experimental work showing that bilateral longitudinal endoscopic myotomies have the ability to significantly lengthen the esophagus with selective division of only the circular muscular fibers. We postulate that preservation of the longitudinal fibers may allow lengthening and native organ reconstruction with less long-term dilatation.

Today, the availability of sophisticated endoscopic tools and techniques in addition to physiology and imaging modalities should allow us to perform truly minimally invasive and precise image-guided treatments to go further than laparoscopic or endoscopic replications of open surgical techniques. The future of NOTES lies not just in the reduction of the invasiveness of selected surgical procedures, but more in the development of innovative surgical concepts and revisitation of old surgical dogmas.

3. Flexible endoscopic mediastinoscopy and esophageal surgery

Erwin Rieder, Christy M. Dunst, and Lee L. Swanström
lswanstrom@orclinic.com

Flexible endoscopy has evolved from a purely diagnostic to an important therapeutic intervention and is continuously replacing traditional surgical procedures. Common bile duct stones, esophageal stenosis or large colon polyps are only few examples where standard or laparoscopic surgery already has been displaced. Recent interest and efforts in the development of NOTES has again pushed the boundaries of the flexible endoscopic approach. Used within the abdominal cavity, however, current flexible endoscopes have problems due to their flexibility and missing strength, which makes appropriate maneuvering difficult to achieve and demanding even for

highly experienced endoscopists. With the esophagus being difficult to reach by open or laparoscopic approaches and the narrowness of the mediastinum, flexibility seems not a burden but even desirable. Although breaching the intact esophageal wall still seems provocative for some and goes against standard surgical paradigms, several working groups have already evaluated future applications of flexible endoscopy for mediastinal or esophageal surgery.[16] Some of these are still experimental, but bear the potential to enhance therapeutic options for patients, particularly those with early cancer. Other esophageal interventions have already been transferred into the clinical setting and have shown favorable results.

Transesophageal endoscopic surgery

Compared to other access routes for NOTES, only a few reports have been published on the transesophageal approach so far. Traditional surgical principles and the fear of catastrophic complications due to esophageal perforation discourage many. However, in at least experimental animal studies, the feasibility of breaching the intact esophageal wall has already been proven. Techniques such as creating a mucosal flap have been successfully described for secure access and allow easy subsequent closure with standard endoscopic clips or T-tag sutures. Transesophageal mediastinoscopy or thoracoscopy as well as several surgical procedures such as paraesophageal lymph node harvest have been demonstrated.[17,18] Whether these favorable results in the animal can be easily transferred to the human setting still remains unanswered.

Paraesophageal/transcervical endoscopic surgery

Concerns regarding possible complications of a full thickness esophagotomy for access led to the development of a single incision/transcervical endoscopic approach. Although rigid mediastinoscopy has been an established procedure, reaching the posterior and distal paraesophageal mediastinum currently still requires a transthoracic or trans hiatal approach with its inherent associated morbidity. Using flexible endoscopy via a small suprasternal notch incision has been demonstrated to be safe and allows mediastinal dissection down to the diaphragm and beyond. Connective tissue tunnels thereby provide sufficient stability and allow the entire visceral mediastinum to be explored. Procedures such as Heller myotomies or biopsy of premarked lymph nodes have been described by us and others.[19]

Flexible endoscopic mediastinoscopy could technically even enable the implementation of a sentinel node concept for early esophageal cancer. As the incidence of tumor involved lymph nodes is significantly related to tumor cell invasion, endoscopic treatment of early esophageal cancer, such as endoscopic mucosal resection, is currently limited to patients, where malignant cells have not exceeded the first two mucosal layers. However, esophagus-preserving treatment could be extended to more patients, if there was documentation of true negative node status. The problem so far has been accurately identifying patients without lymph node involvement due to limitations on the accuracy of endoscopic ultrasound and computed tomography or anatomical access difficulties. Even though, a high frequency of esophageal sentinel nodes in more than one nodal station has been observed, the surgical endoscopic approach described above might facilitate more accurate staging of early adenocarcinoma of the distal esophagus (Fig. 1). Experimental attempts to identify esophageal sentinel lymph nodes have shown favorable results and might provide a more patient tailored therapy in the near future.

Intraesophageal endoscopic surgery

The impact of minimally invasive surgery has significantly changed the treatment of esophageal achalasia in the last decade. Flexible endoscopy seems poised to initiate another paradigm shift in treating this pathology of the lower esophageal sphincter. Initially described by Pasricha *et al.* in 2007, a

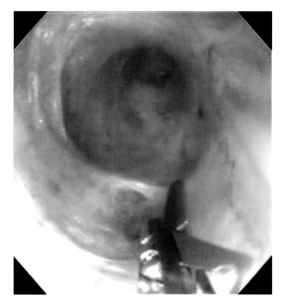

Figure 2. Peroral esophageal myotomy using flexible endoscopic scissors in the pig.

peroral endoscopic myotomy already has been successfully transferred into the clinical setting[20] and might again soon replace the current standard approach of laparoscopic Heller myotomy. Using a flexible endoscopic approach for submucosal access and tunneling the "third space" down to the lower esophageal sphincter, provides the possibility of dividing only the internal layer of circular muscle fibers—presumably the only affected LES component in achalasia (Fig. 2). This may even obviate the need of an otherwise necessary antireflux procedure. So far, short-term clinical results are more than promising.

Conclusion

Driven by attempts to enhance the invasiveness of flexible endoscopy, as well as recent developments in NOTES, we are now experiencing an exciting period in esophageal and mediastinal surgery. As technology advances, simplified techniques facilitated by a flexible endoscopic approach will allow improved access to the mediastinum for a multitude of diagnostic and therapeutic applications. It appears that fundamental surgical principles and traditional paradigms have to be adapted and surgical textbooks will have to be rewritten in the near future.

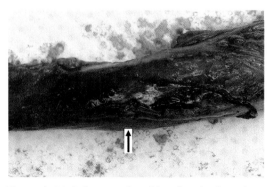

Figure 1. Marked paraesophageal lymph node after submucosal blue-dye injection in the pig.

References

1. Kalloo, A.N., V.K. Singh, S.B. Jagannath, *et al.* 2004. Flexible transgastric peritoneoscopy: a novel approach to diagnostic and therapeutic interventions in the peritoneal cavity. *Gastrointest. Endosc.* **60:** 114–117.

2. ASGE/SAGES. 2006. Working Group on Natural Orifice Translumenal Endoscopic Surgery. White Paper October 2005. *Gastrointest. Endosc.* **63:** 199–203.

3. Swanstrom, L., P. Swain & P. Denk. 2009. Development and validation of a new generation of flexible endoscope for NOTES. *Surg. Innov.* **16:** 104–110.

4. Spaun, G.O., B. Zheng, D.V. Martinec, *et al.* 2010. A comparison of early learning curves for complex bimanual coordination with open, laparoscopic, and flexible endoscopic instrumentation. *Surg. Endosc.* [Epub ahead of print]PMID: 20174939.

5. Spaun, G.O., B. Zheng, D.V. Martinec, *et al.* 2009. Bimanual coordination in natural orifice transluminal surgery: comparing the conventional dual-channel endoscope, the R-Scope, and a novel direct-drive system. *Gastrointest. Endosc.* **69:** e39–e45.

6. Willingham, F.F., D.W. Gee, G.Y. Lauwers, *et al.* 2008. Natural orifice trans- esophageal mediastinoscopy and thoracoscopy. *Surg. Endosc.* **22:** 1042–1047.

7. Woodward, T., D. McCluskey, 3rd, M.B. Wallace, *et al.* 2008. Pilot study of trans-esophageal endoscopic surgery: NOTES esophagomyotomy, vagotomy, lymphadenectomy. *J. Laparoendosc. Adv. Surg. Tech. Part A* **18:** 743–745.

8. Fritscher-Ravens, A., K. Patel, A. Ghanbari, *et al.* 2007. Natural orifice transluminal endoscopic surgery (NOTES) in the mediastinum: long-term survival animal experiments in trans-esophageal access, including minor surgical procedures. *Endoscopy* **39:** 870–875.

9. Fritscher-Ravens, A. & B.L. Davidson. 2006. Targeting the mediastinum: one-stop shopping at all times? *Gastrointest. Endosc.* **63:** 221–222.

10. Inoue, H.M., Kobayashi, Y. Sato, *et al.* 2010. Peroral endoscopic myotomy (POEM) for esophageal achalasia. *Endoscopy* **42:** 265–271.

11. Pasricha, P.J., R. Hawari, I. Ahmed, *et al.* 2007. Submucosal endoscopic esophageal myotomy: a novel experimental approach for the treatment of achalasia. *Endoscopy* **39:** 761–764.

12. Cahill, R.A., M. Asakuma, S. Perretta, *et al.* 2009. Gastric lymphatic mapping for sentinel node biopsy by natural orifice transluminal endoscopic surgery (NOTES). *Surg. Endosc.* **23:** 1110–1116.

13. Cahill, R.A., S. Perretta, J. Leroy, *et al.* 2008. Lymphatic mapping and sentinel node biopsy in the colonic mesentery by Natural Orifice Transluminal Endoscopic Surgery (NOTES). *Ann. Surg. Oncol.* **15:** 2677–2683.

14. Perretta, S., P. Allemann, B. Dallemagne & J. Marescaux. 2009. Natural orifice transluminal endoscopic surgery (N.O.T.E.S.) for neoplasia of the chest and mediastinum. *Surg. Oncol.* **18:** 177–180.

15. Takeuchi, H., H. Fujii, N. Ando, *et al.* 2009. Validation study of radio-guided sentinel lymph node navigation in esophageal cancer. *Ann. Surg.* **249:** 757–763.

16. Swanström, L.L., C.M. Dunst & G. Spaun. 2010. Future applications of flexible endoscopy in esophageal surgery. *J. Gastrointest. Surg.* **14:** S127–S132.

17. Gee, D.W., F.F. Willingham, G.Y. Lauwers, *et al.* 2008. Natural orifice transesophageal mediastinoscopy and thoracoscopy: a survival series in swine. *Surg. Endosc.* **22:** 2117–2122.

18. Fritscher-Ravens, A., K. Patel, A. Ganbari, *et al.* 2007. Natural orifice transluminal endoscopic surgery (NOTES) in the medastinum: long- term survival animal experiments in transesophageal access, including minor surgical procedures. *Endoscopy* **39:** 870–875.

19. Spaun, G.O., C.M. Dunst, D.V. Martinec, *et al.* 2010. Mediastinal surgery in connective tissue tunnels using flexible endoscopy. *Surg. Endosc.* **24:** 2120–2127.

20. Inoue, H., H. Minami, Y. Kobayashi, *et al.* 2010. Peroral endoscopic myotomy (POEM) for esophageal achalasia. *Endoscopy* **42:** 265–271.

Author Index

A

Abrams, J.A., 156–174
Altomare, A., 369–375
Amano, Y., 53–75, 93–113
Amenta, P.S., 76–92
Appelman, H.D., 53–75, 140–155, 156–174, 292–308
Armstrong, D., 76–92, 114–139
Atasoy, A., 248–264, 392–400
Aziz, Q., 341–348

B

Ba-Ssalamah, A., 248–264
Badaloni, A., 175–195
Bajpai, M., 18–35, 76–92
Barr, H., 18–35, 76–92
Beales, I.L.P., 210–229
Bechi, P., 18–35, 53–75, 76–92, 93–113, 114–139
Behar, J., 369–375
Bellizzi, A.M., 53–75, 210–229
Bennett, A., 76–92
Biancani, P., 369–375
Bonavina, L., 140–155, 175–195
Braghetto, I., 175–195
Brasseur, J.G., 323–330
Braverman, A.S., 323–330
Brücher, B., 248–264, 265–291
Burke, Z.D., 309–315

C

Canon, C.L., 175–195
Cao, W., 210–229, 369–375
Casini, V., 114–139
Castiglione, F., 18–35, 53–75, 76–92, 93–113, 114–139
Caygill, C.P.J., 196–209, 405–410
Ceolin, M., 175–195
Chang, A.C., 18–35
Chejfec, G., 1–17
Chen, H., 309–315, 381–391
Chen, X., 309–315, 381–391
Chuttani, R., 53–75, 156–174
Cicala, M., 36–52, 369–375
Clarke, J.O., 349–357
Collard, J.-M., 248–264

D

Das, K.M., 18–35, 76–92, 210–229
De-la-Torre-Bravo, A., 140–155
Degl'Innocenti, D.R., 18–35, 53–75, 76–92, 93–113, 114–139
del Genio, G., 175–195
Deprez, P.H., 248–264
DeVault, K.R., 53–75, 114–139
Diaz-Cervantes, E., 140–155
Dillon, J.F., 93–113
Drewes, A.M., 1–17, 331–340, 341–348
Dua, K.S., 175–195
Dvorak, K., 1–17, 93–113, 114–139, 140–155, 196–209, 230–247, 381–391

E

El-Serag, H., 36–52
El-Zimaity, H., 1–17, 292–308

F

Falk, G.W., 1–17, 53–75, 196–209
Fang, D., 210–229, 230–247
Farmer, A.D., 341–348
Feith, M., 248–264, 265–291
Felix, V.N., 93–113, 196–209, 210–229
Foxwell, T., 392–400
Freschi, G., 18–35, 53–75, 76–92, 93–113, 114–139
Frøkjær, J.B., 331–340, 341–348
Fujimura, T., 392–400

G

Gamboa-Robles, J., 140–155
Gatenby, P.A.C., 405–410
Gerson, L.B., 53–75, 196–209
Gibson, M.K., 392–400
Giuli, R., vii–viii
Going, J.J., 76–92
Goldman, A., 1–17, 93–113, 114–139, 140–155, 230–247, 381–391

Gore

Gore, R.M., 36–52
Greenwald, B.D., 156–174
Gregersen, H., 331–340, 341–348
Gyawali, C.P., 175–195, 349–357

H

Hardie, L.J., 210–229
Harnett, K.M., 369–375
Hattori, T., 392–400
Heeg, P., 365–368
Hejazi, R.A., 175–195
Herrmann, I.F., 365–368
Herzig, S.J., 114–139
Hobson, A.R., 341–348
Hofmann, G., 248–264
Hofstetter, W.L., 265–291
Horwhat, J.D., 53–75, 156–174, 196–209
Houghton, J.M., 381–391
Huang, Q., 53–75
Hunt, R.H., 114–139
Hutchinson, L., 381–391
Hwang, J.H., 196–209

I

Ilson, D.H., 265–291
Ishimura, N., 53–75, 93–113

J

Jacobson, B.C., 1–17, 36–52, 175–195, 230–247
Jadcherla, S.R., 401–404
Jenkins, G., 1–17
Jobe, B., 392–400
Johnson, L.F., 53–75

K

Kamiya, T., 114–139
Kandioler, D., 265–291
Komanduri, S., 156–174, 248–264
Kong, J., 381–391
Krarup, A.L., 331–340, 341–348
Krasna, M.J., 265–291
Krishnadath, K.K., 18–35, 381–391
Kwiatek, M.A., 331–340